Preterm Infants: Interventions for Persisting Ductus Arteriosus

Preterm Infants: Interventions for Persisting Ductus Arteriosus

Editor: Kristle Mitchell

AMERICAN
MEDICAL PUBLISHERS
www.americanmedicalpublishers.com

AMERICAN
MEDICAL PUBLISHERS
www.americanmedicalpublishers.com

Cataloging-in-Publication Data

Preterm infants : interventions for persisting ductus arteriosus / edited by Kristle Mitchell.
p. cm.
Includes bibliographical references and index.
ISBN 979-8-88740-389-2
1. Premature infants. 2. Patent ductus arteriosus. 3. Ductus arteriosus. 4. Pediatric cardiology.
5. Infants--Diseases. 6. Newborn infants--Diseases. I. Mitchell, Kristle.
RJ250 .P74 2023
618.920 11--dc23

American Medical Publishers,
41 Flatbush Avenue,
1st Floor, New York,
NY 11217, USA

ISBN 979-8-88740-389-2 (Hardback)

Contents

Preface

Every book is initially just a concept; it takes months of research and hard work to give it the final shape in which the readers receive it. In its early stages, this book also went through rigorous reviewing. The notable contributions made by experts from across the globe were first molded into patterned chapters and then arranged in a sensibly sequential manner to bring out the best results.

Patent ductus arteriosus (PDA) is a medical condition, wherein the ductus arteriosus blood vessel fails to close after birth. This causes a portion of oxygenated blood from the left heart to flow back to the lungs by flowing through the aorta (which has a higher pressure) to the pulmonary artery. Symptoms become visible towards the end of the first year of life. The common symptoms of PDA include dyspnea (shortness of breath), failure to gain weight at a normal rate, cardiomegaly, and tachycardia. If PDA is not treated at the appropriate time, it may lead to pulmonary hypertension followed by right-sided heart failure. The diagnosis is performed using non-invasive techniques such as echocardiography and chest X-ray. The administration of intravenous indomethacin on the first day of life to all preterm infants lowers the risk of infants developing PDA and the complications associated with PDA. The treatment of this disease comprises both surgical and non-surgical methods. This book includes a detailed explanation of the various interventions for persisting ductus arteriosus. It will provide comprehensive knowledge to the readers.

It has been my immense pleasure to be a part of this project and to contribute my years of learning in such a meaningful form. I would like to take this opportunity to thank all the people who have been associated with the completion of this book at any step.

Editor

1

Echocardiographic Diagnosis and Hemodynamic Evaluation of Patent Ductus Arteriosus in Extremely Low Gestational Age Newborn (ELGAN) Infants

Yogen Singh[1,2*], *Alain Fraisse*[3,4], *Omer Erdeve*[5] *and Begum Atasay*[5]

[1] *Department of Pediatrics - Pediatric Cardiology and Neonatal Medicine, Cambridge University Hospitals NHS Foundation Trust, Cambridge, United Kingdom,* [2] *University of Cambridge Clinical School of Medicine, Cambridge, United Kingdom,* [3] *Pediatric Cardiology Services, Royal Brompton Hospital, London, United Kingdom,* [4] *Imperial College London, National Heart and Lung Institute, London, United Kingdom,* [5] *Division of Neonatology, Department of Pediatrics, Ankara University School of Medicine, Ankara, Turkey*

***Correspondence:**
Yogen Singh
yogen.singh@nhs.net

Persistent Patent ductus arteriosus (PDA) is a common finding in extremely low gestational age newborn infants and its prevalence is inversely proportional to the gestational age. The presence of a persistent PDA is associated with increased mortality and several significant morbidities including intraventricular hemorrhage, pulmonary hemorrhage, necrotizing enterocolitis, and chronic lung disease or bronchopulmonary dysplasia. However, treating PDA has not been demonstrated to have beneficial impact on the long term outcomes. Currently there is no consensus on whether to treat the PDA or not, and if treat, when to treat and how to treat. The echocardiography is the investigation of choice to diagnose PDA, estimating the magnitude of shunt volume and assessing its hemodynamic significance, and to exclude/diagnose any associated congenital heart defect before any intervention. Various echocardiographic parameters and staging/scoring systems have been described to help the clincians making the clinical decisions and some of theses scoring systems are quite complex to apply in a busy day to day clinical practice. This concised review paper is focused to help the clinicians in making a clinical decision based upon clincial and echocardiography parameters. Hence, only the parameters which are commonly used and helpful in making the clinical decisions in day to day clincial practice have been described in this paper.

Keywords: patent ductus arteriosus (PDA), extreme preterm infants, clinical decision making, echocardiographic evaluation of PDA, ELGAN extremely low gestational age newborn

INTRODUCTION

Patent ductus arteriosus (PDA) is an essential component of the fetal circulation and in most of the term infants it closes soon after birth. However, PDA is known to remain persistent in large proportion of extremely low gestational age newborn (ELGAN) infants and its prevalence is inversely proportional to the gestational age (1). The incidence of a persistent PDA in infants born <1,000 g or those under 28 weeks of gestation is around 66% (1, 2).

The important risk factors for persistent PDA include lower gestational age, lack of antenatal steroids, and need for mechanical ventilation. The risk of persistent PDA increases with decreasing gestational age (GA) and lower birth weight (3)[1] (4). Closure is also less likely to occur in infants who have neonatal respiratory distress syndrome needing mechanical ventilation and in those who did not receive antenatal corticosteroids (4, 5).

The presence of a persistent PDA is associated with increased mortality and several significant morbidities including intraventricular hemorrhage (IVH), pulmonary hemorrhage, necrotizing enterocolitis (NEC), and chronic lung disease (CLD) or bronchopulmonary dysplasia (BPD) (6–8). Despite large number of trials, research studies and scientific efforts in making an evidence based consensus on how best to manage the PDA in this vulnerable group of patients, there has been no agreement on how best to treat or even how best to assess the PDA and its impact (9). There continues to be a clinical dilemma who should we treat, how to treat and what the best strategy in the ELGAN infants is. Different treatment strategies have been studied over the years. These include prophylactic treatment, early targeted treatment, treatment of a clinically symptomatic PDA, the conservative approach of "wait and watchful policy," surgical ligation and recently described percutaneous transcatheter closure of PDA (9–12).

This review focuses at clinical decision making in managing PDA in the ELGAN infants. The aim of the paper is not to advice on the type of treatment, but primarily looking on the role of echocardiography in hemodynamic evaluation of PDA which can help in making clinical decision on the bedside.

CLINICAL DIAGNOSIS OF PDA

The clinical signs of PDA depend upon amount of the shunt volume passing across the ductus arteriosus; which primarily depends upon the systemic and pulmonary vascular resistance, ability of the myocardium to adapt to increased shunt volume and size of the ductus arteriosus (13–15) (**Figure 1**).

Infants with even a large PDA often have no clinical signs in the first few days after birth because of persistently high pulmonary vascular resistance (PVR) leading to decreased amount of PDA shunt volume. As PVR drops, shunt volume increases and infant develops the signs and symptoms of PDA. Initially, heart murmur may be heard and often the infant is noted to have fleeting desaturations. As PDA persists then further signs such as hyperactive precordium, bounding pulses and widened pulse pressure are recognized and when myocardium fails to adapt to this increased shunt volume the signs of heart failure develop (15, 16). However, a small proprotion of ELGAN infants with decreased myocardial adaptability may develop hypotension and acidosis even during first few days (16).

Clinical factors and biomarkers can be used both to diagnose PDA and assess its hemodynamic significance In hemodynamically significant PDA (hsPDA), signs and symptoms of pulmonary overcirculation and systemic hypoperfusion are rated by looking at the oxygenation difficulty, number and severity of apnea and desaturations, need and extent of non-invasive or invasive respiratory support, feeding intolerance, radiologic evidence of cardiomegaly and pulmonary edema, presence of oliguria, low mean or diastolic hypotension with or without metabolic acidosis requiring cardiotropic or vassopressor drugs (17). However, most clinical signs have limited sensitivity in the first day of life and hence, there is a few days lag in clinical diagnosis of PDA as compared to echocardiography (15, 17).

Moreover, it is very difficult to diagnose or rule out underlying congenital heart defect on clincial examination alone (18). Hence, echocardiographic diagnosis is mandatory before any clincial intervention.

ECHOCARDIOGRAPHIC EVALUATION OF PDA: DIAGNOSIS AND ASSESSMENT OF HEMODYNAMIC IMPACT OF SHUNT VOLUME

The echocardiography is the gold standard bedside investigation to diagnose PDA. In addition to make a confirmative diagnosis of PDA and exclude/diagnose any associated congenital heart defect (CHD), it can help in estimating the magnitude of shunt volume and assessing its hemodynamic significance—it can be used to assess the hemodynamic impact from pulmonary overcirculation and systemic hypoperfusion due to shunt volume (13–15). This could be systematically achieved by studying: (a) ductal characteristics, (b) parameters of pulmonary overcirculation, and (c) signs of systemic hypoperfusion (**Figure 2**).

Various echocardiographic parameters have been described in the research setting and complex staging/scoring systems (17, 19). This review paper is focused to help the clinicians in making a clinical decision on the bedside and hence the parameters which are commonly used and helpful in day to day common clinical practice have been described.

Echocardiographic Assessment of Ductal Characteristics

The echocardiography can be used to assess the size of PDA by measuring transductal diameter, interrogate shunt direction, and velocity of blood flow across the ductus arteriosus can be measured by using Doppler technique.

Measuring Transductal Diameter

Although the PDA can be visualized from many windows, the high left-sided parasternal "ductal" view is the preferred window to obtain a clear 2D image and accurately measure size of the ductus arteriosus. PDA size is measured from the transductal diameter at the site of maximum constriction (narrowest dimension), which is usually at the pulmonary end (20). Most studies have described measuring PDA size using color Doppler, although with new ultrasound machines and through proper training it can be easily measured on 2D image. If color Doppler is used to measure the duct size the gain setting should

[1]Available online at: https://www.uptodate.com/contents/patent-ductus-arteriosus-in-preterm-infants-pathophysiology-clinical-manifestations-and-diagnosis/abstract/55.

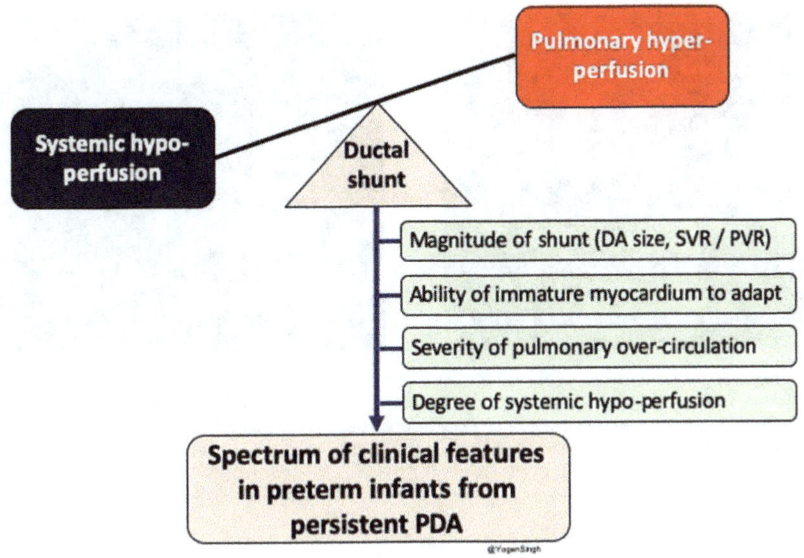

FIGURE 1 | Diagram showing impact of significant left to right shunt across ductal arteriosus (DA) leading to pulmonary over-circulation and systemic hypoperfusion. Spectrum of clinical features in preterm infants depends upon magnitude of ductal shunt, which depends upon DA size and balance between systemic and pulmonary vascular resistance, and inability of immature myocardium to adpat to circulatory disturbance. PDA, patent ductus arteriosus; SVR, systemic vascular resistance; PVR, pulmonary vascular resistance.

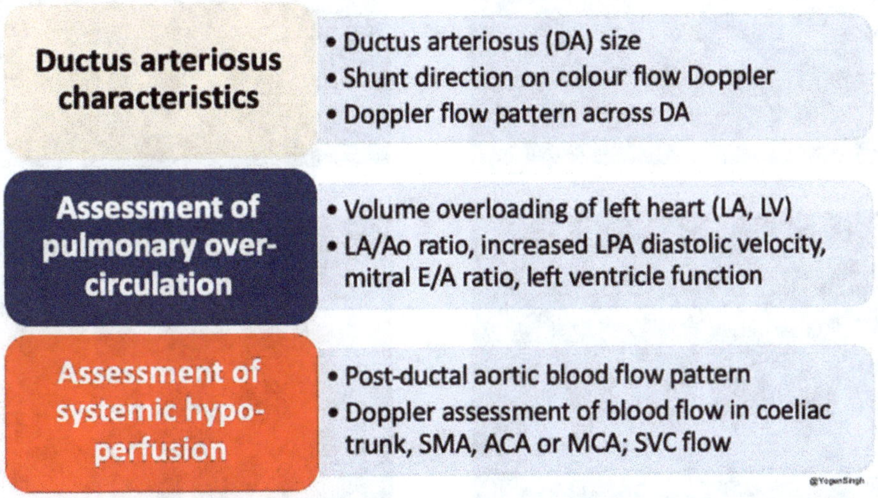

FIGURE 2 | Summary of an approach to echocardiographic assessment of PDA and hemodynamic evaluation; LA, left atrium; LV, left ventricle; DA, ductus arteriosus; Ao, aorta; SMA, superior mesenteric artery; ACA, anterior cerebral artery; MCA, middle cerebral artery; SVC, superior vena cava.

be adequately optimized to minimize the risk of over-estimation. Color compare or simultaneous mode, which allows putting 2D and color Doppler image side by side, can be applied to measure ductal size in both modes using frame by frame technique (**Figure 3**).

Direction of Shunt Across Ductus Arteriosus

The direction of the ductal shunt depends upon the relationship between the pulmonary and systemic pressures. It is assessed using color Doppler and direction of blood flow across ductus arteriosus is normally left to right, from the aorta (high systemic pressure) to the pulmonary artery (low pulmonary pressure) but it can be right to left or bi-directional when there is high pulmonary vascular resistance or when there is anatomical cause (due to certain CHDs). With conventional setting left to right shunt is seen as red jet while right to left shunt is seen as blue (21). A right-to-left shunt across the PDA is more difficult to see because color Doppler will show it as a blue jet, blood going toward aorta from pulmonary end, similar to branch pulmonary arteries. Color compare or simultaneous mode can be very helpful in such situation. Bi-directional flow is often seen during transitional circulation or when the pulmonary

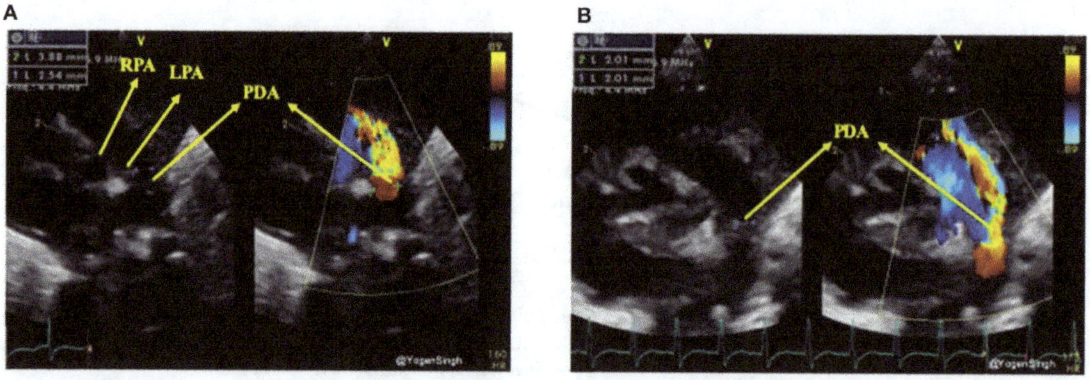

FIGURE 3 | Measurement of ductal size on 2D and color Doppler on high left parasternal "ductal view." **(A)** Showing significant discrepency between ductal diameter measurement on 2D and color Doppler—over-estimation of ductal size on color Doppler because of gain setting; **(B)** showing no significant discrepency between ductal diameter measurement on 2D and color Dopple after optimisation of gain setting. LPA, left pulmonary artery; RPA, right pulmonary artery; PDA, patent ductus arteriosus.

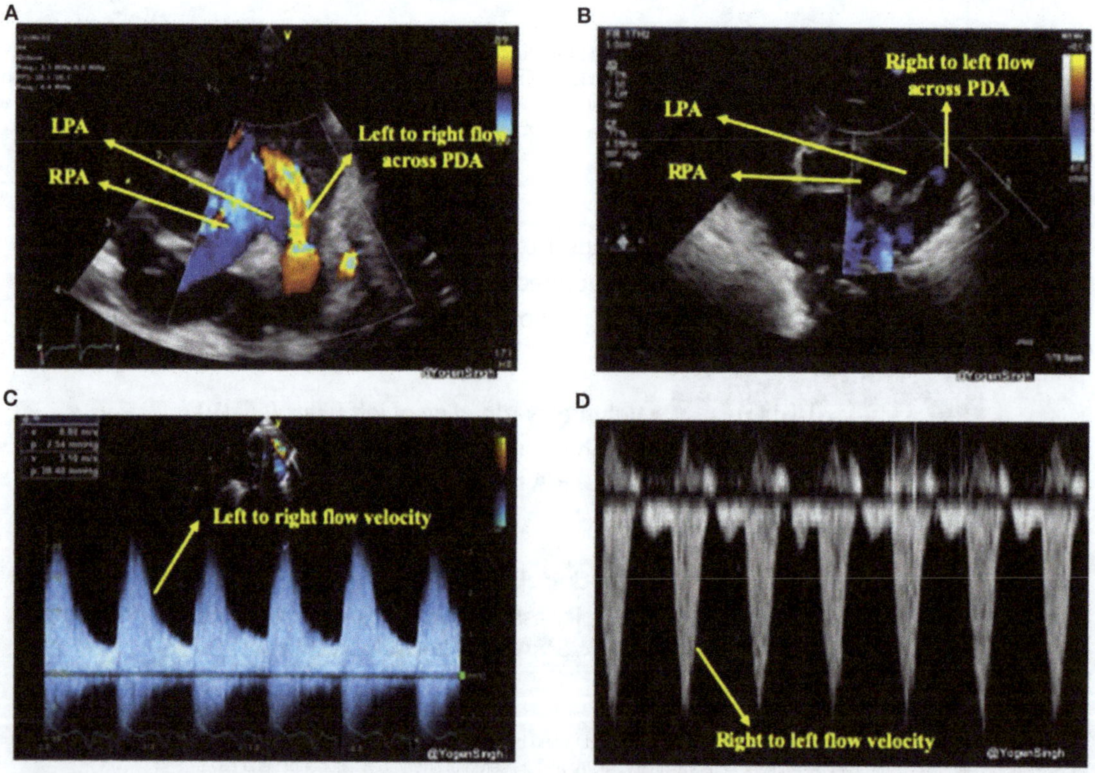

FIGURE 4 | Assessment of PDA shunt direction on color flow and with Doppler application. **(A)** Left to right shunt seen as red (blood coming toward probe) while blood in branch pulmonary arteries seen as blue (blood going away from probe); **(B)** showing right to left shunt seen as blue color—similar to branch pulmonary arteries in a view "three legged trouser;" **(C)** Doppler assessment showing left to right shunt (above the baseline as blood coming toward the probe); and **(D)** Doppler assessment showing right to left shunt (below the baseline as blood going away from the probe). LPA, left pulmonary artery; RPA, right pulmonary artery; PDA, patent ductus arteriosus.

artery pressures are equal to systemic pressures (21). Shunt direction can also be assessed using pulse or continuous wave Doppler where left to right shunt is seen above the baseline (blood coming toward the probe) while right to left shunt is seen below the baseline (blood going away from the probe) (15, 21) (**Figure 4**).

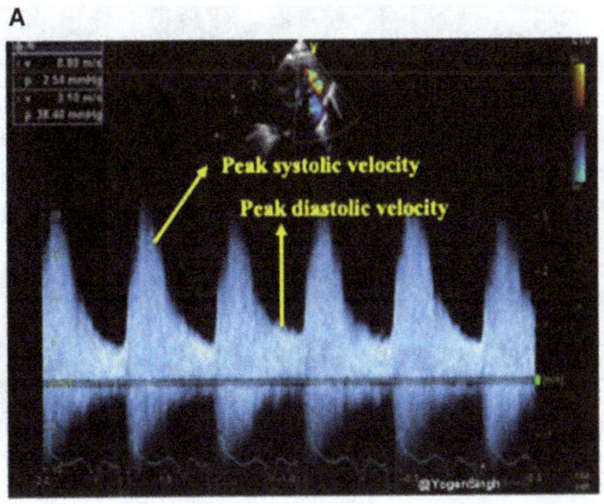

FIGURE 5 | Assessment of restrictive and non-restrictive (pulsatile) flow pattern on Doppler assessment of PDA. **(A)** Showing non-restrictive (pulsatile) flow pattern with end-diastolic velocity (EDV) less than half of the peak systolic velocity; and **(B)** showing restrictive flow pattern with end-diastolic velocity (EDV) more than half of the peak systolic velocity.

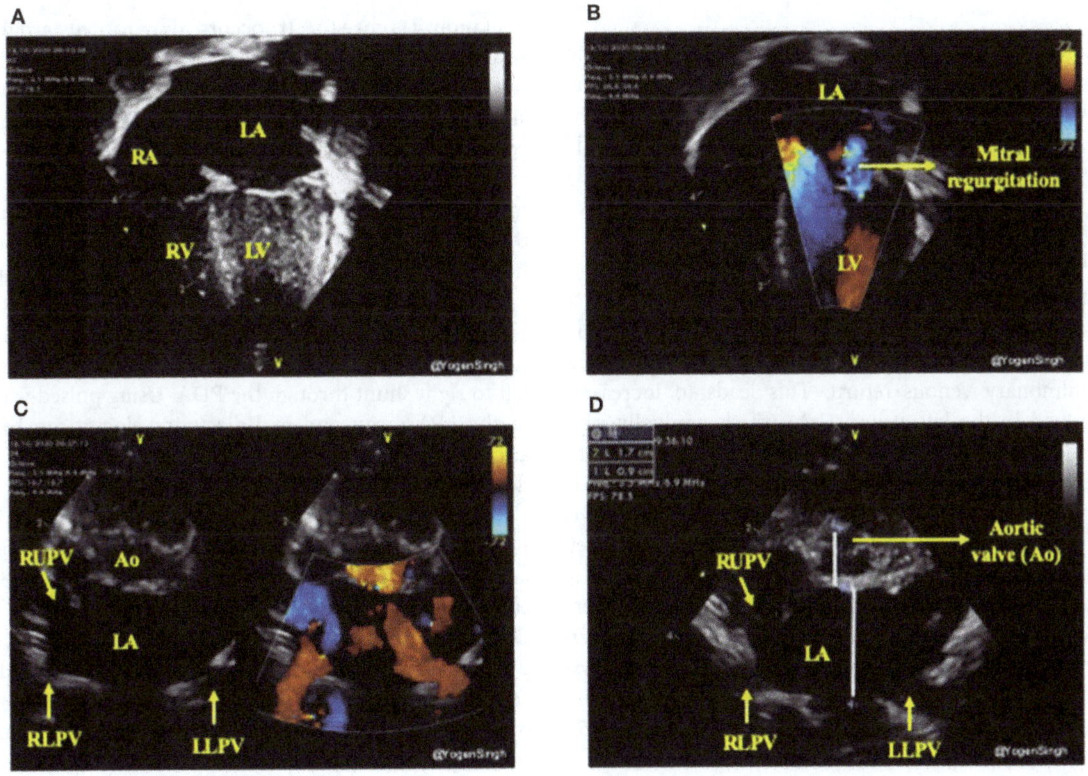

FIGURE 6 | Assessment of left heart volume overloading on visual inspection "eyeballing." **(A)** Apical 4 chamber view in 2D showing dilated left side of the heart (dilated left atrium and left ventricle); **(B)** Mitral regurgitation on color flow mapping as blue jet going back to left atrium (see explanation in text); **(C)** "Crab view" showing dilated pulmonary veins reflecting increased pulmonary venous return and **(D)** Dilated left atrium in parasternal short axis view—on visual inspection LA looks almost the double the size of aortic valve (Ao). LA, left atrium; LV, left ventricle; RA, right atrium; RV, right ventricle; Ao, aortic valve; RUPV, right upper pulmonary vein; RLPV, right lower pulmonary vein; LLPV, left lower upper pulmonary vein.

Velocity of Shunt Across PDA and Its Significance

The shunt velocity across the PDA during the cardiac cycle can be obtained by applying pulse or continuous wave Doppler in the ductus arteriosus. The maximum velocity during systole and diastole can be measured. Non-restrictive shunts have a low peak systolic velocity with a high systolic to end-diastolic

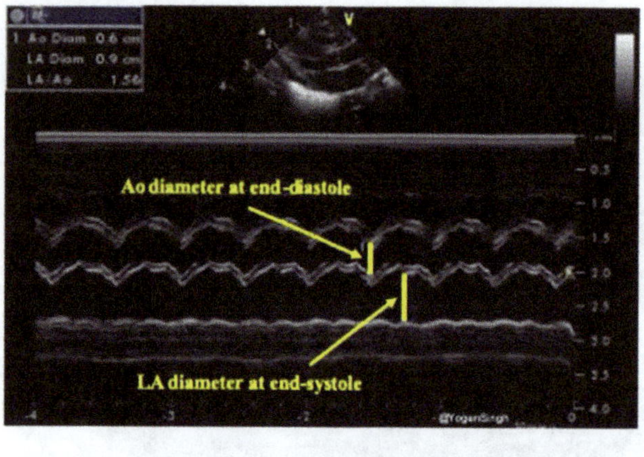

Left atrium (LA) / Aorta (Ao) ratio measurement

FIGURE 7 | Assessment of left atrium (LA) to aorta (Ao) ratio in parasternal long axis view. LA and Ao diameter measurement shown using M-mode and cartoon schematic diagram.

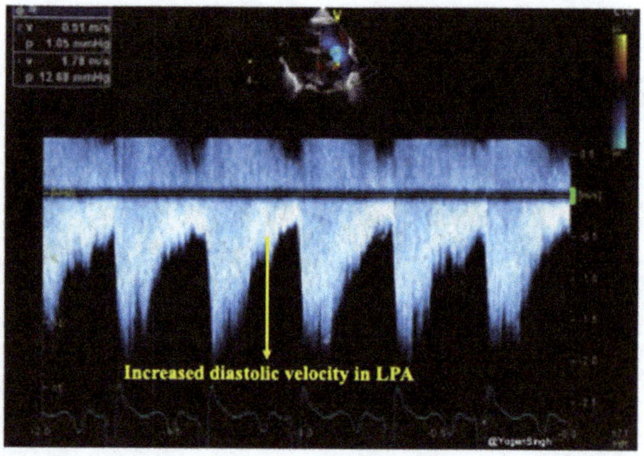

FIGURE 8 | Doppler assessment of blood flow in left pulmonary artery (LPA) showing increased diastolic velocity indicative of significant ductal shunt in diastole leading to turbulence and increased velocity.

velocity gradient while restrictive shunts have a high peak systolic velocity and a low systolic to diastolic velocity gradient. If the ratio between peak systolic and end-diastolic velocity is >2 then it is considered as a pulsatile flow pattern while a ratio of <2 is described as restrictive shunt suggestive of a closing PDA (22, 23) (**Figure 5**).

Echocardiographic Evaluation of Pulmonary Overcirculation

The increased pulmonary blood flow from a significant left-to-right ductal shunt leads to pulmonary blood flow and hence increased pulmonary venous return. This leads to increased volume overload in the left atrium (LA) which gradually gets dilated and if this process of significant left to right shunt persists then it leads to dilatation of left ventricle from increased preload, especially in absence of a large intra-atrial shunt. As aortic valve annulus (Ao) is a relatively fixed structure and it does not get dilated due to left heart overloading. Hence, a ratio of LA/Ao can be used as a surrogate of increased pulmonary venous return (24, 25). Similarly, the left ventricular end diastolic diameter (LVEDD) can be used as surrogate markers for pulmonary venous return. In clinical practice the volume overloading of the left heart can be subjectively assessed by "eyeballing" (15) (**Figure 6**).

Both LA/Ao ratio and LVEDD can be measured from the parasternal long axis view using M-mode with the cursor perpendicular to the aorta at the level of the aortic valve or at the septum at the tip of the mitral valve leaflets, respectively (**Figure 7**). LA/Ao ratio of >1.4 is considered significant and has been used as a cut-off value in many clinical trials (25). The normal reference ranges for LVEDD in preterm infants in relation to body weight and postnatal age have been published and *z*-scores should be used for LVEDD (26).

Variable degree of mitral valve insufficiency is often seen in infants with persistent large PDA and significant left heart dilatation (**Figure 6**). It occurs due to left atrial dilatation resulting in stretching of mitral valve and left ventricular volume-overloading. The mitral valve regurgitation usually improves significantly with normalization of left atrial size and resolves completely within weeks after PDA closure (14, 26, 27).

While assessing left heart volume overloading one should be mindful of intra-atrial shunt. A large left-to-right shunt through the foramen ovale or septal defect can "offload" the left side of the heart even in the presence of a significant ductal shunt leading to an artificially low/normal LA/Ao ratio or low LVEDD.

The presence of forward pulmonary flow in diastole in the left pulmonary artery (LPA) has been described as a sign of significant left to right shunt through the PDA. Using pulsed wave Doppler in the LPA mean and end-diastolic velocity can be measured and cut-off points of 0.42 and 0.20 m/s, respectively, have been described as indicative of significant ductal shunt (24) (**Figure 8**).

The mitral valve E/A ratio refers to the ratio of the velocity of the early (E) diastolic phase of ventricular filling vs. the late atrial (A) contraction component. Mitral valve E/A ratio can be obtained from apical 4-chamber view with the pulsed Doppler range gate set slightly below the mitral valve annulus. In preterm infants, mitral valve E/A ratio is usually <1 due to poor compliance of the myocardium leading to moderate impairment of diastolic performance and low early diastolic filling velocity. In the presence of a hsPDA, atrial pressure increases because high pulmonary venous return and this leads to a reversal of the E/A ratio >1. Various other echocardiographic parameters have been studied and described to assess pulmonary circulation such as left ventricular output (LVO) to superior vena cava flow (SVC) ratio, and decreased isovolumic relaxation time (IVRT) using tissue Doppler Imaging (TDI) (13, 24, 28). There may be limited expertise in doing TDI assessment accurately on neonatologist performed echocardiography. On the other hand, echocardiographic assessments (such as SVC flow and LVO estimation) needing multiple parameters are not only time consuming but also has potential to make errors in measurement

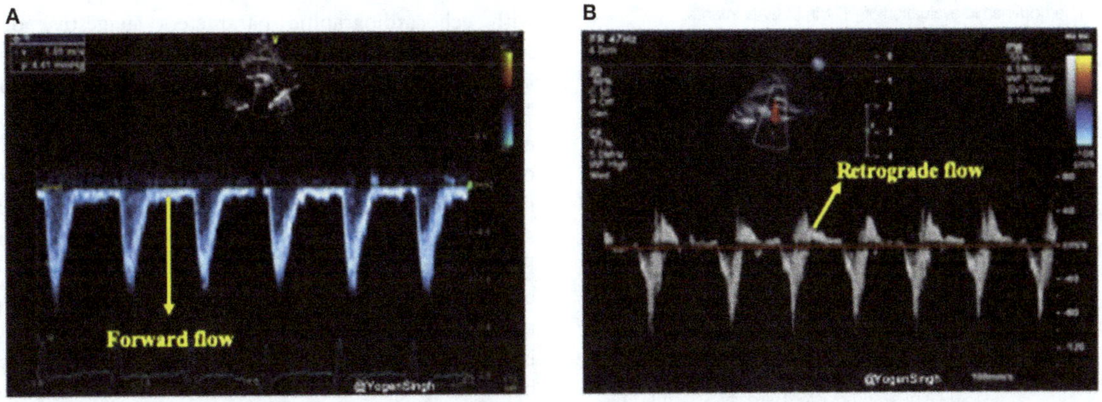

FIGURE 9 | Doppler assessment of blood flow in descending aorta (post-ductal flow). **(A)** Showing forward blood flow during disatole; and **(B)** showing retrograde blood flow during diastole indicating "ductal steal" in presence of a large PDA.

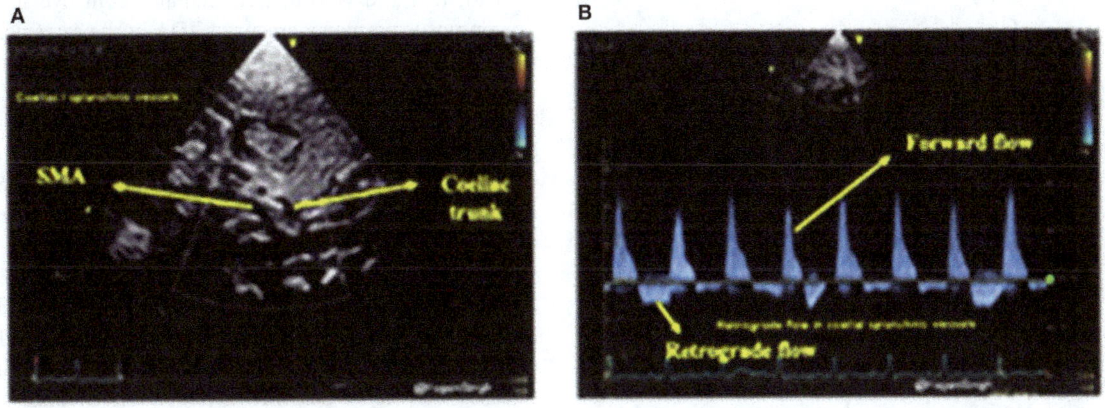

FIGURE 10 | Color flow mapping and Doppler assessment of blood flow in the coeliac trunk and superior mesenteric artery in sub-costal sagittal view. **(A)** Showing color flow mapping of the coeliac and superior mesenteric arteries; and **(B)** showing retrograde blood flow during diastole in the the coeliac and superior mesenteric arteries indicating "ductal steal" in presence of a large PDA.

and significant intra- and inter-observer variability (29–32). Hence, the common echocardiographic parameters often used in clinical decision making on the bedside remain qualitative assessment on visual inspection "eyeballing," LA/Ao ratio and LVEDD measurement. Mitral E/A ratio is easy to measure but one should be mindful that even in preterm infants with no hsPDA E/A ratio gradually become >1 with time as myocardium compliance improves.

Echocardiographic Evaluation of Systemic Hypoperfusion

In the presence of a large PDA, blood shunts away from the systemic circulation throughout the cardiac cycle, however, this becomes more apparent during diastole and it can be studied using Doppler on echocardiography (15, 31). Retrograde or absent blood flow during diastole in descending aorta below the ductal ampulla or in the coeliac axis or superior mesenteric artery have been described as indicator of significant PDA shunt leading to systemic steal (systemic hypoperfusion) (24, 32). Doppler flow patterns from the descending aorta can be obtained from a suprasternal or high parasternal view with the pulsed wave Doppler sample gate placed distal to the origin of ductus arteriosus (ductal ampulla) (**Figure 9**).

Similarly, celiac trunk or superior mesenteric artery can be interrogated using pulsed wave Doppler in the sagittal abdominal view (**Figure 10**). Doppler assessment of the anterior cerebral artery in the mid-sagittal view of brain ultrasound can be performed and retrograde flow during diastole would suggest significant ductal shunt—similar to coeliac or superior mesentery artery Doppler assessment. However, to date the clinical relevance and long term outcomes of the deranged cerebral Doppler flow patterns remain unknown (33).

Based upon the clinical and echocardiographic criteria various staging systems been described and have been shown to help in decision making for intervention (17, 19). However, in authors experience they have not been widely adopted in the clinical practice which could be possibly because of their extensive number of parameters. Recently, van Laere et al.

TABLE 1 | Summary of essential parameters used for echocardiographic assessment and hemodynamic evaluation of PDA in ELGAN infants.

PDA evaluation criteria	Essential echocardiographic parameters for assessment of PDA and hemodynamic evaluation
Ductal characteristics	• PDA size (small <1.5 mm, moderate 1.51–2 mm, large >2 mm) and flow direction (left to right, right to left, or bi-directional) and Doppler assessment with maximum velocity (Vmax) in systole and end-diastole
Assessment of pulmonary over-circulation	• Dilated left side of the heart on visual inspection "eyeballing" and LA/Ao ratio (mild <1.4, moderate 1.41–1.6, severe >1.6) OR LVEDD (correlate with z-scores) OR LPA diastolic velocity, mean velocity >0.42 m/s, end-diastolic velocity >0.2 m/s OR Reversal of mitral E/A ratio *Document presence or absence and magnitude of intra-atrial shunt
Assessment of systemic hypoperfusion	• Retrograde or absent blood flow during diastole in: -descending aorta OR -coeliac trunk or superior mesenteric artery (SMA) OR -anterior or middle cerebral artery

A comprehensive echocardiographic assessment should be performed to rule out any underlying congenital heart defect or pulmonary hypertension and delineate orientation of arch (left or right sidedness) before any intervention to close the PDA.

(13) suggested essential various echocardiographic parameters including measuring left ventricular output in all infants needing assessment of PDA. However, in authors experience these staging systems needing extensive echocardiographic parameters assessment have not been widely adopted in the clinical practice. We have summarized the commonly used parameters which would help the clinicians assessing the PDA and its hemodynamic significance on echocardiography, and in making clinical decisions in the clinical practice.

CLINICAL DECISION MAKING: IS THE PDA HEMODYNAMICALLY SIGNIFICANT?

The above echocardiographic parameters summarized in **Table 1** may help in addressing the issue of whether the PDA is hemodynamically significant or not. However, the definition of an hsPDA continues to evolve. In addition to multiple echocardiographic indices described above, the hemodynamic significance of a persistent PDA should be interpreted by considering the gestational and chronological age, and by assessing the vulnerability of organs at risk for overflow (the lungs), or hypoperfusion (e.g., the brain, intestines, and kidneys). Further work is needed to reach a consensus on how to define and manage a hemodynamically significant persistent PDA in extremely preterm infants (34).

A large PDA with some or all the signs of hemodynamic significance can be seen in a well infant needing no or minimal ventilatory support, and it may not be clinically significant. There is high rate of spontaneous closure of PDA, even in ELGAN infants, if they are left alone (35, 36). On the other hand, a PDA with similar parameters on echocardiography may be associated with significant hemodynamic instability and co-morbidities (5, 6). The debate remains whether well asymptomatic infants with echocardiographic parameters suggestive of large or hemodynamically significant should be treated or not (37–40).

In the last few years, there has been move toward conservative "watchful" approach in infants with no significant clinical signs even when there are echocardiographic parameters suggestive of large hsPDA (9). The published evidence does not support treating an infant with an echocardiographic parameters suggestive of hsPDA without any significant clinical signs of PDA. Large trials have failed to demonstrate any long term benefit (such as death or BPD) from PDA treatment, although they demonstrated short term benefits in terms of decreasing incidence of large intraventricular hemorrhage or pulmonary hemorrhage (39). However, these trials were underpowered to study the long term effects and even more importantly most of these trials used very limited echocardiography dataset to enroll infants (39–43). Hence, in the absence of evidence the debate of whether to treat or not continues and in fact when to treat, how to treat and who to treat remains controversial. There is no consensus on management of PDA in the extremely preterm infants and even there is no consensus on the definition of the commonly used term "hsPDA."

Most clinicians would agree that ductus arteriosus with echocardiographic parameters suggestive of large PDA associated with pulmonary over-circulation and systemic hypoperfusion should be regarded as hsPDA (44). Infants with clinical signs of heart failure and echocardiographic signs of a hsPDA would benefit from treatment. They should be treated with diuretic therapy to offload the heart (decrease preload) and they may benefit from fluid restriction, especially if they are on fluid therapy. This approach would help in cardiovascular stabilization prior to definitive intervention (medical, surgical, or transcatheter approach). Whether all hsPDA should be treated or not, and if treated how best they should be treated, remains debatable. In authors' opinion, infants with echocardiographic signs of hsPDA should be either treated or carefully monitored with low threshold for intervention if clinical condition worsens or does not improve.

The treatment intervention varies from no intervention ("wait and watchful" policy) to treating all PDAs diagnosed on echocardiography. "One size may not fit all"—this truly applies on managing PDA in ELGAN infants with huge variation in clinical course and associated co-morbidities. The lack of evidence on how to best evaluate the PDA in these infants probably results in lack of consensus among the scientific bodies, or even among the clinicians within the same unit (45). The intervention options are: no intervention (conservative management), pharmacological treatment (prophylactic medication, early targeted intervention and treatment of symptomatic infants), transcatheter closure and surgical ligation of PDA.

Studies of prophylactic treatments using indomethacin show reduced rates acute pulmonary hemorrhage, intracranial hemorrhage, and surgical ligation (39). It does however expose large proportion of infants to indomethacin who do not need treatment because of spontaneous closure. Studies on prophylactic use of ibuprofen failed to show the benefits reported

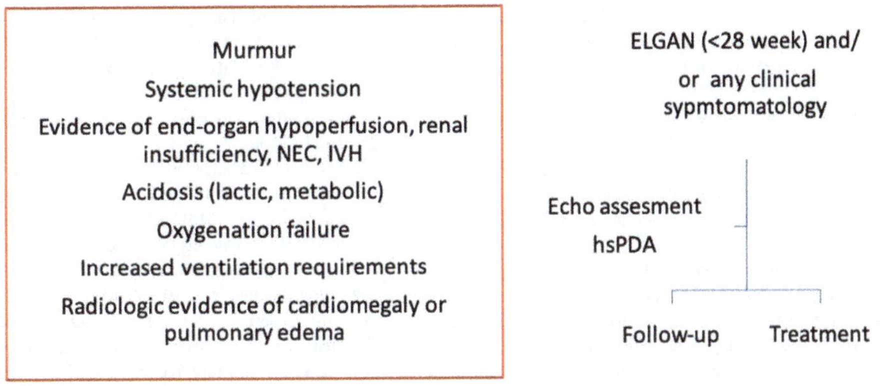

FIGURE 11 | A simple algorithm to clinical decision making in extremely low gestational age newborn infants (ELGAN). Clinical decision whether to treat or follow up should be made based upon both clinical and echocardiography assessment. NEC, necrotizing enterocolitis; IVH, intraventricular hemorrhage; ELGAN, extremely low gestational age newborn infants; hsPDA, hemodynamically significant patent ductus arteriosus.

on using indomethacin (46). Many ongoing studies (BabyOSCAR trial, French TRIOCAPI trial, Dutch BeNEDuCTUS trial, and Australian U-PDA trial focused on the short term and long term outcomes of early targeted treatment approaches[2].

With advances in technologies and expertise, PDA can be closed via transcatheter route with faster recovery and avoiding the risk of complications from surgery. This can now be safely done in ELGAN infants weighing over 700 g (47, 48). A detailed discussion about the evidence for various treatment options is beyond the scope of this review article.

The authors recommend a comprehensive assessment of PDA and its hemodynamic significance before making any clinical decision to treat or not and the clinical decision making should be made in clinical context of the individual infant. A simple algorithm to clinical decision making based upon clinical and echocardiographic assessment, whether to treat or follow up, has been summarized in **Figure 11**. Moreover, this can be dynamic decision, especially in infants with conservative management and serial assessment on neonatologist performed echocardiography can help in making timely individualized decision making.

CONCLUSION

While the best treatment option to treat the PDA in the extremely low gestational age newborn infants remains debatable and lacks consensus at this stage, there has been significant progress in assessing hemodynamic significance of the ductal shunt. Before making a clinical decision to treat a PDA or not, all infants should have a comprehensive structural assessment to rule out any underlying CHD and a meticulous hemodynamic evaluation to assess the impact of PDA shunt on the pulmonary over-circulation and systemic hypoperfusion. In absence of clear evidence, the clinical decision should be individualized based upon clinical concerns and echocardiographic assessment. While in some infants a careful "wait and watchful" strategy may be the best option, other infants may need early intervention to minimize the co-morbidities. There is an urgent need of studying the long term outcomes in the sub-set of infants with hsPDA identified on meticulous echocardiographic assessment.

AUTHOR CONTRIBUTIONS

YS conceptualized the idea and prepared initial manuscript including all images. AF, OE, and BA edited the manuscript and helped in finalizing the manuscript. All authors contributed to the article and approved the submitted version.

[2]Available online at: https://clinicaltrials.gov/ct2/results?term=pDA&Search=Apply&recrs=a&age.

REFERENCES

1. Koch J, Hensley G, Roy L, Brown S, Ramaciotti C, Rosenfeld CR. Prevalence of spontaneous closure of the ductus arteriosus in neonates at a birth weight of 1000 grams or less. *Pediatrics.* (2006) 117:1113–21. doi: 10.1542/peds.2005-1528
2. Bose CL, Laughon MM. Patent ductus arteriosus: lack of evidence for common treatments. *Arch Dis Child Fetal Neonatal Ed.* (2007) 92:F498–502. doi: 10.1136/adc.2005.092734
3. Pourarian S, Farahbakhsh N, Sharma D, Cheriki S, Bijanzadeh F. Prevalence and risk factors associated with the patency of ductus arteriosus in premature neonates: a prospective observational study from Iran. *J Matern Fetal Neonatal Med.* (2017) 30:1460–4. doi: 10.1080/14767058.2016.1219991
4. Costa S, Zecca E, De Luca D, De Carolis MP, Romagnoli C. Efficacy of a single dose of antenatal corticosteroids on morbidity and mortality of preterm infants. *Eur J Obstet Gynecol Reprod Biol.* (2007) 131:154–7. doi: 10.1016/j.ejogrb.2006.05.006
5. Noori S, McCoy M, Friedlich P, Bright B, Gottipati V, Seri I, et al. Failure of ductus arteriosus closure is associated with increased mortality in preterm infants. *Pediatrics.* (2009) 123:e138–44. doi: 10.1542/peds.2008-2418
6. Jaillard S, Larrue B, Rakza T, Magnenant E, Warembourg H, Storme L. Consequences of delayed surgical closure of patent ductus arteriosus in very premature infants. *Ann Thorac Surg.* (2006) 81:231–4.

doi: 10.1016/j.athoracsur.2005.03.141

7. Schena F, Francescato G, Cappelleriet A, Picciolli I, Mayer A, Moscaet F, et al. Association between hemodynamically significant patent ductus arteriosus and bronchopulmonary dysplasia. *J Pediatr.* (2015) 16:1488–92. doi: 10.1016/j.jpeds.2015.03.012
8. Express-Group. Incidence of and risk factors for neonatal morbidity after active perinatal care: extremely preterm infants study in Sweden (EXPRESS). *Acta Paediatr.* (2010) 99:978–92. doi: 10.1111/j.1651-2227.2010.01846.x
9. Benitz WE. Learning to live with patency of the ductus arteriosus in preterm infants. *J Perinatol.* (2011) 31(Suppl. 1):S42–8. doi.org/10.1038/jp.2010.175 doi: 10.1038/jp.2010.175
10. Clyman RI, Liebowitz M, Kaempf J, Erdev O, Bulbul A, Håkansson S, et al. PDA-TOLERATE trial: an exploratory randomized controlled trial of treatment of moderate-to-large patent ductus arteriosus at 1 week of age. *J Pediatr.* (2019) 205:41–8.e6. doi: 10.1016/j.jpeds.2018.09.012
11. Heuchan AM, Clyman RI. Managing the patent ductus arteriosus: current treatment options. *Arch Dis Child Fetal Neonatal Ed.* (2014) 99:F431–6. doi: 10.1136/archdischild-2014-306176
12. Sathanandam S, Balduf K, Chilakala S, Washington J, Allen K, Knott-Craig C, et al. Role of transcatheter patent ductus arteriosus closure in extremely low birth weight infants. *Catheter Cardiovasc Interv.* (2019) 93:89–96. doi: 10.1002/ccd.27808
13. van Laere D, van Overmeire B, Gupta S, El Khuffash A, Savoia M, McNamara PJ, et al. Application of NPE in the assessment of a patent ductus arteriosus. *Pediatric Res.* (2018) 84:S46–56. doi: 10.1038/s41390-018-0077-x
14. Hebert A, Lavoice PM, Giesinger RE, Ting JY, Finan E, Singh Y, et al. Evolution of training guidelines for echocardiography performed by the neonatologist: toward hemodynamic consultation. *J Am Soc Echocardiogr.* (2019) 32:785–90. doi: 10.1016/j.echo.2019.02.002
15. Singh Y, Katheria A, Tissot C. Functional echocardiography in the neonatal intensive care unit. *Indian Pediatr.* (2018) 14:417–25. doi.org/10.1007/s13312-018-1286-4 doi: 10.1007/s13312-018-1286-4
16. Rolland A, Shankar-Aguilera S, Diomandé D, Zupan-Simunek V, BoileauP, et al. Natural evolution of patent ductus arteriosus in the extremely preterm infant. *Arch Dis Child Fetal Neonatal Ed.* (2015) 100:F55–8. doi: 10.1136/archdischild-2014-306339
17. McNamara PJ, Sehgal A. Towards rational management of the patent ductus arteriosus: the need for disease staging. *Arch Dis Child Fetal Neonatal Ed.* (2007) 92:F424–7. doi: 10.1136/adc.2007.118117
18. Singh Y. Evaluation of a child with suspected congenital heart disease. *Paediatr Child Health.* (2018) 28:556–61. doi: 10.1016/j.paed.2018.10.002
19. El-Khuffash A, James AT, Corcoran JD, Dicker P, Franklin O, Elsayed YN, et al. A patent ductus arteriosus severity score predicts chronic lung disease or death before discharge. *J Pediatr.* (2015) 167:1354–61. doi: 10.1016/j.jpeds.2015.09.028
20. Tschuppert S, Doell C, Arlettaz-Mieth R, Baenziger O, Rousson V, Balmer C, et al. The effect of ductal diameter on surgical and medical closure of patent ductus arteriosus in preterm neonates: size matters. *J Thorac Cardiovasc Surg.* (2008) 135:78–82. doi: 10.1016/j.jtcvs.2007.07.027
21. Singh Y, Tissot C. Echocardiographic evaluation of transitional circulation for the neonatologists. TINEC research article. *Front Pediatr.* (2018) 6:79. doi: 10.3389/fped.2018.00140
22. Condo M, Evans N, Bellu R, Kluckow M. Echocardiographic assessment of ductal significance: retrospective comparison of two methods. *Arch Dis Child Fetal Neonatal Ed.* (2012) 97:F35–8. doi: 10.1136/adc.2010.207233
23. Smith A, Maguire M, Livingstone V, Dempsey EM. Peak systolic to end diastolic flow velocity ratio is associated with ductal patency in infants below 32 weeks of gestation. *Arch Dis Child Fetal Neonatal Ed.* (2015) 100:F132–6. doi: 10.1136/archdischild-2014-306439
24. El Hajjar M, Vaksmann G, Rakza T, Kongolo G, Storme L. Severity of the ductal shunt: a comparison of different markers. *Arch Dis Child Fetal Neonatal Ed.* (2005) 90:F419–22. doi: 10.1136/adc.2003.027698
25. Iyer P, Evans N. Re-evaluation of the left atrial to aortic root ratio as a marker of patent ductus arteriosus. *Arch Dis Child Fetal Neonatal Ed.* (1994) 70:F112–7. doi: 10.1136/fn.70.2.F112
26. Abushaban L, Vel MT, Rathinasamy J, Sharma P. Normal reference ranges for left ventricular dimensions in preterm infants. *Ann Pediatr Cardiol.* (2014) 7:180–6. doi: 10.4103/0974-2069.140832
27. Kheiwa A, Ross RD, Kobayashi D. Reversal of severe mitral regurgitation by device closure of a large patent ductus arteriosus in a premature infant. *Cardiol Young.* (2017) 27:189–92. doi: 10.1017/S1047951116000998
28. Walther FJ, Kim DH, Ebrahimi M, Siassi B. Pulsed Doppler measurement of left ventricular output as early predictor of symptomatic patent ductus arteriosus in very preterm infants. *Biol Neonate.* (1989) 56:121–8. doi: 10.1159/000243112
29. Lee A, Liestøl K, Nestaas E, Brunvand L, Lindemann R, Fugelseth D. Superior vena cava flow: feasibility and reliability of the off-line analyses. *Arch Dis Child Fetal Neonatal Ed.* (2010) 95:F121–5. doi: 10.1136/adc.2009.176883
30. Singh Y. Hemodynamic evaluation on echocardiography in neonates and children. TINEC research paper. TINEC research paper. *Front Pediatr.* (2017) 5:201. doi: 10.3389/fped.2017.00201
31. Mertens L, Seri I, Marek J, Arlettaz R, Barker P, McNamara P, et al. Targeted neonatal echocardiography in the neonatal intensive care unit: practice guidelines and recommendations for training. Writing Group of the American Society of Echocardiography (ASE) in collaboration with the European Association of Echocardiography (EAE) and the Association for European Pediatric Cardiologists (AEPC). *J Am Soc Echocardiogr.* (2011) 24:1057–78. doi: 10.1016/j.echo.2011.07.014
32. Broadhouse KM, Price AN, Durighel G, Cox DJ, Finnemore AE, Edwards AD, et al. Assessment of PDA shunt and systemic blood flow in newborns using cardiac MRI. *NMR Biomed.* (2013) 26:1135–41. doi: 10.1002/nbm.2927
33. Ecury-Goossen GM, Raets MMA, Camfferman FA, Vos RHJ, van Rosmalen J, Reiss IRM, et al. Resistive indices of cerebral arteries in very preterm infants: values throughout stay in the neonatal intensive care unit and impact of patent ductus arteriosus. *Pediatr Radiol.* (2016) 46:1291–300. doi: 10.1007/s00247-016-3615-x
34. Shepherd JL, Noori S. What is a hemodynamically significant PDA in preterm infants? *Congen Heart Dis.* (2019) 14:21–6. doi: 10.1111/chd.12727
35. Semberova J, Sirc J, Miletin J, Kucera J, Berka I, Sebkova S, et al. Spontaneous closure of patent ductus arteriosus in infants ≤1500 g. *Pediatrics.* (2017) 140:e20164258. doi: 10.1542/peds.2016-4258
36. Herrman K, Bose C, Lewis K, Laughon M. Spontaneous closure of the patent ductus arteriosus in very low birth weight infants following discharge from the neonatal unit. *Arch Dis Child Fetal Neonatal Ed.* (2009) 94:F48–50. doi: 10.1136/adc.2007.129270
37. Noori S. Patent ductus arteriosus in the preterm infant: to treat or not to treat? *J Perinatol.* (2010) 30:S31–7. doi: 10.1038/jp.2010.97
38. Abdel-Hady H, Nasef N, Shabaan AE, Nour I. Patent ductus arteriosus in preterm infants: do we have the right answers? *Biomed Res Int.* (2013) 2013:676192. doi: 10.1155/2013/676192
39. Schmidt B, Davis P, Moddemann D, Ohlsson A, Roberts RS, Saigal S, et al. Long-term effects of indomethacin prophylaxis in extremely low birth-weight infants. *N Engl J Med.* (2001) 344:1966–72. doi: 10.1056/NEJM200106283442602
40. Kluckow M, Jeffery M, Gill A, Evans N. A randomised placebo-controlled trial of early treatment of the patent ductus arteriosus. *Arch Dis Child Fetal Neonatal Ed.* (2014) 99:F99–104. doi: 10.1136/archdischild-2013-304695
41. Mosalli R, Alfaleh K. Prophylactic surgical ligation of patent ductus arteriosus for prevention of mortality and morbidity in extremely low birth weight infants. *Cochrane Database Syst Rev.* (2008) 1:CD006181. doi: 10.1002/14651858.CD006181.pub2
42. Malviya MN, Ohlsson A, Shah SS. Surgical versus medical treatment with cyclooxygenase inhibitors for symptomatic patent ductus arteriosus in preterm infants. *Cochrane Database Syst Rev.* (2013) 3:CD003951. doi: 10.1002/14651858.CD003951.pub3
43. Ohlsson A, Walia R, Shah SS. Ibuprofen for the treatment of patent ductus arteriosus in preterm or low birth weight (or both) infants. *Cochrane Database Syst Rev.* (2015) 2:CD003481. doi: 10.1002/14651858.CD003481.pub6
44. Zonnenberg I, de Waal K. The definition of a haemodynamic significant duct in randomized controlled trials: a systematic literature review. *Acta Paediatr.* (2012) 101:247–51. doi: 10.1111/j.1651-2227.2011.02468.x
45. Sathanandam S, Whiting S, Cunningham J, Zurakowski D, Apalodimas L, Waller BR, et al. Practice variation in the management of patent ductus arteriosus in extremely low birth weight infants in the United States: survey

results among cardiologists and neonatologists. *Congenit Heart Dis.* (2019) 14:6–14. doi: 10.1111/chd.12729

46. Dani C, Bertini G, Pezzati M, Poggi C, Guerrini P, Martano C, et al. Prophylactic ibuprofen for the prevention of intraventricular hemorrhage among preterm infants: a multicenter, randomized study. *Pediatrics.* (2005) 115:1529–35. doi: 10.1542/peds.2004-1178
47. Backes CH, Cheetham SL, Deyo GM, Leopold S, Ball MK, Smith CV, et al. Percutaneous patent ductus arteriosus (PDA) closure in very preterm infants: feasibility and complications. *J Am Heart Assoc.* (2016) 5:e002923. doi: 10.1161/JAHA.115.002923
48. Regan W, Benbrik N, Sharma SR, Auriau J, Bouvaist H, Bautista-Rodriguez C, et al. Improved ventilation in premature babies after transcatheter versus surgical closure of patent ductus arteriosus. *Int J Cardiol.* (2020) 311:22–7. doi: 10.1016/j.ijcard.2020.03.040

2

Plasma Amino Acid Concentrations at Birth and Patent Ductus Arteriosus in Very and Extremely Preterm Infants

*Maurice J. Huizing[1], Moreyba Borges-Luján[2], Giacomo Cavallaro[3], Gema E. González-Luis[2], Genny Raffaeli[3,4], Pilar Bas-Suárez[5], Jaap A. Bakker[6], Rob M. Moonen[7] and Eduardo Villamor[1]**

[1] Department of Pediatrics, Maastricht University Medical Centre (MUMC+), School for Oncology and Developmental Biology (GROW), Maastricht, Netherlands, [2] Department of Neonatology, Complejo Hospitalario Universitario Insular Materno-Infantil (CHUIMI) de Canarias, Las Palmas de Gran Canaria, Spain, [3] Neonatal Intensive Care Unit, Fondazione IRCCS Cà Granda Ospedale Maggiore Policlinico, Milan, Italy, [4] Department of Clinical Sciences and Community Health, Università degli Studi di Milano, Milan, Italy, [5] Department of Pediatrics, Hospital Vithas Santa Catalina, Las Palmas de Gran Canaria, Spain, [6] Department of Clinical Chemistry and Laboratory Medicine, Leiden University Medical Center, Leiden, Netherlands, [7] Department of Pediatrics, Zuyderland Medical Center, Heerlen, Netherlands

Correspondence:
Eduardo Villamor
e.villamor@mumc.nl

Background: Amino acids are increasingly recognized as bioactive molecules in numerous physiological and pathophysiological pathways. The non-essential amino acid glutamate is vasoactive in the rat ductus arteriosus (DA) and a decrease in its levels within the 1st days of life has been associated with the presence of patent DA (PDA) in extremely preterm infants. However, these findings have not been confirmed in other studies.

Objective: To investigate the possible association between amino acid concentrations in the 1st day of life and the presence of PDA in a cohort of 121 newborns with gestational age (GA) below 30 weeks and birth weight (BW) below 1,500 g.

Methods: Plasma samples were collected 6–12 h after birth and amino acid concentrations were determined by tandem mass spectrometry. Besides PDA, we analyzed the potential association of amino acid concentrations with infant sex, small for GA (SGA, defined as BW<third percentile), antenatal corticosteroids, chorioamnionitis, and preeclampsia. Group differences were analyzed by ANOVA adjusted for GA and BW. A Bonferroni significance threshold of $P < 0.0024$ was used to correct for multiple testing.

Results: PDA was found in 48 of the 121 infants examined. We observed higher mean levels of glutamate in infants with PDA (147.0 μmol/L, SD 84.0) as compared with those without (106.7 μmol/L, SD 49.1, $P = 0.0006$). None of the other amino acid concentrations in the PDA group reached the level of statistical significance that was pre-set to correct for multiple comparisons. Glutamate levels were not significantly affected by infant sex, being SGA, or by exposure to antenatal corticosteroids, clinical chorioamnionitis, or preeclampsia.

Conclusion: Our study not only does not confirm the previous findings of low glutamate levels in preterm infants with PDA, but we have even found elevated glutamate concentrations associated with PDA. Nevertheless, despite the high statistical significance, the difference in glutamate levels may lack clinical significance or may be an epiphenomenon associated with the particular clinical condition of infants with PDA.

Keywords: amino acids, ductus arteriosus [MeSH], glutamate, preterm (birth), metabolomic analysis

INTRODUCTION

Failed or delayed closure of the ductus arteriosus (DA) after birth leads to patent DA (PDA), a common condition among very preterm infants (1–6). The two most relevant vasoactive factors that maintain the DA open during fetal life and mediate its closure after birth are oxygen tension and prostaglandins (4, 5). However, the DA responds to numerous vasoactive agents and its closure is finally the result of a complex interaction of mediators and pathways (4, 5).

In a recent study, Fujita et al. proposed a role for the non-essential amino acid glutamate in the postnatal closure of the DA (7). They reported that plasma glutamate concentration was significantly lower in extremely preterm infants (gestational age <28 weeks) with PDA compared to those without the condition (7). In addition, they observed that intraperitoneal injection of glutamate to pregnant rats induced ductal contraction in the fetus. Moreover, they showed that the mRNA of the glutamate ionotropic receptor α-amino-3-hydroxy-5-methyl-4-isoxazolepropionate (AMPA) type subunit one was highly expressed in rat DA compared to the aorta, and was co-localized with autonomic nerve terminals in the human and rat DA. In agreement with these results, microarrays comparing the genetic profiles of the DA and ascending aorta from mice and rats showed significant changes in the ductal expression of both ionotropic and metabotropic glutamate receptors (8, 9). Altogether, these data suggest a role for glutamatergic signaling in the physiology and/or pathobiology of the DA. Nevertheless, more studies are needed to confirm this hypothesis.

Between 2007 and 2012, our group conducted a prospective study to analyze the association between polymorphisms of the *carbamoyl phosphate synthetase* (*CPS*) gene and necrotizing enterocolitis (NEC) (10–12). In that research, plasma levels of amino acids were determined in the 1st day of life in order to correlate them with the primary outcome of the study. One of the secondary outcomes of the study was PDA. Our aim was to use these unpublished data to investigate the association between glutamate, as well as other amino acids, and the presence of PDA in infants with a gestational age (GA) below 30 weeks.

METHODS

Study Population

This study was performed in a previously described cohort of 121 preterm infants (GA ≤30 weeks and birth weight ≤1,500 g) admitted to the level III neonatal intensive care units of the Maastricht University Medical Center (Maastricht, The Netherlands), Hospital Universitario Materno-Infantil de Canarias (Las Palmas de Gran Canaria, Spain), and Carlo Poma Hospital (Mantova, Italy) between July 2007 and October 2008. All infants had been enrolled in the study "Carbamoyl Phosphate Synthetase (CPS) Polymorphisms as Risk Factor for NEC" (NCT00554866). The institutional review board (IRB) of the three participating centers approved the use of the clinical data of the patients for the present study (IRB numbers: Maastricht MEC-07-2-018; Las Palmas CEIC- 276; Mantova 21366/2007). Written informed consent was obtained from the parents for inclusion in the study. Infants exposed to a blood transfusion, enteral or parenteral proteins/amino acids, or inhaled NO before blood sampling were excluded from the study. The correlation between arginine, citrulline and dimethylarginine levels and CPS polymorphisms and NEC in the same group of patients has been the subject of another publications of our group (10, 11).

PDA Assessment and Other Clinical Variables

The perinatal and neonatal data of enrolled infants (**Table 1**) were extracted from the database of the NCT00554866 trial. At the time of inclusion of the children in the cohort (2007–2008), the three participating centers had very similar protocols for detection and treatment of PDA. These protocols included the performance of a screening echocardiogram by a pediatric cardiologist on postnatal day 2 to 5. As previously described, hemodynamically significant PDA was defined by a transductal diameter >1.5 mm with unrestrictive (<1 m/s) left to right transductal flow on pulse wave Doppler and clinical signs of pulmonary overcirculation (e.g., increasing ventilation, oxygenation problems) and/or systemic hypoperfusion (e.g., abdominal distension, oliguria) (13). In the absence of clear clinical signs, ascertainment of hemodynamic significance was made on the basis of any of the following echocardiographic characteristics: left atrial/aortic root ratio >1.4, mean velocity in the left pulmonary artery >0.6 m/s, or diastolic backflow in the abdominal aorta (13).

GA was determined by the last menstrual period and early ultrasounds (before 20 weeks of gestation). Besides the presence of PDA, the following demographic and clinical characteristics were collected and correlated with the amino acid concentrations: infant sex; small for GA (SGA, defined as birth weight for GA below the sex-specific third percentile); antenatal corticosteroids (defined as two doses of betamethasone administered 24 h apart); clinical chorioamnionitis (defined as every clinical suspicion of infection of the chorion, amnion, amniotic fluid, placenta, or a combination as judged by the obstetrician); and preeclampsia (based on the obstetrician's diagnosis).

Plasma Amino Acid Analysis

One blood sample (500 μL) was obtained between 6 and 12 h after birth from an umbilical artery or peripheral artery catheter. When not available, the blood sample was obtained from venous puncture. Immediately after collection, heparinized blood samples were put on ice and centrifuged within 10 min (4,000 rpm, 10 min, 4°C) to obtain plasma. The plasma was deproteinized with 6 mg of solid 5-sulfosalicylic acid (SSA; Sigma, St. Louis, MO, USA) per 100 μL plasma, and stored at −80°C until further analysis. The samples obtained in Las Palmas and Mantova were transported on dry ice to Maastricht where all the analyses were performed (10).

Concentrations of (underivatized) amino acids in plasma were determined using an ultra-performance liquid chromatography (UPLC) separation module coupled to an electrospray ionization tandem mass spectrometry (ESI-MS/MS, Quattro Premier, Waters, Etten-Leur, The Netherlands). Stable isotope labeled

TABLE 1 | Baseline characteristics and neonatal complications in preterm infants with and without PDA.

	PDA-yes (*n* = 48)	*n* data missing	PDA-no (*n* = 73)	*n* data missing	*P*-value
Birth weight (g)	967 (SD 238)	0	1,069 (SD 238)	0	0.023
Gestational age (wks)	27.5 (SD 1.5)	0	28.6 (SD 1.5)	0	0.000
Male sex	26 (54.2)	0	43 (58.9)	0	0.607
Prenatal steroids	39 (81.2)	0	55 (77.5)	2	0.159
Preeclampsia	5 (10.6)	1	20 (28.2)	2	0.023
Clinical chorioamnionitis	2 (4.2)	0	9 (12.3)	0	0.127
Vaginal delivery	16 (33.3)	0	24 (32.9)	0	0.958
Apgar (1 min)	5 (4–7)	1	7 (5–8)	0	0.079
Apgar (5 min)	8 (6–9)	1	9 (7–9)	0	0.109
RDS	36 (75.0)	0	40 (55.6)	1	0.030
Mechanical vent.	15 (83.3)	0	40 (56.3)	2	0.002
BPD	19 (45.2)	6	14 (21.2)	7	0.008
Hypotension	26 (54.2)	0	27 (37.5)	1	0.072
Sepsis	29 (63.0)	2	34 (46.6)	0	0.080
NEC	5 (10.9)	2	2 (2.9)	5	0.084
IVH	18 (37.5)	0	17 (23.6)	1	0.101
PVL	5 (10.4)	0	4 (5.5)	0	0.311
ROP	4 (10.0)	8	5 (7.5)	6	0.647
Mortality	7 (14.6)	0	9 (12.3)	0	0.720

Results are expressed as mean (SD). median [interquartile range] or absolute numbers of patients (percentage). PDA, patent ductus arteriosus; RDS, respiratory distress syndrome; BPD, bronchopulmonary dysplasia (defined as oxygen at 36 weeks postmenstrual age); NEC, necrotizing enterocolitis (≥stage II); IVH, intraventricular hemorrhage (≥grade 2); PVL, periventricular leukomalacia; ROP, retinopathy of prematurity (≥stage II).

amino acids were used as internal standards for quantification of plasma amino acids. All analyses were performed in one laboratory (Department of Clinical Genetics, Maastricht University Medical Center, Maastricht, The Netherlands) (10).

Statistical Analysis

Results for continuous variables are expressed as mean (SD) or, if variables were not normally distributed, as median (interquartile range). Standardized residuals were examined for outliers, and measurements that were <-3.0 or >3.0 SD from the mean were removed. The possible relationship between amino acid concentrations and PDA was evaluated by ANOVA with adjustment for gestational age, and birth weight. Analysis included 21 ANOVA models (one clinical variable × 21 amino acid measurements) and a Bonferonni significance threshold of $P < 0.0024$ (0.05 divided by 21) was used to correct for multiple testing (14). We performed a power analysis to determine the minimum amino acid concentration ratio (PDA-yes:PDA-no) that would be reach statistical significance ($P < 0.0024$) with our sample size (15). The results of the power analysis are shown in **Supplementary Table 1**. All analyses were performed using IBM SPSS Statistics for Windows (Version 22.0; Armonk, NY, USA).

RESULTS

PDA was found in 48 of the 121 infants examined. The characteristics of the cohort are summarized in **Table 1**. The plasma concentrations of the different amino acids and their relation to PDA are shown in **Table 2**. Glutamate was the only amino acid whose concentration was significantly different ($P < 0.0006$) when the groups with and without PDA were compared. None of the clinical or perinatal characteristics, including sex, BW below third percentile, use of antenatal corticosteroids, history of chorioamnionitis, or history of preeclampsia, led to significant differences in glutamate concentrations (**Table 3**). Glutamate concentrations were also not significantly different in infants who developed intraventricular hemorrhage (≥grade 2), NEC (≥stage II), bronchopulmonary dysplasia (defined as supplementary oxygen at 36 weeks postmenstrual age), or retinopathy of prematurity (≥stage II) (**Table 3**).

Changes in amino acid concentrations depending on infant sex, SGA, and exposure to antenatal corticosteroids, chorioamnionitis, or preeclampsia are depicted in **Supplementary Tables 2–6**. SGA infants showed increased plasma concentrations of asparagine, glutamine, glycine and alanine (**Supplementary Table 3**). Tryptophan levels were significantly reduced in infants exposed to preeclampsia (**Supplementary Table 5**) and α-aminobutyric acid levels were significantly increased in infants exposed to antenatal corticosteroids (**Supplementary Table 6**).

DISCUSSION

Along with their fundamental role as elements for protein and peptide synthesis, amino acids are increasingly recognized as bioactive molecules in numerous physiological and pathophysiological pathways (16). Alterations in amino acid levels during the 1st days of postnatal life have been associated with clinical conditions of prematurity such as RDS or NEC (10, 17–20). Closure of the DA at birth is one of the processes in which a participation of amino acids, specifically glutamate, has been proposed. However, data supporting this potential role of glutamate, although provocative, are still scarce (7). In the present study, we analyzed the concentrations of amino acids in plasma samples obtained between 6 and 12 h of life in a group of preterm newborns who had not yet received amino acid supplementation. Interestingly, glutamate was the only amino acid whose concentration was significantly different between the groups with and without PDA. However, in contrast to the previous report by Fujita et al. (7), glutamate levels were higher in the PDA group. None of the other amino acids showed differences in plasma concentrations in the PDA group that reached the level of statistical significance ($P < 0.0024$) preset in our analysis. In addition, neither infant sex nor obstetric or perinatal conditions significantly affected glutamate concentrations.

Glutamate is a pleiotropic molecule acting at the crossroads of metabolism and signaling, and functioning as both substrate and product in many distinct physiological processes (21–24). Glutamate is synthesized from glutamine, α-ketoglutarate and

TABLE 2 | Plasma concentrations of amino acids (μmol/L) in preterm infants with and without PDA.

Amino acid	PDA status	Mean	SD	*N*	*P*-value	Adjusted *P*-value
Glutamate	PDA-no	106.7	49.1	66	0.004	**0.0006**
	PDA-yes	147.0	84.0	47		
Asparagine	PDA-no	60.8	22.6	70	0.870	0.636
	PDA-yes	61.5	25.6	47		
Serine	PDA-no	155.8	45.3	71	0.232	0.092
	PDA-yes	168.4	61.9	48		
Glutamine	PDA-no	481.1	189.9	69	0.189	0.692
	PDA-yes	441.2	176.1	44		
Histidine	PDA-no	72.7	19.6	70	0.311	0.163
	PDA-yes	76.8	23.8	45		
Glycine	PDA-no	313.9	117.2	72	0.614	0.167
	PDA-yes	325.5	129.1	47		
Threonine	PDA-no	247.4	90.3	72	0.257	0.039
	PDA-yes	268.1	105.5	47		
Citrulline	PDA-no	21.3	6.3	68	0.894	0.807
	PDA-yes	21.2	5.5	48		
Arginine	PDA-no	45.2	22.5	73	0.026	0.074
	PDA-yes	35.7	21.9	45		
Alanine	PDA-no	329.8	178.0	69	0.718	0.441
	PDA-yes	342.2	181.5	45		
Taurine	PDA-no	208.0	94.0	73	0.664	0.468
	PDA-yes	200.9	75.6	47		
α-aminobutyric acid	PDA-no	15.9	7.6	72	0.204	0.253
	PDA-yes	18.1	10.0	48		
Tyrosine	PDA-no	109.8	31.5	69	0.015	0.027
	PDA-yes	129.7	48.8	48		
Valine	PDA-no	167.1	49.3	67	0.201	0.216
	PDA-yes	182.8	52.0	45		
Methionine	PDA-no	49.0	28.0	71	0.004	0.023
	PDA-yes	66.8	37.6	48		
Isoleucine	PDA-no	50.2	24.5	70	0.953	0.831
	PDA-yes	49.9	25.2	46		
Phenylalanine	PDA-no	68.8	15.1	70	0.606	0.358
	PDA-yes	70.7	21.2	46		
Tryptophan	PDA-no	27.7	8.2	66	0.204	0.014
	PDA-yes	29.7	7.7	46		
Leucine	PDA-no	69.1	22.7	67	0.578	0.432
	PDA-yes	71.8	27.5	44		
Ornithine	PDA-no	80.7	40.7	71	0.062	0.033
	PDA-yes	95.9	45.9	47		
Lysine	PDA-no	261.1	103.6	72	0.510	0.423
	PDA-yes	274.3	108.6	46		

Results are expressed as mean (SD). Standardized residuals were examined for outliers, and measurements that were <-3.0 or >3.0 SD from the mean were removed. Adjusted for gestational age and birth weight. PDA, patent ductus arteriosus.

TABLE 3 | Plasma concentrations of glutamate (μmol/L) in different characteristics and outcomes of preterm infants.

Characteristic/ outcome	Mean	SD	*N*	*P*-value	Adjusted *P*-value
Female	150.3	85.4	52	0.012	0.019
Male	115.3	57.4	70		
SGA-no	128.2	74.1	101	0.523	0.857
SGA-yes	132.3	59.3	22		
Prenatal steroids-no	120.0	79.6	25	0.574	0.302
Prenatal steroids-yes	130.5	70.5	95		
Preeclampsia-no	126.6	73.7	91	0.687	0.162
Preeclampsia-yes	116.6	45.2	23		
Chorioamnionitis-no	137.1	72.5	111	0.007	0.015
Chorioamnionitis-yes	77.6	56.3	12		
BPD-no	124.4	76.6	74	0.742	0.160
BPD-yes	128.5	49.7	31		
NEC-no	129.3	70.7	105	0.196	0.224
NEC-yes	166.4	106.6	7		
IVH-no	139.4	82.8	85	0.200	0.470
IVH-yes	122.3	57.5	35		
ROP-no	122.1	63.6	93	0.157	0.066
ROP-yes	71.3	32.9	7		

Results are expressed as mean (SD). Standardized residuals were examined for outliers, and measurements that were <-3.0 or >3.0 SD from the mean were removed. Adjusted for gestational age and birth weight. SGA, small for gestational age; BPD, bronchopulmonary dysplasia (defined as oxygen at 36 weeks postmenstrual age); NEC, necrotizing enterocolitis (≥stage II); IVH, intraventricular hemorrhage (≥grade 2); ROP, retinopathy of prematurity (≥stage II).

5-oxoproline and in turn is the precursor for the biosynthesis of amino acids such as L-proline and L-arginine (24). In addition, other neurotransmitters as well as the antioxidant glutathione are also synthesized from glutamate (24). This ubiquity of glutamate and its metabolism greatly complicates the interpretation of our results. Although we have found an association between high levels of glutamate at birth and the presence of PDA, glutamate levels may be reflecting some other aspect of the perinatal clinical condition rather than having a direct effect on DA closure. Many of the maternal pathological conditions that result in preterm birth are accompanied by alterations in the aminogram that can be transferred to the fetus and affect plasma amino acid levels in the 1st h of life (25–27). However, as mentioned above, we did not find significant changes in glutamate in SGA infants or after exposure to clinical chorioamnionitis, preeclampsia, or antenatal steroids. In addition, infection and brain injury, two conditions that are very frequently present among very preterm infants, are known to alter the circulating levels of glutamate and other amino acids (28, 29).

Glutamate receptors are divided into the ligand-gated ion channel receptors (ionotropic receptors) and G protein-coupled metabotropic receptors (30). Ionotropic receptors are further classified into three groups based on their pharmacology and structural properties: *N*-methyl-D-aspartate (NMDA), AMPA and kainate receptors (30). Glutamatergic communication through NMDA receptors is key in the central nervous system where glutamate is the main excitatory neurotransmitter (21, 22). However, glutamatergic signaling may also occur in non-neuronal tissues, including the cardiovascular system (30–42).

Little is known about glutamate signaling in the vascular system even though not only endothelial and smooth muscle cells can release glutamate, but also platelets and immune cells (21, 34, 43). The vascular effects of glutamate may vary depending on the vascular bed studied. Because of its important role in nervous system homeostasis, most studies have focused on brain (micro)circulation where glutamate is a vasodilator. Nitric oxide (39), carbon monoxide (30, 40, 41), and prostaglandins (42) have been involved in glutamate-induced vasodilation in the central nervous system. As regards other vascular territories, Nguyen-Duong showed glutamate-induced relaxation in porcine coronary arteries (33). This relaxation was attenuated by 4-aminopyridine which suggests the involvement of voltage-gated K^+ (K_V) channels. Inhibition of K_V channels by reactive oxygen species is one of the main mechanisms responsible for oxygen-induced contraction of the DA (4, 5). K_V channel inhibition leads to membrane depolarization and increased Ca^{2+} entry through L-type Ca^{2+} channels (4, 5). Interestingly, Dumas et al. have recently reported K_V-mediated, Ca^{2+}-dependent glutamate release from human pulmonary arterial smooth muscle cells (21). Finally, as mentioned elsewhere, Fujita et al. showed glutamate-induced contraction of fetal rat DA and proposed an AMPA receptor-mediated release of noradrenaline as the mechanism underlying this contraction (7). Another interesting vascular effect of glutamate with potential impact on DA biology is its role as platelet activator, which is in part cyclooxygenase-dependent (34, 43). Platelet activation has been identified as a key factor in ductal closure (44, 45) and a potential role of glutamate might be a hypothesis to consider in future research.

The two most important limitations of our study are the relative small sample size and that is based on a single amino acid determination instead of longitudinal samples collected throughout the first days of life. In the study of Fujita et al., the sample is much smaller (16 infants) than in our study but amino acid levels were determined at birth (arterial umbilical cord blood) and on the 2nd day of life (7). Interestingly, glutamate levels were not significantly diminished in the first sample. In addition, not only glutamate but also leucine, lysine, phenylalanine, valine, tryptophan, methionine, isoleucine, arginine, tyrosine and glycine concentrations were decreased in the PDA group on the 2nd day of life (7). This was despite the fact that both the PDA and control groups received a similar regimen of amino acid supplementation. Of note, the amino acid mixture used by Fujita et al., had a much lower concentration of glutamate than the mixtures commonly used in Europe and America (7). However, the decrease in the levels of most amino acids, and not only glutamate, may suggest a general increase in the demand for amino acids in extremely preterm infants with PDA.

To the best of our knowledge, few other studies have evaluated the association between PDA and amino acid concentrations within the 1st days of life. Ryckman et al. analyzed amino acid concentrations in dried blood spot samples taken on day 1–3 in a cohort of 689 preterm infants (GA<37 weeks) of which 133 had PDA. The levels of glutamate were not affected but leucine, methionine, phenylalanine, and valine concentrations were higher in infants with PDA as compared with those without. Nevertheless, the differences did not reach the limit of statistical significance set by the authors to correct for multiple testing ($P < 5 \times 10^{-5}$). The authors reported similar results when the analysis was limited to the infants with GA below 32 weeks. Ryckman et al. also tested the *ex vivo* response of mouse DA to leucine, methionine, phenylalanine, and valine and observed that the amino acids failed to produce a significant change in ductal tone. Unfortunately, the ductal response to glutamate was not investigated. Very recently, Oltman et al. reported in a cohort of 34,969 infants with GA<37 weeks (1,924 infants with GA<32 weeks) that increased risk for morbidity (including PDA) or mortality was associated with increased concentrations of glycine and proline, as well as decreased concentrations of ornithine in dried blood spot samples taken during the 1st week of life (46). Finally, Bardanzellu et al. showed decreased tryptophan urinary levels (samples collected <12 h of life) in preterm infants with PDA (47). Therefore, the association between PDA and amino acid concentrations varies greatly between studies, making difficult to draw conclusions about the specific role of a particular amino acid in DA biology and pathobiology.

In summary, our study not only does not confirm the previous findings of low glutamate levels in preterm infants with PDA, but we have even found elevated glutamate concentrations associated with PDA. However, association does not mean causality. Despite the high statistical significance, the difference in glutamate levels may lack clinical significance or may be an epiphenomenon associated with the particular clinical condition of infants with PDA.

ETHICS STATEMENT

The studies involving human participants were reviewed and approved by Ethics Committees from Maastricht University Medical Center (Maastricht, The Netherlands), Hospital Universitario Materno-Infantil de Canarias (Las Palmas de Gran Canaria, Spain), and Carlo Poma Hospital (Mantova, Italy). Written informed consent to participate in this study was provided by the participants' legal guardian/next of kin.

AUTHOR CONTRIBUTIONS

MH, MB-L, GC, GG-L, GR, and PB-S collected data for the study, contributed to interpretation of results, and reviewed and revised the manuscript. JB performed the amino acid analysis, contributed to interpretation of results, and reviewed and revised the manuscript. RM contributed to the design of the study, collected data and supervised data collection, performed the statistical analysis, contributed to interpretation of results, and reviewed and revised the manuscript. EV conceptualized the study, supervised data collection and statistical analysis, contributed to interpretation of results, and drafted the manuscript. All authors contributed to the article and approved the submitted version.

REFERENCES

1. Hundscheid T, Onland W, Van Overmeire B, Dijk P, van Kaam AH, Dijkman KP, et al. Early treatment versus expectative management of patent ductus arteriosus in preterm infants: a multicentre, randomised, non-inferiority trial in Europe (BeNeDuctus trial). *BMC Pediatr.* (2018) 18:262. doi: 10.1186/s12887-018-1215-7
2. Reese J, Laughon MM. The patent ductus arteriosus problem: infants who still need treatment. *J Pediatr.* (2015) 167:954–6. doi: 10.1016/j.jpeds.2015.08.023
3. Sallmon H, Koehne P, Hansmann G. Recent advances in the treatment of preterm newborn infants with patent ductus arteriosus. *Clin Perinatol.* (2016) 43:113–29. doi: 10.1016/j.clp.2015.11.008
4. Villamor E, Moreno L, Mohammed R, Pérez-Vizcaíno F, Cogolludo A. Reactive oxygen species as mediators of oxygen signaling during fetal-to-neonatal circulatory transition. *Free Radic Biol Med.* (2019) 142:82–96. doi: 10.1016/j.freeradbiomed.2019.04.008
5. Stoller JZ, DeMauro SB, Dagle JM, Reese J. Current perspectives on pathobiology of the ductus arteriosus. *J Clin Exp Cardiol.* (2012) 8:S8-001. doi: 10.4172/2155-9880.S8-001
6. Gillam-Krakauer M, Reese J. Diagnosis and management of patent ductus arteriosus. *Neoreviews.* (2018) 19:e394–402. doi: 10.1542/neo.19-7-e394
7. Fujita S, Yokoyama U, Ishiwata R, Aoki R, Nagao K, Masukawa D, et al. Glutamate promotes contraction of the rat ductus arteriosus. *Circ J.* (2016) 80:2388–96. doi: 10.1253/circj.CJ-16-0649
8. Shelton EL, Ector G, Galindo CL, Hooper CW, Brown N, Wilkerson I, et al. Transcriptional profiling reveals ductus arteriosus-specific genes that regulate vascular tone. *Physiol Genomics.* (2014) 46:457–66. doi: 10.1152/physiolgenomics.00171.2013
9. Hsieh Y-T, Liu NM, Ohmori E, Yokota T, Kajimura I, Akaike T, et al. Transcription profiles of the ductus arteriosus in Brown-Norway rats with irregular elastic fiber formation. *Circ J.* (2014) 78:1224–33. doi: 10.1253/circj.CJ-13-1029
10. Moonen RM, Huizing MJ, Cavallaro G, González-Luis GE, Bas-Suárez P, Bakker JA, et al. Plasma levels of dimethylarginines in preterm very low birth weight neonates: its relation with perinatal factors and short-term outcome. *Int J Mol Sci.* (2015) 16:19–39. doi: 10.3390/ijms16010019
11. Moonen RM, Reyes I, Cavallaro G, González-Luis G, Bakker JA, Villamor E. The T1405N carbamoyl phosphate synthetase polymorphism does not affect plasma arginine concentrations in preterm infants. *PLoS ONE.* (2010) 5:e10792. doi: 10.1371/journal.pone.0010792
12. Moonen RM, Cavallaro G, Huizing MJ, González-Luis GE, Mosca F, Villamor E. Association between the p. Thr1406Asn polymorphism of the carbamoyl-phosphate synthetase 1 gene and necrotizing enterocolitis: a prospective multicenter study. *Sci Rep.* (2016) 6:36999. doi: 10.1038/srep36999
13. Bas-Suárez MP, González-Luis GE, Saavedra P, Villamor E. Platelet counts in the first seven days of life and patent ductus arteriosus in preterm very low-birth-weight infants. *Neonatology.* (2014) 106:188–94. doi: 10.1159/000362432
14. Armstrong RA. When to use the Bonferroni correction. *Ophthalmic Physiol Opt.* (2014) 34:502–8. doi: 10.1111/opo.12131
15. Honkanen RA, Baruah S, Zimmerman MB, Khanna CL, Weaver YK, Narkiewicz J, et al. Vitreous amino acid concentrations in patients with glaucoma undergoing vitrectomy. *Arch Ophthalmol.* (2003) 121:183–8. doi: 10.1001/archopht.121.2.183
16. Hu X, Guo F. Amino acid sensing in metabolic homeostasis and health. *Endocr Rev.* (2020) 42:56–76. doi: 10.1210/endrev/bnaa026
17. Celik IH, Demirel G, Canpolat FE, Dilmen U. Reduced plasma citrulline levels in low birth weight infants with necrotizing enterocolitis. *J Clin Lab Anal.* (2013) 27:328–32. doi: 10.1002/jcla.21607
18. Celik IH, Demirel G, Canpolat FE, Oguz SS, Erdeve O, Dilmen U. Citrulline levels in premature infants. *Clin Chim Acta.* (2011) 21:2007. doi: 10.1016/j.cca.2011.06.037
19. Canpolat FE, Yurdakök M, Yigit S, Korkmaz A, Tekinalp G. Blood L-arginine Levels in Early Respiratory Distress Syndrome. *Pediatr Pulmonol.* (2005) 40:511–4. doi: 10.1002/ppul.20326
20. Manal El, Sayed M, Sherif L, Said RN, El-Wakkad AS, Amira E-R, et al. Endothelin-1 and L-arginine in preterm infants with respiratory distress. *Am J Perinatol.* (2011) 28:129–36. doi: 10.1055/s-0030-1263295
21. Dumas SJ, Bru-Mercier G, Courboulin A, Quatredeniers M, Rücker-Martin C, Antigny F, et al. NMDA-type glutamate receptor activation promotes vascular remodeling and pulmonary arterial hypertension. *Circulation.* (2018) 137:2371–89. doi: 10.1161/CIRCULATIONAHA.117.029930
22. Brosnan JT, Brosnan ME. Glutamate: a truly functional amino acid. *Amino Acids.* (2013) 45:413–8. doi: 10.1007/s00726-012-1280-4
23. Riedijk MA, de Gast-Bakker D-AH, Wattimena JL, Van Goudoever JB. Splanchnic oxidation is the major metabolic fate of dietary glutamate in enterally fed preterm infants. *Pediatr Res.* (2007) 62:468–73. doi: 10.1203/PDR.0b013e31813cbeba
24. Yelamanchi SD, Jayaram S, Thomas JK, Gundimeda S, Khan AA, Singhal A, et al. A pathway map of glutamate metabolism. *J Cell Commun Signal.* (2016) 10:69–75. doi: 10.1007/s12079-015-0315-5
25. Terán Y, Ponce O, Betancourt L, Hernández L, Rada P. Amino acid profile of plasma and cerebrospinal fluid in preeclampsia. *Pregnancy Hypertens.* (2012) 2:416–22. doi: 10.1016/j.preghy.2012.05.001
26. Dessì A, Marincola FC, Fanos V. Metabolomics and the great obstetrical syndromes–GDM, PET, and IUGR. *Best Pract Res Clin Obstet Gynaecol.* (2015) 29:156–64. doi: 10.1016/j.bpobgyn.2014.04.023
27. Zhang Z, Bassam B, Thomas AG, Williams M, Liu J, Nance E, et al. Maternal inflammation leads to impaired glutamate homeostasis and up-regulation of glutamate carboxypeptidase II in activated microglia in the fetal/newborn rabbit brain. *Neurobiol Dis.* (2016) 94:116–28. doi: 10.1016/j.nbd.2016.06.010
28. Hirose T, Shimizu K, Ogura H, Tasaki O, Hamasaki T, Yamano S, et al. Altered balance of the aminogram in patients with sepsis–the relation to mortality. *Clin Nutr.* (2014) 33:179–82. doi: 10.1016/j.clnu.2013.11.017
29. Pregnolato S, Chakkarapani E, Isles AR, Luyt K. Glutamate transport and preterm brain injury. *Front Physiol.* (2019) 10:417. doi: 10.3389/fphys.2019.00417
30. Parfenova H, Fedinec A, Leffler CW. Ionotropic glutamate receptors in cerebral microvascular endothelium are functionally linked to heme oxygenase. *J Cereb Blood Flow Metab.* (2003) 23:190–7. doi: 10.1097/00004647-200302000-00006
31. Hinoi E, Takarada T, Ueshima T, Tsuchihashi Y, Yoneda Y. Glutamate signaling in peripheral tissues. *Eur J Biochem.* (2004) 271:1–13. doi: 10.1046/j.1432-1033.2003.03907.x
32. Hogan-Cann AD, Anderson CM. Physiological roles of non-neuronal NMDA receptors. *Trends Pharmacol Sci.* (2016) 37:750–67. doi: 10.1016/j.tips.2016.05.012
33. Nguyen-Duong H. Effects of glutamate and zinc ions on the contractility of vascular smooth muscle preparations. *J Elementol.* (2010) 15:559–72. doi: 10.5601/jelem.2010.15.3.559-572
34. Sun H, Swaim A, Herrera JE, Becker D, Becker L, Srivastava K, et al. Platelet kainate receptor signaling promotes thrombosis by stimulating cyclooxygenase activation. *Circ Res.* (2009) 105:595–603. doi: 10.1161/CIRCRESAHA.109.198861
35. Kalev-Zylinska ML, Hearn JI, Makhro A, Bogdanova A. N-methyl-D-aspartate receptors in hematopoietic cells: what have we learned? *Front Physiol.* (2020) 11:577. doi: 10.3389/fphys.2020.00577
36. LeMaistre JL, Sanders SA, Stobart MJ, Lu L, Knox JD, Anderson HD, et al. Coactivation of NMDA receptors by glutamate and D-serine induces dilation of isolated middle cerebral arteries. *J Cereb Blood Flow Metab.* (2012) 32:537–47. doi: 10.1038/jcbfm.2011.161

37. Du J, Li X-H, Li Y-J. Glutamate in peripheral organs: biology and pharmacology. *Eur J Pharmacol.* (2016) 784:42–8. doi: 10.1016/j.ejphar.2016.05.009
38. Jiang H, Holm J, Vidlund M, Vanky F, Friberg Ö, Yang Y, et al. The impact of glutamate infusion on postoperative NT-proBNP in patients undergoing coronary artery bypass surgery: a randomized study. *J Transl Med.* (2020) 18:1–11. doi: 10.1186/s12967-020-02351-7
39. Meng W, Tobin JR, Busija DW. Glutamate-induced cerebral vasodilation is mediated by nitric oxide through N-methyl-D-aspartate receptors. *Stroke.* (1995) 26:857–63. doi: 10.1161/01.STR.26.5.857
40. Fiumana E, Parfenova H, Jaggar JH, Leffler CW. Carbon monoxide mediates vasodilator effects of glutamate in isolated pressurized cerebral arterioles of newborn pigs. *Am J Physiol.* (2003) 284:H1073–9. doi: 10.1152/ajpheart.00881.2002
41. Koneru P, Leffler CW. Role of cGMP in carbon monoxide-induced cerebral vasodilation in piglets. *Am J Physiol.* (2004) 286:H304–9. doi: 10.1152/ajpheart.00810.2003
42. Hall CN, Reynell C, Gesslein B, Hamilton NB, Mishra A, Sutherland BA, et al. Capillary pericytes regulate cerebral blood flow in health and disease. *Nature.* (2014) 508:55–60. doi: 10.1038/nature13165
43. Morrell CN, Sun H, Ikeda M, Beique J-C, Swaim AM, Mason E, et al. Glutamate mediates platelet activation through the AMPA receptor. *J Exp Med.* (2008) 205:575–84. doi: 10.1084/jem.20071474
44. Echtler K, Stark K, Lorenz M, Kerstan S, Walch A, Jennen L, et al. Platelets contribute to postnatal occlusion of the ductus arteriosus. *Nat Med.* (2010) 16:75–82. doi: 10.1038/nm.2060
45. Simon SR, van Zogchel L, Bas-Suárez MP, Cavallaro G, Clyman RI, Villamor E. Platelet counts and patent ductus arteriosus in preterm infants: a systematic review and meta-analysis. *Neonatology.* (2015) 108:143–51. doi: 10.1159/000431281
46. Oltman SP, Rogers EE, Baer RJ, Jasper EA, Anderson JG, Steurer MA, et al. Newborn metabolic vulnerability profile identifies preterm infants at risk for mortality and morbidity. *Pediatr Res.* (2020):1–10. doi: 10.1038/s41390-020-01148-0. [Epub ahead of print].
47. Bardanzellu F, Piras C, Atzei A, Neroni P, Fanos V. Early urinary metabolomics in patent ductus arteriosus anticipates the fate: preliminary data. *Front Pediatrics.* (2020) 8:872. doi: 10.3389/fped.2020.613749

3

Late Administration of Surfactant May Increase the Risk of Patent Ductus Arteriosus

Fuat Emre Canpolat[1*†], *Gülsüm Kadıoğlu Şimşek*[1†], *James Webbe*[2], *Mehmet Büyüktiryaki*[1†], *Nazmiye Bengü Karaçağlar*[1†], *Sarkhan Elbayiyev*[1†] and *H. Gözde Kanmaz Kutman*[1†]

[1] NICU, Department of Neonatology, Ankara City Hospital, University of Health Sciences, Ankara, Turkey, [2] Neonatal Medicine, Imperial College London, London, United Kingdom

***Correspondence:**
Fuat Emre Canpolat
femrecan@gmail.com

†ORCID:
Fuat Emre Canpolat
orcid.org/0000-0001-9307-3003
Gülsüm Kadıoglu Şimşek
orcid.org/0000-0003-4831-8950
Mehmet Büyüktiryaki
orcid.org/0000-0001-8937-4671
Nazmiye Bengü Karaçağlar
orcid.org/0000-0001-6733-4871
Sarkhan Elbayiyev
orcid.org/0000-0002-2113-5591
H. Gözde Kanmaz Kutman
orcid.org/0000-0002-3177-9411

Introduction: Early rescue surfactant is the most effective way of administering surfactant but many infants still receive surfactant later. Our aim was to explore the association between timing of surfactant administration and the development of patent ductus arteriosus and other neonatal morbidities.

Materials and method: This retrospective study analyzed 819 preterm infants under 30 weeks of gestational age and under 1,500 g.

Results: Five hundred and ninety three infants received surfactant during the study period, of these 365 received it within 2 h of life (early group) and 228 received it after two h (late group). Patent ductus arteriosus was detected in 175 (48%) of the early group and 168 (74%) of the late group, $p = 0.001$. Multinominal logistic regression analysis demonstrated that receiving surfactant after 2 h of life has a OR 3.5 (2.2–5.64 95 % CI) and a p-value of 0.001 for developing patent ductus arteriosus.

Conclusion: In this study population we observed that late surfactant administration is associated with increased risk of patent ductus arteriosus.

Keywords: surfactant, early rescue, patent ductus arteriosus, respiratory distress syndrome, preterm infant

INTRODUCTION

Respiratory distress syndrome (RDS) is the most common respiratory disease among preterm infants. Surfactant replacement therapy is an effective treatment for respiratory distress syndrome (1). Surfactant therapy has been shown to reduce disease severity and air leaks leading to improved survival (1). Although management has evolved gradually over the years early rescue surfactant administration is superior to late treatment (2). Previous trials showed that surfactant given earlier in the course of disease works better than later in terms of reducing air leaks (2) and avoiding mechanical ventilation if the intubate-surfactant-extubate (INSURE) technique is used (3). European Consensus Guideline 2019 recommended that early rescue surfactant should be standard (1) and there are occasions when surfactant should be given in the delivery suite, such as when intubation is needed for stabilization.

In some previous reports, early administration of surfactant is associated with shorter duration of ventilation, longer duration of continuous positive airway pressure and longer hospital stay but had little or no impact on bronchopulmonary dysplasia and/or mortality (4). There are limited and controversial data about the effect of surfactant timing on patent ductus arteriosus (5, 6).

One recent trial with a large number of patients concluded that neonates in the late surfactant group who received more than one dose of surfactant were at higher risk of bronchopulmonary dysplasia, retinopathy of prematurity and patent ductus arteriosus requiring ligation (7).

Therefore, our aim was to investigate the relationship between timing of surfactant and development of patent ductus arteriosus. A secondary aim was to compare other neonatal morbidities among these groups.

METHOD

We retrospectively analyzed 819 cases of infants hospitalized in our neonatal intensive care unit during the study period (the years 2013–2018): 593 of these babies received surfactant. The infants were born at <30 weeks of gestation and had birth weight ≤1,500 g. We divided the patients into two groups based on timing of surfactant therapy: the early surfactant group (365 infants) receiving surfactant within 2 h of life and the late group (228 infants) receiving it after 2 h.

In this retrospective cohort, preterm infants with major congenital anomalies, infants with futile or palliative care, and missing information about surfactant administration time were excluded from the study.

Although the FiO_2 requirement >30% in infants with respiratory distress syndrome findings is considered to be an important predictor of the severity of respiratory distress syndrome and non-invasive ventilation failure, considering the high surfactant treatment rates in Turkey, we used administering surfactant in infants who require ≥40% FiO_2 during the study period (2013–2018) as our Turkish Guideline recommended (8). All very low birth weight preterm infants received continuous positive airway pressure (CPAP) as initial respiratory support in the delivery room.

Definitions of Outcomes

Echocardiographic criteria for a diagnosis of patent ductus arteriosus (PDA) were duct size >1.5 mm, a left atrium-to aortic root (LA:Ao) >1.5, left-to-right shunting of blood, end-diastolic reversal of blood flow in the aorta or poor cardiac function in addition to signs of PDA. Two-dimensional color Doppler echocardiography was performed using a GE Vivid 7 Pro, 10S transducer (GE Healthcare, Salt Lake City, Utah). Patent ductus arteriosus was defined as the requirement for medical treatment with evidence of echocardiographic findings at least once at any time during the NICU (Neonatal Intensive Care Unit) admission.

Cranial ultrasound imaging results were based on the worst finding at any given time for this patient before discharge: intraventricular hemorrhage grade III/IV was defined as intraventricular hemorrhage with ventricular enlargement as Papile et al. reported (9). Early onset sepsis was defined as isolation of bacterial, fungal, or viral organism from blood or cerebrospinal fluid in a symptomatic infant within 3 day of life and if more than 3 days defined as late onset sepsis. Bronchopulmonary dysplasia was defined as receiving supplemental oxygen at 36 weeks postmenstrual age (10). Retinopathy of Prematurity was defined according to the International Classification of Retinopathy of Prematurity (ICROP) (11). Clinical chorioamnionitis was defined as inflammation of the chorion and amnion evidenced by presence of either maternal fever ≥38.4°C within 24 h before birth (irrespective of epidural analgesia), uterine tenderness, maternal leukocytosis of >15,000/mm^3, or explicitly mentioned obstetric concern at delivery. Information about histologic confirmation was not available. Days of oxygen, continuous positive airway pressure, or mechanical ventilation were counted during the primary NICU stay before discharge. Treatment of respiratory distress syndrome in our center was according to our local guidelines. Our center generally attempts to minimize invasive respiratory support with initiation of continuous positive airway pressure for all infants at risk of respiratory distress syndrome as soon as possible after birth in the delivery room, with the exception of extremely low gestational ages such as those who are <26 weeks. Continuous positive airway pressure support is the first line of respiratory support with the option of nasal intermittent mandatory ventilation or nasal intermittent positive pressure ventilation in case of increasing episodes of apnea and increased oxygen requirements. Intubation and surfactant administration follows the early symptomatic approach supported by large trials, generally with a cut-off of around 0.4 FiO_2 with concomitant radiological changes, increased work of breathing and evidence of respiratory acidosis with pH <7.25 and pCO_2 >60 mmHg, followed by conventional mechanical ventilation with high frequency modes used generally as rescue therapy. We generally use less invasive surfactant administration procedure to give surfactant to spontaneously breathing preterms (12).

Statistical Analysis

Baseline demographics and the neonatal outcomes were compared among two surfactant timing groups: infants with early and late surfactant, using Chi-square test for categorical variables and Student *t*-test for continuous variables. To further examine the effect of late surfactant use, multiple logistic regression models were applied to compare the primary and secondary outcomes between the surfactant timing groups. The odds ratio (95% confidence interval) of outcomes were determined based on the final multiple logistic regression models derived by backward variable selection procedure with inclusion criterion of 0.05. The factors for the full model included gender, cesarean section, antenatal steroid use as factors, gestational age, and birth weight as covariates. The data management and all statistical analyses were performed using SPSS for Windows version 22, IBM (USA). A two-sided significant level of 0.05 was used.

RESULTS

After exclusion, 819 preterm infants were analyzed in this retrospective study. Five hundred and ninety three infants received surfactant during the years 2013–2018, of these 365 received it within 2 h of life (early rescue group, first group) and 228 received it after two h (late group, second group). Mean gestational age was 27 ± 1.7 and 27.3 ± 1.5 ($p = 0.1$) weeks and mean birth weight was 945 ± 248 vs. 974 ± 232 g ($p = 0.25$), respectively. In the first group 186 (51%) and 111 (49%) in second group were boys. Antenatal steroid ratio was 68% in early and 73% in late group. Other obstetric risks were similar and shown in **Table 1**. Patent ductus arteriosus was detected in 175 (48%) of the early group and 168 (74%) of the late group, $p = 0.001$. All other early neonatal outcomes were compared in **Table 2**. Multinominal logistic regression analysis was made with antenatal steroids (even no difference between groups) and receiving surfactant (any time) as risk factors and gestational age and birth weight as covariates. This analysis found that receiving surfactant after 2 h of life has a OR 3.5 (2.2–5.64 95 % CI) and a p-value of 0.001 for developing patent ductus arteriosus. We grouped and analyzed patients according to gestational age and this is demonstrated in **Figure 1**.

TABLE 1 | Basic clinical characteristics of study groups.

	Early surfactant $n = 365$	Late surfactant $n = 228$	p
Gestational age, weeks ± SD	27 ± 1.7	27.3 ± 1.5	0.1
Birth weight, g ± SD	945 ± 248	974 ± 232	0.25
Male gender, n (%)	186 (51)	111 (49)	0.64
Antenatal steroids, n (%)	248 (68)	166 (73)	0.3
Chorioamnionitis, n (%)	43 (12)	20 (9)	0.251
Preeclampsia, n (%)	69 (19)	38 (17)	0.77
Gestational diabetes, n (%)	14 (4)	7 (3)	1.0
Cesarean section, n (%)	292 (80)	175 (77)	0.43
Multiple gestation, n (%)	80 (22)	48 (21)	0.494
Rupture of membranes, n (%)	70 (19)	29 (13)	0.182

TABLE 2 | Comparison of clinical outcomes of study population.

	Early surfactant $n = 365$	Late surfactant $n = 228$	p
Apgar score	5 (2–8)	5 (1–8)	0.827*
Last day of life receiving oxygen	42 ± 24	40 ± 21	0.597
Respiratory support at 28th day			
Supplemental oxygen	186 (51)	120 (53)	0.639
Non-invasive ventilation	76 (21)	45 (20)	
nIMV	55 (15)	38 (16)	
Mechanical ventilation	54 (15)	32 (14)	
Last day of life receiving respiratory support, days ± SD	21 ± 18	19 ± 15	0.373
Duration of CPAP, days ± SD	5.7 ± 6	7.6 ± 7	0.011
Duration of nIMV, days ± SD	3.1 ± 5	3.8 ± 5	0.236
Duration of MV, days ± SD	6.2 ± 10	7.7 ± 15	0.251
Air leaks, n (%)	10 (2.7)	8 (3.5)	0.282
PDA, n (%)	175 (48)	168 (74)	0.001
Surfactant more than 2 doses	95 (26)	68 (30)	0.313
Early neonatal sepsis, n (%)	80 (22)	57 (25)	0.386
Late onset sepsis, n (%)	131 (36)	75 (33)	0.456
BPD, moderate and severe, n (%)	58 (16)	38 (17)	0.8
IVH Grade III and IV, n (%)	58 (16)	27 (12)	0.17
ROP, n (%)	36 (10)	32 (14)	0.12
Day of discharge, days ± SD	69 ± 21	70 ± 22	0.68
Mortality, n (%)	36 (10)	29 (11)	0.182

*CPAP, continuous positive airway pressure; nIMV, nasal intermittent mandatory ventilation; MV, mechanical ventilation; PDA, patent ductus arteriosus; BPD, bronchopulmonary dysplasia; IVH, intraventricular hemorrhage; ROP, retinopathy of prematurity; SD, standard deviation; *non-parametric test.*

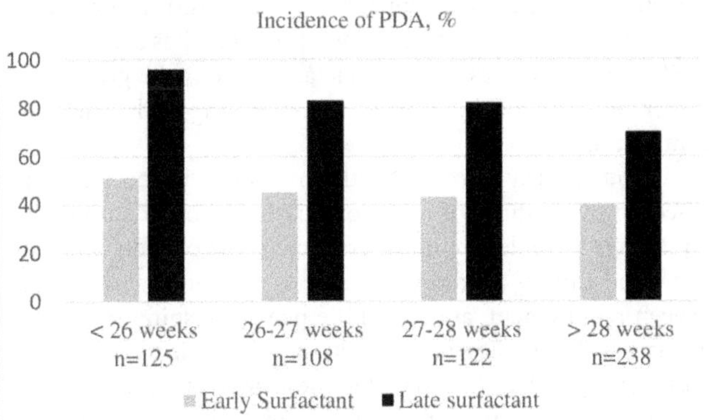

FIGURE 1 | Patent ductus arteriosus incidence among gestational ages compared by early vs. late surfactant timing. PDA, patent ductus arteriosus.

DISCUSSION

According to the results of this study, administering surfactant after the first 2 h of life is associated with higher frequency of patent ductus arteriosus. Although similar studies have been published previously (6, 7), this study is the first in the literature to draw attention to this subject. In addition, the duration of continuous positive airway pressure was slightly but statistically longer in the group with late surfactant administration compared to the group with early administration.

Surfactant therapy is now accepted as the standard treatment method for respiratory distress syndrome and reduces mortality (1, 8). Recommendations for surfactant therapy include preferring natural surfactant preparations, applying it as targeted early rescue therapy, and administering by non-invasive methods if the patient is breathing spontaneously (1, 8).

However, the principles of surfactant administration may vary from country to country or between different guidelines (1, 6, 8, 13, 14). The available evidence suggests that if the patient needs surfactant administering it as early as possible is most beneficial (2, 15). There is also evidence on non-invasive ventilation in the first 72 h of life reduces the need for invasive ventilation and surfactant requirement (16), these all evidences are a part of need for surfactant. The advantages of early surfactant administration over late administration can be summarized as lower incidence of air leaks, less need for mechanical ventilation and a decreased risk of neonatal mortality and bronchopulmonary dysplasia (1, 2). In recent years, decisions regarding whether or not to administer surfactant therapy have been based primarily on an oxygen requirement threshold according to international guidelines (1). This threshold, which is 40% according to old guidelines, has also been applied in Turkey and in the present study (8). In more recent guidelines, this figure has been reduced to 30%, which suggests that surfactant will now be given much earlier and can be interpreted as promoting early surfactant administration (1).

Although early surfactant administration is recommended based on the findings of numerous trials and other studies, it is not always possible in clinical practice. Some patients may have very good clinical condition, normal or near-normal x-rays, low oxygen requirement, and very little need of respiratory support in the first hours. For reasons that are not well-understood, at postnatal age of 6–12 h or later these infants show increased oxygen requirement that cannot be met by pressure support ventilation, and the need for surfactant can arise even though it was not needed before.

This may be attributed to several factors, including the conditions of postnatal care, effectiveness of continuous positive airway pressure, the interface, and depletion and inadequacy of the infant's endogenous surfactant. If continuous positive airway pressure is not effective enough, the infant loses alveolar patency in a matter of hours and has higher tendency toward hypoxia, resulting in lung parenchyma that requires surfactant. With the administration of surfactant in addition to the effects of hypoxia on the lungs, there is a sudden reduction in pulmonary pressure and the ductus arteriosus remains patent. Surfactant administered at a later time causes sudden hemodynamic changes in a lung that has gradually deteriorated and entered this vicious cycle within hours.

This study has certain limitations. One of these is its retrospective nature. Furthermore, the fact that it was conducted at a single center based on a single guideline can also be considered a limitation. Nevertheless, our patient sample is sufficient, and to the best of our knowledge, there is no other study in the literature examining the impact of late surfactant administration on patent ductus arteriosus in a patient group of this size.

In conclusion, our findings support the well-established practice of early surfactant administration from a different angle. Early surfactant administration leads to a lower incidence of patent ductus arteriosus and reduced the need for respiratory support (continuous positive airway pressure duration) in neonates. We did not observe any differences between the groups in terms of bronchopulmonary dysplasia or other morbidities, but prospective studies based on new guidelines may provide stronger evidence as to whether such differences exist.

ETHICS STATEMENT

The studies involving human participants were reviewed and approved by Zekai Tahir Burak Hospital Ethical Committee. Written informed consent to participate in this study was provided by the participants' legal guardian/next of kin.

AUTHOR CONTRIBUTIONS

FC, GK, and MB collected data. NK and SE patient management, data management, and entering data. GK and FC crtitcal review. HK and FC made statistical analysis. JW made review.

REFERENCES

1. Sweet DG, Carnielli V, Greisen G, Hallman M, Ozek E, Te Pas A, et al. European Consensus Guidelines on the Management of Respiratory Distress Syndrome - 2019 upatent ductus arteriosuste. *Neonatology.* (2019) 115:432–51. doi: 10.1159/000499361
2. Bahadue FL, Soll R. Early versus delayed selective surfactant treatment for neonatal respiratory distress syndrome. *Cochrane Database Syst Rev.* (2012) 11:CD001456. doi: 10.1002/14651858.CD001456.pub2
3. Verder H, Albertsen P, Ebbesen F, Greisen G, Robertson B, Bertelsen A, et al. Nasal continuous positive airway pressure and early surfactant therapy for respiratory distress syndrome in newborns of less than 30 weeks' gestation. *Pediatrics.* (1999) 103:E24. doi: 10.1542/peds.103.2.e24
4. Premnath D, Kent AL, Bajuk B, Abdel-Latif ME, NSW and the ACT Neonatal Intensive Care Audit Group. Does timing of initial surfactant treatment make a difference in rates of chronic lung disease or mortality in premature infants? An observational regional study. *J Matern Fetal Neonatal Med.* (2016) 29:91–8. doi: 10.3109/14767058.2014.987747
5. Dilmen U, Özdemir R, Tatar Aksoy H, Uras N, Demirel N, Kirimi E, et al. Early regular versus late selective poractant treatment in preterm infants born between 25 and 30 gestational weeks: a prospective randomized multicenter study. *J Matern Fetal Neonatal Med.* (2014) 27:411–5. doi: 10.3109/14767058.2013.818120
6. Kim SM, Park YJ, Chung SH, Choi YS, Kim CH, Bae CW. Early prophylactic versus late selective use of surfactant for respiratory distress syndrome in very preterm infants: a collaborative study of 53 multi-center trials in Korea. *J Korean Med Sci.* (2014) 29:1126–31. doi: 10.3346/jkms.2014.29.8.1126
7. Stritzke A, Mohammad K, Shah PS, Ye XY, Bhandari V, Akierman A, et al. Use and timing of surfactant administration: impact on neonatal outcomes in extremely low gestational age infants born in Canadian Neonatal Intensive Care Units. *J Matern Fetal Neonatal Med.* (2018) 31:2862–9. doi: 10.1080/14767058.2017.1358266
8. Özkan H, Erdeve Ö, Kutman HGK. Turkish Neonatal Society guideline on the management of respiratory distress syndrome and surfactant treatment. *Turk Pediatri Ars.* (2018) 53:S45–54. doi: 10.5152/TurkPediatriArs.2018.01806
9. Papile LA, Burstein J, Burstein R, Koffler H. Incidence and evolution of subependymal and intraventricular hemorrhage: a study of infants with birth weights less than 1,500 gm. *J Pediatr.* (1978) 92:529–34. doi: 10.1016/S0022-3476(78)80282-0
10. Bancalari E, Jain D. Bronchopulmonary dysplasia: can we agree on a definition? *Am J Perinatol.* (2018) 35:537–40. doi: 10.1055/s-0038-1637761
11. International Committee for the Classification of Retinopathy of Prematurity. The International classification of retinopathy of prematurity revisited. *Arch Ophthalmol.* (2005) 123:991–9. doi: 10.1001/archopht.123.7.991
12. Kanmaz HG, Erdeve O, Canpolat FE, Mutlu B, Dilmen U. Surfactant administration via thin catheter during spontaneous breathing: randomized controlled trial. *Pediatrics.* (2013) 131:e502–9. doi: 10.1542/peds.2012-0603
13. Shah PS, Seidlitz W, Chan P, Yeh S, Musrap N, Lee SK, et al. Internal audit of the Canadian Neonatal Network Data Collection System. *Am J Perinatol.* (2017) 34:1241–9. doi: 10.1055/s-0037-1603325
14. Banerjee S, Fernandez R, Fox GF, Goss KCW, Mactier H, Reynolds P, et al. Surfactant replacement therapy for respiratory distress syndrome in preterm infants: United Kingdom national consensus. *Pediatr Res.* (2019) 86:12–4. doi: 10.1038/s41390-019-0344-5
15. Krause MF, Hoehn T. Timing of surfactant administration determines its physiologic response in a rabbit model of airway lavage. *Biol Neonate.* (2000) 77:196–202. doi: 10.1159/000014216
16. Oncel MY, Arayici S, Uras N, Alyamac-Dizdar E, Sari FN, Karahan S, et al. Nasal continuous positive airway pressure versus nasal intermittent positive-pressure ventilation within the minimally invasive surfactant therapy approach in preterm infants: a randomised controlled trial. *Arch Dis Child Fetal Neonatal Ed.* (2016) 101:F323–8. doi: 10.1136/archdischild-2015-308204

4

Selective Treatment of PDA in High-Risk VLBW Infants with Birth Weight ≤800 g or <27 Weeks and Short-Term Outcome

Thowfique Ibrahim[1,2,3,4*], *Abdul Alim Abdul Haium*[1,2,3,4], *Sarah Jane Tapawan*[1], *Rowena Dela Puerta*[1], *John C. Allen Jr.*[2], *Suresh Chandran*[1,2,3,4†], *Mei Chien Chua*[1,2,3,4] *and Victor Samuel Rajadurai*[1,2,3,4]

[1] Department of Neonatology, KK Women's and Children's Hospital, Singapore, Singapore, [2] Duke-NUS Medical School, Singapore, Singapore, [3] Department of Neonatology, National University of Singapore, Singapore, Singapore, [4] Lee Kong Chian School of Medicine, Singapore, Singapore

***Correspondence:**
Thowfique Ibrahim
thowfique.ibrahim@singhealth.com.sg

†ORCID:
Suresh Chandran
orcid.org/0000-0001-5961-7441

Background: Patent ductus arteriosus (PDA) causing significant left to right shunt can increase key morbidities in preterm infants. Yet, treatment does not improve outcomes and spontaneous closure is the natural course of PDA. The Impact of PDA on 23–26-week gestation infants is uncertain. Selective treatment of such infants would likely balance outcomes.

Objective: To test the hypothesis that treatment of PDA in high-risk VLBW infants [birth weight ≤800 g or gestation <27 weeks, hemodynamically significant, ductal diameter (DD, ≥1.6 mm), and mechanical ventilation] and expectant management in low-risk infants will reduce the need for treatment and surgical ligation, without altering short term morbidities.

Methods: This prospective observational study was initiated subsequent to the introduction of a new treatment protocol in 2016. The 12-months before and after protocol introduction were, respectively, defined as standard and early selective treatment periods. In the early selective treatment cohort, PDA was treated with indomethacin, maximum of two courses, 1 week apart. Surgical ligation was considered after 30 days of age if indicated (DD ≥2 mm, mechanical ventilation). Primary outcomes were need for treatment and rate of ligation. Protocol compliance and secondary outcomes were documented.

Results: 415 infants were studied, 202 and 213 in the standard treatment and early selective treatment cohorts, respectively. Numbers treated (per protocol) in the standard treatment and early selective treatment cohorts were 27.7 and 19.3% (56/202 and 41/213) ($p = 0.049$), and the respective ligation rates were 7.54 and 2.96% ($P = 0.045$). Secondary outcomes were comparable.

Conclusion: The early selective treatment protocol reduced the rates of treatment and surgical ligation of PDA, without altering key morbidities. Further studies under a randomized control trial setting is warranted.

Keywords: PDA, VLBW, prematurity, ductal diameter, Indomethacin

INTRODUCTION

Patent ductus arteriosus (PDA) is a congenital cardiac condition found in 31% of very low birth weight (VLBW) infants (1). Opinion among neonatologists on how to approach the condition is divided, with treatment strategies lacking consensus (2). PDA acts as a shunt by diverting blood from systemic circulation to pulmonary circulation in preterm infants. This ductal steal phenomenon leads to complex circulatory consequences in pulmonary and systemic circulation. These hemodynamic instabilities have been postulated to cause morbidities in preterm infants in several studies (3, 4). Contrary to the expectations, closure of PDA has failed to improve key morbidities in VLBW infants as a whole, and both medical and surgical treatments have been associated with adverse effects (5). On the other hand, even if left untreated, there is usually spontaneous closure, especially in infants of higher gestational ages (6, 7). However, the impact of hemodynamically significant PDA on very high risk infants from 23 to 26 weeks of gestation could be significant due to morbidities like massive pulmonary hemorrhage and intraventricular hemorrhage (8). Current trends in PDA management indicate diminishing rates of aggressive treatment in VLBW infants with selective and delayed treatment of the condition being advocated (9), but this approach has not been methodically tested. The aim of this prospective cohort study with historical control was to evaluate the benefits and disadvantages of selectively treating high-risk infants with a significant PDA. PDA was tolerated in low-risk infants, allowing spontaneous closure, unless the infant demonstrated evidence of early organ failure such as congestive heart failure secondary to the PDA or a rising creatinine level, indicative of early kidney injury.

MATERIALS AND METHODS

This study was approved by the SingHealth Centralized Institutional Review Board (2019/CIRB 2693). All procedures performed in this study involving human participants were in accordance with the ethical standards of the institutional and national research committees and with the 1964 Helsinki declaration and its later amendments or comparable ethical standards. Informed consent was waived for all parents. This was a prospective case control study with a historical control conducted in a level III C neonatal unit of a teaching hospital. All VLBW infants born between 1 April 2016 and 31 March 2017 were included in the early selective treatment cohort. All VLBW infants born between 1 April 2015 and 31 March 2016 were included in the historical standard treatment cohort.

Management of PDA in Early Selective Treatment Period: Protocol Design

A consensus protocol for PDA management was prepared based on published literature, including a review article published by our department (6) with our own patient outcomes. The protocol defined screening, diagnosis, treatment, discharge and follow-up procedures for infants with a PDA (**Figure 1**).

Diagnosis

All high-risk infants (high-risk group) with birth weight ≤800 g and or ≤27 weeks gestational age (GA) at birth, on mechanical ventilation and with significant clinical symptoms or signs of PDA underwent echocardiogram examination (echo) at 12–24 h of age. Significant clinical symptoms or signs were defined as follows: a grade ≥2 systolic murmur, an active precordium, hypotension, wide pulse pressure or metabolic acidosis deemed to be secondary to PDA. VLBW infants who fell outside the high-risk category (low-risk group) had an echocardiogram after 72 h of age if they were on intubated respiratory support with significant clinical symptoms or signs. For treatment purposes, a PDA was defined as significant if the infant fell into the high-risk group, required mechanical ventilation, had clinical symptoms or signs, and had a ductal diameter of ≥1.6 mm on echocardiogram.

Management of PDA in the Early Selective Treatment Period

All the infants in high-risk group with a significant PDA were treated after 24 h of age. The main objective of the treatment was to reduce complications like pulmonary hemorrhage and intraventricular hemorrhage, apart from PDA closure. All other infants who did not belong to a high-risk group (>27 w and or >800 g) but met the criteria for significant PDA were treated at or after 14 days of life (infants between 800 and 1,000 g were considered for earlier echo and treatment at the discretion of the physician if there were significant concerns). In low-risk infants, PDA treatment was delayed to allow for spontaneous closure. VLBW infants on non-invasive breathing support were not treated unless they were showing early evidence of organ dysfunction such as congestive cardiac failure or renal impairment.

All infants with birth weight ≤1 kg, who required treatment for PDA received intravenous (IV) indomethacin. Infants with birth weight ≥1 kg were treated with oral Ibuprofen if the infant was tolerating >50% oral feeds. IV Indomethacin was preferred over IV ibuprofen because of lower cost and fewer GI complications (local experience). A maximum of two courses of indomethacin was used. All infants with a significant PDA were also treated with conservative measures, i.e., fluid restriction, for a duration at the discretion of treating physicians (≤130 ml/kg/day in a ≥5 days old infant). A follow-up echocardiogram was performed 72 h after completion of an Indomethacin course or on Day 7 of life, whichever was later. All high risk infants with a significant PDA and duct diameter >2 mm, despite two courses of indomethacin, were considered for surgical ligation if they required mechanical ventilation support by day 28 of life. PDA ligation was not recommended if an infant had been extubated to CPAP/NIMV. Infants whose PDA remained open underwent an echocardiogram at discharge and at 3–6 months intervals following discharge.

IVH Prophylaxis and PDA Management

In accordance with the protocol implemented in April 2016, all infants born at gestational ages of ≤28 weeks or weights <1,000 g whose mothers had not received a full course of antenatal corticosteroid were given prophylactic indomethacin

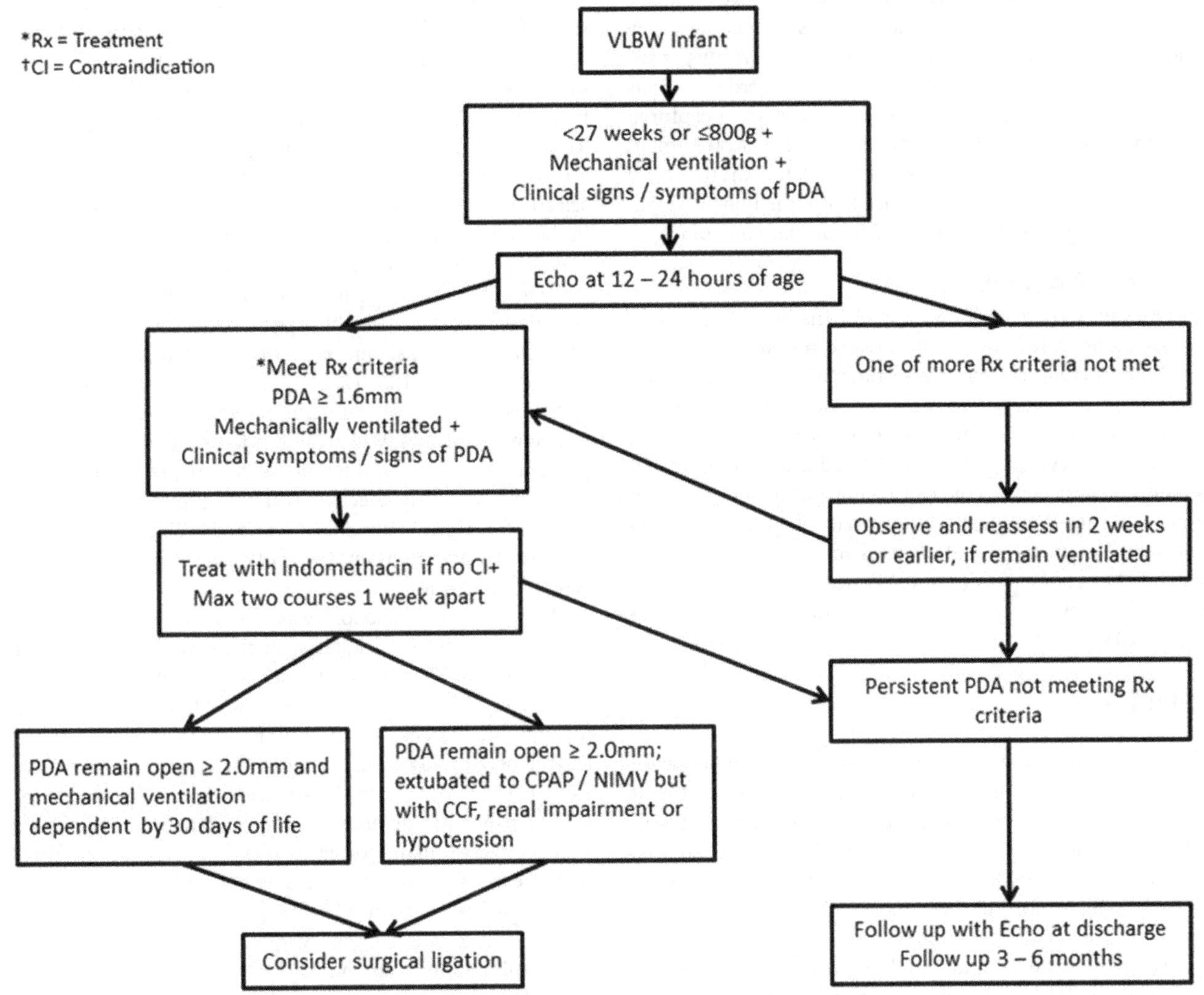

FIGURE 1 | Algorithm for management of PDA in infants with birth weight ≤800 g/<27 weeks gestation. Rx, Treatment; CI, Contraindication; CPAP, Continuous positive airway pressure; PDA, Patent ductus arteriosus; NIMV, Nasal intermittent mandatory ventilation; CCF, Congestive cardiac failure.

to prevent IVH (**Figure 2**, 0.1 mg/kg/day 24 h × 3 doses), with the first dose administered within 6 h of giving birth. A follow-up echocardiogram was performed 72 h following completion of treatment. If the PDA criteria for treatment were met, high-risk infants were eligible to receive one additional course of indomethacin, at least after first week of life.

Management of PDA in the Standard Treatment Period

Treatment decisions were made on a case by case basis by individual consultants, and in doubtful cases the opinion of a senior consultant was sought before initiating treatment. Most consultants considered aggressive and early treatment in the presence of a hemodynamically significant PDA. The review manuscript (6) published by the specialists from the department prior to the introduction of the new protocol may have influenced treatment decisions. All infants with birth weight ≤1 kg, who required treatment for PDA were given intravenous (IV) indomethacin. Indomethacin doses were administered at 24 h intervals and dose varied with postnatal age of the baby. A dose schedule of 0.2, 0.1, and 0.1 mg/kg/dose was used in infants ≤48 h of age. In infants with age ≤7 days of age, a dose schedule of 0.2, 0.2, 0.2 mg/kg/dose were used. When infants were ≥7 days of age, a dose schedule of 0.2, 0.25, 0.25 mg/kg/dose were used. Infants with a birth weight ≥1 kg were treated with oral Ibuprofen if on >50% oral feeds. Three doses, at 24 h intervals were used for a course. Initial stat dose of 10 mg/kg/dose was followed by two 5 mg/kg doses.

Data Collection

Data was collected from a prospectively maintained VLBW electronic data base, which forms part of the Vermont oxford (VON) and Australia New Zealand (ANZNN) network databases, to which our department contributes. Data collected included antenatal characteristics of the mother, delivery details, and key infant characteristics such as gestational age, key morbidities and mortality. Detailed data on PDA diagnosis, treatment and outcome of treatment were also recorded. Details of the COX-inhibitor agents used for treatment were captured for both the early selective treatment and the standard treatment cohort. Compliance data for high risk infants in the early selective treatment cohort was captured. Stratified birth weight and gestational age data were recorded for primary outcomes.

Statistical Analysis

Data were analyzed using SAS 9.1 (SAS Institute, Cary, NC). For continuous variables, results are expressed as mean ± SD, and categorical variables were summarized as counts and percentages. Outcomes before and after instituting the protocol were compared using *t*-tests for continuous variables and Fisher's exact test for categorical variables. We adjusted for potential confounding covariates on the effect of our protocol on rate of treatment and ligation using a multivariable logistic regression model. In the stepwise algorithm used to select predictors, all non-significant predicators ($p \geq 0.20$) were excluded from the final model. Unless otherwise stated, statistical significance was set at $p < 0.05$.

RESULTS

Four hundred and fifteen VLBW infants were studied with 213 and 202 in the intervention and standard treatment cohorts, respectively. The flow diagram of subject recruitment of all 415 infants is shown in the **Figure 3**. Maternal and infant characteristics of early selective and standard treatment cohorts are summarized in **Table 1**. Comparison of primary, secondary outcomes and morbidities of the early selective treatment and standard treatment cohorts are summarized in **Table 2**. Stratified post-conceptional age and birth weight comparisons of treatment rates are summarized in **Table 3**. Detailed birth weight and post-conceptional age-based ligation rates, age at treatment, and ligation comparisons are summarized in **Supplementary Tables 1–7** which are provided as Supplementary Material. Infants who received indomethacin IVH prophylaxis and subsequent PDA treatment are included in the PDA early selective treatment cohort. The percentages of infants diagnosed with a PDA was 33.3% (71/213) in the early selective treatment cohort and 36.1% (73/202) in the standard treatment group ($p = 0.606$). Indomethacin was used as the sole cox inhibitor agent in the treatment of PDA in 82.2% (37/45) of treated early selective treatment cohort and 76.8% (43/56) of treated standard treatment cohort infants, respectively ($p = 0.624$). Ibuprofen was used as the sole cox inhibitor agent in 11.1% (5/45) and 12.5% (7/56) of treated early selective treatment cohort and standard treatment cohort infants, respectively ($p = 1.000$).Three of 45 infants in the early selective treatment cohort and six of 56 infants in the standard treatment cohort received more than one COX-inhibitor agents (viz., Indomethacin, Ibuprofen or Paracetamol) ($p = 0.513$).

Compliance data for high-risk infants in the early selective treatment cohort (37/45) was analyzed. There were 65 high-risk infants in the early selective treatment cohort with 31 having an echocardiogram examination at ≤24 h of age. Forty of high risk infants met the criteria for PDA treatment of which 32(80%) received treatment for PDA closure. The number of high-risk infants who received PDA closure treatment in the early selective treatment (32/65) and standard treatment (32/65) groups were identical at 49.2%. The percentage of low- risk infants who received PDA closure treatment was 9.4% (14/148) in the selective early treatment group and 17.5% (24/137) ($p = 0.055$) in the standard treatment group, respectively.

Comparison of the standard treatment cohort to the standard treatment cohort revealed no significant differences in gender, gestational age, birth weight, Apgar scores and mode of delivery, antenatal steroid use and ethnicity. Mortality, excluding labor room death, was 11.7% (25/213) and 9.9% (20/202) ($p = 0.636$) in the early selective treatment and standard treatment cohort, respectively. Mortality in treated infants was 11/41 and 4/56 in the treated and standard treatment cohorts, respectively. Causes of death in the early selective treatment group were CLD (6/11), sepsis (4/11) and pulmonary hemorrhage (1/11), and in the standard treatment group causes of death were sepsis (2/4), NEC (1/4) and CLD (1/4).

A significant reduction was observed in the number of infants requiring PDA ligation in the early selective treatment cohort compared with the standard treatment cohort, i.e., 2.9% (6/213) vs. 7.5% (15/202) ($p = 0.042$). One infant underwent ligation after discharge. The number of infants requiring PDA treatment was lower in the early selective treatment cohort [56/202 (21.6%)] than in the standard treatment cohort [46/213 (27.7%)], but the difference was not statistically significant ($p = 0.171$). Five infants received treatment outside the protocol in the early selective treatment cohort. Median (IQR) weight for infants treated outside the protocol was 1,230 g (1,018, 1,360) and gestational age 29 w + 4 d (27 w + 5 d, 30 w + 6 d). All infants were on CPAP support. After five infants were deducted from the early selective treatment group, the treatment rate was decreased to 19.3% (41/213) compared to the standard treatment 21.6% (56/202) ($p = 0.049$). The indication was borderline in another four infants for which median birth weight and gestational age were 1,290 g (950, 1,476) and 28 w + 4 d (26 w + 5 d, 30 w + 3 d), respectively. None of the latter four infants showed evidence of congestive heart failure or rising creatinine, and three were on CPAP support. There was no difference in treatment outcomes when the high-risk group was defined as ≤26 or 28 weeks. The treatment rate difference was more pronounced in low-risk infants (26/146 vs. 12/156 $p = 0.009$ in ≤26 weeks infants and 9/100 vs. 2/144 $p = 0.008$, ≤28 weeks in standard treatment and early selective treatment group, respectively). Similar outcomes were observed when the high-risk group was defined as ≤800 or 1,000 g. The median (IQR) time from birth to treatment of PDA was 67 (43, 157) and 83.5 (32.5, 288.5) ($p = 0.804$) hrs in the respective standard and early selective treatment groups. The median (IQR) postnatal age in days for PDA ligation was 36 (27, 48) and 40.5 (36, 62) ($p = 0.352$) for standard treatment and early selective treatment groups, respectively. A statistically significant difference in ligation rate was found between standard treatment and early selective treatment groups in ≤25 weeks/≤800 g infants.

TABLE 1 | Maternal and infant characteristics.

Characteristic	Standard treatment ($n = 202$)	Early selective treatment ($n = 213$)	*P*-value[a]
Maternal age (yr), Mean (SD)	32.2 (5.76)	31.4 (5.14)	0.161
Ethnicity, *n* (%)			0.483
Chinese	104 (51.5)	102 (47.9)	
Malay	52 (25.7)	67 (31.5)	
Indian	22 (10.9)	17 (7.98)	
Other	24 (11.9)	27 (12.7)	
Pregnancy-induced hypertension (PIH), *n* (%)	45 (22.3)	52/213 (24.4)	0.643
Antenatal steroid (complete course), *n* (%)	129 (63.9)	137/213 (64.3)	0.918
Chorioamnionitis, *n* (%)	64 (31.7)	68/213 (31.9)	1.000
Mode of delivery NVD, *n* (%)	59 (29.2)	56 (26.3)	0.512
Apgar score at 5 min <6, *n* (%)	21 (10.4)	19 (8.92)	0.622
Male gender, *n* (%)	109 (54.0)	101 (47.4)	0.202
Gestational age (wk), Mean (SD)	28.8 (3.03)	29.0 (2.97)	0.547
Birth weight (g), Mean (SD)	1,055 (296)	1,072 (296)	0.556

[a] *Two-sample t-test (mean) or Wilcoxon rank sum test (median), Fisher's exact test (counts).*
IQR, Interquartile range; NVD, Normal vaginal delivery.

TABLE 2 | Comparison of primary, secondary outcomes and morbidities.

Characteristic	Standard treatment ($n = 202$)	Early selective treatment ($n = 213$)	*P*-value[a]
Number infants treated with cox inhibitors, *n* (%)	56/202 (27.7)	46/213 (21.6) 41/213 (19.3)*	0.171 **0.049**
PDA ligation, *n* (%)	15/199† (7.54)	6/203† (2.96)	**0.045** 0.059*
Pulmonary hemorrhage, *n* (%)	4/199† (2.01)	7/209† (3.35)	0.544
Severe Intraventricular hemorrhage (IVH), *n* (%)	11/199† (5.53)	10/203† (4.93)	0.825
Spontaneous intestinal perforation (SIP), *n* (%)	3/199† (1.51)	7/196† (3.57)	0.337
Necrotizing Enterocolitis (NEC), *n* (%)	4/199† (2.01)	3/209† (1.44)	0.718
Sepsis, *n* (%)	15/199† (7.43)	21/209† (9.86)	0.390
Retinopathy of prematurity (ROP) stage ≥3, *n* (%)	13/185† (7.03)	19/194† (9.79)	0.360
Any respiratory support at 36 weeks (CLD) *n* (%)	47/185† (25.4)	58/194† (29.9)	0.359
Assisted Ventilation duration (days)	$n = 197$	$n = 198$	
Mean ± SD	30.3 ± 43.8	32.1 ± 45.2	0.694
Median (IQR)	12 (2, 40)	12.5 (3, 40)	0.414
CPAP duration (days)			
Mean ± SD	20.9 ± 30.1	23.5 ± 33.8	0.396
Median (IQR)	8 (1, 32)	8 (1, 33)	0.466
NICU duration (days)			
Mean ± SD	39.1 ± 42.6	47.0 ± 54.7	0.100
Median (IQR)	22.5 (12, 48)	28 (1, 33)	0.197
Death			0.554
Labor Ward, *n*	3	4	
Neonatal death, *n*	14	15	
In hospital (post-neonatal), *n*	6	10	
Total, *n* (%)	23 (11.4)	29 (13.6)	

[a] *Two-sample t-test (mean) or Wilcoxon rank sum test (median), Fisher's exact test (counts).*
† *Excludes death before assessment, IQR, interquartile range.* **After adjusting for gestational age.*
PDA, Patent ductus arteriosus; CPAP, Continuous positive airway pressure.

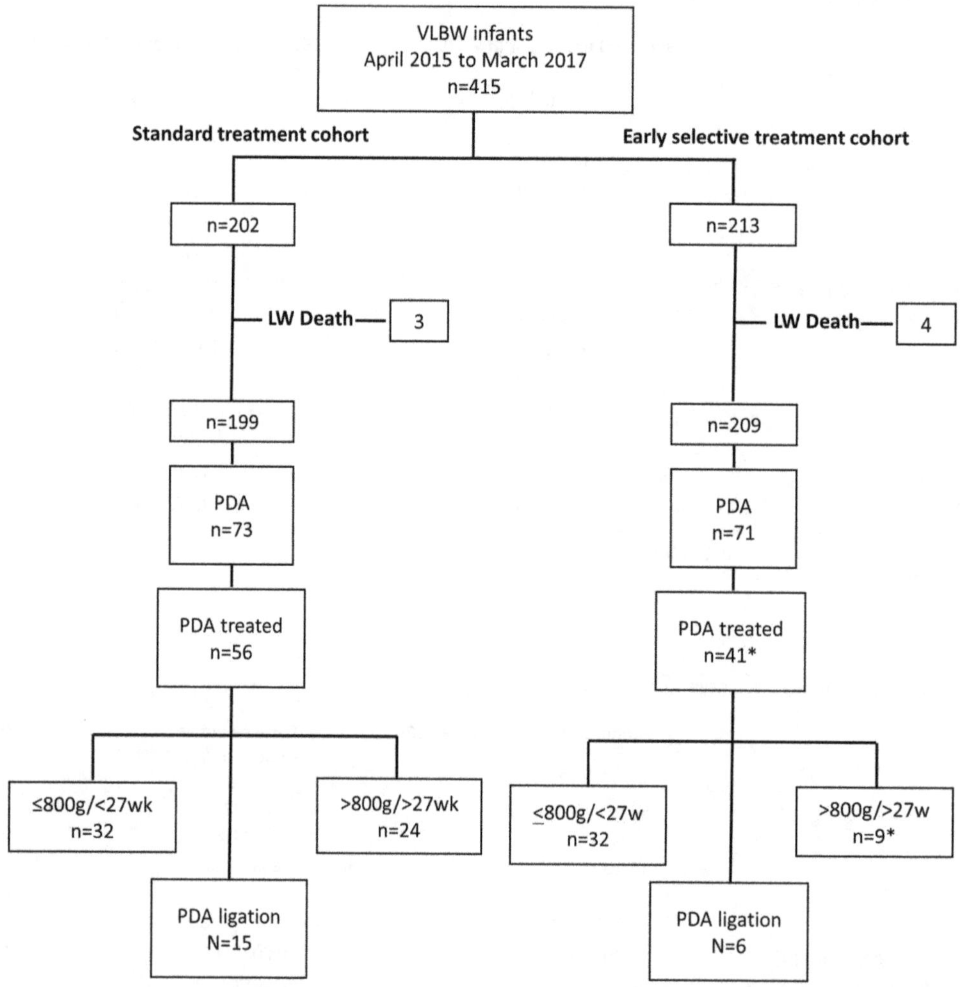

FIGURE 2 | Flow diagram of study cohort representing the number of VLBW infants diagnosed with PDA, received treatment, and underwent PDA ligation in subgroups <800 g/<27 w and >800 g/>27 w infants in control and intervention periods, April 2015 to March 2016 and April 2016 to March 2017, respectively. LW, Labor ward; VLBW, Very low birth weight; PDA, Patent ductus arteriosus. *Excluding five infants treated out of protocol.

Major morbidity rates, including solitary intestinal perforation (SIP) and intraventricular hemorrhage, did not differ significantly between the early selective treatment and standard treatment groups.11 (5.2%) infants in the early selective treatment cohort and 4 (1.88%) infants in the standard treatment cohort who received PDA treatment also received IVH prophylaxis ($p = 0.114$). 16/65 and 11/65 infants ($p = 0.387$), respectively, in the high-risk infants of earl and standard treatment cohorts received IVH prophylaxis. The incidence of pulmonary hemorrhage was comparable between groups (7 vs. 4; $p = 0.545$). Incidence of chronic lung disease (requiring supplemental Oxygen or any form of respiratory support at 36 weeks) was 29.9% (58/194) in the early selective treatment group and 25.4% (47/185) in the standard treatment group ($p = 0.359$).

DISCUSSION

In this study, we selectively treated VLBW infants who were at high- risk for PDA related morbidity, based on gestational age, birth weight, hemodynamic instability, PDA ductal diameter and ventilator support. Low- risk infants were treated only if they demonstrated early evidence of organ failure such as rising creatinine or congestive cardiac failure. Intervention reduced the PDA ligation rate to less than half, and reduction in treatment rate (per protocol). Results show that other key neonatal morbidities during the treatment period were comparable to the standard treatment period, thereby establishing the protocol safety. Mortality rates were comparable in the early selective and standard treatment cohorts. The authors concluded that the increase in mortality rate seen in the treated subgroup of infants was not related to the PDA protocol. Overall mortality in the VLBW infants (including labor room deaths) was reduced to 8.2% (18/219) and 8.1% (14/173) in 2018 and 2019, respectively, without modifying the protocol (10).

Treatment strategies for managing a PDA in VLBW infants vary among neonatologists and lack of uniformity is compounded by lack of agreement on the Echocardiogram characteristics that define a significant PDA (11). Management policies can be broadly summarized as three approaches, (a)

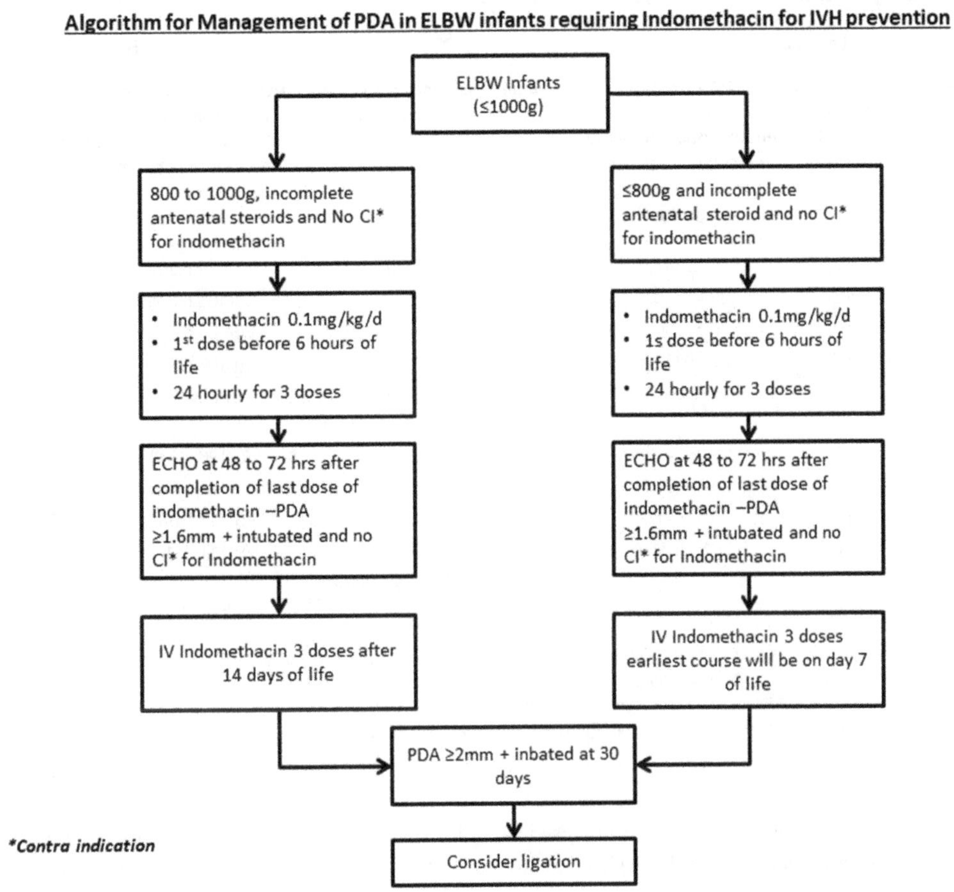

FIGURE 3 | Management of PDA infants who received IVH prophylaxis. PDA, Patent ductus arteriosus; ELBW, Extreme low birth weight; IV, Intravenous.

expectant management with late treatment if the PDA fails to close spontaneously (b) a risk-based approach where risks are scored, tabulated and infants meeting a predefined threshold score are treated for PDA (7) and (c) conservative management defined as allowing spontaneous closure of PDA with no provision for the use of Cyclo oxygenase inhibitors (COX) or ligation. Prophylactic treatment of PDA with indomethacin or Ibuprofen lacks evidence of benefit, with near consensus on this issue in the published literature (9). The expectant approach has the disadvantage of potentially undertreating the condition, which could lead to complications such as pulmonary hemorrhage and prolonged ventilator dependency. The risk-based approach offers a more logical strategy to resolve the issue, but if not well-defined or made rigorous the process has the risk of becoming impractical. In addition, a uniform approach would be required to allow bench marking and quality assurance. With this background, we have introduced a protocol in April 2016. The primary aim of the present study was an initial assessment of this protocol. Our study provides evidence that selective treatment of PDA using a relatively simple risk-based algorithm in VLBW infants is feasible and can significantly reduce the PDA ligation rate. In addition, we found reductions in treatment rates with COX inhibitors, but no adverse impact for increasing major morbidities such as severe IVH, CLD and assisted ventilation days. The literature is divided on the issue of conservative management. A recent meta-analysis has shown no difference in morbidity or mortality when PDA is either treated with placebo or not treated (12, 13). Comparison of a large neonatal network of composite outcomes between two countries has shown a lower composite outcome defined as mortality or major morbidity with aggressive management. A safe approach is required to address this question, especially in 22- to 26-week infants (14). The outcomes of large RCTs with no treatment or placebo treatment arms—with no provision for open label treatment, is required to answer this clinical question.

Indomethacin was the therapeutic agent used for ductal closure in the majority of our infants. Moderate to low-quality evidence suggests that the efficacy of acetaminophen is equivalent to that of Indomethacin and ibuprofen, with fewer side effects (15). Nonetheless, the efficacy of paracetamol in high-risk infants is not clear, especially in infants with post-conceptional age of ≤26 weeks. Available evidence supports the use of indomethacin in high-risk infants (16). The late use of acetaminophen in persistent PDA in high-risk infants reduces the need for surgical ligation but increases the incidence of CLD and duration of respiratory support. However, acetaminophen alone

TABLE 3 | Post conceptional age and birth weight based comparison for rate of treatment.

Low risk				High risk			
Gestation age (GA) group (mos.)	**PDA treated control infants[a]/full-year standard cohort in Gestation age group (%)**	**PDA treated treatment infants[b]/full-year early selective treatment cohort in Gestation age group (%)**	***P*-value**	**Gestation age (GA) group (mos.)**	**PDA treated control infants/full-year standard cohort in Gestation age group (%)**	**PDA treated treatment infants/full-year early selective treatment cohort in Gestation age group (%)**	***P*-value**
≤24	15/28 (53.7)	10/21 (47.6)	0.776	>24	41/174 (23.5)	31/192 (16.1)	0.087
≤25	22/40 (55.0)	22/41 (53.6)	1.000	>25	34/162 (20.9)	19/172 (11.0)	0.016
≤26	30/56 (53.5)	29/57 (50.8)	0.851	>26	26/146 (17.8)	12/156 (7.6)	0.009
≤28	47/102 (46.0)	39/99 (39.3)	0.392	>28	9/100 (9.0)	2/144 (1.38)	0.008
≤30	55/153 (35.9)	46/156 (29.4)	0.274	>30	1/49 (2.0)	0/57 (0.0)	0.462
Weight group (g)				**Weight group (g)**			
≤600	6/16 (37.5)	9/16 (56.2)	0.479	>600	50/186 (26.8)	32/197 (16.2)	0.012
≤800	25/50 (50.0)	25/49 (51.0)	1.000	>800	31/152 (20.3)	16/164 (9.7)	0.007
≤1000	40/87 (45.9)	35/84 (41.1)	0.644	>1000	16/115 (13.9)	6/118 (5.08)	0.0251
≤1,200	47/91 (51.6)	41/129 (31.7)	0.003	>1200	9/111 (8.1)	0/84 (0.0)	0.011
GA/weight group				**GA/weight group**			
≤26/≤800	32/65 (49.2)	22/65 (49.2)	0.851	>26/>800	24/146 (17.5)	14/156 (9.4)	0.055

[a]*The numerators of the High and Low Risk PDA Treated Control Infants sum to N = 56, which is the total number of PDA Treated Control Infants; the denominators sum to N = 202, which is the number of Low Risk + High Risk Full-year Control cohort.*
[b]*The numerators of the High and Low Risk PDA Treated early selective treatment Infants sum to N = 41, which is the total number of PDA Treated treatment Infants (five were excluded PP); the denominators sum to N = 213, which is the number Low Risk + High Risk Full-year treatment infants.*
PDA, Patent ductus arteriosus.

or acetaminophen in combination with ibuprofen can be used as a late treatment to avoid the risk associated with surgical closure of PDA (17–19).

Our findings were comparable to those of the published literature. In a study involving 4,001 infants in a recent cohort of VLBW infants, 21.7% received intervention for a PDA in the form of either COX inhibitors or ligation. In this study the percentage of infants who underwent ligation was high, especially primary ligation (20). Although available evidence suggests improved short and long term outcomes in VLBW infants with reduced PDA treatment (21), it has not been conclusively proven, primarily due to the lack of adequate well-designed studies. Our criteria defining high- risk infants on the basis of birth weight and gestational age as essential elements is supported by the published literature (21, 23). This study combines the principle of expectant management in low-risk infants with relatively aggressive management of PDA in high-risk infants. The study used lower post-conceptional age and higher levels of respiratory support to define high-risk infants. The study also defined the criteria for identifying a small group of low-risk infants who benefit from PDA treatment. As compared to the current study, published studies testing risk-based approaches to identify infants benefitting from PDA treatment used either Echocardiogram (ECHO) based criteria alone or ECHO features combined with lower levels of respiratory support and higher gestational age to define high-risk infants (21, 24). The authors were unable to identify other published studies in the English literature that combine principles of relatively aggressive management in high-risk infants with expectant management in low-risk infants, and which incorporate defined criteria for identifying the small number of infants in the low-risk group who require treatment. Implementation of guidelines employing a conservative approach to PDA management has shown a reduction in treatment rate similar to that observed in the current study (25).

Our study has limitations. Compliance is a significant issue in the implementation of any clinical protocol. Based on the data collected, we observed 90% protocol adherence in study treatment decisions. The study is an observational study—not an RCT, and the treatment in the retrospective standard treatment group is heterogenous and not protocol based. Authors made a systematic effort to analyze the data from the period to mitigate the impact of the absence of a defined protocol in the standard treatment period. Authors have provided the additional data as Supplementary Tables that would aid sample size calculation in a future randomized controlled trial. The protocol relied on measured ductal diameter as the sole Echocardiogram feature to represent ductal significance in the treatment decision algorithm. Addition to the protocol of absence or reversal of flow in diastole would likely better characterize the magnitude of ductal shunt in VLBW infants. Following completion of this study, the IVH prophylaxis criteria were modified in our department to include only infants with GA ≤26 weeks with incomplete antenatal steroid. The number of infants who received indomethacin prophylaxis was higher (11 vs. 16) in the early selective treatment cohort. The difference was not statistically significant, although it may have some beneficial impact on the treatment rate outcome of the protocol.

Our study provides preliminary evidence that selective treatment of PDA in high risk infants is feasible without altering short term outcomes. However, the protocol needs to be validated in a large randomized control trial (RCT) with long-term follow up to obtain further evidence. Inclusion or exclusion of 26-week infants in the high- risk group is a point of contention, and inclusion with the provision of subgroup analysis is probably a pragmatic approach in designing a future study. We would consider a RCT in high- risk infants with a no treatment placebo control arm as a radical and ethically questionable approach given the current state of knowledge. The authors estimate that in a RCT setting, the need for treatment would range from 15 to 17% of VLBW infants.

CONCLUSION

Our study provides preliminary evidence that selective treatment of high- risk VLBW infants with significant PDA is efficacious. Such a policy would eliminate unnecessary exposure to COX inhibitors and PDA ligation, without significantly affecting the rate of major morbidities in this vulnerable population.

ETHICS STATEMENT

The studies involving human participants were reviewed and approved by SingHealth CIRB Singapore. Written informed consent for participation was not provided by the participants' legal guardians/next of kin because: exempted from written consent by the CIRB.

AUTHOR CONTRIBUTIONS

TI conceptualized and designed the study, drafted the initial manuscript, and reviewed and revised the manuscript. AA, ST, JA, SC, MC, and RD designed the data collection instruments, collected data, carried out the initial analyses, and reviewed and revised the manuscript. VR designed the study and critically reviewed the manuscript for important intellectual content. All authors approved the final manuscript as submitted and agree to be accountable for all aspects of the work.

ACKNOWLEDGMENTS

We thank Ann Wright (KKH) and Kristine Calinao (KKH) for her contribution to the publication of the study.

REFERENCES

1. Investigators V-OTNDP. The Vermont-Oxford Trials Network: very low birth weight outcomes for 1990. *Pediatrics.* (1993) 91:540–5.
2. Noori S. Patent ductus arteriosus in the preterm infant: to treat or not to treat? *J Perinatol.* (2010) 30:S31–S7. doi: 10.1038/jp.2010.97
3. Pawar S, Sharma D, Murki S, Subramaniam S, Kandraju H. Construction of ductal diameter centiles in the first 24 h of life and their relation to cerebral blood flow in neonates weighing less than 1250 g in the first 24 h of life. *J Trop Pediatrics.* (2017) 63:476–82. doi: 10.1093/tropej/fmx016
4. Rios DR, Bhattacharya S, Levy PT, McNamara PJ. Circulatory insufficiency and hypotension related to the ductus arteriosus in neonates. *Front Pediatrics.* (2018) 6:62. doi: 10.3389/fped.2018.00062
5. Noori S, McCoy M, Friedlich P, Bright B, Gottipati V, Seri I, et al. Failure of ductus arteriosus closure is associated with increased mortality in preterm infants. *Pediatrics.* (2009) 123:e138–44. doi: 10.1542/peds.2008-2418
6. Ibrahim TK, Haium AA, Chandran S, Rajadurai VS. Current controversies in the management of patent ductus arteriosus in preterm infants. *Indian Pediatrics.* (2014) 51:289–94. doi: 10.1007/s13312-014-0403-2
7. Sankar MN, Bhombal S, Benitz WE. PDA: to treat or not to treat. *Cong Heart Dis.* (2019) 14:46–51. doi: 10.1111/chd.12708
8. Berry MJ, Saito-Benz M, Gray C, Dyson RM, Dellabarca P, Ebmeier S, et al. Outcomes of 23-and 24-weeks gestation infants in Wellington, New Zealand: a single centre experience. *Sci Rep.* (2017) 7:1–8. doi: 10.1038/s41598-017-12911-5
9. Benitz WE. Patent ductus arteriosus in preterm infants. *Pediatrics.* (2016) 137:e20153730. doi: 10.1542/peds.2015-3730
10. Vermont Oxford Network. Available online at: https://nightingale.vtoxford.org (accessed December 4, 2020).
11. Condò M, Evans N, Bellù R, Kluckow M. Echocardiographic assessment of ductal significance: retrospective comparison of two methods. *Arch Dis Childhood Fetal Neonatal Ed.* (2012) 97:F35–8. doi: 10.1136/adc.2010.207233
12. Mitra S, Florez ID, Tamayo ME, Mbuagbaw L, Vanniyasingam T, Veroniki AA, et al. Association of placebo, indomethacin, ibuprofen, and acetaminophen with closure of hemodynamically significant patent ductus arteriosus in preterm infants: a systematic review and meta-analysis. *JAMA.* (2018) 319:1221–38. doi: 10.1001/jama.2018.1896
13. Okulu E, Erdeve O, Arslan Z, Demirel N, Kaya H, Gokce IK, et al. An observational, prospective, multicenter, registry-based cohort study comparing conservative and medical management for patent ductus arteriosus. *Front Pediatr.* (2020) 8:434. doi: 10.3389/fped.2020.00434
14. Isayama T, Mirea L, Mori R, Kusuda S, Fujimura M, Lee SK, et al. Patent ductus arteriosus management and outcomes in Japan and Canada: comparison of proactive and selective approaches. *Am J Perinatol.* (2015) 1087–94. doi: 10.1055/s-0035-1548727
15. Ohlsson A, Shah PS. Paracetamol (acetaminophen) for patent ductus arteriosus in preterm or low birth weight infants. *Cochrane Database Syst Rev.* (2020) 4:CD010061. doi: 10.1002/14651858.CD010061.pub4
16. Liebowitz M, Kaempf J, Erdeve O, Bulbul A, Håkansson S, Lindqvist J, et al. Comparative effectiveness of drugs used to constrict the patent ductus arteriosus: a secondary analysis of the PDA-TOLERATE trial (NCT01958320). *J Perinatol.* (2019) 39:599–607. doi: 10.1038/s41372-019-0347-4
17. Mashally S, Nield LE, McNamara PJ, Martins FF, El-Khuffash A, Jain A, et al. Late oral acetaminophen versus immediate surgical ligation in preterm infants with persistent large patent ductus arteriosus. *J Thorac Cardiovasc Surg.* (2018) 156:1937–44. doi: 10.1016/j.jtcvs.2018.05.098
18. Yurttutan S, Bozkaya A, Hüdayioglu F, Oncel MY. The effect of combined therapy for treatment of monotherapy-resistant PDA in preterm infants. *J Matern Fetal Neonatal Med.* (2019) 32:3662–5. doi: 10.1080/14767058.2018.1481043
19. Weisz DE, Martins FF, Nield LE, El-Khuffash A, Jain A, McNamara PJ. Acetaminophen to avoid surgical ligation in extremely low gestational age neonates with persistent hemodynamically significant patent ductus arteriosus. *J Perinatol.* (2016) 36:649–53. doi: 10.1038/jp.2016.60
20. Ngo S, Profit J, Gould JB, Lee HC. Trends in patent ductus arteriosus diagnosis and management for very low birth weight infants. *Pediatrics.* (2017) 139:e20162390. doi: 10.1542/peds.2016-2390
21. Lokku A, Mirea L, Lee SK, Shah PS, Network CN. Trends and outcomes of patent ductus arteriosus treatment in very preterm infants in Canada. *Am J Perinatol.* (2017) 34:441–50. doi: 10.1055/s-0036-1593351
22. Clyman RI, Liebowitz M, Kaempf J, Erdeve O, Bulbul A, Håkansson S, et al. PDA-TOLERATE trial: an exploratory randomized controlled trial of treatment of moderate-to-large patent ductus arteriosus at 1 week of age. *J Pediatrics.* (2019) 205:41–8. e6. doi: 10.1016/j.jpeds.2018.09.012

23. Hagadorn JI, Bennett MV, Brownell EA, Payton KS, Benitz WE, Lee HC. Covariation of neonatal intensive care unit-level patent ductus arteriosus management and in-neonatal intensive care unit outcomes following preterm birth. *J Pediatrics.* (2018) 203:225–33. e1. doi: 10.1016/j.jpeds.2018.07.025
24. Fink D, El-Khuffash A, McNamara PJ, Nitzan I, Hammerman C. Tale of two patent ductus arteriosus severity scores: similarities and differences. *Am J Perinatol.* (2018) 35:55–8. doi: 10.1055/s-0037-1605576
25. Pavageau L, Brion LP, Rosenfeld CR, Brown LS, Ramaciotti C, Burchfield PJ, et al. Decrease in the frequency of treatment for patent ductus arteriosus after implementation of consensus guidelines: a 15-year experience. *J Perinatol.* (2019) 39:1569–76. doi: 10.1038/s41372-019-0432-8

5

Isoprostanes as Biomarker for Patent Ductus Arteriosus in Preterm Infants

Caterina Coviello[1], *Maria Luisa Tataranno*[2], *Iuri Corsini*[1], *Valentina Leonardi*[1], *Mariangela Longini*[3], *Francesco Bazzini*[3], *Giuseppe Buonocore*[3] *and Carlo Dani*[1,4*]

[1] *Division of Neonatology, Careggi University Hospital of Florence, Florence, Italy,* [2] *Department of Neonatology, University Medical Center Utrecht, Utrecht, Netherlands,* [3] *Department of Pediatrics, Obstetrics and Reproductive Medicine, University of Siena, Siena, Italy,* [4] *Department of Neurosciences, Psychology, Drug Research and Child Health, Careggi University Hospital of Florence, Florence, Italy*

***Correspondence:**
Carlo Dani
cdani@unifi.it

Context: It has been reported that isoprostanes (IPs) have a role in the pathophysiology of ductus arteriosus during the fetal and neonatal period. Our aim in this study was to assess if urinary IPs (uIPs) levels correlate with the risk of developing a hemodynamically significant patent ductus arteriosus (hsPDA) in preterm infants.

Materials and methods: Infants with 23 + 0 – 33 + 6 weeks of gestational age and respiratory distress syndrome (RDS) were consecutively enrolled. Urine samples were collected on the 2nd and 10th day of life (DOL) for uIPs measurement. Echocardiography for hsPDA diagnosis was performed between 24 and 48 h of life. Regression analysis was performed to assess the correlation between uIPs and hsPDA. Receiver operating characteristic (ROC) curve analysis was used to evaluate the accuracy of the uIPs in predicting the occurrence of hsPDA.

Results: Sixty patients were studied: 33 (55%) developed a hsPDA, 27 (45%) had ibuprofen hsPDA closure, and six (10%) required surgical closure. uIPs levels decreased from the 2nd to the 10th DOL. Adjusted regression analysis demonstrated that uIPs on the 2nd DOL were associated ($p = 0.02$) with the risk of developing a hsPDA. A cut-off level of 1627 ng/mg of creatinine of uIPs predicted the development of a hsPDA with a sensitivity of 82% and a specificity of 73%.

Conclusion: Early measurement of uIPs on the 2nd DOL is a reliable biomarker of hsPDA development and, alone or combined with other markers, might represent a non-invasive tool useful for planning the management of PDA in preterm infants.

Keywords: isoprostanes, patent ductus arteriosus, oxidative stress, ibuprofen, preterm infants

INTRODUCTION

Patent ductus arteriosus (PDA) is a frequent complication in preterm infants with respiratory distress syndrome (RDS) and 60–70% of preterm infants of <28 weeks' gestation receives medical and/or surgical treatment for PDA (1). The proper management of PDA is the subject of lively debate because randomized controlled trials (RCTs) of PDA closure using non-steroidal anti-inflammatory drugs (NSAIDs) have often failed to demonstrate relevant benefits in preterm infants (2). However, a persistent left-to-right shunt through the ductus complicating RDS has been associated with a worsening of respiratory failure, lowering of survival rate, and increased risk of intraventricular hemorrhage (IVH) and bronchopulmonary dysplasia (BPD) (1, 3–6). Therefore, pharmacological closure of PDA is indicated before significant left-to-right shunting occurs.

Currently, functional echocardiography is the best tool to diagnose PDA in preterm infants, to monitor its progress, and to determine its treatment (7). In fact, biomarkers, such as brain-type natriuretic peptide (BNP) and N-terminal pro-BNP (NTpBNP), have a significant range concentration overlap between neonates with no PDA, or small, moderate, and large PDA which limits their clinical application (8).

Recently, it was reported that isoprostanes (IsoPs) have a role in DA closure. IsoPs derive from the free radical-mediated peroxidation of phospholipid-bound arachidonate and, although they are mainly known as a biomarker of oxidative stress, they might induce physiological effects during the fetal and neonatal period, such as DA vascular constriction mediated by stimulation of thromboxane receptors (9). Van der Sterren et al. studied the vasoactive effects of IsoPs in chicken embryo isolated DA and demonstrated that they can induce a strong DA constriction (9). These results were confirmed by Chen et al. who found that oxygen exposure increases IsoPs levels in newborn mouse lung which induce constriction of the isolated term DA through the activation of thromboxane A2 (TxA2) receptor (10). Moreover, Longini et al. found that urinary IsoPs (uIPs) levels decreased after PDA closure with ibuprofen in preterm infants (11).

On the basis of these considerations we hypothesized that uIPs level might predict the development of a hemodynamically significant PDA (hsPDA). Thus, our aim was to assess uIPs levels in a cohort of very preterm infants and correlate them with the risk of hsPDA development.

MATERIALS AND METHODS

Population and Sample Collection

A prospective center-based study was carried out from June 2014 to December 2014 at the neonatal intensive care unit of Careggi University Hospital of Florence. The study was approved by the local ethics committee. Infants with gestational age from 23 + 0 to 33 + 6 weeks with respiratory distress syndrome (RDS) were consecutively enrolled after written parental informed consent. Exclusion criteria were major congenital malformations, chromosomal disorders, inborn errors of metabolism, and acute renal failure.

Urine samples of 2 ml were collected from each infant on the 2nd and 10th day of life (DOL) by placing a gauze in the infants' diaper. The samples were frozen and maintained at −80°C until analysis, which was performed at the Laboratory of Oxidative Stress of the University of Siena, Italy. Urinary isoprostanes (uIPs) were measured using tandem mass spectrometry (GC-MS) according to the methodology described by Casetta et al. (12). Urinary creatinine levels were measured at the two time points using a spectrophotometer method (Creatinine Diacron Kit®, Diacron International, Grosseto, Italy). Isoprostane values were corrected for intersubject differences in renal function and were expressed as nanograms of isoprostanes/mg of urinary creatinine.

Management of PDA

All enrolled infants underwent echocardiography between 24 and 48 h of life. The diagnosis of hsPDA requiring pharmacological treatment was made by echocardiographic demonstration of a ductal left-to-right shunt, with a left atrium to aortic root ratio >1.3 or a ductal size >1.5 mm (13), excluding the cases in which the closing flow pattern suggested a restrictive PDA (14). All ultrasound studies were performed by pediatric cardiologists or by neonatologists trained in neonatal echocardiography, and the treatment was decided by the neonatologist on duty. Infants with hsPDA received intravenous ibuprofen (Pedea® Orphan Europe, Puteaux, France) at a dose of 10 mg/kg followed by 5 mg/kg after 24 and 48 h. Pharmacological treatment could be repeated at the same dosage. Infants with hsPDA were considered for surgical ligation after failure of the medical therapy.

General Data Recording

The following clinical and demographic data were also collected by reviewing patients' medical records: GA, birth weight, birth weight <10° percentile, gender, mode of delivery, Apgar score at 5 min of life, fraction of inspired oxygen (FiO_2) on 2nd and 10th DOL, occurrence and duration of non-invasive respiratory support [nasal continuous positive pressure (NCPAP), bilevel positive airway pressure (BiPAP), nasal intermittent ventilation (NIV)], and mechanical ventilation [patient-triggered ventilation (PTV), high frequency oscillatory ventilation (HFOV)], sepsis, BPD, necrotizing enterocolitis (NEC), intraventricular hemorrhage (IVH), periventricular leukomalacia (PVL), retinopathy of prematurity, and stay-in-hospital duration. Sepsis was defined as positive blood culture. BPD was defined as oxygen requirement at 36 weeks of PMA (15). NEC was defined as Bell's stage >2 (16). IVH was classified according to Papile et al. (17), and PVL according to de Vries et al. (18).

Statistical Analysis

Patients' characteristics were described as mean and standard deviation (SD), rate and percentage, or median and interquartile range (IQR). The Student's t-test or Mann–Whitney U test were used to compare continuous data, while X^2 test was used to compare categorical data. Median values, including changes in uIPs levels between 2nd and 10th DOL and between infants with and without hsPDA, were compared using Kruskal–Wallis test. A $p < 0.05$ was considered statistically significant.

Univariate regression analyses were performed to assess the correlation between uIPs and PDA. The following variables were entered into the model: GA, BPD, NEC, IVH, mechanical ventilation, and mean FiO_2 at samples collection. In the final multivariable regression model, relevant perinatal and neonatal factors that showed an association with uIPs with alpha level <0.05 were included. Data analysis was performed using IBM SPSS Statistics version 20 (SPSS INC, Chicago, Illinois, USA).

To analyze the impact of the 'uIPs level on the 2nd DOL on the occurrence of hsPDA, we used ROC (receiver operating characteristic) curve analysis. The test's ability to classify patients as those who will develop hsPDA or not is represented by the area under the ROC curve (AUC). The AUC can be in the range of 0.5–1.0, wherein an AUC of 0.5 indicates that the classification model is of no value, and a value of 1.0 indicates perfect diagnostic accuracy. In turn, the cut-off point of the ROC curve indicates the uIPs level that gives the most true and the

TABLE 1 | Clinical characteristics of the study population.

	No PDA ($n = 27$)	hsPDA ($n = 33$)	*P*
Gestational age (weeks)	31 ± 2	27 ± 2	0.007
Birth weight (gr)	1645 ± 335	878 ± 368	0.949
<10th percentile	0 (0)	7 (21)	
Male	15 (57)	16 (48)	0.301
Cesarean section	19 (73)	22 (66)	0.062
Apgar score at 5 min	9 (8–9)	8 (6–9)	0.004
FiO_2 on 2nd DOL	0.24 ± 0.09	0.27 ± 0.06	0.943
on 10th DOL	0.21 ± 0.02	0.23 ± 0.03	0.063
Mechanical ventilation	3 (11)	20 (60)	<0.001
Duration (day)	0.3 ± 1.4	9.7 ± 22.0	0.003
Non-invasive ventilation	20 (76)	32 (96)	<0.001
Duration (day)	4 ± 4	23 ± 22	<0.001
Sepsis	2 (7)	11 (33)	<0.001
BPD	0 (0)	11 (33)	<0.001
NEC	0 (0)	3 (9)	0.002
IVH	1 (3)	8 (24)	0,005
≥ grade 3	1 (3)	4 (12)	0.367
PVL	0 (0)	2 (6)	0.002
ROP	0 (0)	7 (21)	<0.001
≥ grade 3	0 (0)	2 (6)	N/A
Mortality	0 (0)	3 (9)	<0.001
Stay in hospital (day)	33 ± 2	72 ± 49	<0.001

Mean ± SD, rate and (%), or median and (IQR).
GA, gestational age; hsPDA, hemodynamically significant patent ductus arteriosus; BPD, bronchopulmonary dysplasia; NEC, necrotizing enterocolitis; IVH, intraventricular hemorrhage; PVL, periventricular leukomalacia; ROP, retinopathy of prematurity.

least false indications of hsPDA development, and therefore has the best predictive power.

Post hoc analyses demonstrated that the population size of our study allows an 85% statistical power to detect as significant ($p < 0.05$) the difference between uIPs levels measured on the 2nd and the 10th DOL.

RESULTS

Clinical characteristics of enrolled infants ($n = 60$) are summarized in **Table 1**. We observed a decrease of uIPs levels from the 2nd to the 10th DOL [1627.2 (842.0–4882) vs. 486.1 (292.8–1467.8)] ng/mg of creatinine ($p < 0.01$) (**Figure 1**). Significant changes of uIPs from the 2nd to the 10th DOL were also found in the sub-groups of infants who had ibuprofen closure of hsPDA (**Table 2**).

Fifty-five percentage ($n = 33$) of patients developed a hsPDA, 45% ($n = 27$) had ibuprofen hsPDA closure, and 10% ($n = 6$) failed pharmacological treatment and underwent surgical closure. Eleven patients (18%) received two courses of ibuprofen. Infants with hsPDA had lower GA and Apgar score at 5 min, higher incidence of IVH, PVL, CLD, ROP, NEC, sepsis, mortality, and lengthier stay in NICU compared to infants without PDA (**Table 1**).

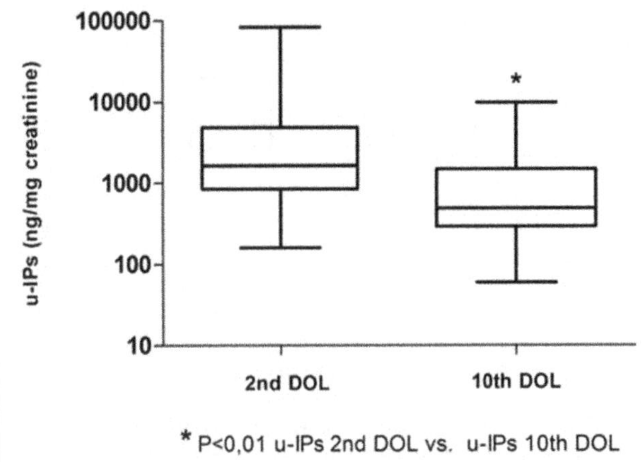

FIGURE 1 | Urinary levels of isoprostanes (uIPs) on the 2nd and 10th DOL. Median values and IQR.

TABLE 2 | Urinary levels of isoprostanes (uIPs, ng/mg of creatinine) on the 2nd and 10th DOL in infants without PDA.

	uIPs on 2nd DOL	uIPs on 10th DOL	*P*
No PDA ($n = 27$)	969.9 (541.0–1470.6)	410.5 (226.0–1027.5)	0.742
Ibuprofen treated PDA ($n = 27$)	2700.0 (1205.7–6688.0)*	535.0 (314.0–1791.9)#	0.001
Surgical closed PDA ($n = 6$)	5028.7 (1233.0–17770.0) **^	1689.0 (198.5–5541.8)	0.974

With hsPDA treated with ibuprofen, or who underwent surgical ligation after failure of pharmacological treatment. Median and IQR.
**P < 0.01 no PDA vs. ibuprofen treated PDA; **P = 0.01 no PDA vs. surgical closure.*
^ P < 0.01 ibuprofen treated PDA vs. surgical closure.
 # These patients had PDA closed on 10th DOL.

Isoprostanes and PDA on the 2nd DOL

Infants without PDA showed a significantly lower uIPs in comparison with infants with ibuprofen-treated hsPDA and who needed surgical closure (after failure of ibuprofen therapy) ($p < 0.01$) (**Table 2** and **Figure 2**). Univariate regression analyses demonstrated that uIPs sampled on the 2nd DOL were associated ($p < 0.05$) with a lower GA and a higher occurrence of hsPDA. After adjusting for GA, BPD, IVH, NEC, and mean FiO_2 the association between uIPs and hsPDA remained significant ($r = 0.38$, B = 2729.8, CI = 416.4–5043,3, $p = 0.02$).

In ROC analysis, uIPs in the 2nd DOL significantly predicted hsPDA development, with an AUC of 0.78 and 95% CI 0.65–0.71 ($p < 0.0001$), showing the best prognostic cutoff point at uIPs = 1627 ng/mg of creatinine, with a sensitivity of 82% and a specificity of 73% (**Figure 3**).

Isoprostanes and PDA on 10th DOL

Six infants (10%) had hsPDA on the 10th DOL. Urinary IPs were similar in infants with or without hsPDA (**Table 2**). Univariate regression analyses did not demonstrate any association on the

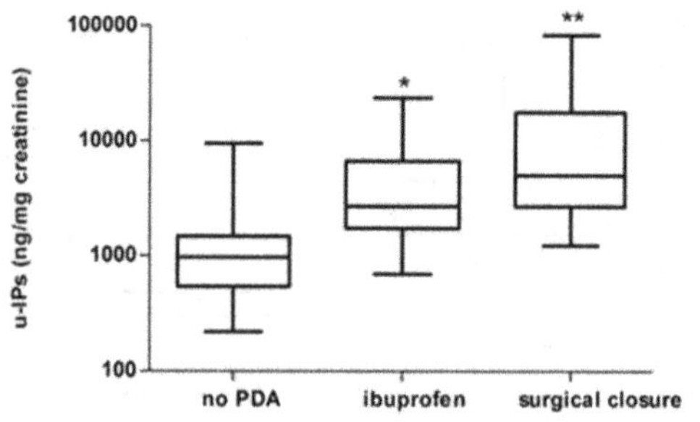

* P<0,01 no PDA vs. ibuprofen treated PDA;** P=0,01 no PDA vs. surgical closure; P=NS ibuprofen treated PDA vs. surgical closure

FIGURE 2 | Urinary levels of isoprostanes (uIPs) on the 2nd DOL in infants without PDA, with hsPDA treated with ibuprofen, or who underwent surgical ligation after failure of pharmacological treatment. Median and IQR.

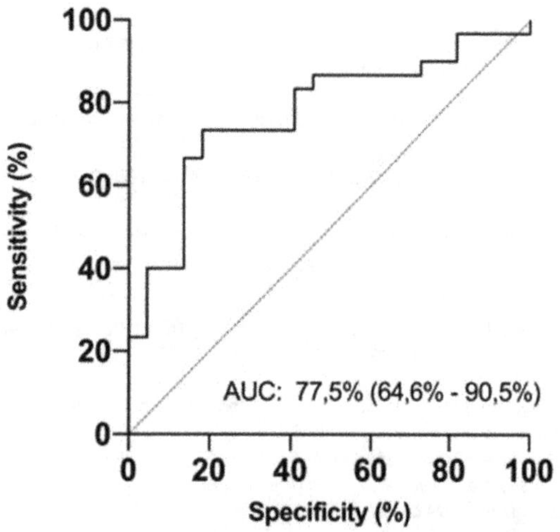

FIGURE 3 | ROC curve analysis for urinary isoprostanes (uIPs) concentration on the 2nd DOL. The area under the curve is 0.775, 95% CI 0.646–0.905. The iPls levels plotted curve indicated 1,627 ng/mg of creatinine as the best predictive threshold with a sensitivity of 82% and a specificity of 73%. ROC curve discriminates newborns with hsPDA from newborns without it.

10th DOL between uIPs and hsPDA. After adjusting for GA, BPD, IVH, NEC, and mean FiO_2 none of the evaluated variables showed a correlation with uIPs.

DISCUSSION

This is the first study to investigate the possible predictive role of uIPs levels on the development of hsPDA. We found that uIPs on the 2nd DOL were higher in infants who developed hsPDA than in infants who did not, and were higher in infants who had hsPDA refractory to drug therapy requiring surgical closure than in infants who had pharmacological closure of hsPDA. It is noteworthy that the correlation between uIPs levels on the 2nd DOL and the development of hsPDA remained statistically significant after adjusting for the main potential confounding factors. Thus, uIPs levels might be a valuable biomarker of hsPDA, as confirmed by ROC analysis which demonstrated that a uIPs cutoff level of 1627 ng/mg of creatinine on the 2nd DOL predicts a hsPDA with a sensitivity of 82% and a specificity of 73%.

Isoprostanes are a product of free radical-induced injury by peroxidation of lipids and their synthesis can easily occur in preterm newborns due to their limited antioxidant defenses and large production of free-radicals according to several factors, such as hyperoxia, inflammation, infections, free iron release, and activation of arachidonic acid cascade (19). The role of IsoPs in the DA closure has recently been reported (8, 9), suggesting that they might induce a DA vascular constriction during the fetal and neonatal period. In particular, Chen et al. found that IsoPs can induce constriction of DA through the activation of thromboxane A2 (TxA2) receptor (10). However, they found that IsoPs can also induce vasodilation of the preterm, isolated DA mediated by the prostaglandin E2 receptor 4 (EP4) (10). Hence, as they demonstrated, IsoPs can exert both constrictive and dilatory effects on the DA depending on relative predominance of the TxA2 and EP4 receptors (10). With increasing maturity, the balance between EP4 and TxA2 shifted in favor of the contractile effects of TxA2 stimulation at term gestation. Therefore, it can be speculated that the postnatal transition from the relatively low oxygen intrauterine environment to the significantly higher oxygen extrauterine environment can induce oxidative stress and IsoPs synthesis in newborn infants. This effect could favor DA constriction and closure in term infants via activation of TxA2 receptor or DA dilation and hsPDA development in preterm infants via activation of EP4 receptors.

On the 10th DOL uIPs decreased in comparison with the 2nd DOL levels, and differences between infants without hsPDA, with hsPDA responding to pharmacological therapy, or requiring surgical closure disappeared. This reduction might be due to the maturation of infants who achieved a more favorable balance between anti-oxidant and pro-oxidant factors and overcame the acute phase of respiratory distress syndrome, in agreement with previously reported inverse correlation between IPs synthesis and gestational age (20). Moreover, only in patients who had the pharmacological therapy of hsPDA, the decrease of uIPs level might be due to the antioxidant properties of ibuprofen (11) which is able to scavenge the hydroxyl radical and/or chelates iron (21) and has been found to suppress neuronal oxidative damage more potently than naproxen or acetylsalicylic acid (22).

Our results confirmed the findings of Longini et al. who studied 43 infants with gestational age <33 weeks and hsPDA, and found that uIPs decreased after PDA closure with ibuprofen (11). Moreover, they found that uIPs increased 1 week (from 11.5 to 14 DOL) after the closure and explained this increase with the lack of ibuprofen antioxidant effect after its suspension (11). This latter result is interesting but we cannot comment on it because studies differed in terms of times of urine sampling, drugs used, and occurrence of repeated course of hsPDA pharmacological therapy.

Limitations of our study include the small number infants with hsPDA which precludes the possibility of using regression analysis to evaluate the possible correlation between uIPs levels and the risk of undergoing surgical closure of hsPDA. Moreover, our population has a wide range of gestational ages which might affect the range of uIPs levels. However, we are confident that the high quality of data analyses could contribute to minimize the effects of this limit on our results.

In conclusion, we found that uIPs levels measured on the 2nd DOL are significantly correlated with the risk of developing a hsPDA. We demonstrated that a uIPs cutoff level of 1627 ng/mg of creatinine can predict a hsPDA with a sensitivity of 82% and a specificity of 73%. Early measurement of uIPs, alone or combined with other markers, might represent a reliable, non-invasive biomarker useful for planning the management of PDA in preterm infants.

Implications for Practice

We found that early and painless measurement of uIPs levels predicts the development of a hsPDA with a sensitivity of 82% and a specificity of 73%. Since the proper management of PDA is continuously debated between neonatologists, the discovery of reliable biomarkers of hsPDA might be useful in the clinical practice in driving its management together with the findings of echocardiography. Thus, if a rapid method for their dosing might be developed, uIPs could be one of these promising biomarkers.

ETHICS STATEMENT

The studies involving human participants were reviewed and approved by Pediatric ethics committee of Tuscany region. Written informed consent to participate in this study was provided by the participants' legal guardian/next of kin.

AUTHOR CONTRIBUTIONS

CC, MT, IC, VL, ML, FB, GB, and CD have made substantial contributions to conception and design of the study, critically revised the article, and have given their final approval of the version to be published. CC and CD performed the data statistical analyses and wrote the manuscript. CC, MT, IC, and VL collected data. All authors contributed to the article and approved the submitted version.

REFERENCES

1. Hamrick SE, Hansmann G. Patent ductus arteriosus of the preterm infant. *Pediatrics.* (2010) 125:1020–30. doi: 10.1542/peds.2009-3506
2. El-Khuffash A, Weisz DE, McNamara PJ. Reflections of the changes in patent ductus arteriosus management during the last 10 years. *Arch Dis Child Fetal Neonatal Ed.* (2016) 101: F474–8. doi: 10.1136/archdischild-2014-306214
3. Brooks JM, Travadi JN, Patole SK, Doherty DA, Simmer K. Is surgical ligation of patent ductus arteriosus necessary? The Western Australian experience of conservative management. *Arch Dis Child Fetal Neonatal Ed.* (2005) 90:F235–9. doi: 10.1136/adc.2004.057638
4. Kaempf JW, Wu XY, Kaempf AJ, Kaempf AM, Wang L, Grunkemeier G. What happens when the patent ductus arteriosus is treated less aggressively in very low birth weight infants? *J Perinatol.* (2012) 32:344–8. doi: 10.1038/jp.2011.102
5. Liebowitz M, Clyman RI. Prophylactic indomethacin compared with delayed conservative management of the patent ductus arteriosus in extremely preterm infants, effects on neonatal outcomes. *J Pediatr.* (2017) 187:119–26. doi: 10.1016/j.jpeds.2017.03.021
6. Schena F, Francescato G, Cappelleri, A, Picciolli I, Mayer A, Mosca F, et al. Association between hemodynamically significant patent ductus arteriosus and bronchopulmonary dysplasia. *J Pediatr.* (2015) 166:1488–92. doi: 10.1016/j.jpeds.2015.03.012
7. van Laere D, van Overmeire B, Gupta S, El-Khuffash A, Savoia M, McNamara PJ, et al. Application of NPE in the assessment of a patent ductus arteriosus. *Pediatr Res.* (2018) 84:S46–56. doi: 10.1038/s41390-018-0077-x
8. Jain A, Shah PS. Diagnosis, evaluation, and management of patent Ductus Arteriosus in preterm neonates. *JAMA Pediatr.* (2015) 169:863–72. doi: 10.1001/jamapediatrics.2015.0987
9. van der Sterren S, Villamor E. Contractile effects of 15-E2t-isoprostane and 15-F2t-isoprostane on chicken embryo ductus arteriosus. *Comp Biochem Physiol A Mol Integr Physiol.* (2011) 159:436–44. doi: 10.1016/j.cbpa.2011.04.010
10. Chen JX, O'Mara PW, Poole SD, Brown N, Ehinger NJ, Slaughter JC, et al. Isoprostanes as physiological mediators of transition to newborn life, novel mechanisms regulating patency of the term and preterm ductus arteriosus. *Pediatr Res.* (2012) 72:122–8. doi: 10.1038/pr.2012.58
11. Longini M, Perrone S, Vezzosi, P. Isoprostane levels in urine of preterm newborns treated with ibuprofen for patent ductus arteriosus closure. *Pediatr Nephrol.* (2011) 26:105–9. doi: 10.1007/s00467-010-1651-6
12. Casetta B, Longini M, Proietti F, Perrone S, Buonocore G. Development of a fast and simple lc-ms/ms method for measuring the f2-isoprostanes in newborns. *J Matern Fetal Neonatal Med.* (2012) 25:S114–8. doi: 10.3109/14767058.2012.664856
13. Dani C, Poggi C, Fontanelli G. Relationship between platelet count and volume and spontaneous and pharmacological closure of ductus arteriosus in preterm infants. *Am J Perinatol.* (2013) 30:359–64. doi: 10.1055/s-0032-1324702
14. Su BH, Peng CT, Tsai CH. Echocardiographic flow pattern of patent ductus arteriosus: a guide to indomethacin treatment in premature infants. *Arch Dis Child Fetal Neonatal Ed.* (1999) 81:F197–200. doi: 10.1136/fn.81.3.F197
15. Onland W, Debray TP, Laughon MM, Miedema M, Cools F, Askie LM, et al. Clinical prediction models for bronchopulmonary dysplasia: a systematic review and external validation study. *BMC Pediatr.* (2013) 13:207. doi: 10.1186/1471-2431-13-207
16. Bell MJ, Ternberg JL, Feigin RD, Keating JP, Marshall R, Barton L, et al. Neonatal necrotizing enterocolitis: therapeutic decisions based upon clinical staging. *Ann Surg.* (1978) 187:1–12. doi: 10.1097/00000658-197801000-00001
17. Papile LS, Burstein J, Burstein R, Keffler H. Incidence and evolution of the sub-ependymal intraventricular hemorrhage: a study of infants weighing less than 1500 grams. *J Pediatr.* (1978) 92:529. doi: 10.1016/S0022-3476(78)80282-0
18. De Vries LS, Eken P, Dubowitz LM. The spectrum of leukomalacia using cranial ultrasounds. *Behav Brain Res.* (1992) 49:1–6. doi: 10.1016/S0166-4328(05)80189-5
19. Helmersson J, Basu S. F2-Isoprostanes and prostaglandin F2α metabolite excretion rate and day to day variation in healthy humans. *Prostaglandins Leukot Essent Fatty Acids.* (2001) 65:99–102. doi: 10.1054/plef.2001.0295
20. Comporti M, Signorini C, Leoncini S, Buonocore G, Rossi V, Ciccoli L. Plasma F2-isoprostanes are elevated in newborns and inversely correlated to gestational age. *Free Radic Biol Med.* (2004) 37:724. doi: 10.1016/j.freeradbiomed.2004.06.007
21. Hamburger SA, McCay PB. Spin trapping of ibuprofen radicals: evidence that ibuprofen is a hydroxyl radical scavenger. *Free Radic Res Commun.* (1990) 9:337–42. doi: 10.3109/10715769009145692
22. Milatovic D, Zaja-Milatovic S, Montine KS, Shie FS, Montine TJ. Neuronal oxidative damage and dendritic degeneration following activation of CD14-dependent innate immune response in vivo. *J Neuroinflammation.* (2004) 1:20. doi: 10.1186/1742-2094-1-20

6

An Observational, Prospective, Multicenter, Registry-Based Cohort Study Comparing Conservative and Medical Management for Patent Ductus Arteriosus

Emel Okulu [1], Omer Erdeve [1], Zehra Arslan [2], Nihal Demirel [3], Huseyin Kaya [4], Ismail Kursad Gokce [4], Sabahattin Ertugrul [5], Merih Cetinkaya [6], Gokhan Buyukkale [6], Ferda Ozlu [7], Huseyin Simsek [7], Yalcin Celik [8], Hilal Ozkan [9], Nilgun Köksal [9], Baris Akcan [10], Munevver Turkmen [10], Kiymet Celik [11], Didem Armangil [12], Ali Bulbul [13], Kadir Serafettin Tekgunduz [14], Mehmet Yekta Oncel [15], Funda Tuzun [16], Ebru Ergenekon [17], Hacer Ergin [18], Saadet Arsan [1] and Turkish Neonatal Society INTERPDA Study Group*

[1] Division of Neonatology, Department of Pediatrics, Ankara University School of Medicine, Ankara, Turkey, [2] Department of Neonatology, Etlik Zubeyde Hanim Women's Health Teaching and Research Hospital, University of Health Sciences, Ankara, Turkey, [3] Division of Neonatology, Department of Pediatrics, Ankara Yildirim Beyazit University School of Medicine, Ankara, Turkey, [4] Division of Neonatology, Department of Pediatrics, Inonu University School of Medicine, Malatya, Turkey, [5] Division of Neonatology, Department of Pediatrics, Dicle University School of Medicine, Diyarbakir, Turkey, [6] Department of Neonatology, University of Health Sciences, Kanuni Sultan Suleyman Training and Research Hospital, Istanbul, Turkey, [7] Division of Neonatology, Department of Pediatrics, Cukurova University School of Medicine, Adana, Turkey, [8] Division of Neonatology, Department of Pediatrics, Mersin University School of Medicine, Mersin, Turkey, [9] Division of Neonatology, Department of Pediatrics, Uludag University School of Medicine, Bursa, Turkey, [10] Division of Neonatology, Department of Pediatrics, Adnan Menderes University School of Medicine, Aydin, Turkey, [11] Neonatal Intensive Care Unit, Diyarbakir Gazi Yasargil Training and Research Hospital, Diyarbakir, Turkey, [12] Neonatal Intensive Care Unit, Koru Hospital, Ankara, Turkey, [13] Department of Neonatology, University of Health Sciences, Sisli Etfal Hamidiye Training and Research Hospital, Istanbul, Turkey, [14] Division of Neonatology, Department of Pediatrics, Ataturk University School of Medicine, Erzurum, Turkey, [15] Division of Neonatology, Department of Pediatrics, Izmir Katip Celebi University School of Medicine, Izmir, Turkey, [16] Division of Neonatology, Department of Pediatrics, Dokuz Eylul University School of Medicine, Izmir, Turkey, [17] Division of Neonatology, Department of Pediatrics, Gazi University School of Medicine, Ankara, Turkey, [18] Division of Neonatology, Department of Pediatrics, Pamukkale University School of Medicine, Denizli, Turkey

***Correspondence:**
Omer Erdeve
omererdeve@yahoo.com

No consensus has been reached on which patent ductus arteriosus (PDAs) in preterm infants require treatment and if so, how, and when they should be treated. A prospective, multicenter, cohort study was conducted to compare the effects of conservative approaches and medical treatment options on ductal closure at discharge, surgical ligation, prematurity-related morbidities, and mortality. Infants between $24^{0/7}$ and $28^{6/7}$ weeks of gestation from 24 neonatal intensive care units were enrolled. Data on PDA management and patients' clinical characteristics were recorded prospectively. Patients with moderate-to-large PDA were compared. Among the 1,193 enrolled infants (26.7 ± 1.4 weeks and 926 ± 243 g), 649 (54%) had no or small PDA, whereas 544 (46%) had moderate-to-large PDA. One hundred thirty (24%) infants with moderate-to-large PDA were managed conservatively, in contrast to 414 (76%) who received medical treatment. Eighty (62%) of 130 infants who were managed conservatively did not receive any rescue treatment and the PDA closure rate was 53% at discharge. There were no differences in the rates of late-onset sepsis, necrotizing enterocolitis (NEC), retinopathy of prematurity, intraventricular hemorrhage (≥Grade 3), surgical ligation, and presence of PDA at discharge between conservatively-managed and medically-treated infants ($p > 0.05$). Multivariate analysis including perinatal factors showed that medical treatment was associated with increased risk for mortality (OR 1.68, 95% CI 1.01–2.80, $p = 0.046$), but decreased risk for BPD or death (BPD/death) (OR 0.59, 95%CI 0.37–0.92, $p = 0.022$). The preferred treatment options were ibuprofen (intravenous 36%, oral 31%), and paracetamol (intravenous 26%, oral 7%). Infants who were treated with oral paracetamol had higher rates of NEC and mortality in comparison to other treatment options. Infants treated before postnatal day 7 had higher rates of mortality and BPD/death than infants who were conservatively managed or treated beyond day 7 ($p = 0.009$ and 0.007, respectively). In preterm infants born at <29 weeks of gestation with moderate-to-large PDA, medical treatment did not show any reduction in the rates of open PDA at discharge, surgical or prematurity-related secondary outcomes. In addition to the high incidence of spontaneous closure of PDA in the first week of life, early treatment (<7 days) was associated with higher rates of mortality and BPD/death.

Keywords: patent ductus arteriosus, preterm, conservative, management, morbidity, mortality, ibuprofen, paracetamol

INTRODUCTION

Patent ductus arteriosus (PDA) is the most common cardiovascular condition in preterm infants. Although the ductus arteriosus (DA) is closed spontaneously in most of the infants born at >28 weeks of gestation (i.e., at the end of the first week of life), persistent patency of the DA is observed in 50–70% of infants born at <28 weeks of gestation, and lasts for weeks after birth (1, 2).

PDA is associated with mortality and morbidities including necrotizing enterocolitis (NEC), pulmonary hemorrhage, intraventricular hemorrhage (IVH), retinopathy of prematurity (ROP), bronchopulmonary dysplasia (BPD), and poor neurodevelopmental outcomes. These morbidities are caused by the left-to-right shunt through the DA that may result in pulmonary hyperperfusion and systemic hypoperfusion (3–6). This association has encouraged neonatologists to treat PDA in order to reduce these associated morbidities, but there remains a wide variety of management options for PDA across centers worldwide (7, 8).

Despite PDA's association with prematurity-related morbidities, no randomized controlled trial to date has demonstrated improvements in BPD, long-term neurodevelopmental outcomes or mortality after medical or surgical treatment of PDA (1, 4, 9–11). Therefore, centers have been performing conservative follow-ups for PDA, especially since higher rates of spontaneous closure rates have been reported in the current era (12, 13). A recent study that compared early routine treatment (ERT) of PDA with conservative management showed that ERT did not reduce either PDA ligations or the presence of a PDA at discharge, and did not improve secondary outcomes, However, ERT was associated with higher rates of late-onset sepsis (LOS) and death in infants born at >26 weeks of gestation (14). Therefore, we aimed to establish a prospective online registry database to examine the variations in PDA management for a nationally-based cohort, and evaluate the effects of PDA management strategies on the rates of PDA closure, PDA ligation, associated morbidities, and survival in preterm infants.

MATERIALS AND METHODS

After the establishment of the Experiences in Timing and Choices for Ductal Closure in Patent Ductus Arteriosus (INTERPDA) Study Online Registry in January 2017, a multicenter prospective observational nationally-based cohort study was conducted. Infants who were born at gestational weeks between $24^{0/7}$ and $28^{6/7}$ and underwent echocardiography in first 3 weeks of life after birth were included. Clinical directors in neonatal intensive care units (NICUs) nationwide were made aware of the study, and 24 NICUs participated. The NICUs were asked to add all hospitalized patients per day to the registry database using an online standard, patient-specific electronic case report form (eCRF) for a 2-years period. Data were then collected prospectively and registered by trained neonatologists.

The study was approved by the Online Studies Scientific Steering Committee of the Turkish Neonatal Society and by the Institutional Review Board of Ankara University. Written informed consent was obtained from the parents or guardians of the newborns. The study was registered at ClinicalTrials.gov (NCT02910609).

The eCRF included demographic and clinical findings including gestational age, birth weight, gender, type of delivery, the presence of prolonged premature rupture of

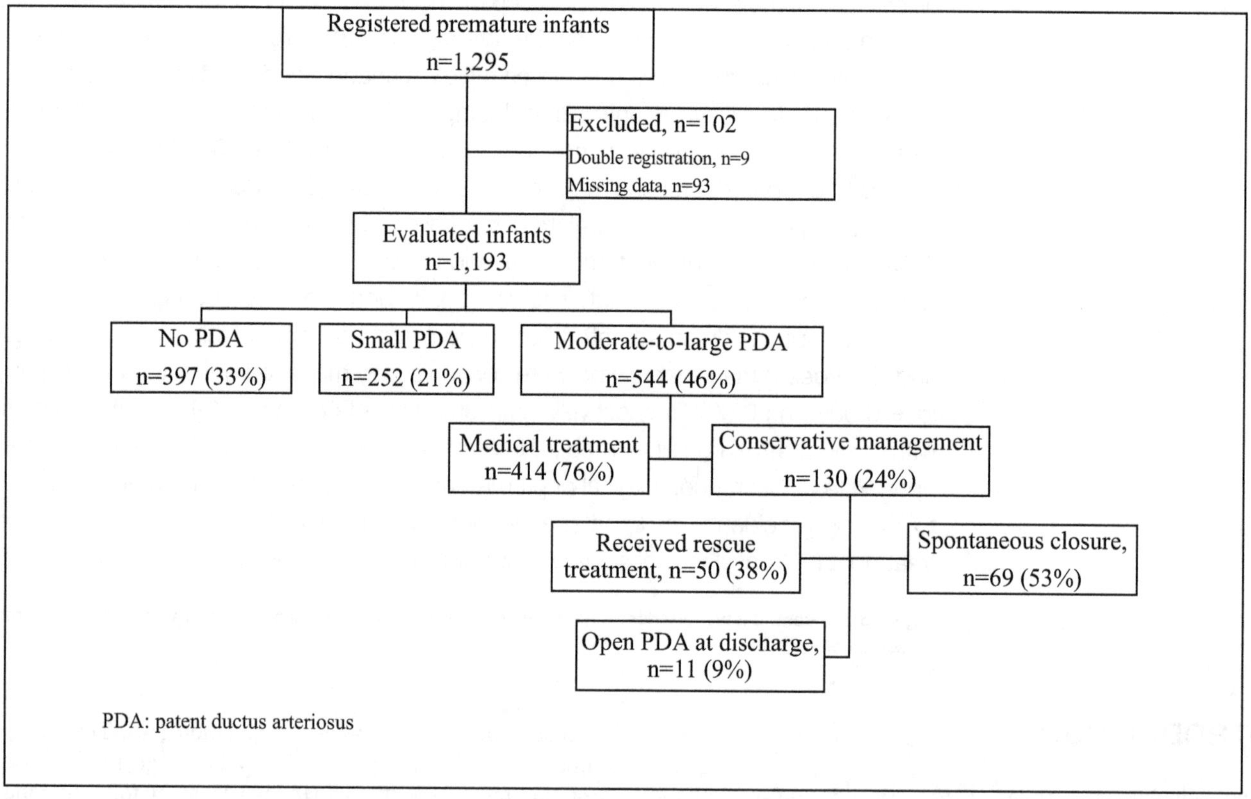

FIGURE 1 | The flow chart of the study.

membranes (PPROM) which was defined as rupture of membranes >18 h before labor and before 37 weeks' gestation, antepartum preeclampsia (15); clinical chorioamnionitis, the use of any antenatal steroid, respiratory distress syndrome (RDS) (16), clinical or culture proven early-onset sepsis in addition to echocardiographic assessment results, type of PDA, management provided to the infants (conservative or medical), the timing of any medication used, type of preferred drug, outcomes of management on ductal closure at discharge, surgical ligation, and adverse events. Associated morbidities such as culture proven LOS, NEC (17), IVH (18), ROP (19), BPD (20), and mortality were also recorded.

Echocardiographic Assessment

Diagnosis of PDA was based on clinical and/or echocardiographic studies, which included 2-dimensional imaging, M-mode, color flow mapping, and Doppler interrogation. A moderate-to-large PDA was defined as an internal ductus diameter >1.5 mm, left atrium-to-aortic root ratio >1.5, and reverse diastolic flow in the descending aorta. A ductus that failed to meet these criteria was defined as small PDA.

Management of PDA

The decision for the management of PDA was left up to each center according to their standard practices.

TABLE 1 | The demographic data of the infants included in INTERPDA study.

	No. of patients (*n* = 1,193)
Gestational age (wk)*	26.7 ± 1.4
Birth weight (g)*	926 ± 243
Gender (male), *n* (%)	605 (51)
Type of delivery (C/S), *n* (%)	949 (79)
Multiple gestation, *n* (%)	231 (19)
PPROM, *n* (%)	288 (24)
Preeclampsia, *n* (%)	305 (26)
Chorioamnionitis, *n* (%)	112 (9)
Antenatal steroid, *n* (%)	83 (70)
Delivery room intubation, *n* (%)	555 (46)
Surfactant use, *n* (%)	956 (80)
RDS, *n* (%)	986 (83)
Early-onset sepsis, *n* (%)	436 (36)

C/S, cesarean section; PPROM, prolonged premature rupture of membranes; RDS, respiratory distress syndrome.
**Data given mean ± SD.*

Infants with moderate-to-large PDA were grouped according to their PDA management as conservative approach or medical treatment. Patients' demographic and clinical findings, outcomes of preferred PDA management, rates of associated morbidities,

TABLE 2 | Demographic and clinical findings of the conservatively managed and medically treated groups of the infants with moderate-to-large PDA.

	Conservative (*n* = 130)	Medical (*n* = 414)	*P*
Gestational age (w)*	26.5 ± 1.4	26.5 ± 1.5	0.89
Birth weight (g)*	924 ± 232	877 ± 230	0.06
Gender (male), *n* (%)	65 (30)	202 (49)	0.81
Type of delivery (C/S), *n* (%)	96 (74)	311 (75)	0.77
Multiple gestation, *n* (%)	22 (17)	90 (22)	0.23
PPROM, *n* (%)	40 (31)	94 (23)	0.06
Preeclampsia, *n* (%)	32 (25)	101 (24)	0.96
Chorioamnionitis, *n* (%)	14 (11)	52 (13)	0.58
Antenatal steroid, *n* (%)	88 (68)	288 (70)	0.68
Delivery room intubation, *n* (%)	64 (49)	239 (58)	0.08
Surfactant use, *n* (%)	104 (80)	380 (92)	< 0.001
RDS, *n* (%)	108 (83)	392 (95)	< 0.001
Early-onset sepsis, *n* (%)	48 (37)	166 (40)	0.52
Received respiratory support, *n* (%)	113 (87)	408 (99)	< 0.001
Duration of respiratory support (d)**	18 (1–245)	22 (1–181)	0.001
Discharged with open PDA, *n* (%)	25 (19)	80 (19)	0.98
PDA ligation, *n* (%)	8 (6)	29 (7)	0.73
LOS, *n* (%)	71 (55)	216 (52)	0.62
IVH (≥Grade 3), *n* (%)	5 (4)	15 (4)	> 0.05
NEC, *n* (%)	28 (21)	107 (26)	0.32
Moderate-severe BPD¥, *n* (%)	25 (47)	93 (49)	0.84
Treated ROP‡, *n* (%)	14 (13)	63 (21)	0.06
Mortality, *n* (%)	29 (22)	144 (35)	0.008
BPD/death, *n* (%)	51 (39)	226 (55)	0.002
Duration of hospitalization (d)**	59 (2-253)	62 (2–357)	0.79

BPD, bronchopulmonary dysplasia; C/S, cesarean section; IVH, intraventricular hemorrhage; LOS, late-onset sepsis; NEC, necrotizing enterocolitis; PDA, patent ductus arteriosus; PPROM, prolonged premature rupture of membranes; RDS, respiratory distress syndrome; ROP, retinopathy of prematurity.
‡Infants had at least one eye examination for ROP.
¥Infants survived at PMA 36 weeks' gestation.
**Data given mean ± SD, **Data given as median (range).*

mortality rate, and BPD or death (BPD/death) were compared between the two groups.

Statistical Analysis

Frequency and percentage (*n*, %) were used to describe categorical data. Pearson Chi-squared test was used to assess the relationship between categorical variables when the test requirements were met. Otherwise, Fisher's exact test or Fisher-Freeman-Halton Exact test was used to test independence between categorical variables depending on the table size. For numerical dependent variables Mann-Whitney *U*-test was used for comparisons between groups due to the fact that the parametric test assumptions were not met. Normality of numerical variables was assessed by Kolmogorov-Smirnov test. Homogeneity of group variances were evaluated by Levene test. Descriptive statistics were reported as minimum value, maximum value, median (interquartile range-IQR). In addition, mean ± standard deviation was also given. After conducting univariate analysis to estimate effects of managements for PDA on mortality and BPD/death by using generalized estimating equations (GEE); multivariate models were evaluated with QICC criteria. All regression analysis was based on GEE, we used non-robust standard errors and accounted for the clustering of infants within center (21). Odds ratio are presented with 95% Cl. Statistical analysis was performed using the IBMM SPSS Statistics version 23 for Windows.

RESULTS

Demographic Data of the Study Group

The final study sample included 1,193 infants after exclusion of 102 from a total of 1,295 because of double-record or missing data (**Figure 1**). The mean gestational age and birth weight of infants were 26.7 ± 1.4 weeks and 926 ± 243 g, respectively. Of the 1,193, 523 (44%) infants were born at <27 weeks' gestation, and 730 (62%) weighed <1,000 g. The prenatal and neonatal demographic characteristics of the infants enrolled in the study are displayed in **Table 1**.

The median of the echocardiographic assessment time was 3 days (interquartile range, IQR = 2 days). The incidence of small PDA and no PDA was 252 (21%) and 397 (33%), respectively; whereas 544 (46%) patients had moderate-to-large PDA on echocardiographic evaluation. The incidence of moderate-to-large PDA was 63, 60, 45, 40, and 38% according to a gestational age of 24, 25, 26, 27, and 28 weeks, respectively.

Data of Infants With Moderate-to-Large PDA

One hundred thirty (24%) infants with moderate-to-large PDA were managed conservatively, in contrast to 414 (76%) infants who received medical treatment. The data for these infants are displayed in **Table 2**. Infants with moderate-to-large PDA in both the conservative and medically-treated groups showed similar gestational age, birth weight, incidences of maternal preeclampsia, chorioamnionitis and PPROM, antenatal steroid use, and early onset sepsis (p >0.05). Higher incidences of delivery room intubation, RDS, and surfactant use were present in medically treated infants ($p < 0.05$).

The respiratory support of infants according to gestational age and PDA management is shown in **Figure 2**. More infants received any respiratory support in medical treatment group than infants in conservative group (99 vs. 87%, $p < 0.001$). The rate of non-invasive ventilation use as respiratory support was higher in conservatively-managed infants with moderate-to-large PDA ($p = 0.004$), whereas the number of infants receiving mechanical ventilation was higher among medically-treated patients ($p = 0.011$).

There were no differences in the rates of open PDA at discharge, surgical ligation, LOS, NEC (any stage), ROP (received treatment who had at least one eye examination for ROP), IVH (≥Grade 3), BPD [moderate-to-severe who survived at postmenstrual [PMA] 36 weeks of gestation] between the groups ($p > 0.05$), but infants who were medically treated had higher rates of mortality (OR 1.82, 95% Cl 1.15–2.89, $p = 0.011$), and BPD/death (OR 1.81

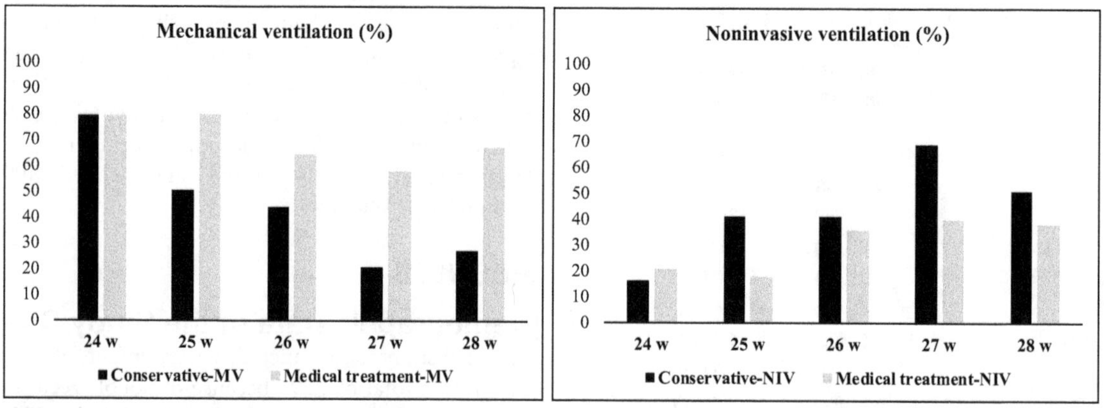

MV: mechanical ventilation; NIV: noninvasive ventilation

FIGURE 2 | The respiratory support of infants and PDA management.

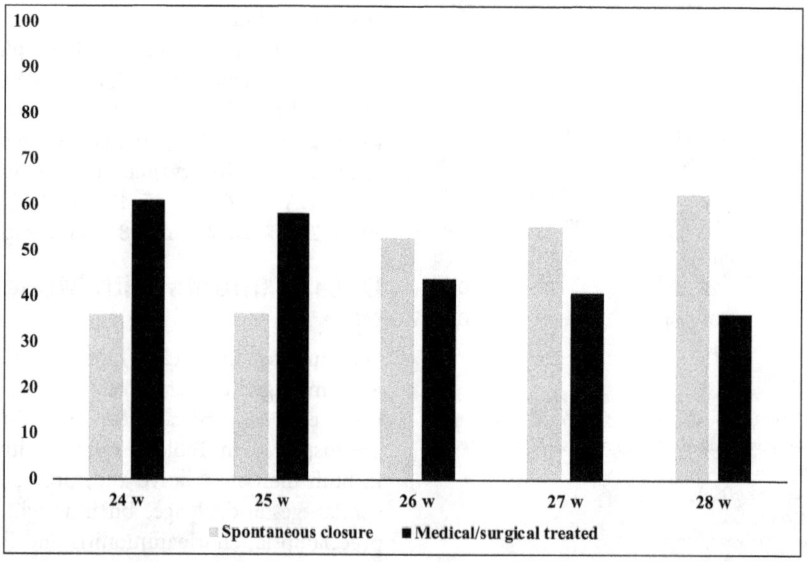

FIGURE 3 | The rates of spontaneous closure or medically/surgical treated ductus according to gestational age.

95% Cl 1.20–2.71, $p = 0.004$) (**Table 2**). However, multivariate analysis including perinatal factors (gestational age, birth weight, chorioamnionitis, delivery room intubation) showed that medical treatment was associated with increased risk for mortality (OR 1.68, 95% Cl 1.01–2.80, $p = 0.046$), but decreased risk for BPD/death (OR 0.59, 95% Cl 0.37–0.92, $p = 0.022$).

Eighty (62%) of the 130 infants who were managed conservatively did not receive any rescue treatment during their hospitalization. PDA closure before hospital discharge was observed in 69 infants. The spontaneous closure rate increased with gestational age and reached a peak level of 63% in infants born at 28 weeks of gestation (**Figure 3**).

We performed a secondary analysis according to gestational age (<27 weeks and ≥27 weeks) to evaluate the effects of PDA management on any of the outcomes (**Table 3**).

Despite similar incidences of open PDA at discharge, PDA ligation, and mortality between groups, higher rates of NEC and BPD/death were observed in medically treated infants born at ≥27 weeks of gestation ($p = 0.026$ and $p = 0.025$, respectively). These infants had higher incidences of RDS and surfactant use, and longer duration of respiratory support (median 24 days vs. 12 days, $p < 0.001$) compared to conservatively managed infants. Univariate analysis showed that medical treatment was associated with an increased the risk of NEC and BPD/death (OR 2.7, 95% Cl 1.09–6.68, $p = 0.031$, and OR 2.12, 95% Cl 1.07–4.20, $p = 0.03$, respectively) in infants born at ≥27 weeks of gestation, however multivariate analysis could not demonstrate the similar effect for BPD/death.

The groups did not differ in duration of respiratory support and rate of mechanical ventilation in infants born at <27 weeks of gestation. The rates of open PDA at discharge,

TABLE 3 | Outcomes of infants born <27 weeks and ≥27 weeks' gestation.

	<27 weeks (n = 282)			≥27 weeks (n = 262)		
	Conservative (n = 68)	Medical (n = 214)	P	Conservative (n = 62)	Medical (n = 200)	P
DEMOGRAPHIC AND CLINICAL DATA						
Gestational age (week)*	25.3 ± 0.9	25.3 ± 0.8	0.37	27.7 ± 0.5	27.8 ± 0.5	0.29
Birth weight (g)*	796 ± 158	754 ± 170	0.06	1,066 ± 219	1,009 ± 212	0.07
Gender (male), n (%)	31 (46)	107 (50)	0.52	34 (55)	95 (47)	0.31
Type of delivery (C/S), n (%)	47 (69)	146 (68)	0.89	49 (79)	165 (82)	0.53
Multiple gestation, n (%)	12 (18)	42 (20)	0.71	10 (16)	48 (24)	0.19
PPROM, n (%)	22 (32)	67 (31)	0.87	18 (29)	27 (13)	0.005
Preeclampsia, n (%)	16 (23)	46 (21)	0.72	16 (26)	55 (27)	0.79
Chorioamnionitis, n (%)	11 (16)	36 (17)	0.90	3 (5)	16 (8)	0.4
Antenatal steroid, n (%)	45 (66)	132 (62)	0.50	43 (69)	156 (78)	0.16
Delivery room intubation, n (%)	40 (59)	154 (72)	0.04	24 (39)	85 (42)	0.59
Surfactant use, n (%)	61 (90)	206 (96)	0.09	44 (71)	177 (88)	0.001
RDS, n (%)	60 (88)	203 (95)	0.05	47 (76)	186 (93)	< 0.001
Early-onset sepsis, n (%)	27 (40)	94 (44)	0.54	21 (34)	72 (36)	0.76
Received respiratory support, n (%)	61 (90)	213 (99)	< 0.001	52 (84)	195 (97)	< 0.001
Duration of respiratory support (d)**	26 (2–245)	23 (1–150)	0.91	14 (1–96)	22 (2–181)	0.001
OUTCOMES						
Discharged with open PDA, n (%)	16 (23)	53 (25)	0.83	9 (14)	27 (13)	0.83
PDA ligation, n (%)	6 (9)	17 (8)	0.81	2 (3)	12 (6)	0.53
LOS, n (%)	44 (65)	24 (55)	0.16	27 (43)	98 (49)	0.45
IVH (≥Grade 3), n (%)	4 (6)	9 (4)	0.52	1 (2)	6 (3)	> 0.05
NEC, n (%)	22 (32)	62 (29)	0.59	6 (10)	45 (22)	0.026
Moderate-severe BPD¥, n (%)	18 (50)	57 (56)	0.50	11 (50)	49 (47)	0.80
Treated ROP‡, n (%)	11 (16)	45 (21)	0.38	3 (5)	18 (9)	0.42
Mortality, n (%)	24 (35)	111 (52)	0.017	5 (8)	33 (16)	0.09
BPD/death, n (%)	37 (54)	150 (70)	0.017	14 (23)	76 (38)	0.025
Duration of hospitalization (d)**	71 (2–253)	54.5 (2–357)	0.34	54 (2–120)	63 (3–180)	0.018

BPD, bronchopulmonary dysplasia; C/S, cesarean section; IVH, intraventricular hemorrhage; LOS, late-onset sepsis; NEC, necrotizing enterocolitis; PDA, patent ductus arteriosus; PPROM, prolonged premature rupture of membranes; RDS, respiratory distress syndrome; ROP, retinopathy of prematurity.
‡Infants had at least one eye examination for ROP.
¥Infants survived at PMA 36 weeks' gestation.
**Data given mean ± SD, **Data given as median (range).*

surgical ligation, and morbidities did not differ significantly in those who were medically treated and those conservatively managed, but medically treated infants had higher rates of mortality and BPD/death. Univariate analysis indicated odds of increased rates of mortality and BPD/death associated with medical treatment in infants born at <27 weeks of gestation (OR 1.97, 95% Cl 1.12–3.47, $p = 0.19$, and OR 1.96, 95% Cl 1.12–3.44, $p = 0.19$), however these were not significant on multivariate analysis.

Data Related to Timing and Preferred Medical Treatment Options

The preferred treatment options were ibuprofen (intravenous 36%, oral 31%), and paracetamol (intravenous 26%, oral 7%) as the initial course; indomethacin was not used in any patient. The median starting time of first-course pharmacological treatment was 3 days (IQR = 2.25 days). The timing of medical treatment was not found to be associated with mortality or morbidities. The most common side effects of drug treatment were impairment of renal function and risk of bleeding, which were mostly reported with ibuprofen treatment.

The incidences of open PDA at discharge, surgical ligation, LOS, BPD, and ROP were similar according to the first-course medication selection. However, infants treated with oral paracetamol had higher rates of NEC and mortality, and infants treated with intravenous paracetamol had a higher rate of BPD/death (**Table 4**).

Ninety-six (26%) of the 362 infants received a second course of treatment with ibuprofen (intravenous 34%, oral 35%) and paracetamol (intravenous 23%, oral 8%), and 29 infants received a third course of treatment mostly with intravenous paracetamol (59%).

Infants who received treatment before postnatal day 7 had higher rates of mortality and BPD/death than infants who were

TABLE 4 | Morbidities and mortality according to treatment options.

	IV ibuprofen (*n* = 148)	Oral ibuprofen (*n* = 129)	IV paracetamol (*n* = 108)	Oral paracetamol (*n* = 29)	*p*
Discharged with open PDA, *n* (%)	28 (19)	19 (15)	24 (22)	9 (31)	0.18
Surgical ligation, *n* (%)	11 (7)	10 (8)	6 (6)	2 (7)	0.91
LOS, *n* (%)	82 (64)	65 (51)	54 (61)	10 (53)	0.08
IVH (≥Gr 3), *n* (%)	3 (2)	6 (5)	5 (5)	1 (3)	0.61
NEC, *n* (%)	40 (27)	32 (25)	20 (18)	15 (52)	0.004
Treated ROP‡, *n* (%)	22 (15)	18 (14)	18 (17)	5 (17)	0.93
Moderate-severeBPD¥, *n* (%)	36 (44)	39 (59)	28 (58)	3 (30)	0.11
Mortality, *n* (%)	46 (31)	34 (26)	48 (44)	16 (55)	0.002
BPD/death, *n* (%)	75 (51)	63 (49)	71 (66)	17 (59)	0.04

BPD, bronchopulmonary dysplasia; IVH, intraventricular hemorrhage; LOS, late-onset sepsis; NEC, necrotizing enterocolitis; PDA, patent ductus arteriosus; ROP, retinopathy of prematurity.
‡Infants had at least one eye examination for ROP.
¥Infants survived at PMA 36 weeks' gestation.

TABLE 5 | Data of mortality, surgical ligation and morbidities in infants who were conservatively managed or medically treated infants (<7 days and ≥7 days).

	Conservative (*n* = 130)	Medical treatment (*n* = 414)		*p*
		<7 days (*N* = 363)	≥7 days (*N* = 51)	
Discharged with open PDA, *n* (%)	25 (19)	72 (20)	8 (16)	0.78
PDA ligation, *n* (%)	8 (6)	24 (7)	5 (10)	0.66
LOS, *n* (%)	71 (55)	188 (52)	28 (55)	0.81
IVH (≥Gr 3), *n* (%)	5 (3.8)	13 (3.6)	2 (3.9)	0.32
NEC, *n* (%)	28 (21)	91 (25)	16 (31)	0.38
Moderate-severe BPD¥, *n* (%)	25 (47)	80 (48)	13 (54)	0.83
Treated ROP‡, *n* (%)	14 (13)	56 (22)	7 (16)	0.12
Mortality, *n* (%)	29 (22)	131 (36)	13 (25)	0.009
BPD/death, *n* (%)	51 (39)	201 (55)	25 (49)	0.007

BPD, bronchopulmonary dysplasia; IVH, intraventricular hemorrhage; LOS, late-onset sepsis; NEC, necrotizing enterocolitis; PDA, patent ductus arteriosus; ROP, retinopathy of prematurity.
‡Infants had at least one eye examination for ROP.
¥Infants survived at PMA 36 weeks' gestation.

conservatively-managed or treated after day 7 ($p = 0.009$ and $p = 0.007$, respectively) (**Table 5**).

DISCUSSION

In this first nationwide study on the management of PDA in preterm infants born at <29 weeks of gestation, we found that there are management variations between NICUs across Turkey. Although most of the patients with moderate-to-large PDA received medical treatment, there was an increasing trend toward the conservative approach. Medical treatment had no effect on the incidence of surgical ligation or prematurity-related morbidities in the overall study group, and early treatment before day 7 of life was associated with higher mortality and BPD/death. Medical treatment was additionally associated with higher rates of NEC in infants who were born at >27 weeks of gestation.

PDA is present in up to 70% of preterm infants born at <28 weeks of gestation (2, 5). The proportion of very low birth weight (VLBW) infants with PDA was reported to be 36% and 38% in Japan and Canadian networks, respectively (22). According to the Korean Neonatal Network 2017 annual report, 45% of VLBW infants had a PDA (23). In the present study, moderate-to-large PDA was present in 46% of preterm infants born at <29 weeks of gestation and increased to 63% in patients born at 24 weeks of gestation.

Management of PDA in extremely preterm infants remains a topic of debate. Treatment to induce ductal closure has been widely practiced until the last decade, despite lack of evidence that it decreases morbidities and mortality. Meta-analyses of trials using non-steroidal anti-inflammatory drugs have shown effectiveness in accelerating ductal closure, but no reduction in neonatal morbidities regardless of the drugs used, indication, timing, gestational age, or route of administration (1). While medical treatment and surgical ligation can close the ductus, such treatment has had side effects (11, 24). The trend toward conservative treatment has been fueled by recent experience with conservative approaches that demonstrated improved neonatal outcomes and a high rate of spontaneous ductal closure at discharge. Lokku et al. demonstrated that an increasing rate of conservative management of PDA occurred alongside a decrease in medical and/or surgical treatment between 2006 and 2012 in Canada (25). An American cohort study with a large population from 280 NICUs showed a significant decrease in diagnosis and medical/surgical treatment of PDA with no evidence of increased morbidities (26). The recent PDA-TOLERATE trial is the only randomized trial that compared routine treatment of a moderate-to-large PDA present at the end of the first week of life in infants born at <28 weeks of gestation to a conservative approach in reducing neonatal morbidities and/or death. It showed that routine treatment of PDA decreased the incidence of PDA at discharge, but failed to decrease the incidence of BPD, BPD/death, and morbidities. Routine treatment of PDA also appeared to increase the incidence of LOS and death among infants born at >26 weeks of gestation (14). Similarly, the present study's results showed a trend toward the conservative approach in our NICUs across Turkey. In this study, although medical treatment of PDA did not show any reduction in the rates of open PDA at discharge, surgical ligation or neonatal morbidities; it was associated with increased mortality among infants born at <29 weeks of gestation. Medical treatment was preferred in more severe cases in which more mature preterm infants were receiving respiratory support by clinicians. However, subgroup analysis in infants born at <27 weeks of gestation showed that conservative management was not inferior to medical treatment in patients with similar characteristics.

The role played by prolonged PDA exposure in the development of morbidities remains unclear. Studies that compared infants who received indomethacin within the first 3 days of life to infants who received indomethacin only if PDA persisted beyond 7 days with specific rescue criteria showed that infants who received early treatment required less ventilatory and inotropic support and experienced a lower rate of BPD and BPD/death (27–29). Jensen et al. reported that prophylactic-used indomethacin reduced the rates of BPD and BPD/death (30). These studies enrolled and treated infants whose PDA may have been spontaneously closed at the end of the first week. A recent PDA-TOLERATE trial showed that no effect was had on the incidence of BPD if either routine treatment of moderate-to-large PDA was given after the first week or if no treatment was given until severe respiratory or hemodynamic symptoms developed (14). Clyman et al. showed that a significant increase in the incidence of BPD/death required at least 7–13 days of untreated moderate-to-large PDA in infants born at <28 weeks; additional exposure did not add an increase to the incidence of BPD/death (31). In the present cohort study of infants born before 29 weeks of gestation, it was found that early treatment before 7 days of life was associated with higher mortality and BPD/death. Treatment at or after 7 days was not associated with an increase in the risk of incidences of any morbidities. Long-term recent studies demonstrated that a conservative approach, even in the case of prolonged PDA, did not increase the risk of neurodevelopmental impairment (13, 32).

The pharmacological agents used to close the DA are prostaglandin synthase inhibitors such as indomethacin and ibuprofen, or a cyclooxygenase inhibitor like acetaminophen (1, 33–35). Meta-analyses on the efficacy of ibuprofen and indomethacin showed no difference in effectiveness; although ibuprofen can have less intestinal and renal side effects (11). Another meta-analysis that evaluated the association between placebo, indomethacin, ibuprofen, and acetaminophen on PDA closure suggested that a high dose of oral ibuprofen was associated with a higher incidence of PDA closure (36). In some randomized controlled trials, oral paracetamol was found to be as effective and safe as ibuprofen in PDA treatment (37–39). According to the Cochrane review, paracetamol was as effective as ibuprofen without showing any difference in neurodevelopmental outcomes (24). Ibuprofen was the most preferred agent followed by paracetamol (67 vs. 33%) in the present study. The choice of medical agent did not affect the incidence of LOS, BPD, ROP, IVH, surgical ligation, or death. But, unlike the other options, paracetamol was associated with higher rates of NEC, mortality and BPD/death which were not reported in previous studies (38, 39).

The present study had a few limitations. First, it was an observational study. However, to the authors' knowledge, the present report represents one of the largest multicenter studies on the outcomes of persistent PDA. Availability of data from a large national prospective cohort of preterm infants who were admitted to tertiary NICUs strengthened these results. Second, this report details the variations and trends in PDA management between NICUs. The design of the study was such that each center used their individual preferences in the decision of PDA management or treatment selection. Potential of unmeasured markers of early severity of illness and the potential for improper adjustment for each subject's observed time in the study which might be attributable to survivor treatment selection could cause bias, and this should be kept in mind when discussing the effect of treatment on the mortality. Although variable practices of PDA management among centers might have affected the natural course of PDA, this afforded the study the chance to compare the different approaches, agents used, timing of treatment, and PDA outcomes. The authors believe that the results of this large clinical database will lead to further studies to improve uniform guidance for the management of PDA.

CONCLUSION

This study provides a summary of the current state of practice for moderate-to-large PDAs in our country, and we think that it will be an important addition to the literature by reporting various treatment and outcome rates. While the majority of NICUs still prefer early symptomatic treatment for moderate-to-large PDA at postnatal 3–5 days of life, there has been a trend toward implementing conservative approaches. As a descriptive study, we observed that medical treatment did not change the incidences of open PDA at discharge, surgical ligation, and morbidities, but was shown to be associated with an increase with mortality. Early medical treatment prior to 7 days of life was not associated with a reduction of the incidences of surgical ligation or morbidities and was associated with higher rates of mortality and BPD/death. Although a conservative approach seems to be preferable option for infants born at <29 weeks of gestation that are suffering from moderate-to-large PDA, we still need well-designed randomized controlled trials to have a final recommendation.

ETHICS STATEMENT

The study was approved by the Online Studies Scientific Steering Committee of the Turkish Neonatal Society and by the Institutional Review Board of Ankara University. Written informed consent was obtained from the parents or guardians of the newborns.

AUTHOR CONTRIBUTIONS

EO and OE contributed substantially to article conception and design and drafted the manuscript. ZA, ND, HK, IG, SE, MC, GB, FO, HS, YC, HO, NK, BA, MT, KC, DA, AB, KT, MO, FT, and EE participated in acquisition of data. SA critically revised it. All authors gave their final approval to this manuscript and agree to be accountable for all aspects of the work, ensuring integrity and accuracy.

ACKNOWLEDGMENTS

We thank the Turkish Neonatal Society for supporting the project, all collaborator NICUs and the following investigators, as the members of the Turkish Neonatal Society INTERPDA Study Group: Begum Atasay (Ankara University School of Medicine, Ankara, Turkey), Esin Koc (Gazi University School of Medicine, Ankara, Turkey), Derya Yalinkilic (Diyarbakir Gazi Yasargil Training and Research Hospital, Diyarbakir, Turkey), Suheyla Ozkutlu (Koru Hospital, Ankara, Turkey), Sinan Uslu (University of Health Sciences, Sisli Etfal Hamidiye Training and Research Hospital, Istanbul, Turkey), Mustafa Kara (Ataturk University School of Medicine, Erzurum, Turkey), Mustafa Kir (Dokuz Eylul University School of Medicine, Izmir, Turkey), Ozmert Ozdemir (Pamukkale University School of Medicine, Denizli, Turkey), Bilge Bayraktar, Yilmaz Yozgat (Bezmialem University School of Medicine, Istanbul, Turkey), Sibel Ozumut, Sertac Aslanoglu (Medeniyet University School of Medicine, Istanbul, Turkey), Kurthan Mert, Selvi Gulasi (Adana Numune Education and Training Hospital, Adana), Oguz Tuncer (Yuzuncu Yil University School of Medicine, Van, Turkey), Sebnem Calkavur, Senem Alkan Ozdemir (University of Health Sciences, Izmir Behcet Uz Children's Hospital, Izmir, Turkey), Tolga Celik (Hacettepe University School of Medicine, Ankara, Turkey), Mahmut Mutlu, Sebnem Kader (Karadeniz Teknik University School of Medicine, Trabzon, Turkey). We would like to thank to Dr. Hatice Yagmur Zengin (Department of Biostatistics, Hacettepe University School of Medicine, Ankara, Turkey) for her assistance with the statistical analysis.

REFERENCES

1. Sankar MN, Bhombal S, Benitz WE. PDA: to treat or not to treat. *Congenital Heart Disease.* (2019) 14:46–51. doi: 10.1111/chd.12708
2. Sung SI, Chang YS, Chun JY, Yoon SA, Yoo HS, Ahn SY, et al. Mandatory closure versus nonintervention for patent ductus arteriosus in very preterm infants. *J Pediatr.* (2016) 177:66–71.e1. doi: 10.1016/j.jpeds.2016.06.046
3. Sosenko IR, Fajardo MF, Claure N, Bancalari E. Timing of patent ductus arteriosus treatment and respiratory outcome in premature infants: a double-blind randomized controlled trial. *J Pediatr.* (2012) 160:929–35. e921. doi: 10.1016/j.jpeds.2011.12.031
4. Mirea L, Sankaran K, Seshia M, Ohlsson A, Allen AC, Aziz K, et al. Canadian Neonatal Network. Treatment of patent ductus arteriosus and neonatal mortality/morbidities: adjustment for treatment selection bias. *J Pediatr.* (2012) 161:689–94 e681. doi: 10.1016/j.jpeds.2012.05.007
5. Clyman RI. The role of patent ductus arteriosus and its treatments in the development of bronchopulmonary dysplasia. *Semin Perinatol.* (2013) 37:102–7. doi: 10.1053/j.semperi.2013.01.006
6. Madan JC, Kendrick D, Hagadorn JI, Frantz ID 3rd; National Institute of Child Health and Human Development Neonatal Research Network. Patent ductus arteriosus therapy: impact on neonatal and 18-month outcome. *Pediatrics.* (2009) 123:674–81. doi: 10.1542/peds.2007-2781
7. Jansen EJS, Dijkman KP, van Lingen RA, de Vries WB, Vijlbrief DC, de Boode WP, et al. Using benchmarking to identify inter-centre differences in persistent ductus arteriosus treatment: can we improve outcome? *Cardiol Young.* (2017) 27:1488–96. doi: 10.1017/S104795111700052X
8. Edstedt Bonamy AK, Gudmundsdottir A, Maier RF, Toome L, Zeitlin J, Bonet M, et al. collaborators from the EPICE Research Group. Patent ductus arteriosus treatment in very preterm infants: a European population-based cohort study (EPICE) on variation and outcomes. *Neonatology.* (2017) 111:367–75. doi: 10.1159/000454798
9. Benitz WE. Committee on fetus and newborn, american academy of pediatrics. Patent ductus arteriosus in preterm infants. *Pediatrics.* (2016) 137:e20153730. doi: 10.1542/peds.2015-3730
10. Kort EJ. Patent ductus arteriosus in the preterm infant: an update on morbidity and mortality. *Curr Pediatr Rev.* (2016) 12:98–105. doi: 10.2174/157339631202160506001621
11. Ohlsson A, Walia R, Shah S. Ibuprofen for the treatment of patent ductus arteriosus in preterm or low birth weight (or both) infants. *Cochrane Database Syst Rev.* (2018) 9:CD003481. doi: 10.1002/14651858.CD0034 81.pub7
12. Letshwiti JB, Semberova J, Pichova K, Dempsey EM, Franklin OM, Miletin J. A conservative treatment of patent ductus arteriosus in very low birth weight infants. *Early Hum Dev.* (2017) 104:45–9. doi: 10.1016/j.earlhumdev.2016.12.008
13. Aldecoa-Bilbao V, García-Catalán MJ, Gaixa M, Clotet Caba J, Teodoro S, Figaró, et al. Neurodevelopmental impairment at two years in premature infants with prolonged patency of ductus arteriosus after a conservative approach. *Am J Perinatol.* (2019). doi: 10.1055/s-0039-1697674. [Epub ahead of print].
14. Clyman RI, Liebowitz M, Kaempf J, Erdeve O, Bulbul A, Håkansson S, et al. PDA-TOLERATE (PDA: TO LEave it alone or Respond And Treat Early) Trial Investigators. PDA-TOLERATE Trial: an-Explaratory randomized controlled trial of treatment of moderate-to-large patent ductus arteriosus at 1 week of age. *J Pediatr.* (2019) 205:41–8.e6. doi: 10.1016/j.jpeds.2018. 09.012
15. Wagner LK. Diagnosis and management of preeclampsia. *Am Fam Physician.* (2004) 15:2317–24. Available online at: www.aafp.org/afp
16. Ozkan H, Erdeve O, Kutman HGK. Turkish Neonatal Society guideline on the management of respiratory distress syndrome and surfactant treatment. *Turk Pediatri Ars.* (2018) 25:45–54. doi: 10.5152/TurkPediatriArs.2018.01806
17. Bell MJ, Ternberg JL, Feigin RD, Keating JP, Marshall R, Barton L, et al. Neonatal necrotizing enterocolitis. Therapeutic decisions based upon clinical staging. *Ann Surg.* (1978) 187:1–7. doi: 10.1097/00000658-197801000-00001
18. Papile LA, Burstein J, Burstein R. Incidence and evolution of subependymal and intraventricular hemorrhage: a study of infants with birth weights less than 1,500 gm. *J Pediatr.* (1978) 92:529–34. doi: 10.1016/s0022-3476(78)80282-0
19. International Committee for the Classification of Retinopathy of Prematurity. The international classification of retinopathy of prematurity revisited. *Arch Ophthalmol.* (2005) 123:991–999. doi: 10.1001/archopht.123.7.991
20. Jobe AH, Bancalari E. Bronchopulmonary dysplasia. *Am J Respir Crit Care Med.* (2001) 163:1723–9. doi: 10.1164/ ajrccm.163.7.2011060
21. Kahan BC. Accounting for centre-effects in multicenter trials with a binary outcome-when, why, and how? *BMC Med Res Methodol.* (2014) 14:20. doi: 10.1186/1471-2288-14-20
22. Isayama T, Mirea L, Mori R, Kusuda S, Fujimura M, Lee SK, et al. On behalf of the neonatal research network of japan and the canadian neonatal network. Patent ductus arteriosus management and outcomes in Japan and Canada: comparison of proactive and selective approaches. *Am J Perinatol.* (2015) 32:1087–94. doi: 10.1055/s-0035-1548727
23. Korea Centers for Disease Control and Prevention. *Korean Neonatal Network*

Annual Report 2017. Cheongju (Korea): Korea Centers for Disease Control and Prevention (2018).

24. Ohlsson A, Shah PS. Paracetamol (acetaminophen) for patent ductus arteriosus in preterm or low birth weight infants. *Cochrane Database Syst Rev.* (2020) 1:CD010061. doi: 10.1002/14651858.CD010061.pub4
25. Lokku A, Mirea L, Lee SK, Shah PS, on behalf of the Canadian Neonatal Network. Trends and outcomes of patent ductus arteriosus treatment in very preterm infants in Canada. *Am J Perinatol.* (2017) 34:441–50. doi: 10.1055/s-0036-1593351
26. Bixler GM, Powers GC, Clark RH, Walker WM, Tolia VN. Changes in the diagnosis and management of patent ductus arteriosus from 2006 to 2015 in United States Neonatal Intensive Care Units. *J Pediatr.* (2017) 189:105–12. doi: 10.1016/j.jpeds.2017.05.024
27. Liebowitz M, Clyman RI. Prophylactic indomethacin compared with delayed conservative management of the patent ductus arteriosus in extremely preterm infants: effects on neonatal outcomes. *J Pediatr.* (2017) 187:119–26. doi: 10.1016/j.jpeds.2017.03.021
28. Kaempf JW, Wu YX, Kaempf AJ, Kaempf AM, Wang L, Grunkemeier G. What happens when the patent ductus arteriosus is treated less aggressively in very low birth weight infants? *J Perinatol.* (2012) 32:344–8. doi: 10.1038/jp.2011.102
29. Liebowitz M, Koo J, Wickremasinghe A, Allen IE, Clyman RI. Effects of prophylactic indomethacin on vasopressor-dependent hypotension in extremely preterm infants. *J Pediatr.* (2017) 182:21–7 e2. doi: 10.1016/j.jpeds.2016.11.008
30. Jensen EA, Dysart KC, Gantz MG, Carper B, Higgins RD, Keszler M, et al. Association between use of prophylactic indomethacin and the risk for bronchopulmonary dysplasia in extremely preterm infants. *J Pediatr.* (2017) 186:34–40.e2. doi: 10.1016/j.jpeds.2017.02.003
31. Clyman RI, Hills NK, Liebowitz M, Johng S. Relationship between duration of infant exposure to a moderate-to-large patent ductus arteriosus shunt and the risk of developing bronchopulmonary dysplasia or death before 36 weeks. *Am J Perinatol.* (2020) 37:216–23. doi: 10.1055/s-0039-1697672
32. Kaga M, Sanjo M, Miura Y, Ono T. Safety of conservative approach for persistent patent ductus arteriosus in preterm infants: neurodevelopmental outcomes at 5 years of age. *Tohoku J Exp Med.* (2019) 249:155–61. doi: 10.1620/tjem.249.155
33. Liebowitz M, Kaempf J, Erdeve O, Bulbul A, Håkansson S, Lindqvist J, et al. Comparative effectiveness of drugs used to constrict the patent ductus arteriosus: a secondary analysis of the PDA-TOLERATE trial (NCT01958320). *J Perinatol.* (2019) 39:599–607. doi: 10.1038/s41372-019-0347-4
34. Oncel MY, Erdeve O. Oral medications regarding their safety and efficacy in the management of patent ductus arteriosus. *World J Clin Pediatr.* (2016) 5:75–81. doi: 10.5409/wjcp.v5.i1.75
35. Oncel MY, Erdeve O. Safety of therapeutics used in management of patent ductus arteriosus in preterm infants. *Curr Drug Saf.* (2015) 10:106–12. doi: 10.2174/1574886309999141030142847
36. Mitra S, Florez ID, Tamayo ME, Mbuagbaw L, Vanniyasingam T, Veroniki AA, et al. Association of placebo, indomethacin, ibuprofen, and acetaminophen with closure of hemodynamically significant patent ductus arteriosus in preterm infants: a systematic review and meta-analysis. *JAMA.* (2018) 319:1221–38. doi: 10.1001/jama.2018.1896
37. El-Farrash RA, El Shimy MS, El-Sakka AS, Ahmed MG, Abdel-Moez DG. Efficacy and safety of oral paracetamol versus oral ibuprofen for closure of patent ductus arteriosus in preterm infants: a randomized controlled trial. *J Matern Fetal Neonatal Med.* (2019) 32:3647–54. doi: 10.1080/14767058.2018.1470235
38. Dang D, Wang D, Zhang C, Zhou W, Zhou Q, Wu H. Comparison of oral paracetamol versus ibuprofen in premature infants with patent ductus arteriosus: a randomized controlled trial. *PLoS ONE.* (2013) 8:e77888. doi: 10.1371/journal.pone.0077888
39. Oncel MY, Yurttutan S, Erdeve O, Uras N, Altug N, Oguz SS, et al. Oral paracetamol versus oral ibuprofen in the management of patent ductus arteriosus in preterm infants: a randomized controlled trial. *J Pediatr.* (2014) 164:510–4.e1. doi: 10.1016/j.jpeds.2013.11.008

7

SIMPLE: A Novel Scoring System for Predicting Hemodynamically Significant Patent Ductus Arteriosus without Echocardiographic Evaluation in Extremely Low Birth Weight Infants

Ilker Gonen [1], Aslan Babayigit [1], Helen Bornaun [2], Beril Yasa [1], Seyma Memur [1], Seda Yilmaz Semerci [1] and Merih Cetinkaya [1]*

[1] Department of Neonatology, Kanuni Sultan Suleyman Training and Research Hospital, Health Sciences University, Istanbul, Turkey, [2] Department of Pediatric Cardiology, Kanuni Sultan Suleyman Training and Research Hospital, Health Sciences University, Istanbul, Turkey

***Correspondence:**
Merih Cetinkaya
drmerih@yahoo.com

Aim: To develop a novel clinical scoring system for predicting hemodynamically significant patent ductus arteriosus (hsPDA) in extremely low birth weight (ELBW) infants.

Methods: A prospective observational study was conducted among ELBW infants born in the study center during a 6-month period. Fourteen items were selected on a literature review basis and weighed by severity on an arbitrary 1–4 scale, the sum of which represented the Scoring preterm Infants for PDA cLinically without Echocardiographic evaluation (SIMPLE) score. The SIMPLE scores were compared at several time points during the first 3 days of life between two groups of patients: those with an hsPDA at echocardiography and those without.

Results: A total of 48 ELBW infants were enrolled, of which 30 infants developed hsPDA. The SIMPLE scores of the infants with hsPDA were significantly greater than those of the infants who did not develop hsPDA. Cut-off SIMPLE scores that were significantly associated with detection of symptomatic hsPDA at each evaluation time point were identified.

Conclusions: SIMPLE is the first scoring system that depends on the risk factors and clinical findings of ELBW infants for early prediction of hsPDA. It is simple, objective and easy to perform, and it does not require any additional tests and/or echocardiographic evaluation. We suggest that SIMPLE can be used as a screening tool for determining the need for echocardiographic evaluation in ELBW infants in order to minimize the number of unnecessary pediatric cardiology consultations.

Keywords: clinical scoring system, echocardigraphy, extremely low birth weight infants, patent ductus arteriosus, SIMPLE

INTRODUCTION

Ductus arteriosus (DA) is an anatomical channel that exists between the pulmonary artery and the aorta. DA is maintained in open conformation throughout fetal life while its persistency after birth is called patent ductus arteriosus (PDA). Although DA closes physiologically within 72 h of life in term infants, it often remains open due to several factors including immaturity, higher prostaglandin levels, respiratory distress, fluid overload, sepsis, and hypoxia in preterm infants (1–3). Spontaneous PDA closure rates for premature infants <28 weeks and/or 1,000 g was reported as 34 and 41%, on the 3rd and 7th days of life, respectively (4). Since PDA produces a left-to-right shunt, clinical findings of systemic stealing and pulmonary overflow develop after completion of the postnatal transition. Clinical findings of PDA include increased respiratory support and precordial pulses, tachycardia, hepatomegaly, accentuated femoral pulses, oliguria, and metabolic acidosis. PDA is also associated with long-term morbidities, such as bronchopulmonary dysplasia (BPD), necrotizing enterocolitis (NEC), focal intestinal perforation, intraventricular hemorrhage (IVH), retinopathy of prematurity (ROP), neurodevelopmental retardation, and death (3, 5, 6).

Although physical examination, clinical findings, and cardiac biomarkers can be used for diagnosis of PDA, echocardiography (echo) is considered the gold standard as a diagnostic tool (1). The scoring systems that have been developed for the PDA diagnosis in preterm infants depend on echo evaluation, and usually they can be used from the 2nd day of life (7–11). As physical examination needs to be performed at two different time points in one of them, this scoring system also comprises the risk of incompatible results in case two different physicians perform the physical examinations (10). Due to these limitations, the previously reported scoring systems may not be useful for the diagnosis of hemodynamically significant PDA (hsPDA) in early days of life, and therefore, are not widely practiced.

Hence, the aim of this study was to establish an easily applied scoring system that allows rapid, standard, and non-invasive evaluation of hsPDA in the early period of life, by combining both the etiology and clinical findings of prematurity without relying on echo findings in extremely low birth weight (ELBW) infants, since the echo evaluation may be challenging at any time point in many neonatal intensive care units (NICUs).

MATERIALS AND METHODS

This prospective observational study was conducted at Kanuni Sultan Suleyman Training and Research Hospital NICU between November 2019 and April 2020. ELBW infants born at the study center with a gestational age of <28 weeks and/or birth weight <1,000 g were eligible for the study. Infants with major congenital anomalies, those who died within the first 24 h of life, and whose parents did not provide signed informed consents were excluded from the study. We established a new scoring system, "SIMPLE" (Scoring preterm Infants for PDA cLinically without Echocardiographic evaluation) for prediction of hsPDA in ELBW infants. The scores were compared at several time points during the first 3 days of life between two groups of patients: those with an hsPDA at echocardiography and those without. The study was approved by the local ethical committee. The flow chart of the study has been presented in **Figure 1**.

The SIMPLE score was elaborated using 14 parameters identified on a literature review basis and weighed by severity on an arbitrary 1–4 scale. These items, which represent established risk factors for PDA, include maternal chorioamnionitis, antenatal steroids, birth weight, cord blood gas, hypotension requiring inotropic support, heart rate, invasive mechanical ventilation (MV) requirement, metabolic acidosis, respiratory acidosis, maximum peak inspiratory pressure (PIP), reduction of PIP, fraction of inspired oxygen (FiO_2) upon admission, FiO_2 decrease over evaluation time points, and surfactant requirement (12, 13). Our team weighted the scores of SIMPLE criteria according to the previously defined PDA risk factors and also their prior subjective clinical experience as our NICU is a tertiary reference center caring for ~70 ELBW infants per year, and some risk factors have already been identified for hsPDA in routine clinical follow-up of these infants. Clinical chorioamnionitis was defined as the presence of fever, uterine fundal tenderness, maternal tachycardia (>100/min), fetal tachycardia (>160/min), and purulent or foul amniotic fluid (14). All these parameters were scored between 0 and 3 points as shown in **Table 1**, and the maximum score is 29. The scores for all patients were recorded at postnatal 6, 12, 18, 24, 48, and at 72 h of life.

The antenatal characteristics of infants, presence of maternal chorioamnionitis, neonatal demographical data, cord blood gas analyses, clinical findings, and neonatal morbidities including neonatal sepsis, NEC, IVH, ROP, BPD, and mortality were all recorded.

Gestational age of the infants was determined according to the last menstrual period of the mother and antenatal ultrasonographic evaluation. Turkish Neonatology Society (TNS) guideline was used for the diagnosis and treatment of respiratory distress syndrome (RDS) (15). BPD was determined according to 2001 National Institute of Child Health and Human Development (NICHD) consensus statement as requirement for supplemental oxygen for the first 28 days of life and was classified into three groups in terms of BPD severity (mild, moderate, and severe), depending on the duration and level of supplemental oxygen and mechanical ventilatory support at 36-week postmenstrual age (16). NEC was diagnosed considering clinical and radiographic findings and was classified according to the modified Bell's criteria (17). The Volpe classification was used for the IVH staging (18). ROP was classified according to The International Classification of Retinopathy of Prematurity (19). Neonatal sepsis was diagnosed according to the criteria of TNS neonatal infection diagnosis and treatment guideline (20).

The echocardiographic evaluations of all infants were performed at postnatal 24, 48, and 72 h of life by the same pediatric cardiologist. The Vivid E BT12 ultrasonography device Vivid E BT12 (General Electrics, MA, US) was used for the echo evaluation. The ultrasonographical evaluation was performed as two-dimensional imaging, M-mode, color flow mapping, diastolic retrograde flow measurement, and Doppler imaging. The ratio of inner diameter of DA to infant weight and the ratio of left atrium to aorta (LA/Ao) were recorded. The

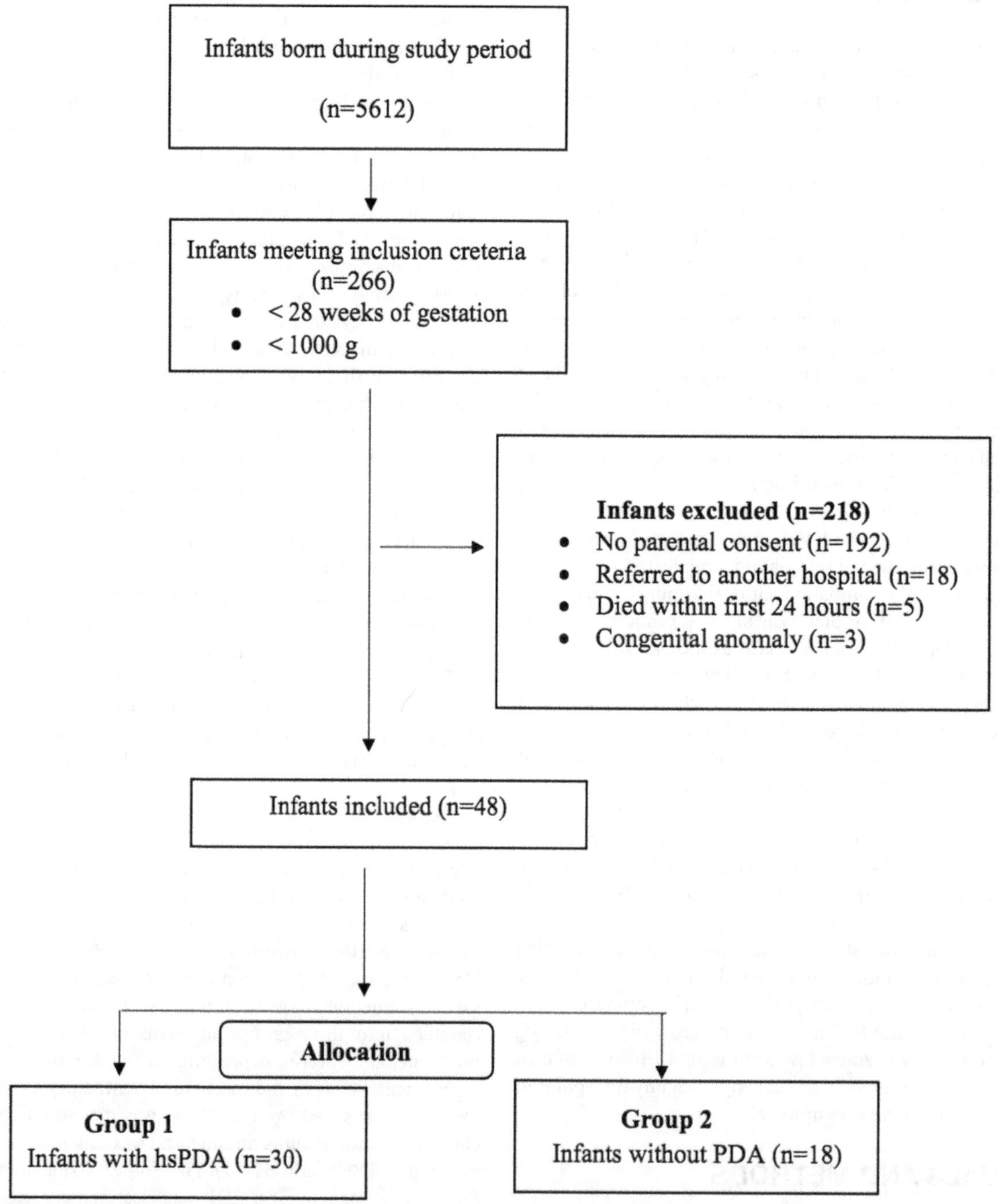

FIGURE 1 | Flow chart of the study population.

criteria for hsPDA were either being the inner diameter of DA > 1.5 mm/kg and/or LA/Ao > 1.5 according to the TNS PDA guideline in preterm infants (21). A medical PDA closure treatment was initiated for infants with hsPDA who had accompanying symptoms including respiratory compromise (requiring persistent mechanical support, increased ventilatory support, and increased oxygen demand), heart failure, metabolic acidosis or large left-to-right ductus shunt with evidence of hemodynamic compromise, such as reversal of flow in the descending aorta during diastole, oliguria or rising serum creatinine concentration, hypotension, or widened pulse pressure (1). Either ibuprofen or paracetamol was given according to clinical findings of the infants and laboratory data. Ibuprofen was used for three consecutive days at a dose of 10 mg/kg/day on the 1st day, 5 mg/kg/day on the 2nd day, and 5 mg/kg/day on the 3rd day (21). The paracetamol treatment was administered

TABLE 1 | Criteria of SIMPLE scoring system.

	0	1	2	3
Presence of maternal chorioamnionitis	No	Yes		
Completed cure of antenatal steroid	Yes	No		
Birth weight, (g)	>1,250	1,000–1,250	750–1,000	<750
Cord blood gas base deficit (mmol/L)	< −12	−12 to −16	> −16	
*Presence of hypotension requiring inotropic support	No	Yes		
*Presence of tachycardia (beat/min)	<160	160–180	>180	
*Need of invasive MV	no	yes		HFOV
*#Presence of metabolic acidosis	pH: >7.35	7.25–7.35	7.10–7.25	<7.1
	BD: < −4	−4 to −10	−10 to −16	< −16
*Presence of respiratory acidosis (PCO_2, mmHg)	35–45	45–55	55–65	>65
*Maximum PIP (cmH_2O)	<18	18–23	>23	
PIP reduction % according to prior assessment	>20%	%10–20	<10%	
FiO_2 at admission (%)	<40	40–60	>60	
FiO_2 reduction % according to prior assessment	>20%	10%–20%	<10%	
Number of surfactant administered	0	1	>1	

*During evaluation episode.
#The highest score will be given according to pH or BD.
BD, base deficit; HFOV, high frequency oscillatory ventilation; MV, mechanical ventilation; PIP, peak inspiratory pressure.

for three consecutive days at a dose of 15 mg/kg q6h in the presence of contraindications for ibuprofen therapy, such as thrombocytopenia (<60.000/mm^3), active bleeding (IVH and gastrointestinal hemorrhage), acute renal failure, or NEC (21).

Statistical analysis was performed by IBM SPSS 22.0 (IBM SPSS for Windows version 22, Armonk, NY, USA). Absolute and relative frequencies were determined for nominal scaled parameters. The consistency of continuous variables to normal distribution was tested using the Shapiro–Wilk test. Descriptive statistics are given as median (range) for continuous variables and *n* (%) for categorical variables. The Mann–Whitney *U*, Pearson's chi-square, and Fisher exact tests were used for appropriate comparisons between groups. To compare the quality of combinations of specific features, receiver operating characteristic (ROC) curves were used to determine the sensitivity and specificity by calculating the area under the curve (depending on the specified cut-off value). The ROC analysis was performed using the MedCalc for Windows, version 19.4 (MedCalc Software, Ostend, Belgium). The ROC curves, cut-off points, and area under curve (AUC) were all compared with each other using the MedCalc statistical software (Ostend, Belgium). A $p < 0.05$ was considered statistically significant.

RESULTS

A total of 48 ELBW infants were included in the study. Within the subjects, 26 (54%) were male. The median gestational age and birth weight of infants were 25 weeks and 730 g, respectively. Thirty-four (70%) infants were intubated at the time of admission to NICU, and the median duration for invasive ventilatory support and oxygen treatment were 13 and 31 days, respectively. The median length of stay at hospital was 52 days (**Table 2**).

A total of 30 (62.5%) infants required medical PDA closure treatment. The median gestational age and birth weight of the infants with hsPDA were 25 weeks and 720 g, whereas the median gestational age and birth weight of infants without PDA were 26 weeks and 760 g, respectively; the difference was not statistically significant. There were no significant differences between infants with and without hsPDA in terms of duration of MV, oxygen treatment, and hospitalization (**Table 2**). The presence of maternal chorioamnionitis, lack of antenatal steroid administration, hypotension, tachycardia, oliguria, and recurrent surfactant requirement and need of high-frequency oscillatory ventilation were all found to be higher in the hsPDA group compared to the no-PDA group (**Table 3**). Both groups were similar in terms of NEC, BPD, late sepsis, and ROP development. The IVH rate was significantly higher in the hsPDA group. A total of 16 (33%) infants died, all of whom had hsPDA (**Table 4**).

The median LA/Ao ratios of all infants were 1.57, 1.55, and 1.5 and the PDA diameter/infant weight ratios were 2.02, 1.9, and 1.9 at 24, 48, and 72 h of life, respectively. The median LA/Ao ratio was significantly higher in the PDA treatment group at 24, 48, and 72 h of life; the median PDA diameter/infant weight ratio was significantly higher in the treatment group at 48 and 72 h of life (**Table 5**).

During NICU hospitalization, 30 infants with symptomatic hsPDA (62%) required intervention. The PDA closure treatments were initiated at 24, 48, and 72 h of life in 13 (43%), 14 (47%), and 3 (10%) infants, respectively. The ibuprofen treatment was initiated in 5 (16%), infants and the paracetamol treatment was initiated in 25 (84%) infants. The Follow-up echocardiographic evaluation showed closure of PDA immediately after the first

TABLE 2 | The demographic data of all infants.

Parameters	All infants (n = 48)	Infants with hsPDA (n = 30)	Infants without PDA (n = 18)	p-value
Gender (male/female, n)	26/22	16/14	10/8	0.34
Gestational age; weeks median (range)	25 (21–29)	25 (21–29)	26 (24–29)	0.06
Birth weight; grams median (range)	730 (340–995)	720 (340–990)	760 (620–995)	0.06
Duration of invasive MV; days median (range)	13 (0–69)	17 (3–69)	9 (0–62)	0.11
Duration of oxygen treatment; days median (range)	31 (2–106)	47 (9–106)	34 (2–69)	0.23
Length of stay at hospital; days median (range)	52 (3–151)	58 (3–142)	43 (34–151)	0.39

hsPDA, hemodynamic significant PDA; MV, mechanical ventilation.

TABLE 3 | Subject characteristics and SIMPLE score items.

Parameters	Infants with hsPDA (n = 30)	Infants without PDA (n = 18)	p-value
Gestational age, weeks, median (range)	25 (21–29)	26 (24–29)	0.06
Birth weight, g, median (range)	720 (340–990)	760 (620–995)	0.06
Maternal chorioamnionitis, n (%)	21 (70)	5 (28)	0.005
Lack of antenatal steroid therapy, n (%)	19 (63)	4 (22)	0.006
Hypotension requiring inotropic support, n (%)	22 (73)	2 (11)	<0.001
Tachycardia, n (%)	16 (53)	3 (17)	0.01
Oliguria, n (%)	11 (37)	1 (5.5)	0.01
Surfactant treatment, n (%)	16 (53)	6 (33)	0.14
Repeated dosage of surfactant (%)	9 (30)	0 (0)	0.001
High frequency ventilation, n (%)	9 (30)	1 (5)	0.003
Cord blood gas deficit ≥ -12 mmol/L, n (%)	7 (14.6)	4 (8.3)	0.92
Need of invasive ventilation, n (%)	26 (54.2)	15 (31.3)	0.75
Metabolic acidosis, pH < 7.35, BD > -4, n (%)	7 (14.6)	4 (8.3)	0.92
Respiratory acidosis, pH < 7.35, $PCO_2 > 45$ mmHg, n (%)	26 (54.2)	15 (31.3)	0.75
Maximum PIP, >18 cm H_2O, n (%)	22 (18–24)	22 (18–24)	0.62
FiO_2 at admission, >40%, n (%)	26 (54.2)	15 (31.3)	0.75

TABLE 4 | Mortality and co-morbidities between study groups.

Parameters	Infants with hsPDA (n = 30)	Infants without PDA (n = 18)	p-value
IVH ≥ Grade 3, 3rd day, n (%)	15 (50)	1 (6)	<0.001
IVH ≥ Grade 3, 7th day, n (%)	17 (57)	1 (6)	<0.001
NEC ≥ stage II, n (%)	7 (23)	2 (11)	0.31
BPD (moderate-severe), n (%)	12 (40)	7 (39)	0.53
Late sepsis, n (%)	12 (40)	12 (67)	0.08
ROP, n (%)	19 (63)	13 (72)	0.26
Mortality, n (%)	16 (53)	0	<0.001

BPD, bronchopulmonary dysplasia; IVH, intraventricular hemorrhage; NEC, necrotizing enterocolitis; ROP, retinopathy of prematurity.

TABLE 5 | Echocardiography indices of the study population.

Parameters	Infants with hsPDA (n = 30)	Infants without PDA (n = 18)	p-value
La/Ao ratio, day 1 median (range)	1.7 (1.2–2.8)	1.3 (1–2.3)	0.009
La/Ao ratio, day 2 median (range)	1.6 (1.3–3.4)	1.2 (0.9–1.8)	<0.001
La/Ao ratio, day 3 median (range)	1.6 (1.2–2.9)	1.2(0.9–1.5)	<0.001
PDA diameter/weight, day 1 median (range)	2.1 (1.1–3.7)	1.9 (1.2–2.7)	0.27
PDA diameter/weight, day 2 median (range)	2.1 (1.1–3.8)	1.6 (1.3–2.3)	<0.001
PDA diameter/weight, day 3 median (range)	2.3 (0.9–3.5)	1.3 (1.1–2.1)	<0.001

La, left atrium; Ao, aorta.

dose in 26 (86%) infants, whereas 4 (14%) infants received repeated doses of the medical treatment. A surgical ligation was performed in three (10%) infants. All cases had permanent closure and no infants revealed symptoms of reopening after effective closure of PDA.

Significantly higher scores were obtained by using SIMPLE in infants with hsPDA compared with those without PDA ($p < 0.05$) (**Table 6**). Hypotension, tachycardia, oliguria, surfactant administration, and high frequency ventilation were significantly higher in the hsPDA group. The SIMPLE scores were similar between two groups of infants who had either medical or surgical

TABLE 6 | SIMPLE scores in infants with/without hemodynamically significant patent ductus arteriosus (hsPDA) by echocardiography.

Evaluation time	SIMPLE scores in infants with hsPDA ($n = 30$) median (range)	SIMPLE scores in infants without PDA ($n = 18$) median (range)	p-value
6 h	12 (5–19)	4 (2–18)	<0.001
12 h	13 (5–20)	4 (2–13)	0.001
18 h	13 (5–22)	4 (2–14)	<0.001
24 h	14 (5–19)	4 (2–14)	<0.001
48 h	15 (10–23)	4 (2–13)	<0.001
72 h	14 (9–21)	4 (2–12)	<0.001

closure. The ROC statistics demonstrated a high sensitivity and specificity of the SIMPLE scores, which did not significantly differ between different time points from 6 to 72 h. The cut-off SIMPLE scores that were found to be statistically significant for the detection of symptomatic hsPDA for each time were identified (**Table 7**, **Figure 2**). However, AUC for established cut-off values did not statistically differ between different time points (data not shown).

DISCUSSION

The utility of a novel scoring system that can be easily applied during the first 3 days of life for prediction of hsPDA in ELBW preterm infants was investigated in this prospective study. The main advantage of SIMPLE consists of the fact that it does not require any echo evaluation. The scoring systems consists of 14 parameters that are related with several risk factors associated with the hsPDA development. SIMPLE was found to predict hsPDA requiring medical intervention from 6 h of life with high specificity and sensitivity. It may also be used as a screening tool to establish the requirement for echo and may prevent unnecessary echo evaluation in NICUs.

The main antenatal risk factors for PDA include maternal chorioamnionitis, maternal pregnancy-induced hypertension, and lack of antenatal steroid administration (1–3, 22). Maternal chorioamnionitis was shown to increase the risk of PDA by 1.43 times (12). Similarly, maternal chorioamnionitis was significantly higher in the hsPDA group in our study. Therefore, chorioamnionitis may be suggested as an important criterion of SIMPLE for early prediction of hsPDA in the ELBW infants. Antenatal steroids had an impact on the incidence of PDA in infants ≤34 weeks of gestational age, whereas its effect in the smallest infants are still conflicting (23). The antenatal steroid treatment reduced the risk of symptomatic PDA (22). Therefore, the antenatal steroid administration status was also included to SIMPLE. As 83% of infants with hsPDA had not received antenatal steroids, we suggest that the lack of antenatal steroid administration is an important risk factor for hsPDA in the ELBW infants. In addition, the requirement of the PDA treatment was significantly lower in infants born to mothers without chorioamnionitis (24). All these data may support the idea of implementation of two important antenatal risk factors in SIMPLE. Also, postnatal risk factors, including prematurity, low birth weight, and gender, were all suggested to be important for the development of PDA in neonates (25). Perinatal asphyxia, respiratory distress, surfactant usage, fluid overload, and sepsis represent common postnatal risk factors of PDA (1–3, 22). The incidence of PDA increases as the gestational age decreases, and 60–70% of infants <28 weeks of gestation receive medical or surgical closure treatment (26). Consistent with the literature, PDA was diagnosed in 95, 93, and 85% of ELBW infants at 24, 48, and 72 h of life, respectively (27). In addition, surfactant use and need for re-dosing were also strongly associated with hsPDA, as previously published (28). Therefore, SIMPLE was found to predictive of hsPDA by including both antenatal and postnatal risk factors.

The most common findings of PDA include widened pulse pressure, systolic murmur, tachycardia, hypotension, pulmonary edema, increased mechanical ventilatory and/or oxygen support, pulmonary hemorrhage, metabolic acidosis, oliguria, and feeding intolerance (5, 10, 25). Similarly, hypotension, tachycardia, oliguria, and requirement of high frequency ventilation were significantly higher in the hsPDA group in our study. Therefore, we suggest that SIMPLE, including common PDA findings in postnatal period, may be used to determine hsPDA. The evaluation of clinical findings objectively from the 1st h of life in a non-invasive manner may offer an important advantage for SIMPLE for early prediction of hsPDA in ELBW infants.

Echocardiography represents the most widespread diagnostic technique, allowing for measurement valuation of the PDA diameter and Doppler flow direction (29). Early ductal diameter of >1.5 mm/kg was found to predict symptomatic PDA with high sensitivity (30). Since significant shunt through PDA may remain clinically "silent" in the 1st days and the development of echocardiographic signs of hsPDA may precede the development of clinical signs by a mean of 2 days, an early selective PDA screening by echo has been recommended in ELBW infants (21, 31, 32). The early echo screening was also shown to be associated with lower in-hospital mortality and likelihood of pulmonary hemorrhage in ELBW infants (33). Therefore, all infants were screened daily with echo in the first 3 days of life in our study to evaluate the efficacy of SIMPLE. However, it may not always be possible to perform echo in every NICU. In contrast to the previous PDA scoring systems, we did not include echo findings in SIMPLE for the purpose of providing an echo -independent scoring system. As minimal handling and maximal comfort are important for the quality of ELBW care, we sought to keep the infants warm, stable, and free from infection by identifying those with hsPDA while avoiding unnecessary, repeated echo examinations (34). In addition, although ELBW infants usually require serial echo evaluation, the number of pediatric cardiologists are not enough to perform all of them at every time point in most of NICUs (35). The SIMPLE scores of infants with hsPDA were higher at all time points. In addition, ELBW infants who received the PDA treatment had also significantly higher SIMPLE scores. Therefore, we suggest that SIMPLE may be used as a time- and cost-effective screening

TABLE 7 | Receiver operating characteristics (ROC) curve statistics for SIMPLE scores at various time points 6–72 h.

Time point	Sensitivity (95% CI)	Specificity (95% CI)	Area under curve (AUC)	Cut-off value	*p*-value*
6 h	92.00 (73.5–98.7)	85.00 (67.7–92.6)	0.926	>8.5	<0.001
12 h	90.00 (73.5–97.9)	94.44 (72.7–99.9)	0.956	>8	<0.001
18 h	93.33 (77.9–99.2)	94.44 (72.7–99.9)	0.949	>8	<0.001
24 h	93.33 (77.9–99.2)	94.44 (72.7–99.9)	0.961	>8	<0.001
48 h	100.00 (88.4–100.0)	94.44 (72.7–99.9)	0.987	>6	<0.001
72 h	100.00 (88.4–100.0)	94.44 (72.7–99.9)	0.991	>6	<0.001

**Each p-value shows the statistical significance of AUC for the given time point.*

tool in ELBW infants who need echo for the confirmation of hsPDA and for the requirement of medical PDA closure. In this context, SIMPLE may prevent unnecessary echo evaluations in ELBW infants and increase the comfort of the infant. It can also guide neonatologists to predict hsPDA without echo findings and may offer an advantage to perform selective echo in ELBW infants in the presence of higher scores, especially in NICUs where it is not possible to perform echo at any time. As studies, such as PDA-Tolerate and INTERPDA which evaluated conservative management in PDA, suggested a new approach for the late echocardiographic evaluation, further randomized controlled studies are required to determine the ideal time of echo screening in ELBW infants (36, 37).

Patent ductus arteriosus is known to be associated with important neonatal morbidities (9, 10). The potential consequences of hsPDA include increased risk for prolonged ventilation, BPD, NEC, IVH, pulmonary hemorrhage, and death (6). However, it is also well-known that all of these are mainly prematurity-associated late morbidities with multifactorial pathogenesis. NEC, BPD, late sepsis, and ROP rates were similar in infants with and without hsPDA in our study. This similarity therefore may suggest validation of SIMPLE for early and accurate prediction of hsPDA in ELBW infants. IVH and mortality rates were significantly higher in the PDA treatment group in this study. As PDA requiring treatment was found to be associated with a higher risk of IVH in a recent study. IVH may be a consequence of hsPDA (38). This finding is in accordance with a previous report indicating an increased risk of death by 3.4 times in the presence of PDA on the 3rd day in ELBW infants (39). In the light of these data, we suggest that hsPDA may be an important contributor for both IVH and mortality in ELBW infants, in spite of medical treatment for closure.

Several severity scores were established for the prediction of PDA depending on the echo findings and seem to be more subjective and usually applied after 2 days of life (7–11, 40). One of them, mainly based on clinical parameters, such as respiratory worsening, acidosis, increased femoral pulses, and precordium pulsatility, from the 2nd to the 10th day of life, reached the highest efficacy and specificity on day 4 (10). However, as this scoring system requires two different physical examination criteria, scoring might be subjective in case two

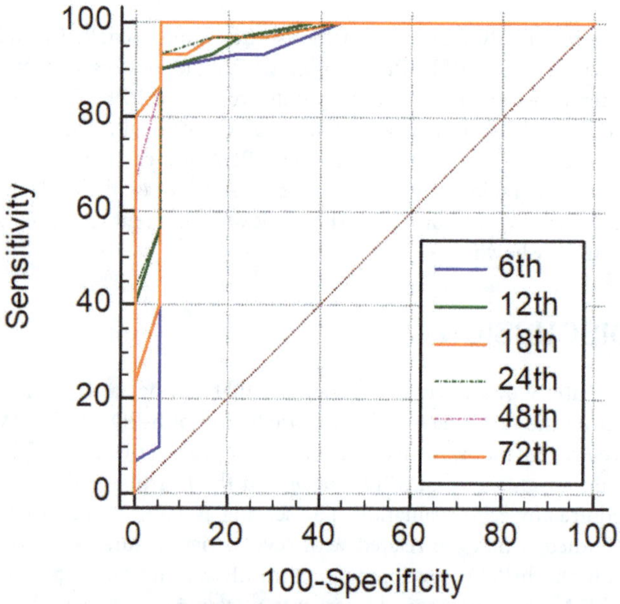

FIGURE 2 | Receiver operating characteristics (ROC) analyses of SIMPLE scoring system at each time point.

different physicians perform physical examinations. Also, the administration of the scoring from the 2nd day of life might be associated with failure of early prediction of PDA. Another PDA scoring system included findings, such as heart rate, murmur, peripheral pulses, precordial pulsation, and cardiothoracic index. However, it is applied initially on the 4th day of life, and it has also to be confirmed with echo (7). The main advantage of SIMPLE was to be performed by objective evaluation of 14 clinical parameters without any dependence of echo compared with the previous scoring systems. SIMPLE scores from 6th h of life at each time point were all higher in infants with hsPDA who required medical intervention. In addition, cut-off scores at each time points for the detection of hsPDA requiring the PDA closure treatment were also established. In SIMPLE, echo might be used for the confirmation of hsPDA diagnosis. As a result, we suggest to use SIMPLE to predict infants who may develop hsPDA from early hours of life and perform the echo evaluation in a more targeted and selective way to confirm PDA diagnosis. This strategy has the potential to decrease unnecessary echo evaluation and maximize the comfort of the ELBW infant. The physician who follows-up the high risk infants for findings of hsPDA may be able to start PDA closure treatment in the most appropriate time period. In addition, in NICUs with limited ability to perform echo at any time, SIMPLE may suggest the neonatologist to identify the ELBW infants for hsPDA and consult with a pediatric cardiologist on the most suitable time period and/or make decision for the medical closure of PDA. However, SIMPLE scores could not predict the response to the PDA closure treatment as they were similar in both medical closure and surgical ligation groups. This may be associated with small number of infants who required surgical ligation.

On the other hand, the present study is limited with the low number of infants enrolled, the single NICU involved in the study and evaluation of the efficacy of SIMPLE only by identification of high-risk infants. We believe that the efficacy of SIMPLE for prediction of long-term outcomes and PDA-associated morbidities, such as NEC, IVH, ROP, and mortality, should also be investigated. Therefore, we aim to evaluate the efficacy of SIMPLE for early prediction of PDA, morbidities associated with PDA, and also mortality in ELBW infants in a larger multicentered prospective observational study. Another limitation of this study is that the incidence of PDA and several comorbidities are higher than in other Western cohorts and registries such as Vermont Oxford Network or NICHD. This is likely to be related to the very low prevalence of antenatal steroid treatment compared to the US (41). This may be due to the fact that our maternal population is mostly underserved, including many migrants with limited or no prenatal care. Thus, SIMPLE should be validated in other populations with standard prenatal care.

In conclusion, to the best of our knowledge, SIMPLE is the first scoring system that relies only on risk factors and clinical findings for the early prediction of hsPDA in ELBW infants. It is simple, objective, and easy to perform. It does not require any additional tests and/or echo during the evaluation. Therefore, we suggest that it can be used as a screening tool for the identification of ELBW infants for their requirement for the echo evaluation. In addition, SIMPLE will probably minimize the unnecessary pediatric cardiology consultations and/or echo evaluation in NICUs with limited sources. It may also lead to early diagnosis and treatment of hsPDA in ELBW infants as it can be performed within the first 24 h of life. However, its efficacy on both early identification of hsPDA- and PDA-associated morbidities, and also mortality should be evaluated in a multicentered prospective study including higher number of premature infants.

ETHICS STATEMENT

The studies involving human participants were reviewed and approved by Kanuni Sultan Suleyman Training and Research Hospital Local Ethical Committee. Written informed consent to participate in this study was provided by the participants' legal guardian/next of kin.

AUTHOR CONTRIBUTIONS

IG and AB conceptualized and designed the study, collected, analyzed, interpreted data, and performed the literature search. HB performed echocardiographic evaluations of infants. BY performed the literature search, carried out initial analyses, interpreted data, and helped to draft article. SM and SS performed literature search and interpreted data. MC designed the study, analyzed the data, and wrote the manuscript. All authors contributed to the article and approved the submitted version.

REFERENCES

1. Gillam-Krakauer M, Reese J. Diagnosis and management of patent ductus arteriosus. *Neoreviews.* (2018) 19:e394–402. doi: 10.1542/neo.19-7-e394
2. Seghal A, McNamara PJ. International perspective on management of a patent ductus arteriosus: Lessons learned. *Semin Fetal Neonatal Med.* (2018) 23:278–84. doi: 10.1016/j.siny.2018.03.002
3. Willis KA, Weems MF. Hemodynamically significant patent ductus arteriosus and the development of bronchopulmonary dysplasia. *Congenit Heart Dis.* (2019) 14:27–32. doi: 10.1111/chd.12691
4. De Klerk JCA, Engbergs AJB, van Beek F, Flint RB, Reiss IKM, Völler S, et al. Spontaneous closure of the ductus arteriosus in preterm infants: a systematic review. *Front Pediatr.* (2020) 8:541. doi: 10.3389/fped.2020.00541
5. Elsayed YN, Fraser D. Patent ductus arteriosus in preterm infants, part 1: understanding the pathophysiologic link between the patent ductus arteriosus and clinical complications. *Neonatal Netw.* (2017) 36:265–72. doi: 10.1891/0730-0832.36.5.265
6. Hamrick SEG, Sallmon H, Rose AT, Porras D, Shelton EL, Reese J, et al. Patent ductus arteriosus of the preterm infant. *Pediatrics.* (2020) 146:e20201209. doi: 10.1542/peds.2020-1209
7. Yeh EF, Raval D. Clinical evaluation of premature infants with patent ductus arteriosus: a scoring system with echocardiogram, acid-base, and blood gas correlations. *Crit Care Med.* (1981) 9:655–7. doi: 10.1097/00003246-198109000-00009
8. Elsayed YN, NICU Hemodynamic Group. A PDA score at 48 to 72 hours of age (Manitoba score) predicts a hemodynamically significant PDA. *Arch Dis Child.* (2012) 97:A228. doi: 10.1136/archdischild-2012-302724.0794
9. El-Khuffash A, James AT, Corcoran JD, Dicker P, Franklin O, Elsayed YN, et al. A patent ductus arteriosus severity score predicts chronic lung disease or death before discharge. *J Pediatr.* (2015) 167:1354–61. doi: 10.1016/j.jpeds.2015.09.028
10. Kindley A, Seipolt B, Heilmann A, Range U, Rudiger M, Hofmann SR. Development of a diagnostic clinical score for hemodynamically significant patent ductus arteriosus. *Front Pediatr.* (2017) 5:280. doi: 10.3389/fped.2017.00280
11. Fink D, El-Khuffash A, McNamara PJ, Nitzan I, Hammerman C. Tale of two patent ductus arteriosus severity scores: similarities and differences. *Am J Perinatol.* (2018) 35:55–8. doi: 10.1055/s-0037-1605576
12. Park HW, Choi YS, Kim KS, Kim SN. Chorioamnionitis and patent ductus arteriosus: a systematic review and meta-analysis. *PLoS ONE.* (2015) 10:e0138114. doi: 10.1371/journal.pone.0138114
13. Chen YY, Wang HP, Chang JT, Chiou YH, Huang YF, Hsieh KS. Taiwan premature infant development collaborative study group. *Pediatr Int.* (2014) 56:72–6. doi: 10.1111/ped.12199
14. Newton ER. Chorioamnionitis and intraamniotic infection. *Clin Obstet Gynecol.* (1993) 36:795. doi: 10.1097/00003081-199312000-00004
15. Ozkan H, Erdeve O, Kutman HGK. Turkish Neonatal Society guideline on the

management of respiratory distress syndrome and surfactant treatment. *Turk Pediatri Ars.* (2018) 53:S45–54. doi: 10.5152/TurkPediatriArs.2018.01806
16. Jobe AH, Bancalari E. Bronchopulmonary dysplasia. *Am J Respir Crit Care Med.* (2001) 163:1723–9. doi: 10.1164/ajrccm.163.7.2011060
17. Walsh MC, Kliegman RM. Necrotizing enterocolitis: treatment based onstaging criteria. *Pediatr Clin North Am.* (1986) 33:179–201. doi: 10.1016/S0031-3955(16)34975-6
18. Volpe JJ. Intracranial hemorrhage: germinal matrix-intraventricular hemorrhage of the premature infant. In: Volpe JJ, editor. *Neurology of the newborn. 5th edition.* Philadelphia, PA: Elsevier (2008). p. 517–88. doi: 10.1016/B978-1-4160-3995-2.10011-1
19. International Committee for the Classification of Retinopathy of Prematurity. The international classification of retinopathy of prematurity revisited. *Arch Opthalmol.* (2005) 123:991–9. doi: 10.1001/archopht.123.7.991
20. Satar M, Arisoy AE, Celik IH. Turkish Neonatal Society guideline on neonatal infections-diagnosis and treatment. *Turk Pediatri Ars.* (2018) 53:S88–100. doi: 10.5152/TurkPediatriArs.2018.01809
21. Koksal N, Aygun C, Uras N. Turkish Neonatal Society guideline on the management of patent ductus arteriosus in preterm infants. *Turk Pediatri Ars.* (2018) 53:S76–87. doi: 10.5152/TurkPediatriArs.2018.01808
22. Lee JA, Sohn SA, Oh S, Choi BM. Perinatal risk factors of symptomatic preterm patent ductus arteriosus and secondary ligation. *Pediatr Neonatol.* (2020) 61:439–46. doi: 10.1016/j.pedneo.2020.03.016
23. Bartholomew J, Kovacs L, Papageorgiou A. Review of the antenatal and postnatal use of steroids. *Indian J Pediatr.* (2014) 81:466–72. doi: 10.1007/s12098-014-1376-9
24. Ryu YH, Oh S, Sohn J, Lee J. The associations between antenatal corticosteroids and in-hospital outcomes of preterm singleton appropriate for gestational age neonates according to the presence of maternal histologic chorioamnionitis. *Neonatology.* (2019) 116:269–375. doi: 10.1159/000502650
25. Kluckow M, Lemmers P. Hemodynamic assessment of the patent ductus arteriosus: beyond ultrasound. *Semin Fetal Neonatal Med.* (2018) 23:239–44. doi: 10.1016/j.siny.2018.04.002
26. Clyman RI. Ibuprofen and patent ductus arteriosus. *N Engl J Med.* (2000) 343:728–30. doi: 10.1056/NEJM200009073431009
27. Mitra S, Rønnestad A, Holmstrøm H. Management of patent ductus arteriosus in preterm infants- where do we stand? *Congenit Heart Dis.* (2013) 8:500–12. doi: 10.1111/chd.12143
28. Kumar A, Lakkundi A, McNamara PJ, Sehgal A. Surfactant and patent ductus arteriosus. *Indian J Pediatr.* (2010) 77:51–5. doi: 10.1007/s12098-009-0299-3
29. Singh Y, Fraisse A, Erdeve O, Atasay B. Echocardiographic diagnosis and hemodynamic evaluation of patent ductus arteriosus in extremely low gestational age newborn (ELGAN) infants. *Front Pediatr.* (2020) 8:573627. doi: 10.3389/fped.2020.573627
30. Kwinta P, Rudzinski A, Kruzcek P, Kordon Z, Pietrzyk J. Can early echocardiographic findings predict patent ductus arteriosus? *Neonatology.* (2009) 95:141–8. doi: 10.1159/000153098
31. Van Laere D, van Overmeire B, Gupta S, El-Khuffash A, Savoia M, McNamara PJ, et al. Application of neonatologist performed echocardiography in the assesment of a patent ductus arteriosus. *Pediatr Res.* (2018) 84:45–56. doi: 10.1038/s41390-018-0077-x
32. Miyata M, Toyoshima K, Yoda H, Murase M, Kawato H, Yamamoto K, et al. Extensive use of vasodilator agents and functional echocardiography to monitor extremely-low-birth-weight infants in Japan. *J Neonatal Perinatal Med.* (2016) 9:261–9. doi: 10.3233/NPM-16915113
33. Rozé JC, Cambonie G, Marchand-Martin L, Gournay V, Durrmeyer X, Durox M, et al. EPIPAGE 2 Study Group. Association between early screening for patent ductus arteriosus and in-hospital mortality among extremely preterm infants. *JAMA.* (2015) 313:2441–8. doi: 10.1001/jama.2015.6734
34. Groves AM, Singh Y, Dempsey E, Molnar Z, Austin T, El-Khuffash A, et al. Introduction to neonatologist-performed echocardiography. *Pediatr Res.* (2018) 84(Suppl. 1):1–12. doi: 10.1038/s41390-018-0076-y
35. Katumba-Lunyenya JL. Neonatal/infant echocardiography by the non-cardiologist: a personal practice, past, present, and future. *Arch Dis Child Fetal Neonatal Ed.* (2002) 86:F55–7. doi: 10.1136/fn.86.1.F55
36. Clyman RI, Liebowitz M, Kaempf J, Erdeve O, Bulbul A, Hakansson S, et al. PDA-TOLERATE trial: an exploratory randomized controlled trial of treatment of moderate-to-large patent ductus arteriosus at 1 week of age. *J Pediatr.* (2019) 205:41–8. doi: 10.1016/j.jpeds.2018.09.012
37. Okulu E, Erdeve O, Arslan Z, Demirel N, Kaya H, Gokce IH, et al. An observational, prospective, multicenter, registry-based cohort study comparing conservative and medical management for patent ductus arteriosus. *Front Pediatr.* (2020) 8:434. doi: 10.3389/fped.2020.00434
38. Khanafer-Larocque I, Soraisham A, Stritzke A, Awad EA, Thomas S, Murthy P, et al. Intraventricular hemorrhage: risk factors and association with patent ductus arteriosus treatment in extremely preterm neonates. *Front Pediatr.* (2019) 7:408. doi: 10.3389/fped.2019.00408
39. Sellmer A, Bjerre JV, Schmidt MR, McNamara PJ, Hjortdal VE, Host B, et al. Morbidity and mortality in preterm neonates with patent ductus arteriosus on day 3. *Arch Dis Child Fetal Neonatal Ed.* (2013) 98:F505–10. doi: 10.1136/archdischild-2013-303816
40. Sehgal A, Paul E, Menahem S. Functional echocardiography in staging for ductal disease severity: role in predicting outcomes. *Eur J Pediatr.* (2013) 172:179–84. doi: 10.1007/s00431-012-1851-0
41. Stoll BJ, Hansen NI, Bell EF, Walsh MC, Carlo WA, Shankaran S. Trends in care practices, morbidity, and mortality of extremely preterm neonates, 1993-2012. *JAMA.* (2015) 314:1039–51. doi: 10.1001/jama.2015.10244

8

Related Factors of Patent Ductus Arteriosus in Preterm Infants

Chang Liu[1,2,3], *Xingwang Zhu*[1,2,3], *Dinggang Li*[1,2,3] *and Yuan Shi*[1,2,3,4*]

[1] Department of Neonatology, Children's Hospital of Chongqing Medical University, Chongqing, China, [2] National Clinical Research Center for Child Health and Disorders, Chongqing, China, [3] Ministry of Education Key Laboratory of Child Development and Disorders, Chongqing, China, [4] Chongqing Key Laboratory of Pediatrics, Chongqing, China

***Correspondence:**
Yuan Shi
shiyuan@hospital.cqmu.edu.cn

Background: Patent ductus arteriosus (PDA) is a dramatically harmful disease in the neonatal period, in particular common in preterm infants, and our study was to determine related factors of PDA in preterm infants.

Methods: A comprehensive literature review was conducted in PubMed, EMBASE, and Web of Science. The pooled odds ratio and standard mean difference were calculated to compare dichotomous and continuous variables, respectively. In addition, we also assessed the heterogeneity and publication bias and carried out sensitivity analysis for each related factor.

Results: We included 45 studies with 87,419 individuals. After the primary analysis and a series of adjustments, results showed chorioamnionitis, lower gestational age, lower birth weight, bronchopulmonary dysplasia, intraventricular hemorrhage, necrotizing enterocolitis, respiratory distress syndrome, sepsis, surfactant treatment, ventilation, and lower platelet count had a positive correlation with PDA, while small for gestational age decreased the incidence of PDA in preterm infants. Besides, premature rupture of membranes, preeclampsia, antenatal steroids, male gender, mean platelet volume, and platelet distribution width were found to have no statistically significant relationship with PDA.

Conclusion: Preterm infants with more immature characteristics generally have a higher likelihood to develop PDA. The prevention, diagnosis, and management of PDA may depend on these results, and effective measures can be taken accordingly.

Keywords: patent ductus arteriosus, preterm infants, related factors, systematic review, meta-analysis

INTRODUCTION

Ductus arteriosus (DA), an essential component of the circulatory system during fetal life, connecting the main pulmonary artery to the descending aorta, diverts ventricular output away from the lungs and toward the placenta *in utero* (1, 2). At term, the spontaneous functional closure of DA normally occurs within 24 to 48 h after delivery due to an increase in partial arterial oxygen tension and a decrease in circulating prostaglandins and prostaglandin receptors in the DA's wall.

Generated by "hypoxic zone," the DA will anatomically close within the next 2 to 3 weeks (1–4). Nevertheless, the DA sometimes fails to close, leading to a condition called patent ductus arteriosus (PDA), which affects 57 of every 100,000 full-term neonates (2). Furthermore, failure to close is strikingly more common in preterm infants (5), and it is estimated that approximately 65% of infants <28 weeks still have an unclosed DA by day 7 after birth (6).

Not only does PDA have a rather high morbidity in preterm infants, but also it has a high severity. The hemodynamic consequence of PDA is a left-to-right shunt (5), resulting in a combination of pulmonary overcirculation and reduced organ perfusion (1, 3–5), which will further entail a series of harmful clinical outcomes such as intraventricular hemorrhage (IVH), bronchopulmonary dysplasia (BPD), necrotizing enterocolitis (NEC), feeding intolerance, decreased glomerular filtration rate, and even mortality (1, 4, 5, 7–10). Therefore, PDA is one of the major causes of long hospitalization duration and poor prognosis for preterm infants and has a seriously damaging effect on the growth and development of newborns, on account of which the early diagnosis and management of PDA are definitely essential. Taking the above into consideration, identifying related factors clearly is worthy of more attention because it can provide numerous helpful insights to develop diagnosis, management, and treatment consensuses to prevent PDA for preterm infants.

A growing body of evidence from recent articles has suggested that a few variables have a causal impact on PDA, notwithstanding some of which are still controversial (11–19). Although there have been several meta-analyses endeavoring to address these conflicting disputes, unfortunately, they focus only on certain one related factor of PDA (20–23), while it is a multifactorial disease, and many factors play different roles in the pathophysiological process. Accordingly, there is an increasingly urgent need to summarize a comprehensive conclusion containing multiple related factors at the same time, and the present study aims to resolve the issue and to evaluate as many potential related factors as possible for PDA.

TABLE 1 | PubMed search strategy.

No.	Search items
#1	((((((((Factor, Risk [Title/Abstract]) OR Factors, Risk [Title/Abstract]) OR Risk Factor [Title/Abstract]) OR Factors [Title/Abstract]) OR Factor [Title/Abstract])) OR relationship [Title/Abstract])) OR "Risk Factors" [Mesh]))
#2	(((((((((((((Infants, Premature[Title/Abstract]) OR Preterm Infant[Title/Abstract]) OR Premature Infant[Title/Abstract]) OR Preterm Infants[Title/Abstract]) OR Infant, Preterm[Title/Abstract]) OR Infants, Preterm[Title/Abstract]) OR Premature Infants[Title/Abstract]) OR Neonatal Prematurity[Title/Abstract]) OR Prematurity, Neonatal[Title/Abstract])) OR "Infant, Premature"[Mesh]) OR ((((((Neonates[Title/Abstract]) OR Infants, Newborn[Title/Abstract]) OR Newborn Infant[Title/Abstract]) OR Newborn Infants[Title/Abstract]) OR Newborns[Title/Abstract]) OR Newborn[Title/Abstract]) OR Neonate[Title/Abstract])) OR "Infant, Newborn"[Mesh]))
#3	(("Ductus Arteriosus, Patent"[Mesh]) OR (((((Patency of the Ductus Arteriosus[Title/Abstract]) OR Patent Ductus Arteriosus[Title/Abstract]) OR Patent Ductus Arteriosus Familial[Title/Abstract]) OR PDA[Title/Abstract]) OR ductus arteriosus[Title/Abstract])))
#4	#1 AND #2 AND #3

PDA, patent ductus arteriosus.

METHODS

Search Strategy

We adhered to the recommendations made by the Preferred Reporting Items for Systematic Reviews and Meta-Analyses (PRISMA) guidelines (24). The study was registered in PROSPERO, number CRD42020171459. PubMed, EMBASE, and Web of Science were systematically searched until March 2020, and only those studies written in English or Chinese were included. The search strategy used in PubMed is shown in **Table 1**, and similar search strategies were also taken in EMBASE and Web of Science.

Study Selection

We included eligible studies that compared infants with PDA to infants without PDA. Articles were included if they belonged to case-control studies, cohort studies, or retrospective cohort studies. We excluded studies if they enrolled infants with gestational age (GA) ≥37 weeks or/and birth weight (BW) ≥2,500 g. Meanwhile, studies without control group data were excluded, too. Two reviewers (C.L. and X.Z.) independently assessed the titles and abstracts of studies that we found through the search strategies. Then, the full texts were retrieved, and the eligibility according to the inclusion criteria was evaluated. Any disagreement was resolved through a discussion with a third reviewer (Y.S.). The PRISMA flow diagram of the search is shown in **Figure 1**.

Data Extraction and Quality Assessment

The following information was extracted from each study: name of the first author, publication year, country/region, study type (case-control or cohort, prospective or retrospective), the number of included infants, mean BW and GA of included infants, definition of PDA, the time of PDA assessment after birth, and aim of study, which is illustrated in **Supplementary Table 1**. Then, we analyzed these related factors that were mentioned in at least three articles, and both adjusted and unadjusted results were compiled and compared if included articles could provide sufficient data.

The Newcastle–Ottawa Scale (25) was applied to observational studies to review the risk of bias. We evaluated included studies by scoring them, with a maximum of nine points, consisting of four points in selection of the study groups, two points in comparability of the groups, and three points in assessment of outcome/exposure. The detailed results are displayed in **Supplementary Table 2**.

Data Synthesis and Analysis

We combined and analyzed studies using Comprehensive Meta-Analysis v. 3.0 software. The pooled odds ratio (OR) and

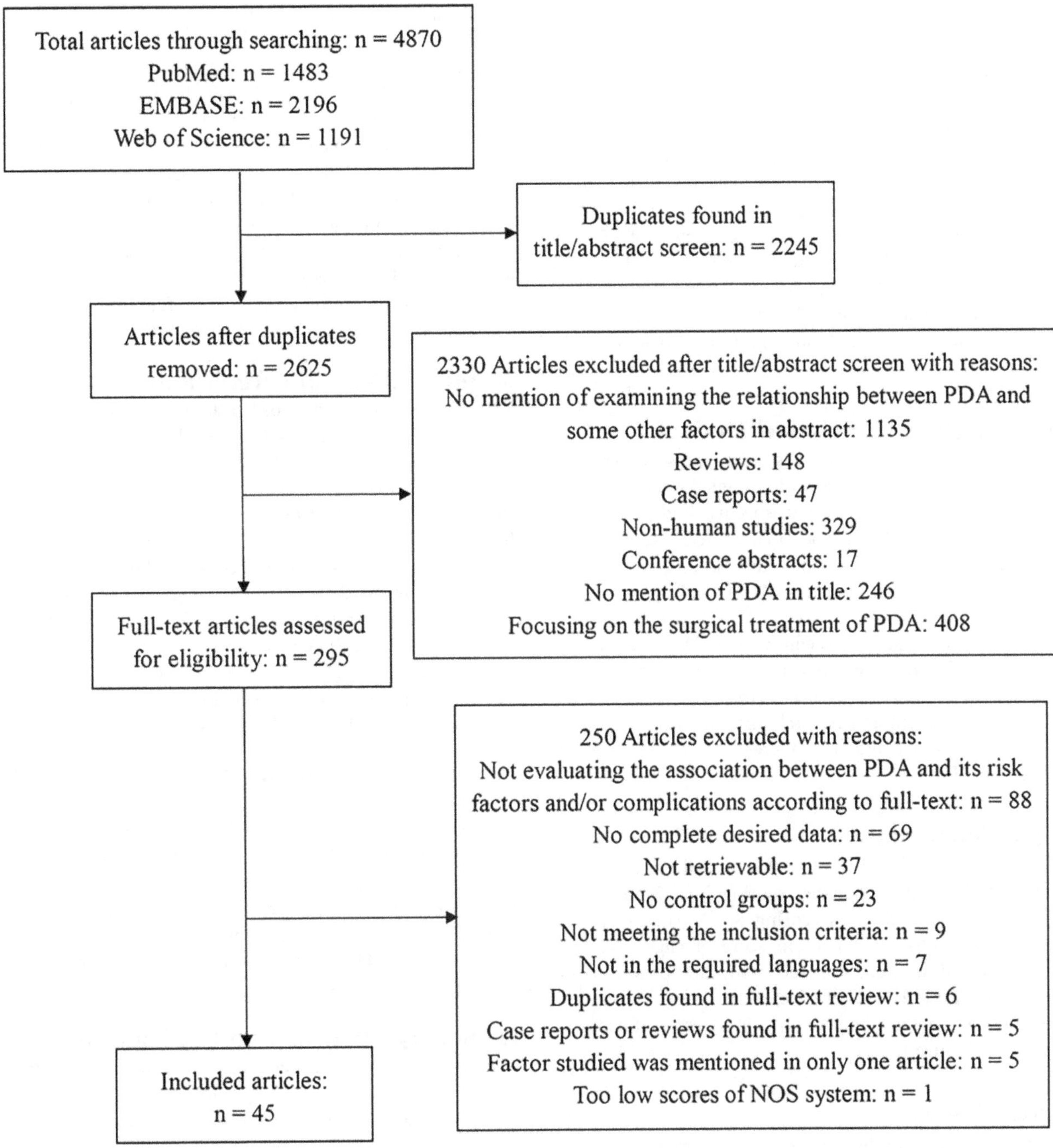

FIGURE 1 | Flow diagram describing the systematic review of related factors of patent ductus arteriosus in preterm infants.

standard mean difference (SMD) were calculated to compare dichotomous and continuous variables, respectively. The method of Wan et al. was used to estimate the mean and standard deviation when continuous variables were reported as median and range/interquartile range in studies (26). The I^2 statistic and P-value of heterogeneity test were used for testing the heterogeneity. Once there was no significant heterogeneity ($P > 0.10$, $I^2 < 50\%$), the fixed-effects model was adopted; otherwise, the random-effects model was applied. We also analyzed publication bias when more than 10 studies were available for one related factor (27). The publication bias was assessed through funnel plot and Egger's test. When $P < 0.10$ in Egger's test, we considered it had a significant publication bias and used trim-and-fill computation to adjust the result. Sensitivity analysis was performed by removing the articles one by one, then we compared the ORs (SMDs) before and after the removal. When the OR (SMD) changed significantly, we excluded that article in final analysis.

RESULTS

Literature Search

The electronic database search yielded 4,870 articles in total. After removing 2,245 duplicates, we examined 2,625 article titles and abstracts. After independent review by two reviewers, 2,330 studies were deemed not relevant to related factors of PDA in preterm infants. The full-text versions were evaluated for the remaining 295 articles, of which 250 were excluded because of various reasons. Finally, we included 45 studies, and the flow diagram summarizing the study identification and selection is shown in **Figure 1**.

Characteristics of Included Studies

The baseline characteristics of the 45 studies representing a total of 87,419 preterm infants are shown in **Supplementary Table 1**. Among the 45 studies, 25 were retrospective studies, 18 were prospective studies, and two had unclear designs. These 45 included studies comprised 34 cohort studies and 11 case-control studies. The sample sizes ranged from 31 to 43,576 participants, with mean GA ranging from 25.7 to 31.1 weeks and mean BW ranging from 761 to 1,852 g. The definitions of PDA in each study varied significantly, from hemodynamically significant PDA to echocardiogram or whether receiving treatment or not. The time of PDA assessment and research aims of each study were also markedly different and the concrete details are listed in **Supplementary Table 1**.

Quality Assessment

The methodological quality of the enrolled studies was satisfactorily high, with 13 studies scoring 9 of 9 points on the Newcastle-Ottawa Scale, 4 scoring 8, 23 scoring 7, and 5 scoring 6, which is the minimum score of eligibility, and the reasons for downgrade of each study are presented in **Supplementary Table 2**. However, one article was excluded because it scored only five points in quality assessment process, as described in **Figure 1**.

Maternal Factors

In the primary analysis, infants whose mothers were diagnosed with chorioamnionitis (CA) were more likely to develop PDA than those whose mothers were not diagnosed with CA [OR = 1.317, 95% confidence interval (CI) = 1.081–1.604; I^2 = 41.578%] (**Figures 2A,B**). We did not find any significant association between PDA and premature rupture of membranes (PROM) (OR = 0.757; 95% CI = 0.568–1.009; I^2 = 47.358%) (**Figure 2C**) and preeclampsia (OR = 0.890; 95% CI = 0.677–1.171; I^2 =72.730%) (**Figure 2D**). There was also no association between PDA and antenatal steroids according to both pooled unadjusted data (OR = 0.931; 95% CI = 0.822–1.054; I^2 = 36.655%) (**Figures 2E,F**) and adjusted data (OR = 0.727; 95% CI = 0.479–1.102; I^2 = 66.286%) (**Figure 2G**).

Neonatal Characteristics

We obtained an expected result that infants with lower GA (SMD = −0.698; 95% CI = −0.831 to −0.565; I^2 = 93.794 %) (**Figures 3A,B**) and lower BW (SMD = −0.528; 95% CI = −0.669 to −0.387; I^2 = 94.896 %) (**Figures 3C,D**) developed PDA more easily. The meta-analysis indicated that small for gestational age (SGA) could decrease the incidence of PDA (OR = 0.739; 95% CI = 0.591–0.923; I^2 = 85.495%) (**Figures 4A,B**). Male infants were more likely to develop PDA compared to female infants in the light of the unadjusted data (OR = 1.071; 95% CI = 1.027–1.118; I^2 = 26.025%) (**Figures 4C,D**), but pooled OR after adjustment for confounders showed no significant association between gender of infants and PDA (OR = 0.969; 95% CI = 0.763–1.232; I^2 = 0%) (**Figure 4E**).

Complications and Treatment

We found that PDA had a positive association with BPD (OR = 3.066; 95% CI = 2.471–3.804; I^2 = 0%) (**Figures 5A,B**), IVH (OR = 1.774; 95% CI = 1.494–2.108; I^2 = 0%) (**Figures 5C,D**), NEC (OR = 1.939; 95% CI = 1.343–2.801; I^2 = 0%) (**Figures 5E,F**), and sepsis (OR = 1.994; 95% CI = 1.462–2.721; I^2 = 54.919%) (**Figure 6A**). Both unadjusted (OR = 4.518; 95% CI = 3.160–6.460; I^2 = 82.053%) (**Figures 6B,C**) and adjusted (OR = 3.954; 95% CI = 2.394–6.530; I^2 = 78.081%) (**Figure 6D**) pooled data indicated that respiratory distress syndrome (RDS) was a clear risk factor of PDA. PDA was also significantly associated with surfactant treatment (OR = 4.399; 95% CI = 3.248–5.958; I^2 = 80.788%) (**Figures 7A,B**) and ventilation (OR = 3.983; 95% CI = 2.591–6.122; I^2 = 89.534%) (**Figure 7C**).

Laboratory Examination

No significant association was discovered between the PDA and mean platelet volume (MPV) (SMD = −0.144; 95% CI = −0.425, 0.136; I^2 = 89.011%) (**Figure 8A**) and platelet distribution width (PDW) (SMD = 0.060; 95% CI = −0.126 to 0.245; I^2 = 67.558%) (**Figure 8B**). Meanwhile, pooled data demonstrated that low platelet count (SMD = −0.190; 95% CI = −0.320 to −0.061; I^2 = 58.469%) (**Figure 8C**) improved the incidence of PDA among preterm infants.

Sensitivity Analysis and Publication Bias

A sensitivity analysis was performed to evaluate the robustness of the conclusions by omitting each study sequentially and comparing the effects of the eliminations of each study on the pooled ORs or SMDs. We found that the exclusion of Thompson et al. (28) obviously changed the OR and 95% CI value for male gender to 0.951 (0.883–1.024), and the difference in OR and 95% CI value after the removal was statistically substantial. Therefore, we came to a revised conclusion that the gender of preterm infants had no effect on the occurrence of PDA (OR = 0.951; 95% CI = 0.883–1.024; I^2 = 0%), and the detailed information is shown in **Supplementary Table 4**.

For every studied related factor mentioned in at least 10 articles, we not only drew a funnel plot, but also conducted Egger's test to evaluate its publication bias. If $P < 0.10$ in Egger's test, statistically significant publication bias was determined, and we carried out trim-and-fill computation to adjust the results.

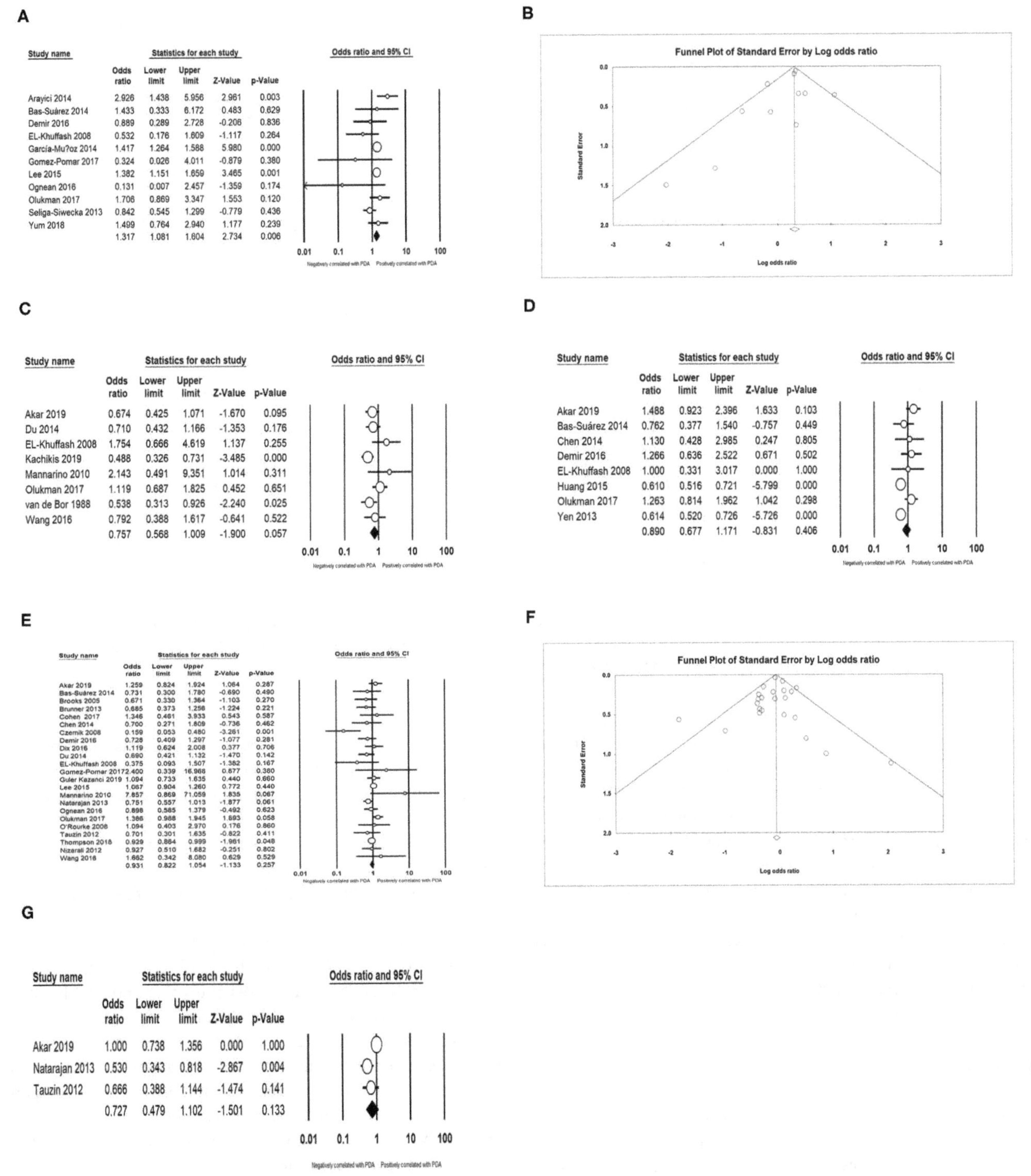

FIGURE 2 | Results of maternal factors in primary analysis. **(A)** Forest plot of association between PDA and chorioamnionitis; **(B)** funnel plot for publication bias of the association between PDA and chorioamnionitis; **(C)** forest plot of association between PDA and premature rupture of membranes; **(D)** forest plot of association between PDA and preeclampsia; **(E)** forest plot of association between PDA and antenatal steroids (according to unadjusted data); **(F)** funnel plot for publication bias of the association between PDA and antenatal steroids (according to unadjusted data); **(G)** forest plot of association between PDA and antenatal steroids (according to adjusted data). PDA, patent ductus arteriosus.

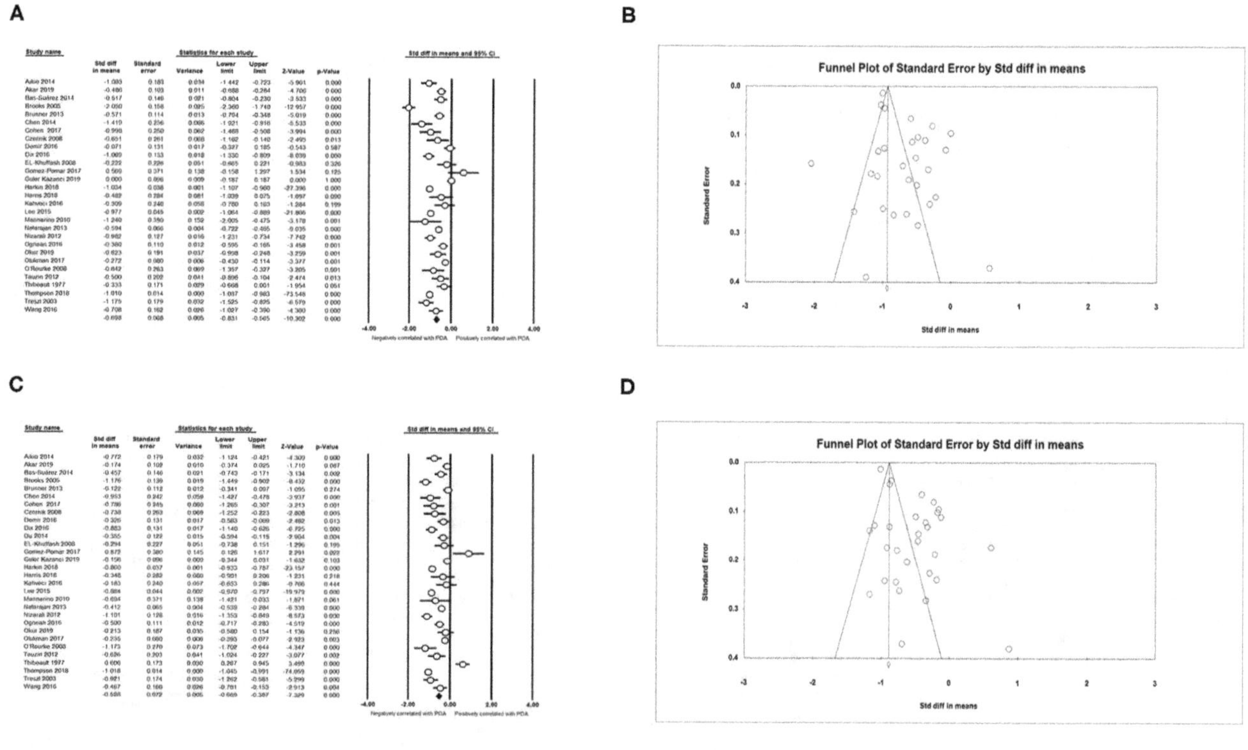

FIGURE 3 | Results of neonatal characteristics in primary analysis. **(A)** Forest plot of association between PDA and gestational age; **(B)** funnel plot for publication bias of the association between PDA and gestational age; **(C)** forest plot of association between PDA and birth weight; **(D)** funnel plot for publication bias of the association between PDA and birth weight. PDA, patent ductus arteriosus.

The results of the Egger's test suggested that the publication biases of IVH, BW, and GA were statistically significant ($P < 0.10$). However, the results of trim-and-fill computation showed that the identified biases did not interfere with interpretation of the results. The results of analysis concerning publication bias are recorded in **Supplementary Table 5**.

P-value in Egger's test of male gender was <0.10 in primary analysis. However, it turned to be non-significant after study exclusion of sensitivity analysis. Hence, we did not conduct trim-and-fill computation for male gender in the end, and we discussed the association between gender and PDA according to the results of sensitivity analysis.

DISCUSSION

It is a well-recognized fact that the incidence of PDA is inversely related to GA and BW of infants (15, 18, 29–34). The study of Koch et al. (35) showed that with each additional week of GA, the probability of spontaneous closure of the DA increased by 1.5 times. As noted above, the functional closure of DA is promoted by the increase of oxygen and the reduction of prostaglandins after birth. Nonetheless, preterm smooth muscle cells are more sensitive to circulating prostaglandins and nitric oxide, and even they can produce an increased amount of nitric oxide after birth (34, 36–39), while preterm DA's sensitivity to oxygen decreases, and preterm infants are often accompanied by hypoxemia (15, 17, 34). Besides, the term DA is more muscular and thicker-walled compared to the preterm DA, which is not sufficiently mature for the spontaneous closure after delivery (31, 38).

Our study confirms the results of prior meta-analysis (21), which supported a positive correlation between CA and PDA in preterm infants. On the one hand, CA is a definite risk factor for preterm birth (40, 41), and on the other hand, some cytokines regarding inflammatory process result in some hemodynamic changes (18, 21, 42). Interestingly, another meta-analysis on the same theme revealed that it was the confounders (differences in GA and BW) that considerably influenced the association between CA and PDA, and even CA played a protective role in the occurrence of PDA by facilitating lung maturation and diminishing the use of surfactant and mechanical ventilation (20, 43). It is a pity that the view cannot be proved in present analysis because we found only two studies showing pertinent data adjusted for confounders.

Although antenatal steroids has been reported to shield preterm infants from PDA (44) with an explanation that steroids appear to not only modify DA's sensitivity to prostaglandins, but also enhance the sensitivity of immature DA to oxygen, affect the synthesis of prostaglandins, and decrease the incidence of neonatal RDS (15, 17, 18), this affiliation was not found in this meta-analysis in accordance with both unadjusted and adjusted data. The following reasons probably can explain

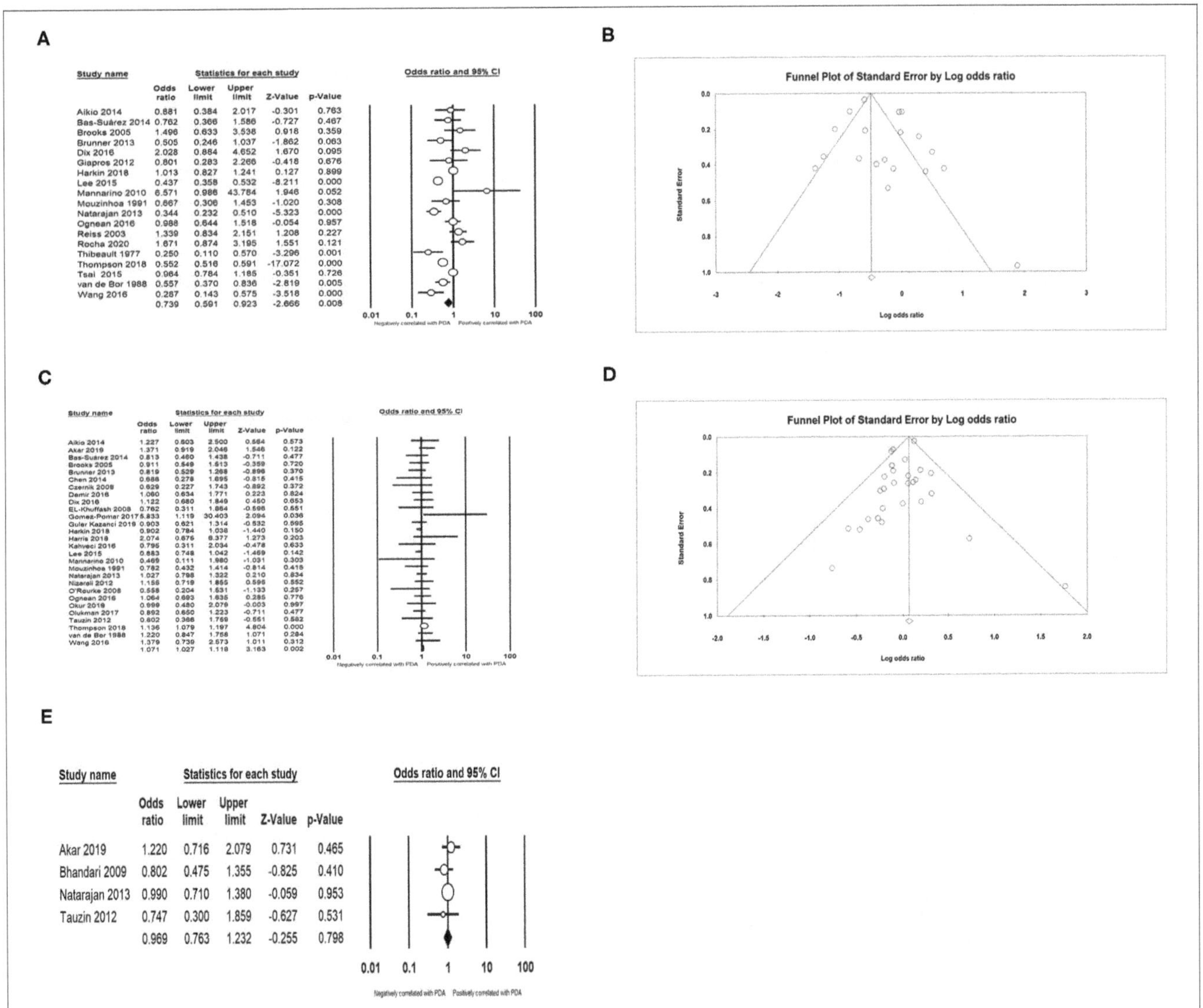

FIGURE 4 | Results of neonatal characteristics in primary analysis. **(A)** Forest plot of association between PDA and small for gestational age; **(B)** funnel plot for publication bias of the association between PDA and small for gestational age; **(C)** forest plot of association between PDA and male gender (according to unadjusted data); **(D)** funnel plot for publication bias of the association between PDA and male gender (according to unadjusted data); **(E)** forest plot of association between PDA and male gender (according to adjusted data). PDA, patent ductus arteriosus.

the surprising result. First, we did not distinguish infants with full course and partial course of treatment in the data synthesis process. Second, the number of included articles was not sufficient, and some valuable articles might be omitted, especially only three articles presenting adjusted data. Third, none of the included articles took the relationship between PDA and antenatal steroids as the main research purpose, and most of these articles had a retrospective design, which would have an impact on the results of these studies. Besides, Shelton et al. found that among infants born at <26 weeks, antenatal steroids could constrict DA apparently only when prostaglandin production had been eliminated. Although they did not observe the phenomenon among infants born at 26–28 weeks, they speculated that the effects of antenatal steroids might be different depending on the GA of infants (45).

Previous literature has indicated that PROM (46) and preeclampsia (47, 48) are predictors for preterm birth, so it seems quite reasonable that they are also risk factors for PDA. Surprisingly, our results manifest that they unexpectedly play a non-promotive role in the occurrence of PDA. In fact, the seemingly irrational results can still be interpreted by the theory that PROM (49) and preeclampsia (18) can exert maturational effects on pulmonary function, and moreover, mothers complicated by these conditions have a higher possibility to obtain more efficient management and more adequate treatment, which prolongs GA and prevents PDA after birth (50, 51).

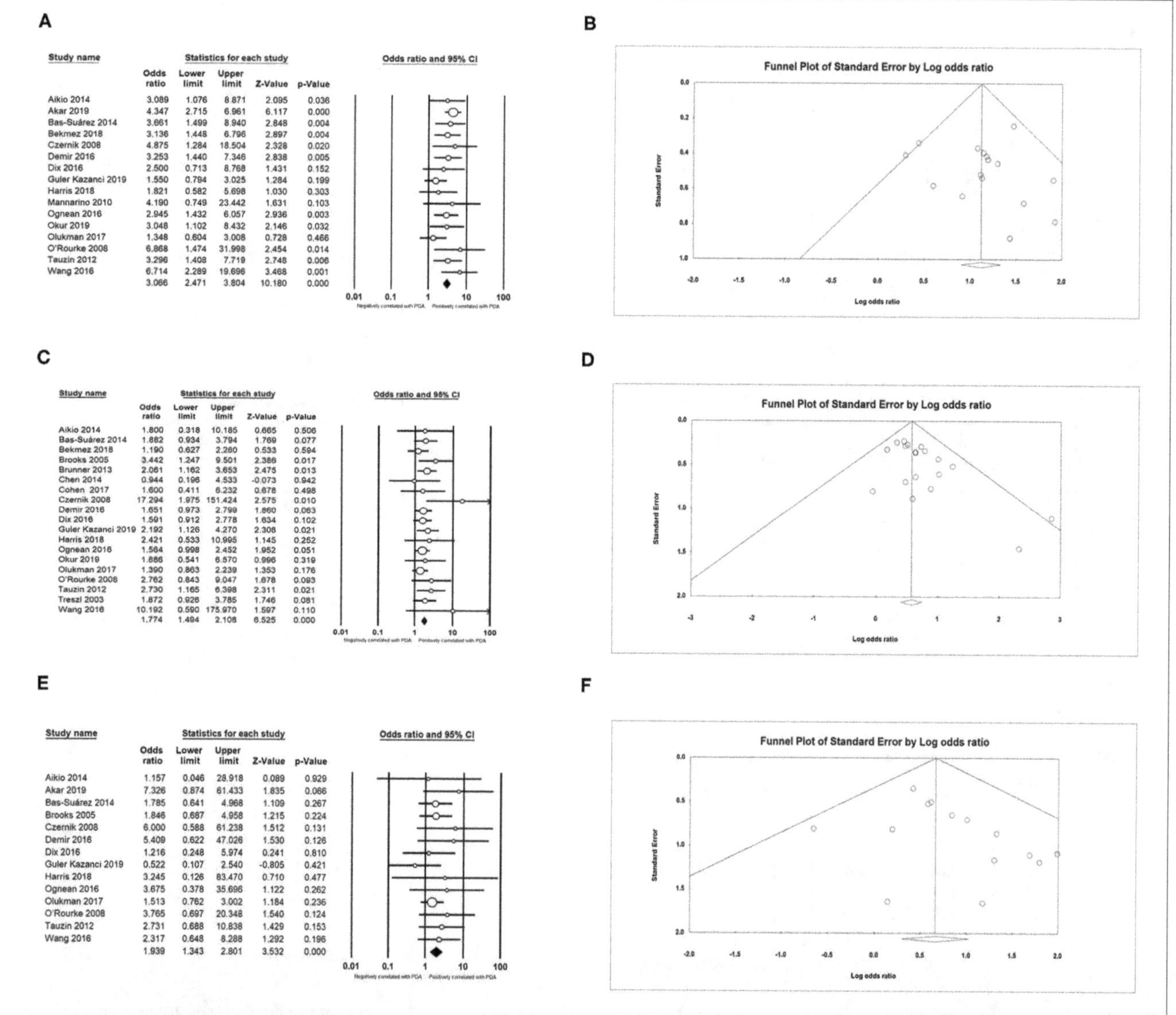

FIGURE 5 | Results of complications in primary analysis. **(A)** Forest plot of association between PDA and bronchopulmonary dysplasia; **(B)** funnel plot for publication bias of the association between PDA and bronchopulmonary dysplasia; **(C)** forest plot of association between PDA and intraventricular hemorrhage; **(D)** funnel plot for publication bias of the association between PDA and intraventricular hemorrhage; **(E)** forest plot of association between PDA and necrotizing enterocolitis; **(F)** funnel plot for publication bias of the association between PDA and necrotizing enterocolitis. PDA, patent ductus arteriosus.

Our results are compatible with the findings of Villamor-Martinez et al., who pointed out that infants diagnosed with SGA were characterized by lower risk for PDA in comparison with those in control group. In their meta-analysis, a noteworthy difference in GA owing to fewer "indicated deliveries" in SGA group than in control group was detected, which could account for the negative association between SGA and PDA (23), and Wang et al. also proposed this hypothesis (19). Hammoud et al. reported male gender was a risk factor for PDA (52). However, both pooled unadjusted results after sensitivity analysis and pooled adjusted results in our study show no association between gender and PDA.

We corroborate that infants with PDA are at a greater risk of various neonatal diseases. Left-to-right shunting across the DA results in pulmonary overcirculation and decreased systemic perfusion. "Diastolic steal" through the DA to the lungs reduces the blood supply to other organs, escalating the rate of IVH and NEC (18, 49, 53–58). The mechanism of RDS causing PDA is mainly related to hypoxemia, and pulmonary hyperperfusion resulting from PDA impairs surfactant production in the alveolar cells, which means the relationship between PDA and RDS is complex and bidirectional (15, 18, 23, 49). PDA can promote an interstitial and alveolar pulmonary edema and decreased lung compliance, and in turn, it gives rise to higher ventilator settings and prolonged ventilation duration, which has been implicated in the pathogenesis of BPD (18, 49, 54, 59–63). In recent studies, Clyman et al. found that exposure to PDA increased risk of BPD only when the infants required at least 10 days of intubation,

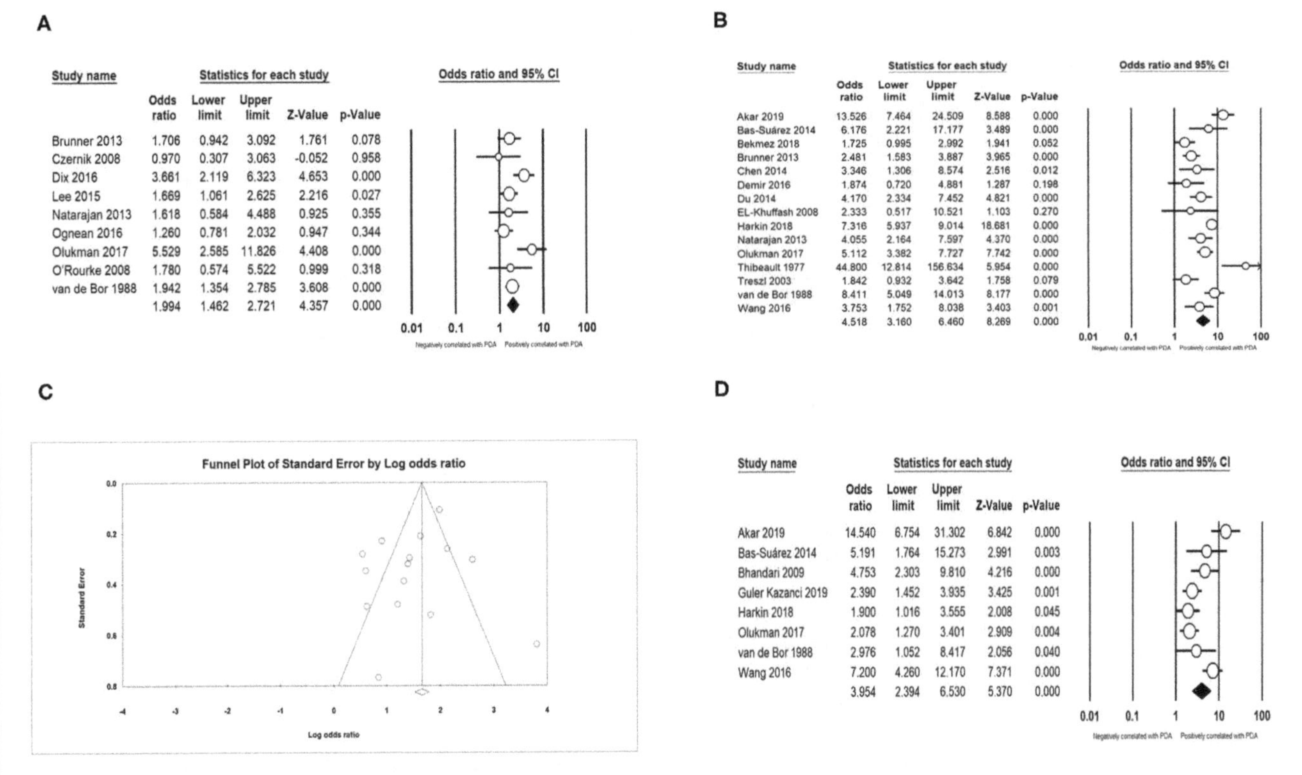

FIGURE 6 | Results of complications in primary analysis. **(A)** Forest plot of association between PDA and sepsis; **(B)** forest plot of association between PDA and respiratory distress syndrome (according to unadjusted data); **(C)** funnel plot for publication bias of the association between PDA and respiratory distress syndrome; **(D)** forest plot of association between PDA and respiratory distress syndrome. PDA, patent ductus arteriosus.

and the incidence of BPD (grades 2 and 3) was low in infants requiring less ventilatory support, regardless of whether PDA constricted or remained open for several weeks (64, 65). The positive correlation between PDA and sepsis can be attributed to elevated prostaglandins in infected infants (18, 49, 66).

Given the tight relationship between PDA and RDS, it can be readily understood that infants with PDA are more likely to receive surfactant and ventilation administration (18, 67). What's more, Nizarali et al. proposed that a significant drop in pulmonary vascular resistance after surfactant administration would cause a larger shunt through DA, indicating that the use of surfactant would aggravate PDA (17).

A number of studies have suggested the compelling relationship between low platelet count and PDA (14, 22, 68–70), and our study further substantiates these results. Echtler et al. identified that platelets were recruited to contract DA within minutes after birth, initiate thrombotic occlusion of DA, and support subsequent anatomical reorganization (68). MPV and PDW are non-significant in predicting PDA in our results despite the statement that they are markers reflecting platelet activity (33, 71).

We conducted an extra analysis focusing only on the included articles in the last 10 years because some of included articles are so outdated that they probably affect the stability of our conclusions as a consequence of the fact that there have been many changes in neonatal intensive care unit such as higher conservative management rates and promotion of advanced prevention and treatment measures of PDA in developing countries. However, the pooled results of articles in the last 10 years were not statistically different from original results for each factor except PROM, and its OR and 95% CI values changed to 0.713 (0.574–0.884), which meant PROM could decrease the risk of PDA. But this change will not contradict our previous explanation, for PROM still plays a non-promotive role in the occurrence of PDA according to the results of included articles in last 10 years.

This meta-analysis has several limitations. First, all the included articles were observational studies, and most of them had a retrospective design, which could arouse inherent bias. Second, there was a significant variability among studies with regard to the definition of PDA, baseline characteristics of neonates, and included confounders. Third, some valuable factors, such as B-type natriuretic peptide level and fluid intake, could not be analyzed in this meta-analysis because of insufficient data. Fourth, most included articles did not make a multivariate regression analysis, so for most factors, we cannot determine their independent effects for PDA.

CONCLUSION

To our best knowledge, this is the first comprehensive meta-analysis taking into account multiple related factors of PDA, and a total of 18 potential related factors were examined.

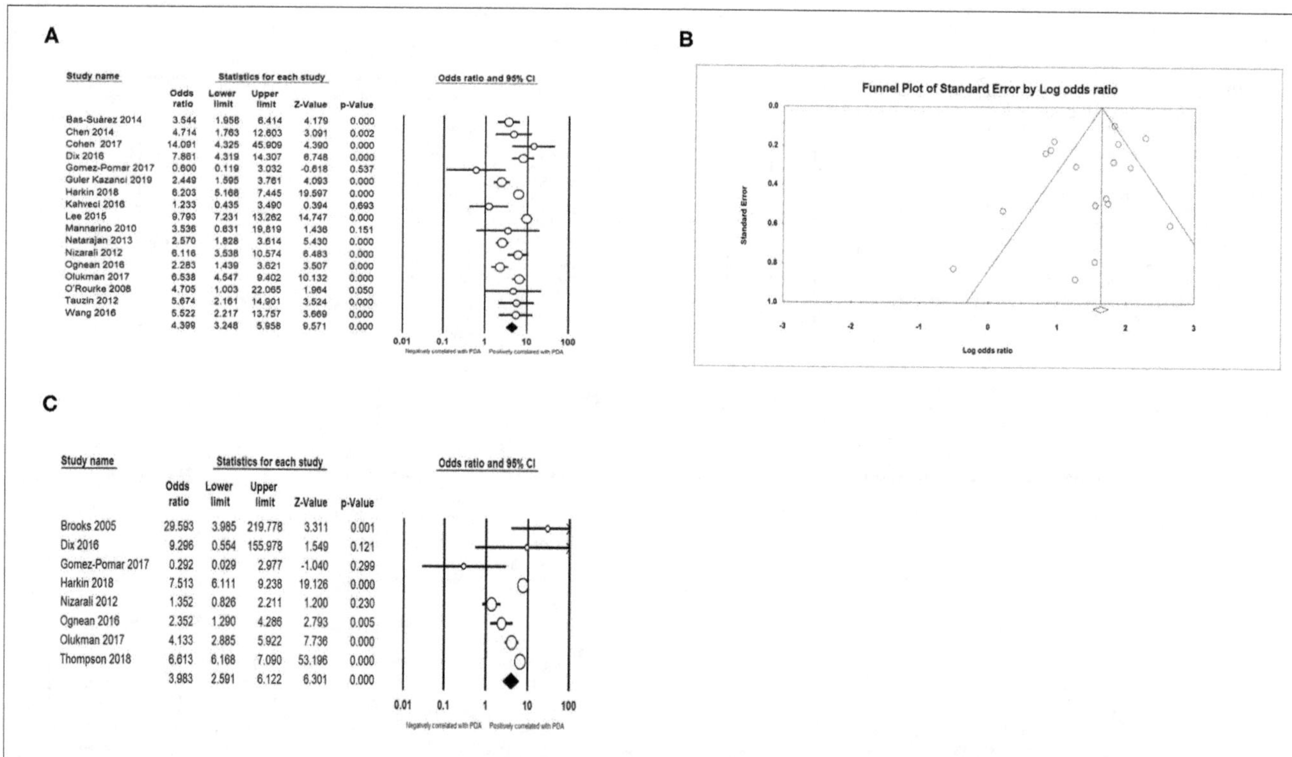

FIGURE 7 | Results of treatment in primary analysis. **(A)** Forest plot of association between PDA and surfactant treatment; **(B)** funnel plot for publication bias of the association between PDA and surfactant treatment; **(C)** forest plot of association between PDA and ventilation. PDA, patent ductus arteriosus.

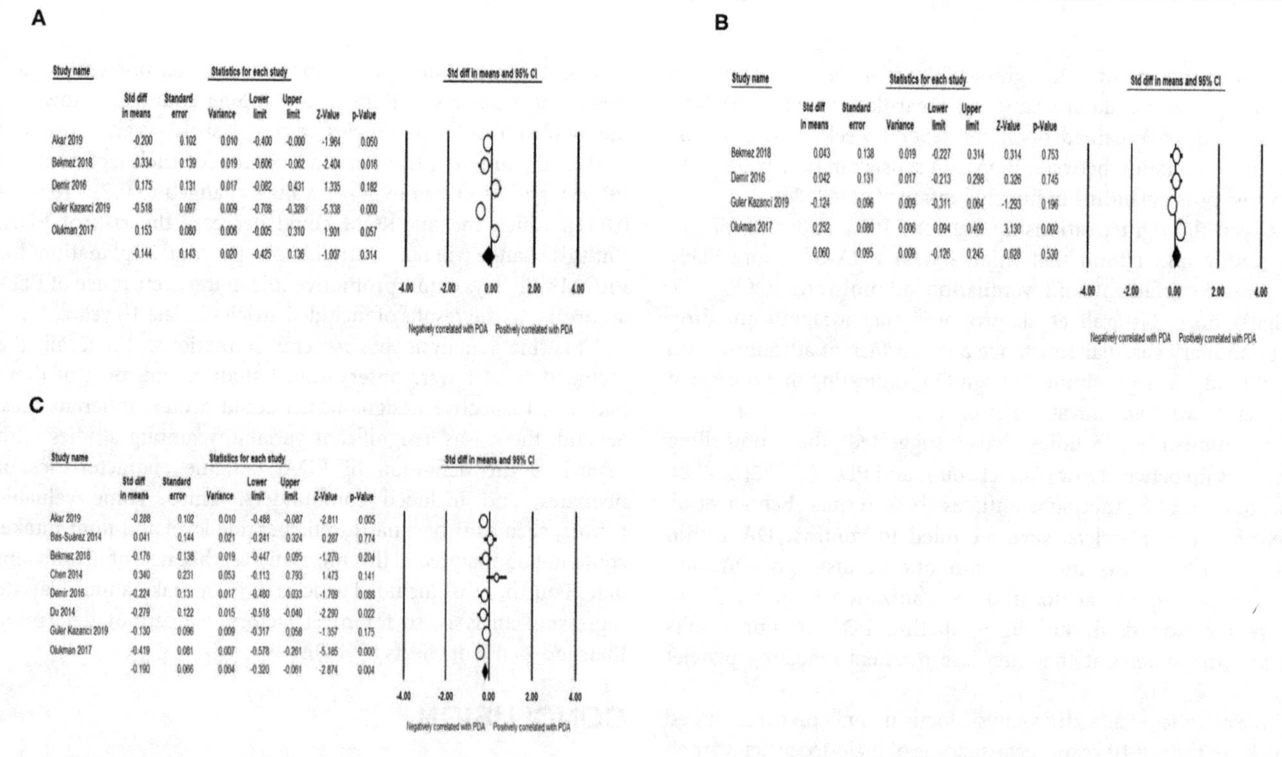

FIGURE 8 | Results of laboratory examination in primary analysis. **(A)** Forest plot of association between PDA and mean platelet volume; **(B)** forest plot of association between PDA and platelet distribution width; **(C)** forest plot of association between patent ductus arteriosus PDA and platelet count. PDA, patent ductus arteriosus.

After a series of data analysis, the final results revealed that CA, lower GA, lower BW, BPD, IVH, NEC, RDS, sepsis, surfactant treatment, ventilation, and lower platelet count were positively related to PDA, whereas SGA exerted a converse effect among preterm infants. Additionally, we also found that PROM, preeclampsia, antenatal steroids, male gender, MPV, and PDW had no statistically significant link with PDA. Our findings can be helpful to design prevention strategies and management standards for PDA. Also, future large prospective studies are strongly demanded to validate the accuracy and reliability of the conclusions.

Requests to access these datasets should be directed to Chang Liu, 1113943180@qq.com.

AUTHOR CONTRIBUTIONS

CL proposed the idea and designed the whole research plan. CL and XZ conducted the database search and extracted the data. CL and DL performed the data analysis and prepared the figures and the tables. CL wrote the manuscript. All authors reviewed the manuscript.

REFERENCES

1. Clyman RI. Ibuprofen and patent ductus arteriosus. *N Engl J Med.* (2000) 343:728–30. doi: 10.1056/NEJM200009073431009
2. Hamrick SEG, Hansmann G. Patent ductus arteriosus of the preterm infant. *Pediatrics.* (2010) 125:1020–30. doi: 10.1542/peds2009-3506
3. Schneider DJ, Moore JW. Patent ductus arteriosus. *Circulation.* (2006) 114:1873–82. doi: 10.1161/CIRCULATIONAHA.105.592063
4. Giliberti P, De Leonibus C, Giordano L, Giliberti P. The physiopathology of the patent ductus arteriosus. *J Matern-Fetal Neo Med.* (2009) 22(Suppl 3):6–9. doi: 10.1080/14767050903198215
5. Rozé J-C, Cambonie G, Marchand-Martin L, Gournay V, Durrmeyer X, Durox M, et al. Association between early screening for patent ductus arteriosus and in-hospital mortality among extremely preterm infants. *JAMA.* (2015) 313:2441–8. doi: 10.1001/jama.2015.6734
6. Benitz WE, Committee on F, Newborn AAoP. Patent ductus arteriosus in preterm infants. *Pediatrics.* (2016) 137:e20153730. doi: 10.1542/peds.2015-3730
7. Waldvogel S, Atkinson A, Wilbeaux M, Nelle M, Berger MR, Gerull R. High dose indomethacin for patent ductus arteriosus closure increases neonatal morbidity. *Am J Perinatol.* (2019). doi: 10.1055/s-0039-3400996. [Epub ahead of print].
8. Slaughter JL, Cua CL, Notestine JL, Rivera BK, Marzec L, Hade EM, et al. Early prediction of spontaneous Patent Ductus Arteriosus (PDA) closure and PDA-associated outcomes: a prospective cohort investigation. *BMC Pediatr.* (2019) 19:333. doi: 10.1186/s12887-019-1708-z
9. Ghaderian M, Barekatain B, Dardashty AB. Comparison of oral acetaminophen with oral ibuprofen on closure of symptomatic patent ductus arteriosus in preterm neonates. *J Res Med Sci.* (2019) 24:96. doi: 10.4103/jrms.JRMS_197_19
10. Dani C, Mosca F, Cresi F, Lago P, Lista G, Laforgia N, et al. Patent ductus arteriosus in preterm infants born at 23–24 weeks' gestation: should we pay more attention? *Early Hum Dev.* (2019) 135:16–22. doi: 10.1016/j.earlhumdev.2019.06.002
11. Akar S, Topcuoglu S, Tuten A, Ozalkaya E, Karatepe HO, Gokmen T, et al. Is the first postnatal platelet mass as an indicator of patent Ductus Arteriosus? *Arch Iran Med.* (2019) 22:687–91.
12. Bas-Suárez MP, González-Luis GE, Saavedra P, Villamor EJN. Platelet counts in the first seven days of life and patent ductus arteriosus in preterm very low-birth-weight infants. *Neonatology.* (2014) 106:188–94. doi: 10.1159/000362432
13. Chen YY, Wang HP, Chang JT, Chiou YH, Huang YF, Hsieh KS. Perinatal factors in patent ductus arteriosus in very low-birthweight infants. *Pediatr Int.* (2014) 56:72–6. doi: 10.1111/ped.12199
14. Demir N, Peker E, Ece I, Agengin K, Bulan KA, Tuncer O. Is platelet mass a more significant indicator than platelet count of closure of patent ductus arteriosus? *J Matern-Fetal Neo Med.* (2016) 29:1915–8. doi: 10.3109/14767058.2015.1067296
15. Du JF, Liu TT, Wu H. Risk factors for patent ductus arteriosus in early preterm infants: a case-control study. *Chin J Contemp Pediatr.* (2016) 18:15–9. doi: 10.7499/j.issn.1008-8830.2016.01.004
16. Harkin P, Marttila R, Pokka T, Saarela T, Hallman M. Morbidities associated with patent ductus arteriosus in preterm infants. Nationwide cohort study. *J Matern Fetal Neonatal Med.* (2018) 31:2576–83. doi: 10.1080/14767058.2017.1347921
17. Nizarali Z, Marques T, Costa C, Barroso R, Cunha M. Patent Ductus Arteriosus: perinatal Risk factors. *J Neonatal Biol.* (2012) 1:3. doi: 10.4172/2167-0897.1000109
18. Ognean ML, Boanta O, Kovacs S, Zgarcea C, Dumitra R, Olariu E, et al. Persistent Ductus Arteriosus in critically Ill preterm infants. *J Crit Care Med.* (2016) 2:175–84. doi: 10.1515/jccm-2016-0026
19. Wang C-H, Shi L-P, Ma X-L, Luo F, Chen Z, Lin H-J, et al. [Factors influencing the prognosis of patent ductus arteriosus in very low birth weight infants]. *Zhongguo dang dai er ke za zhi = Chin J Contemp Pediatr.* (2016) 18:688–93. doi: 10.7499 / j.issn.1008-8830.2016.08.003
20. Behbodi E, Villamor-Martínez E, Degraeuwe PLJ, Villamor E. Chorioamnionitis appears not to be a risk factor for patent ductus arteriosus in preterm infants: a systematic review and meta-analysis. *Sci Rep.* (2016) 6:37967. doi: 10.1038/srep37967
21. Park HW, Choi Y-S, Kim KS, Kim S-N. Chorioamnionitis and Patent Ductus Arteriosus: a systematic review and meta-analysis. *PLoS* ONE. (2015) 10:e0138114. doi: 10.1371/journal.pone.0138114
22. Simon SR, van Zogchel L, Bas-Suárez MP, Cavallaro G, Clyman RI, Villamor E. Platelet counts and patent ductus arteriosus in preterm infants: a systematic review and meta-analysis. *Neonatology.* (2015) 108:143–51. doi: 10.1159/000431281
23. Villamor-Martinez E, Kilani MA, Degraeuwe PL, Clyman RI, Villamor E. Intrauterine growth restriction and patent ductus arteriosus in very and extremely preterm infants: a systematic review and meta-analysis. *Front Endocrinol.* (2019) 10:58. doi: 10.3389/fendo.2019.00058
24. Moher D, Liberati A, Tetzlaff J, Altman DG, med PGJP. Preferred reporting items for systematic reviews and meta-analyses: the PRISMA statement. *PLoS Med.* (2009) 6:e1000097. doi: 10.1371/journal.pmed.1000097
25. Wells GA, O' Connell D, Peterson J, Welch V, Losos M, Tugwell P. *The Newcastle-Ottawa Scale (NOS) for Assessing the Quality of Nonrandomised Studies in Meta-Analyses* (2011). Available online at: www.ohri.ca/programs/clinical_epidemiology/oxford.asp
26. Wan X, Wang W, Liu J, Tong TJBmrm. Estimating the sample mean and standard deviation from the sample size, median, range and/or interquartile range. *BMC Med Res Methodol.* (2014) 14:135. doi: 10.1186/1471-2288-14-135
27. Sterne JA, Sutton AJ, Ioannidis JP, Terrin N, Jones DR, Lau J, et al. Recommendations for examining and interpreting funnel plot asymmetry in meta-analyses of randomised controlled trials. *BMJ.* (2011) 343:d4002. doi: 10.1136/bmj.d4002
28. Thompson EJ, Greenberg RG, Kumar K, Laughon M, Smith PB, Clark RH, et al. Association between furosemide exposure and patent ductus arteriosus in hospitalized infants of very low birth weight. *J Pediatr.* (2018) 199:231–6. doi: 10.1016/j.jpeds.2018.03.067
29. Czernik C, Lemmer J, Metze B, Koehne PS, Mueller C, Obladen M. B-type natriuretic peptide to predict ductus intervention in infants < 28 weeks. *Pediatr Res.* (2008) 64:286–90. doi: 10.1203/PDR.0b013e3181799594
30. Noori S, McCoy M, Friedlich P, Bright B, Gottipati V, Seri I, et al. Failure of ductus arteriosus closure is associated with increased mortality in preterm infants. *Pediatrics.* (2009) 123:e138–e44. doi: 10.1542/peds.2008-2418

31. Deshpande P, Baczynski M, McNamara PJ, Jain A. Patent ductus arteriosus: the physiology of transition. *Semin Fetal Neonatal Med.* (2018) 23:225–31. doi: 10.1016/j.siny.2018.05.001
32. Harris SL, More K, Dixon B, Troughton R, Pemberton C, Horwood J, et al. Factors affecting N-terminal pro-B-type natriuretic peptide levels in preterm infants and use in determination of haemodynamic significance of patent ductus arteriosus. *Eur J Pediatr.* (2018) 177:521–32. doi: 10.1007/s00431-018-3089-y
33. Olukman O, Ozdemir R, Karadeniz C, Calkavur S, Mese T, Vergin C. Is there a relationship between platelet parameters and patency of ductus arteriosus in preterm infants? *Blood Coagul Fibrinolysis.* (2017) 28:8–13. doi: 10.1097/mbc.0000000000000520
34. Tauzin L, Joubert C, Noel AC, Bouissou A, Moulies ME. Effect of persistent patent ductus arteriosus on mortality and morbidity in very low-birthweight infants. *Acta Paediatr.* (2012) 101:419–23. doi: 10.1111/j.1651-2227.2011.02550.x
35. Koch J, Hensley G, Roy L, Brown S, Ramaciotti C, Rosenfeld CR. Prevalence of spontaneous closure of the ductus arteriosus in neonates at a birth weight of 1000 grams or less. *Pediatrics.* (2006) 117:1113–21. doi: 10.1542/peds.2005-1528
36. Liu H, Manganiello V, Waleh N, Clyman RI. Expression, activity, and function of phosphodiesterases in the mature and immature ductus arteriosus. *Pediatr Res.* (2008) 64:477–81. doi: 10.1203/PDR.0b013e3181827c2c
37. Clyman RI, Mauray F, Rudolph AM, Heymann MA. Age-dependent sensitivity of the lamb ductus arteriosus to indomethacin and prostaglandins. *J Pediatr.* (1980) 96:94–8. doi: 10.1016/s0022-3476(80)80338-6
38. Clyman RI. Mechanisms regulating the ductus arteriosus. *Biol Neonate.* (2006) 89:330–5. doi: 10.1159/000092870
39. Hermes-DeSantis ER, Clyman RI. Patent ductus arteriosus: pathophysiology and management. *J Perinatol.* (2006) 26(Suppl 1):S14–8. doi: 10.1038/sj.jp.7211465
40. Galinsky R, Polglase GR, Hooper SB, Black MJ, Moss TJM. The consequences of chorioamnionitis: preterm birth and effects on development. *J Pregnancy.* (2013) 2013:412831. doi: 10.1155/2013/412831
41. Pugni L, Pietrasanta C, Acaia B, Merlo D, Ronchi A, Ossola MW, et al. Chorioamnionitis and neonatal outcome in preterm infants: a clinical overview. *J Matern-Fetal Neo Med.* (2016) 29:1525–9. doi: 10.3109/14767058.2015.1053862
42. Arayici S, Simsek GK, Oncel MY, Eras Z, Canpolat FE, Oguz SS, et al. The effect of histological chorioamnionitis on the short-term outcome of preterm infants <= 32 weeks: a single-center study. *J Matern Fetal Neonatal Med.* (2014) 27:1129–33. doi: 10.3109/14767058.2013.850668
43. Garcia-Munoz Rodrigo F, Galan Henriquez G, Figueras Aloy J, Garcia-Alix Perez A. Outcomes of very-low-birth-weight infants exposed to maternal clinical chorioamnionitis: a multicentre study. *Neonatology.* (2014) 106:229–34. doi: 10.1159/000363127
44. Wright LL, Verter J, Younes N, Stevenson D, Fanaroff AA, Shankaran S, et al. Antenatal corticosteroid administration and neonatal outcome in very low birth weight infants: the NICHD Neonatal Research Network. *Am J Obstet Gynecol.* (1995) 173:269–74. doi: 10.1016/0002-9378(95)90212-0
45. Shelton EL, Waleh N, Plosa EJ, Benjamin JT, Milne GL, Hooper CW, et al. Effects of antenatal betamethasone on preterm human and mouse ductus arteriosus: comparison with baboon data. *Pediatr Res.* (2018) 84:458–65. doi: 10.1038/s41390-018-0006-z
46. Shen ZZ, Wang YW, Ma S, Zhan YL, Wu SS, Feng YH, et al. [Risk factors for preterm birth, low birth weight and small for gestational age: a prospective cohort study]. *Zhonghua liu xing bing xue za zhi = Zhonghua liuxingbingxue zazhi.* (2019) 40:1125–9. doi: 10.3760/cma.j.issn.0254-6450.2019.09.020
47. Li X, Zhang W, Lin J, Liu H, Yang Z, Teng Y, et al. Preterm birth, low birthweight, and small for gestational age among women with preeclampsia: does maternal age matter? *Pregnancy Hypertens.* (2018) 13:260–6. doi: 10.1016/j.preghy.2018.07.004
48. Vogel JP, Chawanpaiboon S, Moller A-B, Watananirun K, Bonet M, Lumbiganon P. The global epidemiology of preterm birth. *Best Pract Res Clin Obstet Gynaecol.* (2018) 52:3–12. doi: 10.1016/j.bpobgyn.2018.04.003
49. Van De Bor M, Verloove-Vanhorick SP, Brand R, Ruys JH. Patent ductus arteriosus in a cohort of 1338 preterm infants: a collaborative study. *Paediatr Perinat Epidemiol.* (1988) 2:328–36. doi: 10.1111/j.1365-3016.1988.tb00227.x
50. Rehan VK, Moddemann D, Casiro OG. Outcome of very-low-birth-weight (< 1,500 grams) infants born to mothers with diabetes. *Clin Pediatr.* (2002) 41:481–91. doi: 10.1177/000992280204100705
51. Kachikis A, Walker CL, McAdams RM, Gyamfi-Bannerman C, Waldorf KMA. Phenotypic overlap in neonatal respiratory morbidity following preterm premature rupture of membranes versus spontaneous preterm labor. *J Matern Fetal Neonatal Med.* (2019) 1–8. doi: 10.1080/14767058.2019.1651280
52. Hammoud MS, Elsori HA, Hanafi E-AM, Shalabi AA, Fouda IA, Devarajan LV. Incidence and risk factors associated with the patency of ductus arteriosus in preterm infants with respiratory distress syndrome in Kuwait. *Saudi Med J.* (2003) 24:982–5.
53. Evans N, Kluckow M. Early ductal shunting and intraventricular haemorrhage in ventilated preterm infants. *Arch Dis Child Fetal Neonatal Ed.* (1996) 75:F183–6. doi: 10.1136/fn.75.3.f183
54. Capozzi G, Santoro G. Patent ductus arteriosus: patho-physiology, hemodynamic effects and clinical complications. *J Matern-Fetal Neo Med.* (2011) 24(Suppl 1):15–6. doi: 10.3109/14767058.2011.607564
55. Noerr B. Current controversies in the understanding of necrotizing enterocolitis. Part 1. *Adv Neo Care.* (2003) 3:107–20. doi: 10.1016/s1536-0903(03)00072-9
56. Ryder RW, Shelton JD, Guinan ME. Necrotizing enterocolitis: a prospective multicenter investigation. *Am J Epidemiol.* (1980) 112:113–23. doi: 10.1093/oxfordjournals.aje.a112960
57. Dollberg S, Lusky A, Reichman B. Patent ductus arteriosus, indomethacin and necrotizing enterocolitis in very low birth weight infants: a population-based study. *J Pediatr Gastroenterol Nutr.* (2005) 40:184–8. doi: 10.1097/00005176-200502000-00019
58. Sarkar S, Dechert R, Schumacher RE, Donn SM. Is refractory hypotension in preterm infants a manifestation of early ductal shunting? *J Perinatol.* (2007) 27:353–8. doi: 10.1038/sj.jp.7211749
59. Brown ER. Increased risk of bronchopulmonary dysplasia in infants with patent ductus arteriosus. *J Pediatr.* (1979) 95(5 Pt 2):865–6. doi: 10.1016/s0022-3476(79)80454-0
60. Clyman RI, Chorne N. Patent ductus arteriosus: evidence for and against treatment. *J Pediatr.* (2007) 150:216–9. doi: 10.1016/j.jpeds.2006.12.048
61. Sellmer A, Bjerre JV, Schmidt MR, McNamara PJ, Hjortdal VE, Høst B, et al. Morbidity and mortality in preterm neonates with patent ductus arteriosus on day 3. *Arch Dis Child Fetal Neo Ed.* (2013) 98:F505–10. doi: 10.1136/archdischild-2013-303816
62. Marshall DD, Kotelchuck M, Young TE, Bose CL, Kruyer L, O'Shea TM. Risk factors for chronic lung disease in the surfactant era: a North Carolina population-based study of very low birth weight infants. North Carolina Neonatologists Association. *Pediatrics.* (1999) 104:1345–50. doi: 10.1542/peds.104.6.1345
63. Abdel-Hady H, Nasef N, Shabaan AE, Nour I. Patent ductus arteriosus in preterm infants: do we have the right answers? *Biomed Res Int.* (2013) 2013:676192. doi: 10.1155/2013/676192
64. Clyman RI, Hills NK. The effect of prolonged tracheal intubation on the association between patent ductus arteriosus and bronchopulmonary dysplasia (grades 2 and 3). *J Perinatol.* (2020) 40:1358–65. doi: 10.1038/s41372-020-0718-x
65. Clyman RI, Kaempf J, Liebowitz M, Erdeve O, Bulbul A, Håkansson S, et al. Prolonged tracheal intubation and the association between patent ductus arteriosus and bronchopulmonary dysplasia: a secondary analysis of the PDA-TOLERATE trial. *J Pediatr.* (2020). doi: 10.1016/j.jpeds.2020.09.047. [Epub ahead of print].
66. Gonzalez A, Sosenko IR, Chandar J, Hummler H, Claure N, Bancalari EJTJop. Influence of infection on patent ductus arteriosus and chronic lung disease in premature infants weighing 1000 grams or less. (1996) 128:470–8. doi: 10.1016/s0022-3476(96)70356-6
67. Gomez-Pomar E, Makhoul M, Westgate PM, Ibonia KT, Patwardhan A, Giannone PJ, et al. Relationship between perfusion index and patent ductus arteriosus in preterm infants. *Pediatr Res.* (2017) 81:775–9. doi: 10.1038/pr.2017.10
68. Echtler K, Stark K, Lorenz M, Kerstan S, Walch A, Jennen L, et al. Platelets contribute to postnatal occlusion of the ductus arteriosus. *Nat Med.* (2010) 16:75–82. doi: 10.1038/nm.2060

69. Dani C, Poggi C, Fontanelli G. Relationship between platelet count and volume and spontaneous and pharmacological closure of ductus arteriosus in preterm infants. *Am J Perinatol.* (2013) 30:359–64. doi: 10.1055/s-0032-1324702
70. Alyamac Dizdar E, Ozdemir R, Sari FN, Yurttutan S, Gokmen T, Erdeve O, et al. Low platelet count is associated with ductus arteriosus patency in preterm newborns. *Early Hum Dev.* (2012) 88:813–6. doi: 10.1016/j.earlhumdev.2012.05.007
71. Guler Kazanci E, Buyuktiryaki M, Unsal H, Tayman C. Useful platelet indices for the diagnosis and follow-up of patent ductus arteriosus. *Am J Perinatol.* (2019) 36:1521–7. doi: 10.1055/s-0039-1688821

9

Early Urinary Metabolomics in Patent Ductus Arteriosus Anticipates the Fate

Flaminia Bardanzellu[1*], *Cristina Piras*[2], *Alessandra Atzei*[1], *Paola Neroni*[1] and *Vassilios Fanos*[1]

[1] *Neonatal Intensive Care Unit, Department of Surgical Sciences, Azienda Ospedaliero-Universitaria and University of Cagliari, Cagliari, Italy,* [2] *Department of Biomedical Sciences, University of Cagliari, Cagliari, Italy*

Correspondence:
Flaminia Bardanzellu
bardanzellu.flaminia@virgilio.it

Introduction: In premature neonates, the persistence of hemodynamically significant ductus arteriosus (hsPDA) can be associated with short- and long-term consequences, impairing their outcome. The correct strategy of management for such condition is under debate, especially regarding contraindications and/or side effects. In recent years, metabolomics was applied to several perinatal, pediatric, and adult conditions to investigate potential biomarkers of disease, which have become useful for early diagnosis and/or therapeutic management.

Aim of the Study: The main purpose of our exploratory study was to asses, through ^{1}H-NMR metabolomics analysis of urinary samples at birth, possible metabolic pathways differentiating, with a significant predictive power, those preterm neonates who will subsequently develop hsPDA and neonates of comparable gestational age (GA) who will undergo spontaneous ductal closure or the persistence of an irrelevant PDA (no-hsPDA). Moreover, we investigated potential prenatal or perinatal clinical factors potentially influencing the development of hsPDA.

Materials and Methods: We enrolled $n = 35$ preterm neonates with GA between 24 and 32 weeks; urinary samples were collected within the first 12 h of life. Patients were closely monitored regarding intensive care, respiratory support, fluid balance and administered drugs; an echocardiogram was performed at 48–72 h.

Results: Our results reported a significant correlation between lower GA at birth and the development of hsPDA. Moreover, neonates with GA $\leq$ 30 w developing hsPDA were characterized by lower Apgar scores at 1′ and 5′, higher rates of perinatal asphyxia, higher need of delivery room resuscitation and subsequent surfactant administration. Interestingly, metabolomics analysis at birth detected a clear separation between the ^{1}H-NMR urinary spectra of subjects GA $\leq$ 30 w not developing hsPDA ($n = 19$) and those of subjects born at GA $\leq$ 30 w in which hsPDA was confirmed at 48–72 h of life ($n = 5$).

Conclusions: This is the first study applying metabolomics to investigate the PDA condition. Although preliminary and conducted on a limited sample, our results reveal that metabolomics could be a promising tool in the early identification of hsPDA, potentially superior to the clinical or laboratory predictive tools explored to date and even to the clinical observations and correlations in our sample, through the detection of specific urinary metabolites.

Keywords: metabolomics, PDA, prematurity, biomarkers, ^{1}H-NMR

INTRODUCTION

Ductus arteriosus (DA) or ductus Botalli, one of the fetal shunts allowing oxygenation during intrauterine life (1, 2), physiologically undergoes spontaneous functional closure within the first 72 h of postnatal life, through molecular mechanisms that have been extensively discussed (3–5).

In preterm neonates, ductal closure can fail or delay, mostly due to reduced response to oxygen-induced vasoconstriction, lower activity of vasavasorum, higher levels of prostaglandin E2 (PGE2) and increased sensitivity to prostaglandins and nitric oxide (NO) compared to full term neonates (2, 3). A low-grade inflammatory status and oxidative stress could also take part in maintaining PDA, *via* increasing prostaglandin levels (1, 6).

The risk of developing a persistence of ductal patency (PDA) increases with decreasing gestational age (GA), with relevant short- and long-term consequences in term of morbidity, especially in case of hemodynamically significant PDA (hsPDA) (1, 7, 8).

PDA closure can be performed pharmacologically or, in case of failure or contraindication, with surgical ligation or transcatheter closure (8–18).

However, all these strategies can have side effects and potential risks and, as evidenced by current literature, the ideal strategy of management is still under debate, especially regarding if, when and how to treat or not PDA.

Several predisposing factors have been associated to PDA condition, sometimes with contrasting results, such as genetic factors (19–21), maternal pregnancy induced hypertension (PIH) (22), chorioamnionitis (23, 24), maternal antepartum hemorrhage, respiratory distress syndrome (RDS), lower birth weight (BW), Apgar score and GA, female gender (22, 25), dopamine administration and eccessive intravenous fluid administration (26), neonatal sepsis (27, 28), need for surfactant (22, 25, 26, 29), maternal and neonatal drug assumption (2, 30–38), platelet number, function and other platelet-related parameters (4, 5, 39–47).

Objects of study have also been the factors that can influence therapy response, as reported for male gender (48), polymorphisms influencing drug metabolism (19, 49), and GA (48).

The full comprehension of all the molecular and genetic mechanisms underlying ductal closure or patency maintenance could help in identifying serum or urinary biomarkers potentially associated with PDA condition, especially hsPDA, supporting or anticipating ultrasound or clinical diagnosis.

HsPDA determines ductal diastolic steal, leading to systemic hypoperfusion (cerebral, renal, pulmonary, gastro-intestinal etc...) and the subsequent hypoxia can affect tissues and endothelium with variable impact on hemodynamics. Identifying early markers of this condition could help in the precocious identification of those newborns at high risk of hsPDA, orienting clinical strategy, and avoiding overtreatment of subjects who would undergo spontaneous ductal closure, improving diagnosis and treatment.

Up to now, several literature studies have tried to associate different biomarkers to hsPDA, such as serum B-type Natriuretic Peptide (BNP), segment of the amino terminal B-type Natriuretic Peptide (NT-proBNP) (1, 50–59), cardiac Troponin T (cTnT) (57), lactate levels (60), ions (61), osmolality (62), base excess or hematocrit (63), platelets count and functions (64–66), perfusion index (67), proteomics (68), and among urinary markers, isoprostans, u-ngal (69), proBNP and NT-proBNP-to-creatinine ratio (70–73), also with potential associations with PDA diameter and therapy response, often with contrasting results (74, 75).

Systemic inflammation (76–78) and oxidative stress (79, 80) have also been associated with PDA and therapy response, through urinary and serum markers.

Finding biomarkers that are able to predict therapy response could be useful to avoid unnecessary treatment and potentially perform a targeted therapy, choosing and treating only those infants that could respond to the treatment.

Metabolomics is one of the "omics" technologies that, in the last years, emerged as a promising tool to be applied in several fields of neonatology and pediatrics to characterize and describe pathophysiological processes (81, 82).

Due to its ability in dynamically detecting, in a non-invasive way, the whole set of low molecular weight molecules (including sugar, aminoacids, lipids etc...) in cells, tissues and biological fluids, it can help in describing, in a highly individualized way, the exact response of an organism to environmental stimuli and pathophysiological conditions, including drugs, nutrition, lifestyle, diseases and others, as recently reviewed by our group (81).

Metabolomics biomarkers, if accurately identified and confirmed through repeated studies and validation tests, could be investigated to obtain, in a precocious and non-invasive way, information regarding disease onset, progression and, potentially, therapy response.

Our research group has been interested in metabolomics for many years, carrying many promising studies on several prenatal, perinatal, infant, and adult conditions and diseases, with the aim of achieving a personalized medicine. More details can be found in our reviews on the topic (81, 82).

Even if, to date, the exact meaning of each metabolite variation and its pathophysiological implication was not completely defined, we strongly believe that the clinical interpretation of the promising results obtained could be completed by creating a specific and updated atlas.

Due to these reasons, we hypothesize that metabolomics could provide useful biomarkers even in the condition of PDA. Thus, we decided to perform an exploratory study analyzing urinary samples at birth in a cohort of preterm neonates, to assess, among the complete overview of possible prenatal or perinatal factors taken into account, if some metabolites could result as predictive of hsPDA, highlighting substantial differences among those neonates who subsequently will develop hsPDA and those who will undergo spontaneous closure, or in which PDA will not determine hemodynamic consequences.

To the best of our knowledge, this is the first metabolomics study in the investigation of PDA disease. A previous preliminary report by our group was performed few years ago (83) and a preliminary investigation on metabolomics differences between urinary profiles of responders and non-responders to ibuprofen therapy was performed by Castell-Miñana et al. (84).

AIM OF THE STUDY

Our hypothesis was to identify, through potential early metabolic perturbations in the group of newborns that will develop hsPDA, different urinary pathways compared to those newborns in which the duct will undergo spontaneous closure or minimal patency without impact on hemodynamics.

Thus, the principal aim of the exploratory study was to investigate, for the first time, the possible predictive role of ^{1}H-NMR metabolomics analysis of urinary samples at birth regarding the development of hsPDA. In fact, we investigated possible metabolic differences between urinary pathways of those preterm neonates who will subsequently develop hsPDA confirmed at 48–72 h of life, rather than neonates of comparable GA who will undergo spontaneous closure or the persistence of irrelevant PDA at the same time point (no-hsPDA).

We also aimed to evaluate whether the predictive role of urinary metabolomics may be superior to the clinical criteria or biomarkers considered up to now. Therefore, we investigated potential prenatal or perinatal clinical factors potentially influencing the development of hsPDA in our sample group.

Finally, we tried to find a potential link correlating metabolic variation in the two groups and pathogenesis of hsPDA; in our opinion, the early identification of specific metabolites suggestive of PDA could be a fundamental and complementary tool to be used, alongside the clinic, for applying a personalized approach to the treatment of PDA.

MATERIALS AND METHODS

Study Population

A population of $n = 35$ preterm neonates admitted to Neonatal Intensive Care Unit of Duilio Casula Hospital, University of Cagliari, with GA included between 24 and 32 weeks, was enrolled between October 2019 and June 2020.

In all the newborns, a urinary sample of 3 mL was collected until 12 h after birth, through the non-invasive technique of the cotton wad.

All the subjects underwent cardiologic evaluation performed by the neonatal cardiologist of our neonatal intensive care unit (NICU) within the first 24 h and successively at 48–72 h and 120 h after birth. Echocardiography and Color-doppler aimed to evaluate cardiac anatomy and functionality and to assess the presence and the hemodynamic features of PDA. In subjects with a persistent PDA or hsPDA, an echocardiography was performed in the subsequent days, according to the clinical indication.

Each echocardiography aimed to asses PDA diameter (indexed for body weight expressed in kilograms), left atrium/Aortic Root Ratio (LA/Ao), patent ductus arteriosus/left branch of pulmonary artery ratio (PDA/LPA), systolic and diastolic velocity of duct flow to assess the restrictive or non-restrictive pattern. Additional cardiological evaluations were performed according to clinical necessities. PDA was considered hemodynamically significant in case of a PDA diameter/neonatal weight $\geq$ 1.5 mm/Kg and LA/Ao $>$ 1.4 in addition to an eventual PDA/LPA $>$ 0.8 and/or a peak diastolic velocity lower than 50% of the peak systolic velocity measured at ductal level 48–72 h after birth.

Echocardiography was performed using Esaote MyLab^{TM}Twice EVO 13.0/13.0 m, and the images' acquisition was obtained with 8 MHz two-dimensional probe.

During hospitalization, all the newborns underwent instrumental exams (chest radiography, cerebral ultrasound, abdominal ultrasound, hearing screening, fundus oculi exam) and hematic exams (complete blood count, hepatic and renal function, infection indexes, and blood culture in case of suspected sepsis), eventually repeated according to the clinical needs.

All demographic data and the information regarding pregnancy, birth, neonatal management in delivery room, assistance in NICU, invasive and non-invasive ventilation, oxygen needs, surfactant administration, fluid balance, nutrition, and drugs were recorded.

The Ethics Committee of University of Cagliari gave its approval for this study (Protocol NP/2017/470) and the parents signed an informed consent and gave their approval for this study.

Sample Analysis

Urine Sample Preparation

Urine samples were thawed in ice. An aliquot of 800 μL of urine was transferred into a tube together with 8 μL of a 1% aqueous solution of NaN3 in order to inhibit bacteria growth and stored at −80°C. The sample was centrifuged at 12,000 g for 10 min at 4°C to remove solid particles. Then, 630 μL of the supernatant solution was mixed with 70 μL of potassium phosphate buffer in D2O (1.5 M, pH 7.4) containing sodium 3-trimethylsilyl-propionate-2,2,3,3,-d4 (TSP) as an internal standard (98 atom% D, Sigma-Aldrich, Milan). The mixture was vortexed and an aliquot of 650 μL was transferred to 5-mm NMR glass tubes for ^{1}H-NMR analysis (85).

^{1}H-NMR Spectroscopic Analysis and Data Pre-processing

^{1}H-NMR spectra were recorded at 300 K using a Varian UNITY INOVA 500 spectrometer operating at 499.839 MHz for proton and equipped with a 5 mm double resonance probe (Agilent Technologies, CA, USA). The acquisition parameters of the ^{1}H-NMR spectra are reported in our previous article (85). NMR spectra were processed using an ACDlab Processor Academic Edition (Advanced Chemistry Development, 12.01, 2010). After Fourier transformation with 0.3 Hz line broadening, ^{1}H-NMR spectra were phased and baseline corrected and chemical shifts referenced to the signal of internal standard TSP at $\delta = 0.0$ ppm. The spectral region comprising the signal of residual water and urea (4.7–4.9 ppm) was removed. The ACD Labs intelligent bucketing method was used for spectral integration (86). A 0.04 ppm bucket has been applied. The area of bucket regions were normalized to the total spectral area to compensate the different dilutions of original urine samples. Finally, the spectral data was imported into the SIMCA software (Version 15.0, Sartorius Stedim Biotech, Umea, Sweden) for statistical multivariate analysis. All imported data were then pre-processed using Pareto scaling (87).

Statistical Analysis

The data were collected and analyzed with Microsoft Excel 2019 program; the results were expressed as the mean value ± the standard deviation (SD). For statistical analysis, Student's T-test was applied to compare the means of each variable analyzed in the study. A p-value < 0.05 was considered as statistically significant, and a p-value < 0.001 as highly significant.

A Chi-Square-test was used for testing relationships on categorical variables and to evaluate tests of independence.

Multivariate Statistical Analysis

Principal component analysis (PCA), Partial Least-Squares Discriminant Analysis (PLS-DA) and Orthogonal Partial Least-Squares Discriminant Analysis (OPLS-DA) were used for multivariate statistical analyses of NMR data (88). Principal component analysis is an unsupervised analysis and is applied to identify unusual clusters, anomalies, or trends in the samples based on the similarities of their metabolic profiles. Supervised PLS-DA and OPLS-DA methods were used to reduce model complexity and to better highlight variables responsible for the discrimination of predefined classes. The models quality expressed as R2Y (goodness of classification) and Q2Y (goodness of prediction) and the over-fitting were evaluated through the default leave-1/7th-out cross validation test and "permutation test" (400 times) respectively. The intercept is a measure of the overfit, Q2Y intercept value <0.05 is indicative of a valid model. To identify potential metabolites that mainly contributed to group separation, an S-line plot for the OPLS-DA models was built (89).

Univariate Statistical Analysis

GraphPad Prism software (version 7.01, GraphPad Software, Inc., San Diego, CA, USA) was used to perform the univariate statistical analysis. The potential significant metabolites identified were quantified using Chenomx NMR Suite 7.1 (Chenomx Inc., Edmonton, Alberta, Canada) (90). The statistical significance of the differences in metabolite concentrations was calculated by using the Mann-Whitney U-test and a p-value < 0.05 was considered statistically significant. The Benjamini-Hochberg method was subsequently applied to the obtained p-values to acquire the level of significance for multiple testing (91). Finally, to further evaluate the diagnostic power of the potential biomarkers the ROC (receiver operator characteristic) curve was constructed to test the sensitivity, specificity and calculate area under the ROC curve (AUC) to only metabolites with p-values < 0.01. AUC indicates the accuracy of a test for correctly distinguishing No-hsPDA from hsPDA. The 95% CI (Confidence Interval) for the AUC curves were also calculated.

RESULTS

Clinical Analysis

Our study population was composed by $n = 35$ newborns with GA included between 24^{+2} and 32^{+4} weeks. Mean GA was 29.92 ± 2.06 weeks. Mean birth weight was 1,346 ± 367 g and $n = 23/35$ subjects were males.

All the information regarding pregnancy characteristics, complications and outcome are reported in **Table 1**.

In our sample of preterm neonates, $n = 4/35$ were born by vaginal delivery (VD) and $n = 31/35$ by urgent cesarean section (UCS). On a total of $n = 29$ pregnancies, $n = 3$ deliveries were vaginal, while $n = 26$ were UCS. The causes of preterm birth through UCS have been represented by intrauterine growth restriction (IUGR) and flux alteration (23%), cardiotocography (CTG) alterations/neonatal bradycardia (23%), placental abruption (19.2%), preterm labor/other maternal causes (19.2%), preeclampsia (8%), twin-to-twin transfusion (3.8%), and fetal tachycardia (3.8%).

All the information regarding perinatal characteristics of our group of newborns have been reported in **Table 2** and neonatal outcomes, as well as the information regarding the development of hsPDA and the needs for treatment are reported in **Table 3**. In $n = 5/35$ neonates (14.3%) hsPDA was confirmed at echocardiographic examination at 48–72 h of life. All the newborns developing hsPDA were born at GA $\leq$ 30 weeks. Thus, to make the sample more homogeneous, we decided to report our results excluding those neonates of GA > 30 weeks, since hsPDA resulted as being highly dependent on GA at birth and was absent in neonates > 30 weeks. However, all the results obtained by the analysis of the whole population can be found in **Tables 1–3**.

Our group on neonates born at GA $\leq$ 30 weeks was composed by $n = 24$ neonates. All the information on pregnancy, perinatal characteristics and neonatal early outcome regarding this subpopulation of newborns were analyzed and statistical comparisons were made between those newborns with GA $\leq$ 30 weeks subsequently undergoing spontaneous closure of PDA or maintaining an hemodynamically irrelevant PDA (no-hsPDA) and those neonates developing hsPDA (**Tables 1–3**).

The first group, ($\leq$30 w no-hsPDA) was composed by $n = 19/24$ neonates, while the second group ($\leq$30 w hsPDA) included $n = 5/24$ neonates, $p < 0.01$.

TABLE 1 | Maternal and pregnancy characteristics and complications.

		Total sample (≤32 w)	≤30 w	≤30 w no-hsPSA	≤30 w hsPDA	*p*-value* (calculated comparing no-hsPDA and hsPDA)
Chorioamnionitis	Yes	2/35 (5.71%)	2/24 (8.33%)	2/19 (10.53%)	0/5 (0%)	0.3
	No	33/35 (94.29%)	22/24 (91.67%)	17/19 (89.47%)	5/5 (100%)	
Altered glucose load curve	Yes	1/35 (2.86%)	1/24 (4.17%)	1/19 (5.26%)	0/5 (0%)	-
	No	16/35 (45.71%)	8/24 (33.33%)	6/19 (31.58%)	2/5 (40%)	
	N.p.	18/35 (51.43)	15/24 (62.5%)	12/19 (63.16%)	3/5 (60%)	
Placental abruption	Yes	6/35 (17.14%)	6/24 (25%)	4/19 (21%)	2/5 (40%)	0.4
	No	29/35 (82.86%)	18/24 (75%)	15/19 (79%)	3/5 (60%)	
Hypertension (in treatment)	Yes	4/35 (11.43%)	4/24 (16.67%)	2/19 (10.53%)	2/5 (40%)	0.11
	No	31/35 (88.57%)	20/24 (83.33%)	17/19 (89.47%)	3/5 (60%)	
PROM > 18 hours	Yes	5/35 (14.29)	5/24 (20.3%)	5/19 (26.31%)	0/5 (0%)	0.19
	No	30/35 (85.71%)	19/24 (79.17%)	14/19 (73.69%)	5/5 (100%)	
Antenatal Steroids	Yes	24/35 (68.57%) 2 doses: 22/24 1 dose: 2/24	15/24 (62.5%) 2 doses: 14/15 1 dose: 1/15	12/19 (63.16%) 2 doses: 11/12 1 doses: 1/12	3/5 (60%) 2 doses: 3/5	0.9
	No	11/35 (31.43%)	9/24 (37.5)	7/19 (36.84%)	2/5 (40%)	

w, Weeks; hsPDA, hemodinamically significant patent ductus arteriosus; n.p., not performed; PROM, premature rupture of membranes (>18 h).
**Statistically significant if p < 0.05.*
-, Not calculated because the authors do not believe it could be useful for statistical analysis.

Maternal/pregnancy complications were analyzed, including chorioamnionitis, placental abruption, hypertension in treatment, premature rupture of membranes (PROM > 18 h), and not statistically significant differences occurred in the two groups ≤30 w no-hsPDA vs. ≤30 w hsPDA (**Table 1**).

Maternal administration of steroids occurred in $n = 15/24$ mothers, $n = 12/19$ in the group ≤30 w no-hsPDA vs. $n = 3/5$ in the group ≤30 w hsPDA, $p = 0.9$.

Information regarding maternal glucose load was available only for a few patients, since such a test is performed between 26 and 28 GA and many of the women delivering preterm were not able to perform it. Thus, statistical evaluations were not performed regarding eventual alteration in glucose tolerance or pregnancy induced diabetes mellitus.

In the group of neonates ≤30 w, mean GA was 29 ± 1.85 weeks and mean BW was 1239.92 ± 329 g; $n = 14/24$ were males.

Twins were $n = 9/24$; twins are not even in number, since one of them was excluded by the study because we could not collect the urinary sample.

GA was significantly higher in the ≤30 w no-hsPDA group (29.63 ± 1.03) vs. ≤30 w hsPDA (26.62 ± 2.46), with statisticalsignificance $p < 0.001$ and even BW was higher in the fist group 1,302 ± 261 g vs. 1,004 ± 476 g, without statistical significance ($p = 0.069$).

Twins were more frequent in the group ≤30 w no-hsPDA $n = 9/19$ vs. ≤30 w hsPDA $n = 0/5$, $p < 0.05$.

Information regarding length, weight, and head circumference percentiles at birth were not statistically significant in terms of number of patients large for GA (LGA), appropriate (AGA) or small for GA (SGA) ($p = 0.75$). Moreover, even delivery mode in terms of VD or UCS was not statistically different in the two groups ($p = 0.6$).

Significant differences occurred, taking into account the Apgar score in the two groups of patients. Apgar score was significantly higher in the ≤30 w no-hsPDA group (6.58 ± 1.74) vs. ≤30 w hsPDA (3.8 ± 3.11), at the first minute of life (1′), with statistical significance $p < 0.01$ and at 5 min of life (5′) (7.48 ± 1.21) vs. (6 ± 2.45), $p < 0.05$. The incidence of perinatal asphyxia was higher in the ≤30 w hsPDA group than ≤30 w no-hsPDA group ($p < 0.05$); in detail, severe asphyxia was more frequent in the first group ($p < 0.01$).

The needs for delivery room resuscitation was higher in the ≤30 w hsPDA group ($p < 0.05$), especially regarding the needs of endotracheal intubation, chest compressions, or adrenaline,

TABLE 2 | Perinatal characteristics.

		Total sample (≤32 w)	**≤30 w**	**≤30 w no-hsPSA**	**≤30 w hsPDA**	***p*-value* (calculated comparing no-hsPDA and hsPDA)**
Number of subjects		35	24	19/24 (79.2%)	5/24 (20.8%)	**<0.01***
Sex		M 23/35 (65.7%)	M 14/24 (58.33%)	M 11/19 (57.9%)	M 3/5 (60%)	0.93
Gestational age	w ± SD	29.92 ± 2.06	29 ± 1.85	29.63 ± 1.03	26.62 ± 2.46	**<0.001***
Birth weight g ± SD		1,346 ± 367	1239.92 ± 329	1,302 ± 261	1,004 ± 476	0.069
Twins	Yes	13/35 (37.14%)	9/24** (37.5%)	9/19 (47.4%)	0/5 (0%)	**<0.05***
	No	22/35 (62.86%)	15/24 (62.5%)	10/19 (52.6%)	5/5 (100%)	
Antropometry (percentiles)	LGA	4/35 (11.4%)	3/24 (12.5%)	2/19 (10.5%)	1/5 (20%)	0.75
	AGA	29/35 (82.9%)	20/24 (83.3%)	16/19 (84.2%)	4/5 (80%)	
	SGA	2/35 (5.7%)	1/24 (4.2%)	1/19 (5.3%)	0/5 (0%)	
Mode of delivery	VD	4/35 (11.43%)	1/24 (4.2%)	1/19 (5.26%)	0/5 (0%)	0.6
	UCS	31/35 (88.57%)	23/24 (95.8%)	18/19 (94.74%)	5/5 (100%)	
Apgar Score Mean ± SD	1′	5.83 ± 2.25	6 ± 2.32	6.58 ± 1.74	3.8 ± 3.11	**<0.01***
	5′	7.34 ± 1.97	7.46 ± 1.67	7.48 ± 1.21	6 ± 2.45	**<0.05***
Apgar Score (Median)	1′	6	6	7	3	-
	5′	8	8	8	5	-
Delivery room resuscitation	No	2/35 (5,7%)	1/24 (4,17)	1/19 (5,26%)	0/5 (0%)	**<0.05***
	n.i. ventilation + O_2	25/35 (71.4%)	18/24 (75%)	16/19 (84.21%)	2/5 (40%)	**e.t intubation: <0.05***
	e.t. intubation + O_2 ± chest compressions or adrenaline	8/35 (22.9%)	5/24 (20.83%)	2/19 (10.53%)	3/5 (60%)	
Perinatal asphyxia	No	18/35 (51.4%)	12/24 (50%)	10/19 (52.64%)	1/5 (20%)	**<0.05***
	Mild	12/35 (34.3%)	9/24 (37.5%)	8/19 (42.1%)	1/5 (20%)	**Severe: <0.01***
	Severe	5/35 (14.3%)	3/24 (62.5%)	1/19 (5.26%)	3/5 (60%)	

w, Weeks; hsPDA, hemodinamically significant patent ductus arteriosus; g, grams; SD, standard deviation; LGA, lrge for gestational age; AGA, appropriate for gestational age; SGA, small for gestational age; VG, vaginal delivery; UCS, urgent cesarean section; n.i., non-invasive; e.t., endotracheal.
**Statistically significant if $p < 0.05$.*
***Twins are not even in number, since one of them was excluded by the study because we could not collect the urinary sample. Bold values are statistically significant.*

occurring in $n = 2/19$ (10.53%) in the ≤30 w no-hsPDA group, vs. 3/5 (60%) in the ≤30 w hsPDA group ($p < 0.05$).

RDS occurred in the whole sample of newborns ≤30 w $n = 24/24$ (100%).

The need for one or more doses of surfactant was $n = 10/19$ in the ≤30 w no-hsPDA group and $n = 5/5$ in the ≤30 w hsPDA group ($p < 0.05$).

In the group ≤30 w hsPDA group, $n = 4/5$ (80%) were pharmacologically treated for hsPDA closure.

HsPDA closure was achieved in the whole ≤30 w hsPDA group. In $n = 4$ (20%) it occurred with treatment, while $n = 1/5$ underwent spontaneous closure (20%).

In our sample, early onset sepsis (EOS) was detected through blood culture in $n = 2/19$ among the ≤30 w no-hsPDA neonates vs. $n = 2/5$ among the ≤30 w hsPDA ($p = 0.11$); late onset sepsis (LOS) occurred in $n = 5/19$ vs. $n = 1/5$ ($p = 0.77$) and the co-occurrence of EOS + LOS in 2/19 and 2/5 ($p = 0.11$) in the same groups.

Early aminoglicosydes administration to treat EOS was administered in $n = 5/19$ among neonates ≤30 w no-hsPDA vs. $n = 2/5$ in the ≤30 w hsPDA group ($p = 0.5$), not statistically significant. Serum creatinine values at 3–5 days of life were 0.57 ± 0.21 mg/dl in the ≤30 w no-hsPDA vs. 0.65 ± 0.21 mg/dl in the ≤30 w hsPDA group ($p = 0.46$).

None of our patients died.

Metabolomics Analysis

The metabolomics profile of urine samples was investigated using ^{1}H-NMR spectroscopy coupled with multivariate data analysis. Metabolites were identified on the basis of literature information (85) and by using a dedicated library, such as the Human Metabolome Database (HMDB, http://www.hmdb.ca) and the 500 MHz library from Chenomx NMR suite 7.1. Major NMR resonances were originated from free amino acids, organic acids, sugars, small organic compounds and osmolytes. A first unsupervised PCA analysis was conducted to identify potential outliers (outside the 95% confidence limit). The result of the PCA analysis (data not shown) shows a rather homogeneous cohort of samples and no NMR spectrum was excluded from subsequent analyses. To remove potential information not related to the pathology of interest and highlight

TABLE 3 | Neonatal early outcome.

		Total sample (≤32 w)	≤30 w	≤30 w no-hsPSA	≤30 w hsPDA	*p*-value* (calculated comparing no-hsPDA and hsPDA)
RDS		35/35 (100%)	24/24 (100%)	19/19 (100%)	5/5 (100%)	-
Need for surfactant	Yes	22/35 (62.9%)	15/24 (62.5%)	10/19 (52.63%)	5/5 (100%)	**<0.05***
	No	13/35% (37.1%)	9/24 (37.5%)	9/19 (47.37%)	0/5 (0%)	
Surfactant doses (*n*)	1	14/35	8/24	7/19	1/5	-
	2	7/35	5/24	3/19	2/5	-
	4	1/35	1/24	0/19	1/5	-
hsPSA	Yes	5/35 (14.3%)	5/24 (20.83%)	0/19 (0%)	5/5 (100%)	-
	No	30/35 (85.7%)	19/24 (79.17%)	19/19 (100%)	0/5 (0%)	-
Treatment for hsPDA	Yes	4/35 (11.4%)	4/24 (16.67%)	0/19 (0%)	4/5 (80%)	-
	No	31/35 (88.6%)	20/24 (83.33%)	19/19 (100%)	1/5 (20%)	-
hsPDA closure**	Yes (treatment)	4/35 (11.42)	4/24 (16.67%)	-	4/5 (80%)	-
	Yes (no treatment)	1/35 (2.8%)	1/24 (4.17%)	-	1/5 (20%)	-
	No (treatment)	0/35 (0%)	0/24 (0%)	-	0/5 (0%)	-
Sepsis	EOS	7/35 (20%)	4/24 (16.67%)	2/19 (10.53%)	2/5 (40%)	0.11
	LOS	6/35 (17.1%)	6/24 (25%)	5/19 (26.31%)	1/5 (20%)	0.77
	EOS + LOS	4/35 (11.43%)	4/24 (16.67%)	2/19 (10.53%)	2/5 (40%)	0.11
Early aminoglycosides administration		8/35 (22.8%)	7/24 (29.17%)	5/19 (26.31%)	2/5 (40%)	0.5
Creatinine values at 3-5 days of life mean value ± SD		0.56 ± 0.2	0.59 ± 0.21	0.57 ± 0.21	0.65 ± 0.21	0.46
Death		0/35 (0%)	0/24 (0%)	0/19 (0%)	0/5 (0%)	-

w, Weeks; hsPDA, hemodinamically significant patent ductus arteriosus; RDS, respiratory distress syndrome; n, number; EOS, early onset sepsis; LOS, late onset sepsis; SD, standard deviation.

**Statistically significant if $p < 0.05$.*

***When pharmacological treatment for hsPDA was performed, ibuprofen at the standard dose was used as first choice drug, while in case of contraindication, paracetamol was preferred.*

-, Not calculated because the authors do not believe it could be useful for statistical analysis. Bold values are statistically significant.

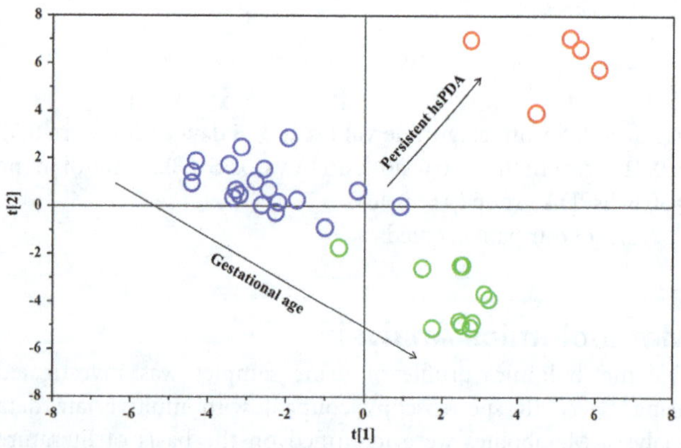

FIGURE 1 | PLS-DA scores plot of ^{1}H NMR spectra of urine samples: ≤30 w No-hsPDA (blue circle), >30 w No-hsPDA (green circle) and ≤30 w hsPDA (red circle).

possible differences in metabolomics urine profile between No-hsPDA (≤ and >30 w) and hsPDA (≤30 w) subjects, a PLS-DA analysis was subsequently conducted on the same dataset.

The PLS-DA scores plot (**Figure 1**) shows a marked separation along t(1) component between No-hsPDA (≤ and >30 w) and hsPDA (≤30 w) subjects, while along t(2) it is possible to observe a separation due to the different gestational age between No-hsPDA (≤30 w) and No-hsPDA (>30 w) subjects. The PLS-DA model was established with two components and showed good values of R2X, R2Y, and Q2 (**Table 4**). The validity of the PLS-DA model was evaluated through a permutation test (**Supplementary Figure 1**) using 400 times. The test results are reported in **Table 4** and indicate the statistical validity of the PLS-DA model. To understand if the hsDPA can be a relevant variable on the urinary metabolomics profile of the studied subjects, an OPLS-DA model was constructed by considering the No-hsPDA (≤ and >30 w) subjects as a single class. OPLS-DA scores plot (**Supplementary Figure 2**) shows that the No-hsPDA (≤ and >30 w) subjects are clearly separate from hsPDA (≤30 w), indicating how the metabolomics profile between the two groups is strongly influenced by the hsPDA. The statistical parameters for the OPLS-DA model are shown in **Table 4**. The validity of the OPLS-DA model was evaluated through a permutation test (**Supplementary Figure 3**) using 400 times. The permutation test results indicate the statistical validity of the OPLS-DA model (**Table 4**). In order to identify potential metabolites closely involved in the separation of samples due to hsPDA, No-hsPDA (>30 w) subjects were excluded from the analysis. An OPLS-DA analysis was conducted by comparing subjects of the same gestational age with or without hsPDA. OPLS-DA scores plot in **Figure 2** shows how subjects with No-hsPDA (≤30 w) are clearly

TABLE 4 | Parameters for PLS-DA and OPLS-DA models.

	PLS-DA and OPLS-DA models			Permutation (400 times)*		
Groups	**Components[a]**	**R2Xcum[b]**	**R2Ycum[c]**	**Q2cum[d]**	**R2 intercept**	**Q2 intercept**
≤30 w No-hsPDA vs. >30 w No-hsPDA vs. ≤30 w hsPDA	2	0.669	0.819	0.501	0.474	−0.508
≤ and >30 w No-hsPDA vs. ≤30 w hsPDA	1P + 2O	0.539	0.862	0.479	0.586	−0.594
≤30 w No-hsPDA vs. ≤30 w hsPDA	1P + 2O	0.512	0.888	0.433	0.511	−0.496

[a] *The number of Predictive and Orthogonal components used to create the OPLS-DA statistical models.*
[b,c] *R2X and R2Y indicated the cumulative explained fraction of the variation of the X block and Y block for the extracted components.*
[d] *Q2 cum values indicated cumulative predicted fraction of the variation of the Y block for the extracted components.*
**An Q2 intercept value <0.05 are indicative of a valid model.*

separated from subjects hsPDA (≤30 w), indicating differences in the metabolomics profile between the two groups. The OPLS-DA model was established with one predictive and two orthogonal components and showed good values of R2X, R2Y, and Q2 (**Table 4**). The permutation test results are reported in **Table 4** and shown in **Supplementary Figure 4**. The S-line plot shown in the **Figure 3**, was used to highlight the potential metabolites that contributed to the urine profile modification in No-hsPDA (≤30 w) subjects compared to hsPDA (≤30 w). A $p(\text{corr}) > 0.5$ was selected as a significance level. The spectral regions identified in the S-line plot characterized by the superimposition of NMR signals corresponding to the different metabolites present in urine, were quantified with Chenomx NMR Suite 7.1. and subjected to the Mann-Whitney U-test to identify significant changes in the of metabolites concentration in the two groups. The result of the univariate statistical analysis showed as 3-Methylxanthine, betaine, glucose, glycylproline, lactate, trimethylamine N-oxide (TMAO), tryptophan, myoinositol and 4-Hydroxyproline changed significantly in No-hsPDA (≤30 w) compared to hsPDA (≤30 w) (**Table 5**). The **Figure 4** shows the relative concentrations of metabolites, where No-hsPDA (≤30 w) subjects were characterized by a higher level of 3-Methylxanthine, betaine, glycylproline, TMAO, tryptophan, myoinositol and 4-Hydroxyproline, and lower of levels glucose and lactate compared to hsPDA (≤30 w). Finally, A ROC curve was constructed by using the only metabolites with p-value < 0.01 (TMAO, tryptophan, and glucose) and the area under the curve of ROC analysis (**Figure 5**) was found to be 0.894 (95% CI: 0.717–1), denoting a high predictive accuracy of the model.

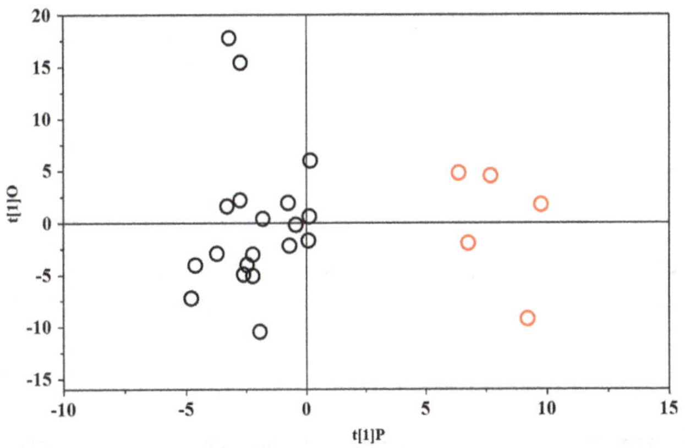

FIGURE 2 | OPLS-DA scores plot of ^{1}H NMR spectra of urine samples: ≤30 w No-hsPDA (black circle) and ≤30 w hsPDA (red circle).

DISCUSSION

Clinical Discussion

Our group confirmed that prematurity influences the occurrence of hsPDA, which resulted as more frequent at a lower GA ($p < 0.001$). BW, although lower in the ≤30 w hsPDA group, did not reach a statistical significance ($p = 0.069$).

First of all, we must underline that our population, although relevant and significant for a metabolomics study, is small for epidemiological consideration and our clinical results should be confirmed on larger samples before deducing significant associations.

In our sample of neonates with GA ≤30 w, the Apgar scores were significantly different in the two groups, with the lowest values in the neonates ≤30 w hsPDA both at 1′ ($p < 0.01$) and at 5′ ($p < 0.05$); therefore, the incidence of perinatal asphyxia was higher in this group ($p < 0.05$), especially severe asphyxia ($p < 0.01$). The association between lower values of the Apgar score and hsPDA have also been observed in the studies of Pourarian et al. and Lee et al. (22, 25), although the significance of the first study is limited by the inclusion of any size of PDA in the analysis.

Due to their worse condition at birth, those neonates subsequently developing hsPDA, also compatible with their aforementioned lower GA, more frequently required delivery room resuscitation ($p < 0.05$).

According to these data, neonates subsequently developing hsPDA showed the worst cardio-respiratory conditions at birth; however, it is not easy to asses with certainty if those neonates show the worst perinatal outcomes and subsequently hsPDA due to their lower GA or if the asphyxia itself could predispose to the development of hsPDA, likely through altered mechanisms of hypoxia-reperfusion, the potential involvement of systemic oxidant stress, vascular impairment and hemodynamic changes.

Surfactant administration was performed in a lower number of subjects in ≤30 w no-hsPDA group vs. ≤30 w hsPDA (p

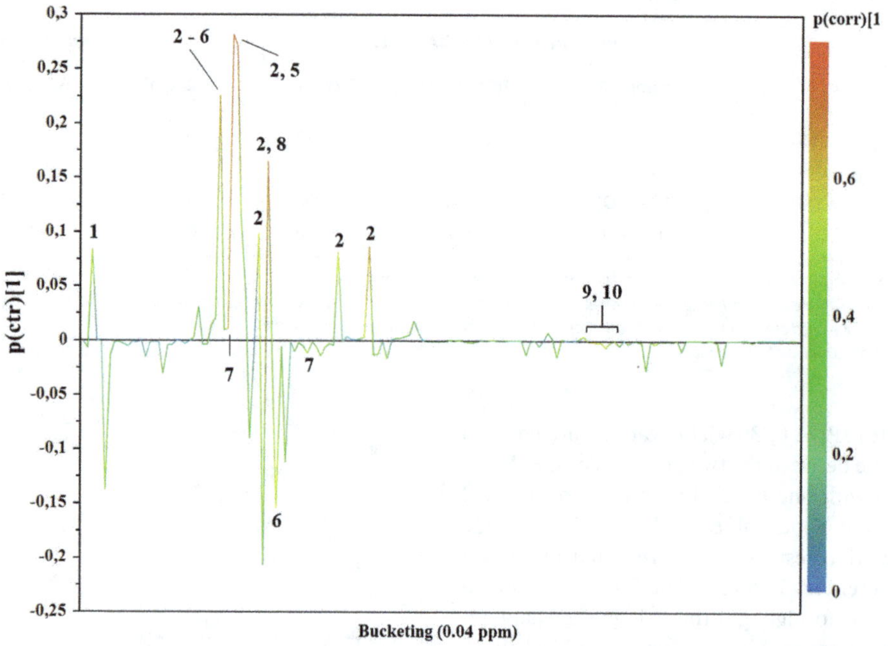

FIGURE 3 | Color-coded coefficient loadings plots of urine metabolomics profiles between ≤30 w No-hsPDA and ≤30 w hsPDA subjects. Peaks: 1, Lactate; 2, Glucose; 3, Betaine; 4, Trimethylamine-N-Oxide (TMAO); 5, Taurine; 6, Myo-Inositol; 7, 4-Hydroxyproline; 8, Creatine; 9, Tryptophan and 10 Hippurate.

TABLE 5 | Discriminant metabolites for OPLS-DA model.

Metabolites	Mean (SD) of group (mM)[a]		*p*-value[b]
	≤30 w No-hsPDA	≤30 w hsPDA	
3-Methylxanthine	0.53 ± 0.34	0.23 ± 0.18	0.05
4-Hydroxyproline	6.39 ± 2.22	3.44 ± 1.72	0.03
Betaine	1.55 ± 0.73	0.69 ± 0.20	0.02
Creatine	1.19 ± 0.82	0.94 ± 0.78	0.31
Glucose	10.8 ± 7.24	37.5 ± 22.1	0.01
Glycylproline	8.55 ± 3.26	4.17 ± 1.97	0.02
Hippurate	0.52 ± 0.29	0.38 ± 0.17	0.44
Lactate	2.87 ± 1.03	6.10 ± 2.5	0.02
Methylhistidine	2.29 ± 1.95	1.18 ± 0.92	0.59
Myo-Inositol	34.6 ± 11.9	19.2 ± 6.03	0.04
Taurine	11.0 ± 4.44	5.78 ± 2.22	0.70
TMAO*	8.15 ± 2.39	4.68 ± 2.20	0.01
Tryptophan	0.76 ± 0.24	0.39 ± 0.17	<0.01

[a] *Relative concentrations were calculated by normalization of the molar concentration of each metabolite to the total molar concentration of all 13 metabolites for each sample.*
[b] *Statistical significance was determined using the Mann-Whitney U-test (two-tailed) and a p-value <0.05 was considered statistically significant. The Benjamini-Hochberg adjustment was applied.*
* *Trimethylamine-N-Oxide.*

< 0.05). Such a result seems in agreement with some recent literature results (22, 25, 26), especially sustaining the association between late surfactant administration (after 2 h of life) and hsPDA, due to the rapid reduction in pulmonary pressure that favors blood flow through PDA (left-to-right shunt), lung hyperflow and ductal persistence (29). Further studies are needed to clarify whether surfactant administration could increase the risk of hsPDA or PDA could have more possibilities to evolve in hsPDA in those preterm neonates with a higher early respiratory impairment at birth, lung hypoxia and alveolar damage, evidenced by an increased need for surfactant and a more severe RDS.

Sepsis and early aminoglycosides administration were not more frequent in one of the two groups of our sample, although in literature neonatal sepsis has been identified as a predisposing factor for hsPDA through systemic inflammation and consequent potential ductal relaxation, both *via* respiratory failure and hypoxia, inflammatory mediators, and eventual aminoglycosides administration (27, 28).

Since aminoglycosides clearance can be reduced in premature neonates, in our NICU we measure the "peak" and "trough" serum levels after administration, to reduce the dose or prolong therapeutic intervals for the following administrations, performing a "tailored" therapeutic regimen (92).

Although renal function could be early impaired by hsPDA (93–95), in our sample, no statistically significant differences in creatinine values within the first 5 days of life occurred in the two groups.

However, serum creatinine increase can be delayed and only occur after a significant kidney injury, not representing a sensible and precocious marker (96).

Metabolomics Discussion

According to our findings, metabolomics pathways characterizing urinary samples collected in the early period after birth seem highly dependent on neonatal probability to develop hsPDA confirmed at 48–72 h of life.

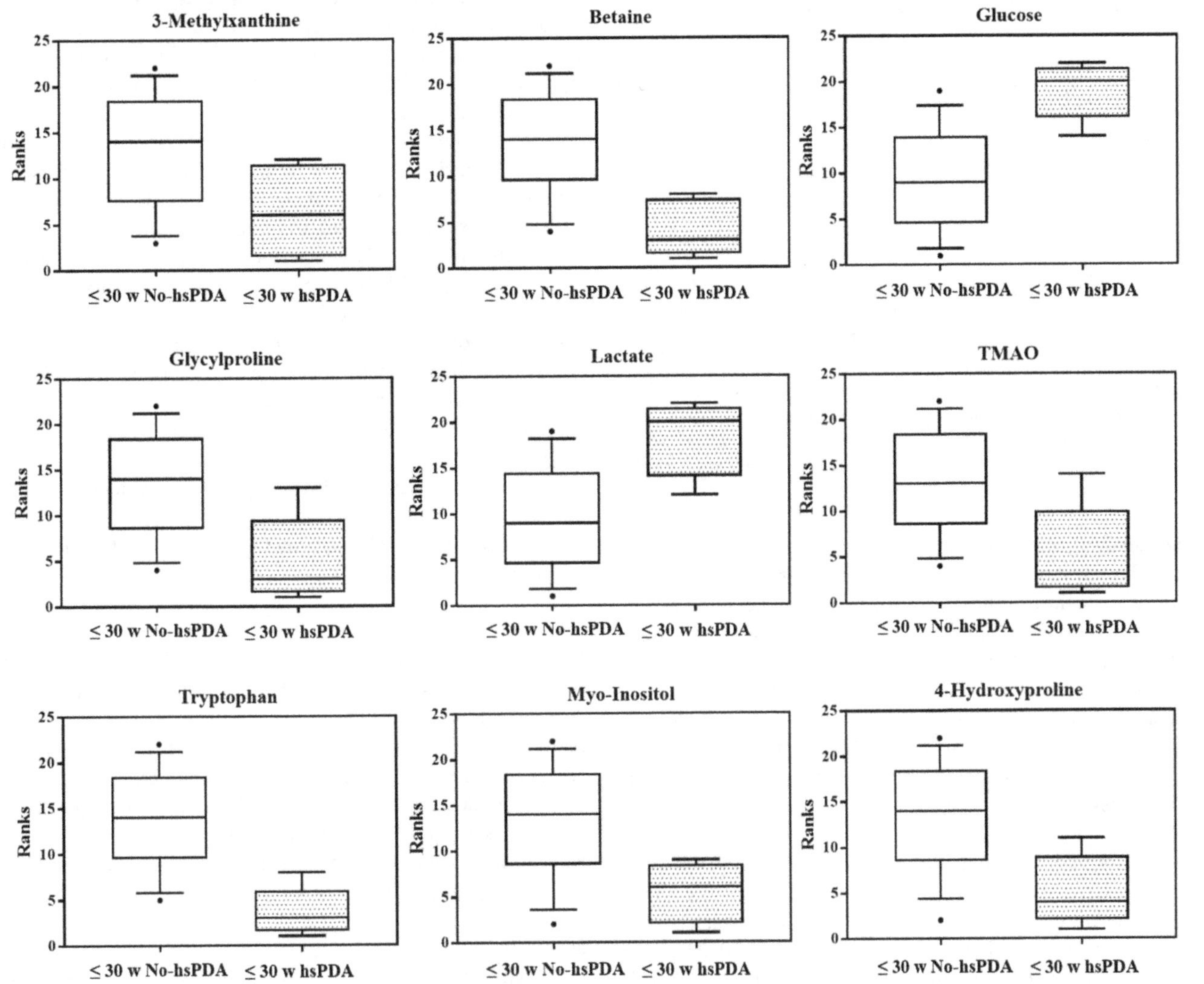

FIGURE 4 | Box-and-whisker plots showing progressive changes of the metabolites concentration on ≤30 w No-hsPDA and ≤30 w hsPDA urine samples. Statistical significance was determined using the Mann-Whitney U-test (two-tailed) and a p-value < 0.05 was considered statistically significant. The Benjamini-Hochberg adjustment was applied.

In detail, analyzing the whole number of urinary samples ($n = 35$) and as evidenced in **Figure 1**, there is a strong separation between the metabolomics profile of those newborns subsequently showing hsPDA ($n = 5/35$, red circles) and neonates no-hsPDA ($n = 30$, blue and green circles). Moreover, this urinary analysis also shows a clear dependence on GA, which increases in the newborns moving from the top to bottom of the plot: in fact, as showed in **Figure 1**, among the neonates no-hsPDA, the subjects represented in blue were born at GA ≤ 30 w ($n = 19/35$), while those represented in green all show GA > 30 w.

From this analysis, it can be deduced that urinary samples at birth are strongly different in neonates subsequently developing hsPDA, all showing GA ≤ 30 w ($n = 5/35$) and therefore well-separated in the plot from the whole sample of the neonates no-hsPDA ($n = 30$, including ≤ 30 w no-hsPDA, $n = 19$, and GA > 30 w, $n = 11$) and even located in the upper half area of the plot with neonates GA ≤ 30 w. In fact, the lower half of the plot is almost exclusively populated by neonates with GA > 30 w and the lower half of the plot is occupied by neonates of GA ≤ 30 w ($n = 24/35$ in total) with the aforementioned clear separation between ≤30 no-hsPDA (blue) and ≤30 w hsPDA.

The clear separation between urinary profiles of neonates hsPDA ($n = 5/35$, in red) and no-hsPDA ($n = 30/35$ if taking into account GA ≤ 30 w and GA > 30 w together, black circles) can be also observed in the plot of **Supplementary Figure 2.**

However, although we initially selected our population study according to the range of GA 24–32 weeks and therefore included in the analysis $n = 35$ subjects, we observed that none of the newborns GA > 30 w developed hsPDA. HsPDA was diagnosed only in newborns GA ≤ 30 w. Thus, observing a metabolomics dependence of our samples on GA, as reported and discussed for **Figure 1**, we decided to exclude those neonates GA > 30 w from

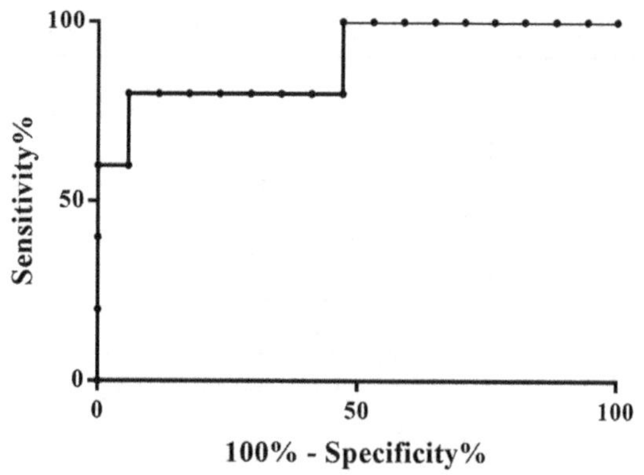

FIGURE 5 | Representative ROC curves based on metabolites with p-value < 0.01 between ≤30 w No-hsPDA and ≤30 w hsPDA subjects. AUC: 0.894; Standard Error: 0.09; 95% CI: 0.717–1; p-value: 0.0087.

further analysis, reducing our sample to those neonates GA ≤ 30 w, to have a more homogeneous population in terms of GA and to improve the significance of our metabolomics comparison between neonates developing hsPDA (≤30 w hsPDA) and those not developing hsPDA (≤30 w no-hsPDA).

By the multivariate analysis of the urine spectra, as evidenced in **Figure 2**, a clear separation between urinary metabolomics profiles between ≤30 w no-hsPDA (black circles) vs. ≤30 w hsPDA (red circles), occurred and represents one of the most important results of our study.

Moreover, in the plot, $n = 2/19$ subjects of the ≤30 w no-hsPDA group, although localized in the appropriate area of the plot (no-hsPDA) seem mildly distant from the other samples. Interestingly, they showed some unique clinical features, represented by a congenital viral infection of the TORCH group in one subject and early pulmonary hypertension treated with NO immediately after birth in the second.

Additionally, we decided to quantify the most characterizing metabolites responsible for sample separation. As reported in the results, the ≤30 w hsPDA group was characterized by lower levels of 3-methylxanthine, betaine, glycylproline, TMAO, tryptophan, myoinositol and 4-hydroxyproline, and higher levels of glucose and lactate.

Firstly, we considered the potential interference of drugs in our group of neonates, by evaluating all the molecules and excipients administered (antibiotics, vitamins, parenteral nutrition, and other eventual drugs). Timing and modality of sampling were standardized and all the newborns underwent the same nutrition regimen.

Then, we tried to give a meaning to metabolomics variations, taking into account that there are not similar studies in literature.

Lactate

The significantly higher levels of urinary lactate observed in hsPDA group could be determined by the increase in anaerobic glycolysis following oxygen reduction and ischemia, with lactate being the end product of anaerobic metabolism (97, 98). We should understand if anaerobic metabolism determining lactate increase could be related to perinatal asphyxia and RDS, as reported by Ma et al. (99), or could be an early consequence of ductal steal and blood flow through PDA determining systemic hypoperfusion or depend on a not fully clarified interplay of these two mechanisms.

Lactate could also represent a compensatory and protective metabolite facing the increase in oxidative stress induced by reperfusion after ischemic damage, potentially lowering the levels of reactive oxygen species and superoxide anion (97, 98).

Lactate increase, following hypoperfusion and lactic acidosis by ductal steal, could also be one of the causes sustaining hsPDA, *via* the effects of acidosis and oxidant mechanisms linked to reperfusion on vasodilation and ductal relaxation (63).

Systemic hypoperfusion involves most organs including the brain; in this regard, the neuroprotective action of lactate, especially facing cerebral ischemia, was recently reported (100–106).

In some experiments involving animal models, hypoxic-ischemic encephalopathy was followed by an increased local level of lactate and glucose, sustaining their potential role as neuroprotectors (107, 108).

Glucose

In our hsPDA neonates, we observed a significant urinary increase in glucose levels. We hypothesized that glucose excretion, following its serum increase, could be determined by an increased stimulation of glucose-alanine cycle, since hypoxia-associated stress and an increased energy request could stimulate cortisol endogenous production (97). In hsPDA patients, a precocious ductal diastolic steal, even at birth, could be associated with an increase in oxygen consumption, also favored by RDS, influencing oxygen and glucose metabolism.

Myoinositol

It is synthesized from glucose-6-phosphate and represents a precursor of inositol (109). Intracellular myoinositol, a second messenger of insulin, was identified as a potential biomarker of impaired glucose metabolism (109–112).

Several factors regulate maternal, cord blood and neonatal myoinositol levels (110). Urinary levels of such metabolite at birth were identified as biomarkers of IUGR (112).

Since maternal myoinositol supplementation was shown to prevent neonatal hypoglycemia (110, 113), we hypothesized that urinary reduction of such metabolite in our hsPDA sample could be related to an increase in energy metabolism and glucose need.

Moreover, we suppose that its reduction could depend on alteration in glucose metabolism, possibly following a higher energy request.

During fetal life, myoinositol can increase to face oxidative stress in a low-oxigen environment (114, 115). Thus, we can also hypothesize that such metabolite is more consumed in hsPDA neonates, and therefore less excreted at urinary level, to improve antioxidant activity.

Finally, since myoinositol can also modify surfactant composition (110), our sampe of hsPDA neonates could have suffered of a more severe RDS at birth due to modifications in surfactant quality.

Betaine and TMAO

Betaine was significantly lower in hsPDA group. This metabolite, involved in several processes, derives from choline oxidation and acts as a methyl groups donor, also taking part in DNA methylation and signal transduction (97). It also serves as methyl donor for homocysteine during convertion into methionine; it can be assumed with diet or be synthesized through choline oxidation (109).

A potential link was observed between betaine ingestion and TMAO circulating levels, with pathways involving gut microbiota (116).

Among the intestinal microbes able to produce TMAO, we cite *A. hydrogenalis, C. asparagiforme, C. hateway* and others (117, 118).

Thus, the reduction in TMAO and betaine levels in our group of preterm hsPDA neonates, instead of no-hsPDA controls, seems to depend on modifications involving gut microbiota, due to the close link between these two metabolites and their interplay influencing intestinal microbes, in a not fully clarified way. This was also previously demonstrated in a metabolomics study on neonates developing BPD (97).

TMAO levels could be significantly influenced by antibiotics, due to their action on intestinal microflora (117).

However, in our group of neonates, no differences occurred in the administered antibiotics and dosages pro kilogram. Moreover, kidney function and creatinine levels did not show significant differences between the two groups, refuting the hypothesis of altered antibiotic metabolism.

TMAO and myoinositol urinary levels have been proposed to increase in case of renal dysfunction (98, 119–123).

Thus, we would have expected an increase in their levels in hsPDA neonates. On the contrary, they were significantly reduced, in disagreement with the hypothesis of a precocious kidney damage following ductal steal and renal hypoperfusion. In addition, the good creatinine levels observed in our hsPDA group, without significant differences instead of no-hsPDA group, would not sustain this hypothesis.

Tryptophan

It is an essential aminoacid taking part in several metabolic processes, such as nitrogen balance, growth, and production of niacin (a precursor of serotonin).

Tryptophan is mostly metabolized through the kynurenine pathway (90%); the 3% is converted into serotonin (5-OH-tryptamine) and the remaining quote undergoes intestinal microbiota degradation with production of indole and its derivatives (124).

Alterations in one of these processes could determine several effects in neuronal metabolic pathways.

Tryptophan and kynurenine could pass the blood-brain barrier and determine anti-inflammatory, immunosuppressive and antioxidant functions with neuroprotective actions (124).

We should also underline that tryptophan is reduced in neuroinflammatory diseases and neuroblastoma (124, 125), Alzheimer's and Parkinson's diseases (126, 127) and increased in neuropsychiatric disorders, such as autism (128).

In our sample, we speculated that reduced levels of such metabolite in the urines of hsPDA neonates could be related to cerebral hypoperfusion; the resulting oxidative/ischemic or inflammatory damage could determine an increase in tryptophan transport to the brain, with a reduced excretion of such metabolite, to improve neuroprotective effects. However, such compensatory mechanisms still need to be verified and eventually clarified.

Finally, the reduction observed in tryptophan level could also be related to microbial alterations, potentially modulating brain function.

4-Hydroxyproline

It is a major constituent of collagen, contributing to its stabilization, and elastin. It is a non-essential aminoacid derived by hydroxylation of proline.

The increase in hydroxyproline levels (serum or urine) can be related to muscle damage (129) and collagen catabolism (bone reabsorption or tissue damage), even in response to oxidant stress. Such metabolite can be found altered in depression, Alzheimer disease and inborn errors of metabolism (130).

Glycylproline

This metabolite is a dipeptide composed by glycine and proline; it is involved in collagen metabolism. It can be mostly found in cytoplasm and it was correlated with Alzheimer's disease and inborn metabolic disorders too (131).

3-Methylxanthine

It is one of the xanthine purine derivatives compounds; it can be mostly found in cytoplasm (132).

In humans, 3-methylxanthine, adenosine agonist, is a metabolite of theophylline (133) and caffeine (134), undergoes renal excretion without modifications (135).

In our sample, urinary 3-methylxantine can derive from the metabolism of caffeine administered to prevent prematurity-related apnea.

This metabolite, although not representing the most significant among our findings, was reduced in urinary samples of hsPDA neonates.

The newborns of the two groups (no-hsPDA and hsPDA) assumed the same dose of caffeine, thus the reason of such different excretions is not clear.

According to literature data, caffeine and theophylline metabolism are influenced by hepathic and renal function, in addition to some cytochrome polymorphisms (136).

The exact meaning of the decrease in 4-hydroxyproline, glycyproline and 3-methylxanthine in our sample of hsPDA neonates still requires clarification.

In conclusion, the early evaluation of neonatal urine to predict at birth the subsequent development of hsPDA should include the three "top metabolites" (glucose, thryptophan, and TMAO), which resulted the most significant in our preliminary results ($p < 0.01$). According to our study, we can affirm that the increase in glucose and the decrease in tryptophan and TMAO resulted the best predictors of hsPDA.

It would be interesting, even if not clinically appropriate, to perform brain magnetic resonance spectroscopy (MRS) to assess if biochemical changes in the brain agree with the urinary variations reported.

According to our results, metabolomics seems to have the unique ability to predict, in a sensible and specific way, those preterm newborns who will undergo physiological closure of DA or will maintain a no-hsPDA, instead of those neonates who will develop a hsPDA confirmed at 48–72 h of life, only through a non-invasive collection of a small urine sample at birth undergoing ^{1}H-NMR evaluation.

We underline that our analysis was performed on the urine of the first 12 h of life and the metabolomics results can be considered a portrait of the metabolic basal status of each newborn. The role in predicting the subsequent development of hsPDA, if confirmed in future studies on a larger cohort of patients, could represent a unique peculiarity of metabolomics, able to individuate those newborns more predisposed to hsPDA before the occurrence of lung hyperflow clinical signs.

Such metabolomics approach could have the promising role to help in predicting those neonates who could develop hsPDA, preventing delay in therapeutic treatment, at the same time avoiding treatment to those who probably would not require it due to the spontaneous ductal closure.

This is the first time that metabolomics was applied in the early detection of hsPDA, and we decided to evaluate urinary samples due to the non-invasiveness of urine collection, being performed in the first hours after birth, and even taking into account the experience of our research group on urinary metabolomics in neonatology (97, 109, 137–140).

In our opinion, this kind of experimental study opens the way for future studies on a greater number of samples, possibly also multicenter studies, and the results, if confirmed, could lead to the individualization of clinical approaches in such field.

The analysis of seriate urinary samples before, during and after treatment, in subjects developing hsPDA, could help in detecting potential biomarkers predicting therapy response or drug toxicity, allowing physicians to choose in a personalized way the drug to administer, and potentially reducing side effects and improving treatment efficacy.

Thus, we strongly believe that, in the near future, such preliminary results could acquire a clinical and therapeutic meaning in improving hsPDA treatment. Such an innovative approach would result very differently from generalized therapeutic prophylaxis, that can determine side effects of complications even in those subjects who will have spontaneously achieved ductal closure.

The exact meaning of the metabolomics variation in our sample still requires a full comprehension since we only made some hypotheses and clinical speculation on the basis of what is currently known oh hsPDA pathophysiology.

In fact, this is the first available study on such a topic and our results, although promising, are preliminary reports on a limited number of samples that should be confirmed on larger groups.

However, despite these limitations, we believe that metabolomics is highly promising in the field of hsPDA, providing a combination of specific metabolites, also considering that, despite years of study on this topic, sensible and specific markers of such a condition are still lacking. In our opinion, the predictive power of metabolomics could result as potentially superior to the clinical or laboratory predictive tools explored to date.

CONCLUSIONS

If our preliminary data will be confirmed, in the future, a simple and non-invasive urinary stick at birth could gave relevant and predictive information on the spontaneous closure or persistence of ductus arteriosus. This could be highly promising, given the great impact of such condition on immediate and long-term health, even taking into account the concept of perinatal programming. Metabolomics approach could help the clinicians to orient their therapeutic strategies in the management of such vulnerable newborns, early identifying those who could develop a hsPDA and therefore avoiding delaying treatment in such subjects, as well as, at the same time, identifying groups of newborns in which this condition is unlikely to occur and the therapy would therefore result in an overtreatment, not exempt from toxicity and side effects.

In our opinion, it could be useful to perform a subsequent study to confirm these data on larger samples and even to evaluate urinary profiles in relation to the kind, timing, and response to the treatment.

If these results will be confirmed, metabolomics could become a good tool in the early detection of hsPSA neonates, showing a stronger predictive power than clinical findings and laboratory parameters investigated to date, to optimize their management thanks to specific and holistic biomarkers in a field currently full of controversies.

ETHICS STATEMENT

The studies involving human participants were reviewed and approved by Ethic Committee University of Cagliari. Written informed consent to participate in this study was provided by the participants' legal guardian/next of kin.

AUTHOR CONTRIBUTIONS

FB selected the patients, collected urinary samples, reviewed literature, and wrote the manuscript. CP performed metabolomics experiments, metabolomics data analysis, and wrote the manuscript. PN and AA contributed in writing the manuscript and performed echocardiograms. VF supervised the whole experiment and critically revised the manuscript. All authors contributed to the article and approved the submitted version.

SUPPLEMENTARY MATERIAL

Supplementary Figure 1 | Validation plots of OPLS-DA model (≤30 w No-hsPDA, >30 w No-hsPDA and ≤30 w hsPDA) using a permutation test. The horizontal axis shows the correlation between the permuted and actual data, while the vertical axis displays the cumulative values of R_2 and Q_2. The intercept gives an estimate of the overfitting phenomenon.

Supplementary Figure 2 | OPLS-DA scores plot of ^{1}H NMR spectra of urine samples: ≤30 w No-hsPDA and >30 w No-hsPDA (black circle), and ≤30 w hsPDA (red circle).

Supplementary Figure 3 | Validation plots of OPLS-DA model (≤ and >30 w No-hsPDA and ≤30 w hsPDA) using a permutation test. The horizontal axis shows the correlation between the permuted and actual data, while the vertical axis displays the cumulative values of R_2 and Q_2. The intercept gives an estimate of the overfitting phenomenon.

Supplementary Figure 4 | Validation plots of OPLS-DA model (≤30 w No-hsPDA and ≤30 w hsPDA) using a permutation test. The horizontal axis shows the correlation between the permuted and actual data, while the vertical axis displays the cumulative values of R_2 and Q_2. The intercept gives an estimate of the overfitting phenomenon.

REFERENCES

1. Bardanzellu F, Neroni P, Dessì A, Fanos V. Paracetamol in patent ductus arteriosus treatment: efficacious and safe? *Biomed Res Int.* (2017) 2017:1438038. doi: 10.1155/2017/1438038
2. Hundscheid T, van den Broek M, van der Lee R, de Boode WP. Understanding the pathobiology in patent ductus arteriosus in prematurity-beyond prostaglandins and oxygen. *Pediatr Res.* (2019) 86:28–38. doi: 10.1038/s41390-019-0387-7
3. Ovali F. Molecular and mechanical mechanisms regulating ductus arteriosus closure in preterm infants. *Front Pediatr.* (2020) 8:516. doi: 10.3389/fped.2020.00516
4. Kahvecioglu D, Erdeve O, Akduman H, Ucar T, Alan S, Çakir U, et al. Influence of platelet count, platelet mass index, and platelet function on the spontaneous closure of ductus arteriosus in the prematurity. *Pediatr Neonatol.* (2018) 59:53–57. doi: 10.1016/j.pedneo.2017.01.006
5. Engur D. Regarding platelets and ductus: is it platelet function rather than number that matters for ductal closure? *Pediatr Neonatol.* (2018) 59:640–1. doi: 10.1016/j.pedneo.2018.08.006
6. Gonzalez A, Sosenko IR, Chandar J, Hummler H, Claure N, Bancalari E. Influence of infection on patent ductus arteriosus and chronic lung disease in premature infants weighing 1000 grams or less. *J Pediatr.* (1996) 128:470–8. doi: 10.1016/S0022-3476(96)70356-6
7. Benitz WE, Committee on Fetus and Newborn, American Academy of Pediatrics. Patent ductus arteriosus in preterm infants. *Pediatrics.* (2016) 137:e20153730. doi: 10.1542/peds.2015-3730
8. de Klerk JCA, Engbers AGJ, van Beek F, Flint RB, Reiss IKM,Völler S, et al. Spontaneous closure of the ductus arteriosus in preterm infants: a systematic review. *Front Pediatr.* (2020) 8:541. doi: 10.3389/fped.2020.00541
9. Cuzzolin L, Dal Cerè M, Fanos V. NSAID-induced nephrotoxicity from the fetus to the child. *Drug Saf.* (2001) 24:9–18. doi: 10.2165/00002018-200124010-00002
10. Mitra S, Florez ID, Tamayo ME, Mbuagbaw L, Vanniyasingam T, Veroniki AA, et al. Association of placebo, indomethacin, ibuprofen, and acetaminophen with closure of hemodynamically significant patent ductus arteriosus in preterm infants: a systematic review and meta-analysis. *JAMA.* (2018) 319:1221–38. doi: 10.1001/jama.2018.1896
11. Farooqui MA, Elsayed YN, Jeyaraman MM, Dingwall O, Tagin M, Zarychanski R, et al. Pre-symptomatic targeted treatment of patent ductus arteriosus in preterm newborns: a systematic review and meta-analysis. *J Neonatal Perinatal Med.* (2019) 12:1–7. doi: 10.3233/NPM-17130
12. Marconi E, Bettiol A, Ambrosio G, Perduca V, Vannacci A, Troiani S, et al. Efficacy and safety of pharmacological treatments for patent ductus arteriosus closure: a systematic review and network meta-analysis of clinical trials and observational studies. *Pharmacol Res.* (2019) 148:104418. doi: 10.1016/j.phrs.2019.104418
13. Ohlsson A, Shah SS. Ibuprofen for the prevention of patent ductus arteriosus in preterm and/or low birth weight infants. *Cochrane Database Syst Rev.* (2019) 6:CD004213. doi: 10.1002/14651858.CD004213.pub4
14. Ohlsson A, Shah PS. Paracetamol (acetaminophen) for patent ductus arteriosus in preterm or low birth weight infants. *Cochrane Database Syst Rev.* (2020) 1:CD010061. doi: 10.1002/14651858.CD010061.pub4
15. de Waal K, Phad N, Stubbs M, Chen Y, Kluckow M. A randomized placebo-controlled pilot trial of early targeted non-steroidal anti-inflammatory drugs in preterm infants with a patent ductus arteriosus. *J Pediatr.* (2020) 25:S0022-3476(20)31098-2. doi: 10.1016/j.jpeds.2020.08.062
16. Clyman RI, Liebowitz M. Treatment and nontreatment of the patent ductus arteriosus: identifying their roles in neonatal morbidity. *J Pediatr.* (2017) 189:13–7. doi: 10.1016/j.jpeds.2017.06.054
17. Ficial B, Corsini I, Fiocchi S, Schena F, Capolupo I, Cerbo RM, et al. Survey of PDA management in very low birth weight infants across Italy. *Ital J Pediatr.* (2020) 46:22. doi: 10.1186/s13052-020-0773-0
18. Dani C, Mosca F, Cresi F, Lago P, Lista G, Laforgia N, et al. Patent ductus arteriosus in preterm infants born at 23-24 weeks' gestation: should we pay more attention? *Early Hum Dev.* (2019) 135:16–22. doi: 10.1016/j.earlhumdev.2019.06.002
19. Lewis TR, Shelton EL, Van Driest SL, Kannankeril PJ, Reese J. Genetics of the patent ductus arteriosus (PDA) and pharmacogenetics of PDA treatment. *Semin Fetal Neonatal Med.* (2018) 23:232–8. doi: 10.1016/j.siny.2018.02.006
20. Dagle JM, Ryckman KK, Spracklen CN, Momany AM, Cotten CM, Levy J, et al. Genetic variants associated with patent ductus arteriosus in extremely preterm infants. *J Perinatol.* (2019) 39:401–8. doi: 10.1038/s41372-018-0285-6
21. Dagle JM, Lepp NT, Cooper ME, Schaa KL, Kelsey KJ, Orr KL, et al. Determination of genetic predisposition to patent ductus arteriosus in preterm infants. *Pediatrics.* (2009) 123:1116–23. doi: 10.1542/peds.2008-0313
22. Lee JA, Sohn JA, Oh S, Choi BM. Perinatal risk factors of symptomatic preterm patent ductus arteriosus and secondary ligation. *Pediatr Neonatol.* (2020) 61:439–46. doi: 10.1016/j.pedneo.2020.03.016
23. Park HW, Choi YS, Kim KS, Kim SN. Chorioamnionitis and patent ductus arteriosus: a systematic review and meta-analysis. *PLoS ONE.* (2015) 10:e0138114. doi: 10.1371/journal.pone.0138114
24. Behbodi E, Villamor-Martínez E, Degraeuwe PL, Villamor E. Chorioamnionitis appears not to be a risk factor for patent ductus arteriosus in preterm infants: a systematic review and meta-analysis. *Sci Rep.* (2016) 6:37967. doi: 10.1038/srep37967
25. Pourarian S, Farahbakhsh N, Sharma D, Cheriki S, Bijanzadeh F. Prevalence and risk factors associated with the patency of ductus arteriosus in premature neonates: a prospective observational study from Iran. *J Matern Fetal Neonatal Med.* (2017) 30:1460–4. doi: 10.1080/14767058.2016.1219991
26. Wu YH, Chang SW, Chen CC, Liu HY, Lai YJ, Huang EY, et al. Differential determinants of patent ductus arteriosus closure for prematurity of varying birth body weight: a retrospective cohort study. *Pediatr Neonatol.* (2020) 5:S1875-9572(20)30091-7. doi: 10.1016/j.pedneo.2020.05.011
27. Vucovich MM, Cotton RB, Shelton EL, Goettel JA, Ehinger NJ, Poole SD, et al. Aminoglycoside-mediated relaxation of the ductus arteriosus in sepsis-associated PDA. *Am J Physiol Heart Circ Physiol.* (2014) 307:H732–40. doi: 10.1152/ajpheart.00838.2013
28. Reese J, Veldman A, Shah L, Vucovich M, Cotton RB. Inadvertent relaxation of the ductus arteriosus by pharmacologic agents that are commonly used in the neonatal period. *Semin Perinatol.* (2010) 34:222–30. doi: 10.1053/j.semperi.2010.02.007
29. Canpolat FE, Kadioglu Simşek G, Webbe J, Büyüktiryaki M, Karaçaglar NB, Elbayiyev S, et al. Late administration of surfactant may increase the risk of patent ductus arteriosus. *Front Pediatr.* (2020) 8:130. doi: 10.3389/fped.2020.00130
30. Fridman E, Mangel L, Mandel D, Beer G, Kapusta L, Marom R. Effects of maternal aspirin treatment on hemodynamically significant patent ductus

arteriosus in preterm infants—pilot study. *J Matern Fetal Neonatal Med* (2020) 6:1–6. doi: 10.1080/14767058.2020.1736028

31. Henderson JT, Whitlock EP, O'Connor E, Senger CA, Thompson JH, Rowland MG. Low-dose aspirin for prevention of morbidity and mortality from preeclampsia: a systematic evidence review for the U.S. Preventive Services Task Force. *Ann Intern Med.* (2014) 160:695–703. doi: 10.7326/M13-2844
32. American College of Obstetricians and Gynecologists, Task Force on Hypertension in Pregnancy. Hypertension in pregnancy. Report of the American College of Obstetricians and Gynecologists' Task Force on Hypertension in Pregnancy. *Obstet Gynecol.* (2013) 122:1122–31. doi: 10.1097/01.AOG.0000437382.03963.88
33. World Health Organization. *WHO Recommendations for Prevention and Treatment of Pre-eclampsia and Eclampsia.* Geneva: World Health Organization (2011).
34. Karlowicz MG, White LE. Severe intracranial hemorrhage in a term neonate associated with maternal acetylsalicylic acid ingestion. *Clin Pediatr (Phila)* (1993) 32:740–3. doi: 10.1177/000992289303201206
35. Di Sessa TG, Moretti ML, Khoury A, Pulliam DA, Arheart KL, Sibai BM. Cardiac function in fetuses and newborns exposed to low-dose aspirin during pregnancy. *Am J Obstet Gynecol.* (1994) 171:892–900. doi: 10.1016/S0002-9378(94)70056-7
36. Qasim A, Jain SK, Aly AM. Antenatal magnesium sulfate exposure and hemodynamically significant patent ductus arteriosus in premature infants. *AJP Rep.* (2019) 9:e353–6. doi: 10.1055/s-0039-3400316
37. Kishibuchi A, Akaike T, Minamisawa S. Standard-dose gentamicin does not increase risk of patent ductus arteriosus. *Pediatr Neonatol.* (2020) 61:45–50. doi: 10.1016/j.pedneo.2019.05.011
38. Thompson EJ, Greenberg RG, Kumar K, Laughon M, Smith PB, Clark RH, et al. Association between furosemide exposure and patent ductus arteriosus in hospitalized infants of very low birth weight. *J Pediatr.* (2018) 199:231–6. doi: 10.1016/j.jpeds.2018.03.067
39. Simon SR, van Zogchel L, Bas-Suárez MP, Cavallaro G, Clyman RI, Villamor E. Platelet counts and patent ductus arteriosus in preterm infants: a systematic review and meta-analysis. *Neonatology.* (2015) 108:143–51. doi: 10.1159/000431281
40. Akar S, Topcuoglu S, Tuten A, Ozalkaya E, Karatepe HO, Gokmen T, et al. Is the first postnatal platelet mass as an indicator of patent ductus arteriosus? *Arch Iran Med.* (2019) 22:687–91.
41. Guler Kazanci E, Buyuktiryaki M, Unsal H, Tayman C. Useful platelet indices for the diagnosis and follow-up of patent ductus arteriosus. *Am J Perinatol* (2019) 36:1521–7. doi: 10.1055/s-0039-1688821
42. Demirel G, Yilmaz A, Vatansever B, Tastekin A. Is high platelet distribution width in the first hours of life can predict hemodynamically significant patent ductus arteriosus in preterm newborns? *J Matern Fetal Neonatal Med.* (2020) 33:2049–53. doi: 10.1080/14767058.2018.1536743
43. Karabulut B, Arcagök BC, Simsek A. Utility of the platelet-to-lymphocyte ratio in diagnosing and predicting treatment success in preterm neonates with patent ductus arteriosus. *Fetal Pediatr Pathol.* (2019) 9:1–10. doi: 10.1080/15513815.2019.1686786
44. Temel MT, Coskun ME, Akbayram S, Demiryürek AT. Association between neutrophil/lymphocyte ratio with ductus arteriosus patency in preterm newborns. *Bratisl Lek Listy.* (2017) 118:491–4. doi: 10.4149/BLL_2017_094
45. Sallmon H, Metze B, Koehne P, Opgen-Rhein B, Weiss K, Will JC, et al. Mature and immature platelets during the first week after birth and incidence of patent ductus arteriosus. *Cardiol Young.* (2020) 30:769–73. doi: 10.1017/S1047951120000943
46. Özer Bekmez B, Tayman C, Büyüktiryaki M, Çetinkaya AK, Çakir U, Derme T. A promising, novel index in the diagnosis and follow-up of patent ductus arteriosus: red cell distribution width-to-platelet ratio. *J Clin Lab Anal.* (2018) 32:e22616. doi: 10.1002/jcla.22616
47. Ghirardello S, Raffaeli G, Crippa BL, Gulden S, Amodeo I, Consonni D, et al. The thromboelastographic profile at birth in very preterm newborns with patent ductus arteriosus. *Neonatology.* (2020) 2:1–8. doi: 10.1159/000507553
48. Kaur S, Stritzke A, Soraisham AS. Does postmenstrual age affect medical patent ductus arteriosus treatment success in preterm infants? *Am J Perinatol.* (2019) 36:1504–9. doi: 10.1055/s-0039-1678555
49. Smith CJ, Ryckman KK, Bahr TM, Dagle JM. Polymorphisms in CYP2C9 are associated with response to indomethacin among neonates with patent ductus arteriosus. *Pediatr Res.* (2017) 82:776–80. doi: 10.1038/pr.2017.145
50. Tan ZH, Baral VR. Principles of clinical management of patent ductus arteriosus in extremely preterm neonates. *Curr Pediatr Rev.* (2016) 12:83–97. doi: 10.2174/1573396312021605060O1309
51. Abdel-Hady H, Nasef N, Shabaan AE, Nour I. Patent ductus arteriosus in preterm infants: do we have the right answers? *Biomed Res Int.* (2013) 2013:676192. doi: 10.1155/2013/676192
52. Liu Y, Huang ZL, Gong L, Zhang Z, Zhang SC, Zhou YX. N-terminal pro-brain natriuretic peptide used for screening hemodynamically significant patent ductus arteriosus in very low birth weight infants: how and when? *Clin Hemorheol Microcirc.* (2020) 75:335–47. doi: 10.3233/CH-190803
53. Oh SH, Lee BS, Jung E, Oh MY, Do HJ, Kim EA, et al. Plasma B-type natriuretic peptide cannot predict treatment response to ibuprofen in preterm infants with patent ductus arteriosus. *Sci Rep.* (2020) 10:4430. doi: 10.1038/s41598-020-61291-w
54. Halil H, Tayman C, Cakir U, Buyuktiryaki M, Serkant U, Oguz SS. Serum endocan level as a predictive marker for hemodynamically significant patent ductus arteriosus in very low birth weight infants. *Am J Perinatol.* (2017) 34:1312–7. doi: 10.1055/s-0037-1603509
55. Rodriguez-Blanco S, Oulego-Erroz I, Gautreaux-Minaya S, Perez-Muñuzuri A, Couce-Pico ML. Early NT-proBNP levels as a screening tool for the detection of hemodynamically significant patent ductus arteriosus during the first week of life in very low birth weight infants. *J Perinatol.* (2018) 38:881–8. doi: 10.1038/s41372-018-0123-x
56. Harris SL, More K, Dixon B, Troughton R, Pemberton C, Horwood J, et al. Factors affecting N-terminal pro-B-type natriuretic peptide levels in preterm infants and use in determination of haemodynamic significance of patent ductus arteriosus. *Eur J Pediatr.* (2018) 177:521–32. doi: 10.1007/s00431-018-3089-y
57. Asrani P, Aly AM, Jiwani AK, Niebuhr BR, Christenson RH, Jain SK. High-sensitivity troponin T in preterm infants with a hemodynamically significant patent ductus arteriosus. *J Perinatol.* (2018) 38:1483–9. doi: 10.1038/s41372-018-0192-x
58. Montaner Ramón A, Galve Pradel Z, Fernández Espuelas C, Jiménez Montañés L, Samper Villagrasa MP, Rite Gracia S. Utilidad del propéptido natriurético cerebral en el diagnóstico y manejo del ductus arterioso permeable (Usefulness of brain natriuretic propeptide in the diagnosis and management of patent ductus arteriosus). *An Pediatr (Barc).* (2017) 86:321–8. doi: 10.1016/j.anpedi.2016.01.007
59. Shin J, Lee EH, Lee JH, Choi BM, Hong YS. Individualized ibuprofen treatment using serial B-type natriuretic peptide measurement for symptomatic patent ductus arteriosus in very preterm infants. *Korean J Pediatr.* (2017) 60:175–80. doi: 10.3345/kjp.2017.60.6.175
60. Okur N, Tayman C, Büyüktiryaki M, Kadioglu Simşek G, Ozer Bekmez B, Altug N. Can lactate levels be used as a marker of patent ductus arteriosus in preterm babies? *J Clin Lab Anal.* (2019) 33:e22664. doi: 10.1002/jcla.22664
61. Cakir U, Tayman C, Buyuktiryaki M, Unsal H, Ozer Bekmez B. Do calcium and potassium levels influence ductal patency in preterm infants? *Am J Perinatol.* (2020) 37:1123–9. doi: 10.1055/s-0039-1692389
62. Cakir U, Tayman C. A mystery of patent ductus arteriosus and serum osmolality in preterm infants. *Am J Perinatol.* (2019) 36:641–6. doi: 10.1055/s-0038-1673397
63. Mydam J, Rastogi A, Naheed ZJ. Base excess and hematocrit predict response to indomethacin in very low birth weight infants with patent ductus arteriosus. *Ital J Pediatr.* (2019) 45:107. doi: 10.1186/s13052-019-0706-y
64. Mitra S, Chan AK, Paes BA; Thrombosis and Hemostasis in Newborns (THIN) Group. The association of platelets with failed patent ductus arteriosus closure after a primary course of indomethacin or ibuprofen: a systematic review and meta-analysis. *J Matern Fetal Neonatal Med.* (2017) 30:127–33. doi: 10.3109/14767058.2016.1163684
65. Sallmon H, Weber SC, Dirks J, Schiffer T, Klippstein T, Stein A, et al. Association between platelet counts before and during pharmacological therapy for patent ductus arteriosus and treatment failure in preterm infants. *Front Pediatr.* (2018) 6:41. doi: 10.3389/fped.2018.00041

66. Kumar J, Dutta S, Sundaram V, Saini SS, Sharma RR, Varma N. Platelet transfusion for PDA closure in preterm infants: a randomized controlled trial. *Pediatrics.* (2019) 143:e20182565. doi: 10.1542/peds.2018-2565
67. Navarro-Guzmán EA, Ledezma-Bautista I, Rubio-Hernández ME, Escalante-Padrón FJ, Lima-Roguel V, Pierdant-Perez M. Correlation of perfusion index with patent ductus arteriosus repercussion in premature newborns. *Arch Cardiol Mex.* (2019) 89:111–7. doi: 10.24875/ACME.M19000033
68. Hou HT, Xi-Zhang, Wang J, Liu LX, Zhang JF, Yang Q, et al. Altered plasma proteins released from platelets and endothelial cells are associated with human patent ductus arteriosus. *J Cell Physiol.* (2019) 234:6842–53. doi: 10.1002/jcp.27433
69. Sellmer A, Bech BH, Bjerre JV, Schmidt MR, Hjortdal VE, Esberg G, et al. Urinary neutrophil gelatinase-associated lipocalin in the evaluation of patent ductus arteriosus and AKI in very preterm neonates: a cohort study. *BMC Pediatr.* (2017) 17:7. doi: 10.1186/s12887-016-0761-0
70. El-Khuffash AF, Slevin M, McNamara PJ, Molloy EJ. Troponin T, N-terminal pro natriuretic peptide and a patent ductus arteriosus scoring system predict death before discharge or neurodevelopmental outcome at 2 years in preterm infants. *Arch Dis Child Fetal Neonatal Ed.* (2011) 96:F133–7. doi: 10.1136/adc.2010.185967
71. Czernik C, Metze B, Müller C, Bührer C. Urinary NT-proBNP and ductal closure in preterm infants. *J Perinatol.* (2013) 33:212–7. doi: 10.1038/jp.2012.86
72. Khan SS, Sithisarn T, Bada HS, Vranicar M, Westgate PM, Hanna M. Urinary NT-proBNP levels and echocardiographic parameters for patent ductus arteriosus. *J Perinatol.* (2017) 37:1319–24. doi: 10.1038/jp.2017.139
73. Vettukattil JJ. Editorial: patent ductus arteriosus in extremely premature neonates. *Curr Pediatr Rev.* (2016) 12:78–82. doi: 10.2174/157339631202160506001001
74. Kulkarni M, Gokulakrishnan G, Price J, Fernandes CJ, Leeflang M, Pammi M. Diagnosing significant PDA using natriuretic peptides in preterm neonates: a systematic review. *Pediatrics.* (2015) 135:e510–25. doi: 10.1542/peds.2014-1995
75. Rostas SE, McPherson CC. Pharmacotherapy for patent ductus arteriosus: current options and outstanding questions. *Curr Pediatr Rev.* (2016) 12:110–9. doi: 10.2174/157339631202160506002028
76. Hillman M, Meinarde L, Rizzotti A, Cuestas E. Inflammation, high-sensitivity C-reactive protein, and persistent patent ductus arteriosus in preterm infants. *Rev Esp Cardiol (Engl Ed).* (2016) 69:84–5. doi: 10.1016/j.rec.2015.09.014
77. Meinarde L, Hillman M, Rizzotti A, Basquiera AL, Tabares A, Cuestas E. C-reactive protein, platelets, and patent ductus arteriosus. *Platelets.* (2016) 27:821–3. doi: 10.1080/09537104.2016.1203398
78. Olsson KW, Larsson A, Jonzon A, Sindelar R. Exploration of potential biochemical markers for persistence of patent ductus arteriosus in preterm infants at 22-27 weeks' gestation. *Pediatr Res.* (2019) 86:333–8. doi: 10.1038/s41390-018-0182-x
79. Inayat M, Bany-Mohammed F, Valencia A, Tay C, Jacinto J, Aranda JV, et al. Antioxidants and biomarkers of oxidative stress in preterm infants with symptomatic patent ductus arteriosus. *Am J Perinatol.* (2015) 32:895–904. doi: 10.1055/s-0035-1544948
80. Coviello C, Tataranno ML, Corsini I, Leonardi V, Longini M, Bazzini F, et al. Isoprostanes as biomarker for patent ductus arteriosus in preterm infants. *Front Pediatr.* (2020) 8:555. doi: 10.3389/fped.2020.00555
81. Bardanzellu F, Fanos V. How could metabolomics change pediatric health? *Ital J Pediatr.* (2020) 46:37. doi: 10.1186/s13052-020-0807-7
82. Fanos V, Pintus R, Dessì A. Clinical metabolomics in neonatology: from metabolites to diseases. *Neonatology.* (2018) 113:406–13. doi: 10.1159/000487620
83. Fanos V, Barberini L, Antonucci R, Atzori L. Pharma-metabolomics in neonatology: is it a dream or a fact? *Curr Pharm Des.* (2012) 18:2996–3006. doi: 10.2174/1381612811209022996
84. Castell Miñana M, Quintás Soriano G, Fernández Tudela B, Vento Torres M. Urinary metabolomics as a new strategy to discriminate response to ibuprofen therapy in preterm neonates with patent ductus arteriosus. In: *Proceedings of the Selected Abstracts of the 8th International Workshop on Neonatology.* Cagliari (2012). p. 111–59.
85. Piras C, Pintus R, Pruna D, Dessì A, Atzori L, Fanos V. Pediatric acute-onset neuropsychiatric syndrome and mycoplasma pneumoniae infection: a case report analysis with a metabolomics approach. *Curr Pediatr Rev.* (2020) 16:183–93. doi: 10.2174/1573396315666191022102925
86. Sousa SAA, Magalhaes A, Ferreira MMC. Optimized bucketing for NMR spectra: three case studies. *Chemometr Intell Lab.* (2013) 122:93–102. doi: 10.1016/j.chemolab.2013.01.006
87. van den Berg RA, Hoefsloot HC, Westerhuis JA, Smilde AK, van der Werf MJ. Centering, scaling, and transformations: improving the biological information content of metabolomics data. *BMC Genomics.* (2006) 7:142. doi: 10.1186/1471-2164-7-142
88. Piras C, Pibiri M, Leoni VP, Cabras F, Restivo A, Griffin JL, et al. Urinary1H-NMR metabolic signature in subjects undergoing colonoscopy for colon cancer diagnosis. *Appl Sci.* (2020) 10:5401. doi: 10.3390/app10165401
89. Piras C, Arisci N, Poddighe S, Liggi S, Mariotti S, Atzori L. Metabolomic profile in hyperthyroid patients before and after antithyroid drug treatment: correlation with thyroid hormone and TSH concentration. *Int J Biochem Cell Biol.* (2017) 93:119–28. doi: 10.1016/j.biocel.2017.07.024
90. Weljie AM, Newton J, Mercier P, Carlson E, Slupsky CM. Targeted profiling: quantitative analysis of 1H NMR metabolomics data. *Anal Chem.* (2006) 78:4430–42. doi: 10.1021/ac060209g
91. Benjamini Y, Hochberg Y. Controlling the false discovery rate: a practical and powerful approach to multiple testing. *J R Stat Soc B (Methodol).* (1995) 57:289–300. doi: 10.1111/j.2517-6161.1995.tb02031.x
92. Testa M, Fanos V, Martinelli V, Stronati M, Mussap M, Del Zompo M. Therapeutic drug monitoring of gentamicin in neonatal intensive care unit: experience in 68 newborns. *J Chemother.* (2007) 19(Suppl. 2):39–41. doi: 10.1080/1120009X.2007.11782443
93. Majed B, Bateman DA, Uy N, Lin F. Patent ductus arteriosus is associated with acute kidney injury in the preterm infant. *Pediatr Nephrol.* (2019) 34:1129–39. doi: 10.1007/s00467-019-4194-5
94. Velazquez DM, Reidy KJ, Sharma M, Kim M, Vega M, Havranek T. The effect of hemodynamically significant patent ductus arteriosus on acute kidney injury and systemic hypertension in extremely low gestational age newborns. *J Matern Fetal Neonatal Med.* (2019) 32:3209–14. doi: 10.1080/14767058.2018.1460349
95. Coffman Z, Steflik D, Chowdhury SM, Twombley K, Buckley J. Echocardiographic predictors of acute kidney injury in neonates with a patent ductus arteriosus. *J Perinatol.* (2020) 40:510–4. doi: 10.1038/s41372-019-0560-1
96. Fanos V, Antonucci R, Zaffanello M, Mussap M. Nenatal drug induced nephrotoxicity: old and next generation biomarkers for early detection and management of neonatal drug-induced nephrotoxicity, with special emphasis on uNGAL and on metabolomics. *Curr Med Chem.* (2012) 19:4595–605. doi: 10.2174/092986712803306439
97. Pintus MC, Lussu M, Dessì A, Pintus R, Noto A, Masile V, et al. Urinary 1H-NMR metabolomics in the first week of life can anticipate BPD diagnosis. *Oxid Med Cell Longev.* (2018) 2018:7620671. doi: 10.1155/2018/7620671
98. Fanos V, Pintus MC, Lussu M, Atzori L, Noto A, Stronati M, et al. Urinary metabolomics of bronchopulmonary dysplasia (BPD): preliminary data at birth suggest it is a congenital disease. *J Matern Fetal Neonatal Med.* (2014) 27(Suppl. 2):39–45. doi: 10.3109/14767058.2014.955966
99. Ma S, Shieh LI, Huang CC. High-resolution proton nuclear magnetic resonance studies of urine from asphyxiated newborn infants. *Appl Biochem Biotechnol.* (1995) 53:37–51. doi: 10.1007/BF02783480
100. Mason S. A novel, multi-faceted perception of lactate in neurology. *Front Neurosci.* (2020) 14:460. doi: 10.3389/fnins.2020.00460
101. Castillo X, Rosafio K, Wyss MT, Drandarov K, Buck A, Pellerin L, et al. A probable dual mode of action for both L- and D-lactate neuroprotection in cerebral ischemia. *J Cereb Blood Flow Metab.* (2015) 35:1561–9. doi: 10.1038/jcbfm.2015.115
102. Mason S. Lactate shuttles in neuroenergetics-homeostasis, allostasis and beyond. *Front Neurosci.* (2017) 11:43. doi: 10.3389/fnins.2017.00043
103. Huang L, Nakamura Y, Lo EH, Hayakawa K. Astrocyte signaling in the neurovascular unit after central nervous system injury. *Int J Mol Sci.* (2019) 20:282. doi: 10.3390/ijms20020282
104. Tauffenberger A, Fiumelli H, Almustafa S, Magistretti PJ. Lactate and pyruvate promote oxidative stress resistance through hormetic ROS

signaling. *Cell Death Dis.* (2019) 10:653. doi: 10.1038/s41419-019-1877-6

105. Vohra R, Kolko M. Lactate: more than merely a metabolic waste product in the inner retina. *Mol Neurobiol.* (2020) 57:2021–37. doi: 10.1007/s12035-019-01863-8
106. Vohra R, Aldana BI, Bulli G, Skytt DM, Waagepetersen H, Bergersen LH, et al. Lactate-mediated protection of retinal ganglion cells. *J Mol Biol.* (2019) 431:1878–88. doi: 10.1016/j.jmb.2019.03.005
107. Zheng Y, Wang XM. Expression changes in lactate and glucose metabolism and associated transporters in basal ganglia following hypoxicischemic reperfusion injury in piglets. *Am J Neuroradiol.* (2018) 39:569–76 doi: 10.3174/ajnr.A5505
108. Oses JP, Müller AP, Strogulski NR, Moreira JD, Böhmer AE, Hansel G, et al. Sustained elevation of cerebrospinal fluid glucose and lactate after a single seizure does not parallel with mitochondria energy production. *Epilepsy Res.* (2019) 152:35–41. doi: 10.1016/j.eplepsyres.2019.03.007
109. Cesare Marincola F, Corbu S, Lussu M, Noto A, Dessì A, Longo S, et al. Impact of early postnatal nutrition on the NMR urinary metabolic profile of infant. *J Proteome Res.* (2016) 15:3712–23. doi: 10.1021/acs.jproteome.6b00537
110. Brion LP, Phelps DL, Ward RM, Nolen TL, Hallman NMK, Das A, et al. Blood myo-inositol concentrations in preterm and term infants. *J Perinatol.* (2020) doi: 10.1038/s41372-020-00799-5. [Epub ahead of print].
111. Dessì A, Fanos V. Myoinositol: a new marker of intrauterine growth restriction? *J Obstet Gynaecol.* (2013) 33:776–80. doi: 10.3109/01443615.2013.831046
112. Dessì A, Marincola FC, Pattumelli MG, Ciccarelli S, Corbu S, Ossicini C, et al. Investigation of the ^{1}H-NMR based urine metabolomic profiles of IUGR, LGA and AGA newborns on the first day of life. *J Matern Fetal Neonatal Med.* (2014) 27(Suppl. 2):13–9. doi: 10.3109/14767058.2014.955674
113. Brown J, Crawford TJ, Alsweiler J, Crowther CA. Dietary supplementation with myo-inositol in women during pregnancy for treating gestational diabetes. *Cochrane Database Syst Rev.* (2016) 9:CD012048. doi: 10.1002/14651858.CD012048.pub2
114. Jauniaux E, Hempstock J, Teng C, Battaglia FC, Burton GJ. Polyol concentrations in the fluid compartments of the human conceptus during the first trimester of pregnancy: maintenance of redox potential in a low oxygen environment. *J Clin Endocrinol Metab.* (2005) 90:1171–5. doi: 10.1210/jc.2004-1513
115. Greene ND, Leung KY, Copp AJ. Inositol, neural tube closure and the prevention of neural tube defects. *Birth Defects Res.* (2017) 109:68–80. doi: 10.1002/bdra.23533
116. Wang Z, Tang WH, Buffa JA, Fu X, Britt EB, Koeth RA, et al. Prognostic value of choline and betaine depends on intestinal microbiota-generated metabolite trimethylamine-N-oxide. *Eur Heart J.* (2014) 35:904–10. doi: 10.1093/eurheartj/ehu002
117. Velasquez MT, Ramezani A, Manal A, Raj DS. Trimethylamine N-oxide: the good, the bad and the unknown. *Toxins (Basel).* (2016) 8:326. doi: 10.3390/toxins8110326
118. Romano KA, Vivas EI, Amador-Noguez D, Rey FE. Intestinal microbiota composition modulates choline bioavailability from diet and accumulation of the proatherogenic metabolite trimethylamine-N-oxide. *mBio.* (2015) 6:e02481. doi: 10.1128/mBio.02481-14
119. Foxall PJ, Mellotte GJ, Bending MR, Lindon JC, Nicholson JK. NMR spectroscopy as a novel approach to the monitoring of renal transplant function. *Kidney Int.* (1993) 43:234–45. doi: 10.1038/ki.1993.37
120. Le Moyec L, Pruna A, Eugène M, Bedrossian J, Idatte JM, Huneau JF, et al. Proton nuclear magnetic resonance spectroscopy of urine and plasma in renal transplantation follow-up. *Nephron.* (1993) 65:433–9. doi: 10.1159/000187525
121. Bairaktari E, Seferiadis K, Liamis G, Psihogios N, Tsolas O, Elisaf M. Rhabdomyolysis-related renal tubular damage studied by proton nuclear magnetic resonance spectroscopy of urine. *Clin Chem.* (2002) 48:1106–9. doi: 10.1093/clinchem/48.7.1106
122. Faure JP, Jayle C, Dutheil D, Eugene M, Zhang K, Goujon JM, et al. Evidence for protective roles of polyethylene glycol plus high sodium solution and trimetazidine against consequences of renal medulla ischaemia during cold preservation and reperfusion in a pig kidney model. *Nephrol Dial Transplant.* (2004) 19:1742–51. doi: 10.1093/ndt/gfh142
123. Foxall PJ, Bewley S, Neild GH, Rodeck CH, Nicholson JK. Analysis of fetal and neonatal urine using proton nuclear magnetic resonance spectroscopy. *Arch Dis Child Fetal Neonatal Ed.* (1995) 73:F153–7. doi: 10.1136/fn.73.3.F153
124. Simonato M, Fochi I, Vedovelli L, Giambelluca S, Carollo C, Padalino M, et al. Urinary metabolomics reveals kynurenine pathway perturbation in newborns with transposition of great arteries after surgical repair. *Metabolomics.* (2019) 15:145. doi: 10.1007/s11306-019-1605-3
125. Adams S, Teo C, McDonald KL, Zinger A, Bustamante S, Lim CK, et al. Involvement of the kynurenine pathway in human glioma pathophysiology. *PLoS ONE.* (2014) 9:e112945. doi: 10.1371/journal.pone.0112945
126. Chatterjee P, Goozee K, Lim CK, James I, Shen K, Jacobs KR, et al. Alterations in serum kynurenine pathway metabolites in individuals with high neocortical amyloid-β load: a pilot study. *Sci Rep.* (2018) 8:8008. doi: 10.1038/s41598-018-25968-7
127. Lim CK, Fernández-Gomez FJ, Braidy N, Estrada C, Costa C, Costa S, et al. Involvement of the kynurenine pathway in the pathogenesis of Parkinson's disease. *Prog Neurobiol.* (2017) 155:76–95. doi: 10.1016/j.pneurobio.2015.12.009
128. Lussu M, Noto A, Masili A, Rinaldi AC, Dessì A, De Angelis M, et al. The urinary 1 H-NMR metabolomics profile of an italian autistic children population and their unaffected siblings. *Autism Res.* (2017) 10:1058–66. doi: 10.1002/aur.1748
129. Nogueira Ade C, Vale RG, Gomes AL, Dantas EH. The effect of muscle actions on the level of connective tissue damage. *Res Sports Med.* (2011) 19:259–70. doi: 10.1080/15438627.2011.608046
130. PubChem. *PubChem Compound Summary for CID 5810, Hydroxyproline.* Bethesda, MD: National Library of Medicine; National Center for Biotechnology Information (2004). Available online at: https://pubchem.ncbi.nlm.nih.gov/compound/Hydroxyproline (accessed October 3, 2020).
131. PubChem. *PubChem Compound Summary for CID 79101, Glycylproline.* Bethesda, MD: National Library of Medicine; National Center for Biotechnology Information (2004). Available online at: https://pubchem.ncbi.nlm.nih.gov/compound/Glycylproline (accessed October 3, 2020).
132. PubChem. *PubChem Compound Summary for CID 70639, 3-Methylxanthine.* Bethesda, MD: National Library of Medicine; National Center for Biotechnology Information (2004). Available online at: https://pubchem.ncbi.nlm.nih.gov/compound/3-Methylxanthine (accessed October 3, 2020).
133. Algharrawi KH, Summers RM, Gopishetty S, Subramanian M. Direct conversion of theophylline to 3-methylxanthine by metabolically engineered *E. coli. Microb Cell Fact.* (2015) 14:203. doi: 10.1186/s12934-015-0395-1
134. Bechtel YC, Lelouët H, Hrusovsky S, Brientini MP, Mantion G, Paintaud G, et al. Caffeine metabolism before and after liver transplantation. *Int J Clin Pharmacol Ther.* (2001) 39:53–60. doi: 10.5414/CPP39053
135. Nadai M, Kato M, Yoshizumi H, Kimura M, Kurono S, Abe F, et al. Possible involvement of organic anion and cation transporters in renal excretion of xanthine derivatives, 3-methylxanthine and enprofylline. *Life Sci.* (2007) 81:1175–82. doi: 10.1016/j.lfs.2007.07.032
136. Sohn JA, Kim HS, Oh J, Cho JY, Yu KS, Lee J, et al. Prediction of serum theophylline concentrations and cytochrome P450 1A2 activity by analyzing urinary metabolites in preterm infants. *Br J Clin Pharmacol.* (2017) 83:1279–86. doi: 10.1111/bcp.13211
137. Barberini L, Noto A, Fattuoni C, Grapov D, Casanova A, Fenu G, et al. Urinary metabolomics (GC-MS) reveals that low and high birth weight infants share elevated inositol concentrations at birth. *J Matern Fetal Neonatal Med.* (2014) 2:20–6. doi: 10.3109/14767058.2014.954786
138. Atzori L, Antonucci R, Barberini L, Locci E, Marincola FC, Scano P, et al. 1H NMR-based metabolomic analysis of urine from preterm and term neonates. *Front Biosci (Elite Ed).* (2011) 3:1005–12. doi: 10.2741/306
139. Dessì A, Atzori L, Noto A, Visser GH, Gazzolo D, Zanardo V, et al.

Metabolomics in newborns with intrauterine growth retardation (IUGR): urine reveals markers of metabolic syndrome. *J Matern Fetal Neonatal Med.* (2011) 2:35–9. doi: 10.3109/14767058.2011.605868

140. Fanos V, Caboni P, Corsello G, Stronati M, Gazzolo D, Noto A, et al. Urinary (1)H-NMR and GC-MS metabolomics predicts early and late onset neonatal sepsis. *Early Hum Dev.* (2014) 90(Suppl. 1):S78–83. doi: 10.1016/S0378-3782(14)70024-6

10

A Matched Case Control Study of Surgically and Non-Surgically Treated Patent Ductus Arteriosus in Extremely Pre-Term Infants

Karl Wilhelm Olsson[1†], *Sawin Youssef*[1†], *Mattias Kjellberg*[1], *Renske Raaijmakers*[2] *and Richard Sindelar*[1*]

[1] *Department of Women's and Children's Health, Uppsala University, Uppsala, Sweden,* [2] *Division of Neonatology, Department of Pediatrics, Sahlgrenska University Hospital, Gothenburg, Sweden*

Correspondence:
Richard Sindelar
richard.sindelar@kbh.uu.se

† *These authors share first authorship*

Introduction: There are still uncertainties about the timing and indication for surgical ligation of patent ductus arteriosus (PDA) in pre-term infants, where lower gestational age (GA) usually is predictive for surgical treatment.

Objective: Our aim was to assess differences in clinical characteristics and outcomes between surgically treated and matched non-surgically treated PDA in extremely pre-term infants.

Methods: All extremely pre-term infants born 2010–2016 with surgically treated PDA (Ligated group; $n = 44$) were compared to non-surgically treated infants (Control group; $n = 44$) matched for gestational age (+/−1 week) and time of birth (+/−1 month). Perinatal parameters, echocardiographic variables, details of pharmacological PDA treatment, morbidity, and mortality were assessed.

Result: Mean GA and birthweight were similar between the Ligated group ($24^{+5} \pm 1^{+3}$ weeks and 668 ± 170 g) and the Control group ($24^{+5} \pm 1^{+3}$ weeks and 704 ± 166 g; $p = 1.000$ and $p = 0.319$, respectively). Infants in the Ligated group had larger ductal diameters prior to pharmacological treatment, and lack of diameter decrease and PDA closure after treatment ($p = 0.022$, $p = 0.043$ and 0.006, respectively). Transfusions, post-natal steroids and invasive respiratory support were more common in the Ligated group. Except for a higher incidence of severe bronchopulmonary dysplasia (BPD) in the Ligated group there were no other differences in outcomes or mortality between the groups.

Conclusion: Early large ductal diameter and reduced responsiveness to pharmacological treatment predicted the need for future surgical ligation in this matched cohort study of extremely pre-term infants where the effect of GA and differences in treatment strategies were excluded. Besides an increased incidence of severe BPD in the Ligated group, no other differences in morbidity or mortality were detected.

Keywords: case-control study, echocardiography, extreme pre-maturity, ligation, patent ductus arteriosus

INTRODUCTION

Patency of the ductus arteriosus in newborn pre-term infants continues to be one of the most challenging problems in neonatal intensive care units. Despite extensive research efforts, there are still uncertainties about the diagnostic criteria and treatment strategies for patent ductus arteriosus (PDA) in pre-term infants, and specifically in extremely pre-term newborn infants (1, 2).

Before pharmacological treatment was available, early surgical ligation was performed to close PDA in pre-term infants (3). As the initial reduction in morbidity after surgical closure did not translate into improved outcomes, pharmacological treatment with cyclooxygenase inhibitors or acetaminophen eventually became the first-hand choice for PDA treatment. Surgery was then reserved for infants with persistent hemodynamically significant PDA where either contraindications for pharmacological treatment were present or for infants that did not respond to pharmacological treatment (4–6). As it has been recognized that there is a high degree of spontaneous closure of ductus arteriosus and a low efficiency of pharmacological treatment, the application of pharmacological treatment has also declined during the last decade (7). Recently, arguments have also been presented in favor of conservative management of PDA with neither pharmacological nor surgical treatment in pre-term infants (8–10).

Never the less, PDA in extremely pre-term infants (<28 weeks gestational age) might lead to significant hemodynamic effects with cardiac and pulmonary complications such as heart failure, prolonged mechanical ventilation and increased incidence of bronchopulmonary dysplasia (BPD) (11). With improved survival of extremely pre-term infants, these infants have a higher risk of developing a symptomatic PDA that either exhibits contraindications for or fails to respond to pharmacological treatment, whereby the need for surgical treatment might increase in this cohort (12, 13).

There are few studies on surgically treated PDA in infants born before 28 weeks gestational age, and results from studies of infants born at a higher gestational age might be difficult to apply in extremely pre-term infants. Also, many studies on surgically treated PDA were conducted during an era where surfactant therapy, antenatal steroids, non-invasive positive pressure ventilation, routine echocardiography, or pharmacological treatment of PDA were not fully established (14, 15). The aim of this matched case control study of PDA was to investigate the differences in peri- and post-natal characteristics, pharmacological PDA treatment, and outcomes between surgically and non-surgically treated extremely pre-term infants. By matching surgically treated infants with infants born within the same month and week of GA, we wanted to exclude the possible effects of maturation and different treatment strategies over time, factors that could interfere with the studied parameters (16).

SUBJECTS AND METHODS

Subjects

From January 2010 to December 2016, 463 infants were born at 22 + 0 to 27 + 6 weeks GA and admitted to the neonatal intensive care unit at Uppsala University Children's Hospital. Forty-four infants were surgically treated for PDA (Ligated group). Each infant in the Ligated group was matched to an infant in the Control group from the Swedish Neonatal Quality Register (44 out of 101 eligible infants), blindly as to any other outcomes except for (1) not having undergone surgery for PDA, (2) being born within +/−1 month of the birthdate, and (3) within +/−1 week of the gestational age of the infant in the Ligated group. Infants with congenital anomalies or heart conditions other than PDA or foramen ovale were excluded from both groups in this study. This retrospective observational study was approved by the Regional Ethical Review Board, D:nr 933-17.

Perinatal Parameters, Post-Natal Treatments, and Outcomes

Medical records were assessed for perinatal parameters: birthweight, sex, prolonged pre-mature rupture of membranes, administration of pre-natal steroids, mode of delivery, and Apgar-scores at 1, 5 and 10 min. Information on number and volume of erythrocyte transfusions, administration of inotropic drugs, post-natal steroid administration, pharmacological PDA treatment, and surgical treatment of PDA were collected. Clinical outcomes data were assessed for BPD [graded mild, moderate or severe according to Higgins et al. (17)], intraventricular hemorrhage (IVH; graded according to Papile's criteria) (18), retinopathy of pre-maturity (ROP; graded according to the International Classification of ROP) (19), necrotizing enterocolitis (NEC; graded according to the modified Bell's criteria) (20), sepsis (defined as positive blood culture with clinical signs of infection; or as negative blood culture with clinical signs of infection and positive laboratory infectious tests), and mortality.

Ventilatory Parameters

The patient data management/monitoring systems IntelliVue Clinical Information Portfolio (ICIP; Philips Healthcare, Eindhoven, Netherlands) and MetaVision (Metavision; iMDsoft, Düsseldorf, Germany) were used at the unit during the studied period. Data obtained from these monitoring systems included total days with ventilatory support, mode of ventilatory support, ventilator settings, and supplementary oxygen administration.

Echocardiography

Infants in the unit routinely underwent echocardiographic examinations during the first day of life with additional examinations if they exhibited clinical signs of PDA. Examinations were also performed within 24 h of treatment completion, if the infant's clinical condition called for it, and before discharge. The initial assessment was carried out by a pediatric cardiologist and the following examinations either by a pediatric cardiologist or neonatologist with appropriate training and experience (21).

Examinations included assessment of the ductal diameter measured at the narrowest point from the parasternal short axis view, ductal flow velocity measured in line with the ductal flow from the parasternal short axis view, left atrium to aortic root ratio measured from the parasternal long axis and flow in the descending aorta assessed above and below the ductal orifice (22).

Ductal closure was defined as absence of identifiable flow in the ductus arteriosus by color Doppler.

Pharmacological Treatment of PDA

Hemodynamically significant PDA (hsPDA) was defined as an open ductus arteriosus with predominantly left-to-right flow after the first day of life and either: (A) ductal diameter of $\geq$1.5 mm; (B) LA/Ao of >1.5; or (C) an appropriate view of the descending aorta showing absent or reversed flow during diastole (22). Pharmacological treatment was initiated if hsPDA was identified before the seventh day of life. Contraindications were renal failure (serum creatinine >120 µmol/L or serum urea >12 mmol/L), thrombocytopenia (platelets $<50 \times 10^9$/L), recent IVH grade II–IV, and NEC. Three doses of Ibuprofen (5 mg/mL, Pedea, Orphan Europe Nordic, Stockholm, Sweden) were administered intravenously with an initial dose of 10 mg/kg infused over 20 min and subsequent doses of 5 mg/kg at 24 and 48 h after the initial dose. No additional pharmacological ductus treatment was administered after the first course.

Surgical Treatment of PDA

Surgical ligation was carried out if pharmacological treatment was contraindicated or failed and hsPDA still persisted in combination with clinical signs of deterioration in pulmonary and systemic circulation, i.e. clinically hemodynamically significant; or if PDA reopened and was found to be clinically hemodynamically significant after pharmacological treatment (23).

Statistical Analysis

Matlab (The Mathworks Inc., Natick, Massachusetts) was used for statistical analysis. Categorical variables were statistically analyzed using Fisher exact test. Continuous variables were analyzed using Student's *t*-test or Mann–Whitney *U*-test. Normal distribution of parameters was tested by Kolmogorov-Smirnov's goodness of fit test. Categorical variables are presented as number and percent, and continuous variables are presented as mean and standard deviation (SD) or median and interquartile range (IQR). All *p*-values presented are two-tailed, and a $p < 0.05$ was considered significant. Multivariate logistic regression was used to examine the relationship between treatments possibly affecting ductal closure (post-natal steroids, transfusions, pharmacological PDA treatment, and ventilatory days), ductal patency/diameter on first examination, and subsequent surgical ligation.

RESULTS

There was no difference in GA or birthweight between the Ligated group and the Control group. Perinatal characteristics for all infants are presented in **Table 1**. Of all infants born at 22–27 weeks GA during the study period, only 9.5% were surgically

TABLE 1 | Perinatal characteristics and treatments.

	Ligated $n = 44$	Control $n = 44$	*p*
Perinatal characteristics			
Gestational age, weeks	$24^{+5} \pm 1^{+3}$	$24^{+5} \pm 1^{+3}$	1.000
Birthweight, grams	668 ± 170	704 ± 166	0.319
Male, *n*	25 (57%)	21 (48%)	0.522
Pre-term pre-mature rupture of membranes, *n*	11 (25%)	12 (27%)	1.000
Pre-natal steroids, *n*	44 (100%)	44 (100%)	1.000
Cesarean section, *n*	26 (59%)	22 (50%)	0.521
Apgar 1	4.0 ± 2.2	5.2 ± 2.4	0.018
Apgar 5	5.8 ± 2.2	6.6 ± 2.0	0.064
Apgar 10	7.4 ± 2.1	8.0 ± 1.5	0.166
Treatment			
Transfusions, *n*	5 (3–6)	3 (1–4)	<0.001
Transfusion volume, ml/kg	75 (45–90)	45 (15–60)	<0.001
Inotropic support, *n*	10 (23%)	6 (14%)	0.408
Post-natal steroids, *n*	11 (25%)	1 (2%)	0.004
Invasive ventilation, days	47 (38–68)	20 (3–36)	<0.001
CPAP, days	14 (8–26)	13 (5–32)	0.729
Invasive and non-invasive ventilation, days	63 (49–99)	40 (13–70)	<0.001
Pharmacological PDA-treatment, *n*	23 (52%)	22 (50%)	1.000
Time of pharmacological treatment, days	5.2 ± 4.7	4.4 ± 6.6	0.654

Continuous variables are presented as mean ± standard deviation or median and interquartile range (IQR), and categorical variables are presented as number and percent. CPAP, Continuous positive airway pressure; PDA, Patent ductus arteriosus.

ligated. Infants in the Ligated group had surgery for PDA at a mean post-natal age of 50 ± 26 days.

Perinatal Parameters

Median Apgar score at 1 min was higher in the Control group but all other perinatal parameters, including birthweight, sex, prolonged pre-mature rupture of membranes, administration of pre-natal steroids, and mode of delivery were similar between the groups (**Table 1**).

Ventilatory Parameters

Infants in the Ligated group needed ventilatory assistance for a longer period, with mainly prolonged invasive ventilation (**Table 1**). Infants in the Ligated group also received more post-natal steroids. On the day before surgery, 35 infants (80%) were on invasive ventilatory support and 9 (20%) were on CPAP.

Inotropic Support and Transfusions

There was no difference in inotropic support between the groups (**Table 1**). Infants in the Ligated group received in average two red blood cell transfusions more than infants in the Control group during their hospital stay, but no infants received transfusion in connection to their surgery for PDA.

Pharmacological Treatment of PDA

The same amount of infants received pharmacological treatment in both groups and during the same time interval (**Table 1**). One infant in the Control group received treatment with indomethacin, whereas all other treated infants received ibuprofen according to the described protocol. Five infants in the Ligated group and seven infants in the Control group received acetaminophen as analgesic (20 mg/kg rectally twice daily for 2–5 days) in connection with surgery for NEC ($p = 0.757$). No other infants received acetaminophen before discharge.

All infants in the Ligated group had hsPDA during the first week of life, compared to 31 infants (70%) in the Control group ($p < 0.001$). Eleven infants in the Control group had a closed ductus arteriosus at the first echocardiographic examination and none in the Ligated group (**Table 2**). All infants were examined at the same time after birth.

All 23 of the pharmacologically treated infants in the Ligated group underwent post-treatment echocardiography, while 19 of 22 (86%) of the treated infants in the Control group were examined (**Table 2**). The success of pharmacological treatment was most limited in the Ligated group where all but one infant had an open PDA after treatment, in comparison to 11 infants in the Control group. The ductal diameter was unchanged in the Ligated group, whereas it was reduced after treatment in the Control group (**Table 2**).

Multivariate Logistical Regression for Surgical Predictive Variables

In a logistical regression analysis of factors associated with persistent PDA (post-natal steroids, transfusions, pharmacological PDA treatment, and ventilatory days) and echocardiographic findings on the first examination, prolonged need for invasive ventilation was the only factor independently associated with surgical ligation (**Table 3**).

TABLE 2 | Echocardiography before and after pharmacological treatment.

	Ligated *n* = 44	Control *n* = 44	*p*
Pre-treatment			
Timing, day	2 (1–3)	2 (1–2)	0.169
Ductus open, *n*	43 (98%)	33 (75%)	0.004
Ductus diameter, mm	1.9 ± 0.7	1.5 ± 0.9	0.022
Ductus Vmax, m/s	1.32 ± 0.42	1.38 ± 0.51	0.640
LA/Ao	1.8 ± 0.4	1.6 ± 0.4	0.213
hsPDA, *n*	35 (80%)	24 (55%)	0.023
Post-pharmacological treatment	***n* = 23**	***n* = 19**	
Timing, day	14 (9-21)	13 (6-30)	0.795
Ductus open, *n*	22 (96%)	11 (58%)	0.006
Ductus diameter, mm	2.0 ± 0.8	0.9 ± 0.9	0.001
Ductus diameter change, mm	0.0 ± 1.1	−0.9 ± 1.2	0.043
Ductus Vmax, m/s	1.32 ± 0.38	1.66 ± 0.57	0.074
LA/Ao	1.7 ± 0.5	1.6 ± 0.4	0.647
hsPDA, *n*	12 (52%)	5 (26%)	0.120

Continuous variables are presented as mean ± standard deviation or median and interquartile range (IQR), and categorical variables are presented as number and percent. Vmax, maximal flow velocity; LA/Ao, Left atrium to aortic root ratio; hsPDA, hemodynamically significant patent ductus arteriosus.

TABLE 3 | Multivariate logistical regression for surgical predictive variables.

	OR (95% CI)	*p*
Ductus open at first echo	3.123 (0.088–111.517)	0.531
Ductus diameter at first echo	1.654 (0.521–5.250)	0.393
Pharmacological treatment	1.056 (0.298–3.751)	0.932
Post-natal steroid treatment	–	1.000
Number of transfusions	1.051 (0.842–1.312)	0.661
Days with invasive ventilation	1.041 (1.003–1.079)	0.018

OR, Odds ratio.

Outcomes

Infants in the Ligated group had a higher incidence of severe BPD, whereas mild and moderate BPD were similar to the Control group. The incidence of IVH, NEC, sepsis, and ROP were the same in both groups and there was no difference in mortality (**Table 4**).

DISCUSSION

This retrospective study investigates indications for surgical treatment of PDA and compares outcome for infants subjected to ligation with non-surgically treated controls matched for gestational age and time of birth in order to exclude maturational aspects and other treatment strategies that might have affected

TABLE 4 | Outcomes.

	Ligated $n = 44$	Control $n = 44$	p
Mild BPD, n	1 (2%)	2 (5%)	1.000
Moderate BPD, n	4 (9%)	7 (16%)	0.521
Severe BPD, n	38 (86%)	28 (64%)	0.025
IVH grade I–II, n	11 (25%)	5 (11%)	0.166
IVH grade III–IV, n	5 (11%)	2 (5%)	0.434
ROP stage III, n	14 (32%)	15 (34%)	0.653
NEC stage IIIa–IIIb, n	5 (11%)	8 (18%)	0.549
Sepsis, n	19 (43%)	21 (48%)	0.831
Mortality, n	5 (11%)	5 (11%)	1.000
Age at death, day	117 ± 72	191 ± 178	0.417

Continuous variables are presented as mean ± standard deviation and categorical variables are presented as number and percent. BPD, Bronchopulmonary dysplasia; IVH, Intraventricular hemorrhage; ROP, Retinopathy of pre-maturity; NEC, Necrotizing enterocolitis.

our data. The cohort was well-matched for GA and the groups did not differ in mean birthweight, sex balance and proportion of pharmacologically treated infants.

Only 9.5% of all infants born at 22–27 weeks gestational age during the studied period were subjected to surgical ligation. Compared to the rate of surgery in cohorts in previous studies, this reflects a conservative approach in line with the general trend during the last decade, where increased survival has been observed with this strategy but also with a trend toward increased BPD, periventricular leukomalacia and ROP (7, 23). In a recent mini-review of conservative treatment for PDA, the authors stated that there do exist evidence for this approach even in the most severe forms of hsPDA and in extremely pre-term infants without a concomitant increase in either mortality or morbidity (24, 25). In addition, more than half of the infants in the Ligated groups in our study had been primarily pharmacologically treated for PDA and did not show any response to this treatment, reflecting the poor effectiveness of pharmacological treatment in extremely pre-term infants, as previously described by our group and others (26–30).

An early large ductal diameter was associated with future need for surgical ligation in this cohort. This is expected, as a large ductal diameter is one of the criteria for hemodynamical significant PDA used at most centers, including ours, and thus part of the indication for both pharmacological treatment and eventual surgical ligation. The decrease in diameter in infants in the Control group but not in the Ligated group during pharmacological treatment confirms the finding of Pees et al. that a reduction in ductal diameter indicates treatment response (31). There was also a trend toward a lower ductal Vmax being associated with surgical ligation, which is in line with previous results from our center (27, 32).

Early identification of infants with a high risk of developing PDA with considerable hemodynamic effects and with a low chance of successful pharmacological closure is likely to minimize the risk for complications and improve outcomes of surgical treatment. Early low ductal flow velocity and lack of reduction in ductal diameter after failed pharmacological treatment might therefore be useful indices for considering future surgical ligation. Prospective studies of these echocardiographic markers and surgical treatment in this subgroup are thus called for.

In these matched cohorts of extremely pre-term infants, differences in outcomes between the Ligated group and the Control group were mainly related to pulmonary complications. Infants in the Ligated group had more days with invasive ventilation, which was also the only factor independently associated with surgical ligation. As failure to come off the ventilator is an important indication for surgical treatment, this could partly be a confounding effect as indicated by a large study by Weisz et al. (11). In a prospective randomized controlled study of infants born <28 weeks' GA (the PDA-TOLERATE Trial Study) there seemed to be an association between maintained intubation beyond 10 days of life and moderate to severe BPD, when moderate to large PDA persisted more than 10 days and deaths were excluded (33). However, in a prospective multicenter study of infants born between 24^{+0} and 28^{+6} weeks' GA (the INTERPDA Study), a possible reduction of PDA exposure by early medical treatment did not reduce either surgical ligation or BPD incidence, but on the contrary, was associated with a higher mortality (34). Even though the total amount of infants included in our study was smaller in view of the matched cohort study characteristic, the Ligated group was larger and had a lower mean GA than in the two cited studies ($n = 44/88$ vs. $n = 22/202$ and $n = 37/444$; mean GA 24 + 5 weeks vs. 25 + 6 and 26 + 3 weeks; matched cohort vs. PDA-TOLERATE and INTERPDA, respectively), implying that maturational and ventilatory aspects could have interfered with the outcomes of our study while still being relevant for this conservatively managed cohort of extremely pre-term infants (33, 34).

Infants in the Ligated group received more red blood cell transfusions than the Control group. The need for red blood cell transfusions has previously been associated with presence of PDA (35), however, in a study by Sellmer et al. there was no difference between infants with small and large PDAs (36). Lower hemoglobin values have also been associated with BPD and the need for transfusions could therefore be a confounder for pulmonary disease (35–37).

There were no other significant differences in morbidity nor mortality between the groups, highlighting the fact that extremely low gestational age and presence of PDA do not necessarily lead to future surgical treatment. Besides the observed longer duration of mechanical ventilation in the Ligated group, surgical ligation did not have any detrimental effects in this cohort and could be considered a valid alternative in the most pre-term infants with considerable hemodynamic effects of their PDA and low chance of spontaneous or pharmacological closure. Nonetheless, the results of this study need to be interpreted cautiously due to its retrospective nature. The lack of randomization also means that it cannot be ruled out that unidentified clinical factors could have influenced the course of PDA and outcomes after surgical ligation.

CONCLUSION

The efficacy of pharmacological treatment was limited in this cohort of extremely pre-term infants. Early large ductal diameter and lack of decrease in ductal diameter during pharmacological PDA treatment predicted future need for surgical ligation. Infants who were surgically treated for PDA needed more respiratory support and had a higher incidence of severe BPD than infants that were not surgically ligated. The compromised pulmonary function might reflect a more pronounced hsPDA and an indicator for surgery in these infants, which was neither associated with increased mortality or other morbidities. With no difference in mortality between our matched surgically and non-surgically treated groups, there is still a need for prospective studies validating the indications for and timing of surgical treatment in extremely pre-term infants, as well as randomized trials to confirm the outcomes of ligation.

ETHICS STATEMENT

The studies involving human participants were reviewed and approved by the Regional Ethical Review Board. Written informed consent from the participants' legal guardian/next of kin was not required to participate in this study in accordance with the national legislation and the institutional requirements.

AUTHOR CONTRIBUTIONS

KO conceptualized and designed the study, supervised data collection, and drafted the initial manuscript. SY conceptualized and designed the study, carried out the data collection, and reviewed the manuscript. MK and RS conceptualized and designed the study, coordinated and supervised data collection, and reviewed and revised the manuscript. RR conceptualized and designed the study and reviewed and revised the manuscript. All authors approved the final manuscript as submitted and agree to be accountable for all aspects of the work.

ACKNOWLEDGMENTS

The authors would like to thank the nurses at the Neonatal Intensive Care Unit, Uppsala University Children's Hospital, Uppsala.

REFERENCES

1. Juszczak E, Gupta S. Continued uncertainty regarding treatment of patent ductus arteriosus in premature infants and the role of clinical trials. *Semin Fetal Neonatal Med.* (2018) 23:267–72. doi: 10.1016/j.siny.2018.03.004
2. Clyman RI, Liebowitz M. Treatment and nontreatment of the patent ductus arteriosus: identifying their roles in neonatal morbidity. *J Pediatr.* (2017) 189:13–7. doi: 10.1016/j.jpeds.2017.06.054
3. El-Khuffash A, Weisz DE, McNamara PJ. Reflections of the changes in patent ductus arteriosus management during the last 10 years. *Arch Dis Child Fetal Neonatal Ed.* (2016) 101:F474–8. doi: 10.1136/archdischild-2014-306214
4. Jhaveri N, Moon-Grady A, Clyman RI. Early surgical ligation versus a conservative approach for management of patent ductus arteriosus that fails to close after indomethacin treatment. *J Pediatr.* (2010) 157:381–7. doi: 10.1016/j.jpeds.2010.02.062
5. Clyman RI, Cassady G, Kirklin JK, Collins M, Philips JB. The role of patent ductus arteriosus ligation in bronchopulmonary dysplasia: reexamining a randomized controlled trial. *J Pediatr.* (2009) 154:873–6. doi: 10.1016/j.jpeds.2009.01.005
6. Mirea L, Sankaran K, Seshia M, Ohlsson A, Allen AC, Aziz K, et al. Treatment of patent ductus arteriosus and neonatal mortality/morbidities: adjustment for treatment selection bias. *J Pediatr.* (2012) 161:689–94. doi: 10.1016/j.jpeds.2012.05.007
7. Hagadorn JI, Brownell EA, Trzaski JM, Johnson KR, Lainwala S, Campbell BT, et al. Trends and variation in management and outcomes of very low-birth-weight infants with patent ductus arteriosus. *Pediatr Res.* (2016) 80:785–92. doi: 10.1038/pr.2016.166
8. Clyman RI, Liebowitz M, Kaempf J, Erdeve O, Bulbul A, Håkansson S, et al. PDA-TOLERATE Trial. An exploratory randomized controlled trial of treatment of moderate-to-large patent ductus arteriosus at 1 week of age. *J Pediatr.* (2018) 205:41–8. doi: 10.1016/j.jpeds.2018.09.012
9. Semberova J, Sirc J, Miletin J, Kucera J, Berka I, Sebkova S, et al. Spontaneous closure of patent ductus arteriosus in infants ≤1500 g. *Pediatrics.* (2017) 140:e20164258. doi: 10.1542/peds.2016-4258
10. Rolland A, Shankar-Aguilera S, Diomandé D, Zupan-Simunek V, Boileau P. Natural evolution of patent ductus arteriosus in the extremely preterm infant. *Arch Dis Child Fetal Neonatal Ed.* (2015) 100:F55–8. doi: 10.1136/archdischild-2014-306339
11. Weisz DE, Mirea L, Rosenberg E, Jang M, Ly L, Church PT, et al. Association of patent ductus arteriosus ligation with death or neurodevelopmental impairment among extremely preterm infants. *JAMA Pediatr.* (2017) 171:443–9. doi: 10.1001/jamapediatrics.2016.5143
12. Dani C, Bertini G, Corsini I, Elia S, Vangi V, Pratesi S, et al. The fate of ductus arteriosus in infants at 23-27 weeks of gestation: from spontaneous closure to ibuprofen resistance. *Acta Paediatr.* (2008) 97:1176–1180. doi: 10.1111/j.1651-2227.2008.00871.x
13. Richards J, Johnson A, Fox G, Campbell M. A second course of ibuprofen is effective in the closure of a clinically significant PDA in ELBW infants. *Pediatrics.* (2009) 124:e287–93. doi: 10.1542/peds.2008-2232
14. Malviya M, Ohlsson A, Shah S. Surgical versus medical treatment with cyclooxygenase inhibitors for symptomatic patent ductus arteriosus in preterm infants. *Cochrane Database Syst Rev.* (2013) 2013:CD00395. doi: 10.1002/14651858.CD003951.pub3
15. Pereira SS, Kempley ST, Shah DK, Morris JK, Sinha AK. Early echocardiography does not predict subsequent treatment of symptomatic patent ductus arteriosus in extremely preterm infants. *Acta Paediatr.* (2018) 107:1909–16. doi: 10.1111/apa.14361
16. de Graaf MA, Jager KJ, Zoccali C, Dekker FW. Matching, an appealing method to avoid confounding? *Nephron Clin Pract.* (2011) 118:c315–8. doi: 10.1159/000323136
17. Higgins RD, Jobe AH, Koso-Thomas M, Bancalari E, Viscardi RM, Hartert TV, et al. Bronchopulmonary dysplasia: executive summary of a workshop. *J Pediatr.* (2018) 197:300–8. doi: 10.1016/j.jpeds.2018.01.043
18. Papile LA, Burstein J, Burstein R, Koffler H. Incidence and evolution of subependymal and intraventricular hemorrhage: a study of infants with birth weights less than 1,500 gm. *J Pediatr.* (1978) 92:529–34. doi: 10.1016/S0022-3476(78)80282-0
19. International Committee for the Classification of Retinopathy of Prematurity. The international classification of retinopathy of prematurity revisited. *Arch Ophthalmol.* (2005) 123:991–9. doi: 10.1001/archopht.123.7.991
20. Lee JS, Polin RA. Treatment and prevention of necrotizing enterocolitis. *Semin Neonatol.* (2003) 8:449–59. doi: 10.1016/S1084-2756(03)00123-4

21. van Laere D, van Overmeire B, Gupta S, El-Khuffash A, Savoia M, McNamara PJ, et al. European special interest group 'neonatologist performed echocardiography' (NPE). Application of NPE in the assessment of a patent ductus arteriosus. *Pediatr Res.* (2018) 84 (Suppl. 1):46–56. doi: 10.1038/s41390-018-0077-x
22. Singh Y, Fraisse A, Erdeve O, Atasay B. Echocardiographic diagnosis and hemodynamic evaluation of patent ductus arteriosus in extremely low gestational age newborn (ELGAN) infants. *Front Pediatr.* (2020) 8:573627. doi: 10.3389/fped.2020.573627
23. Weinberg JG, Evans FJ, Burns KM, Pearson GD, Kaltman JR. Surgical ligation of patent ductus arteriosus in premature infants: trends and practice variation. *Cardiol Young.* (2016) 26:1107–14. doi: 10.1017/S1047951115001869
24. Sung SI, Chang YS, Ahn SY, Jo HS, Yang M, Park WS. Conservative non-intervention approach for hemodynamically significant patent ductus arteriosus in extremely preterm infants. *Front Pediatr.* (2020) 8:605134. doi: 10.3389/fped.2020.605134
25. Sung SI, Lee MH, Ahn SY, Chang YS, Park WS. Effect of nonintervention vs oral ibuprofen in patent ductus arteriosus in preterm infants: a randomized clinical trial. *JAMA Pediatr.* (2020) 174:755–63. doi: 10.1001/jamapediatrics.2020.1447
26. Olsson KW, Sindelar R. Pharmacological ductus arteriosus treatment in infants born at 22-23 gestational weeks. *Pediatr Res.* (2011) 70:268. doi: 10.1038/pr.2011.493
27. Olsson KW, Jonzon A, Sindelar R. A high ductal flow velocity is associated with successful pharmacological closure of patent ductus arteriosus in infants 22–27 weeks gestational age. *Crit Care Res Pract.* (2012) 2012:715265 doi: 10.1155/2012/715265
28. Ohlsson A, Walia R, Shah SS. Ibuprofen for the treatment of patent ductus arteriosus in preterm or low birth weight (or both) infants. *Cochrane Database Syst Rev.* (2020) 2:CD003481. doi: 10.1002/14651858.CD003481.pub8
29. Terrin G, Conte F, Oncel MY, Scipione A, McNamara PJ, Simons S, et al. Paracetamol for the treatment of patent ductus arteriosus in preterm neonates: a systematic review and meta-analysis. *Arch Dis Child Fetal Neonatal Ed.* (2016) 101:F127–36. doi: 10.1136/archdischild-2014-307312
30. Ohlsson A, Shah PS. Paracetamol (acetaminophen) for patent ductus arteriosus in preterm or low birth weight infants. *Cochrane Database Syst Rev.* (2020) 1:CD010061. doi: 10.1002/14651858.CD010061.pub4
31. Pees C, Walch E, Obladen M, Koehne P. Echocardiography predicts closure of patent ductus arteriosus in response to ibuprofen in infants less than 28 week gestational age. *Early Hum Dev.* (2010) 86:503–8. doi: 10.1016/j.earlhumdev.2010.06.012
32. Olsson KW, Jonzon A, Sindelar R. Early haemodynamically significant patent ductus arteriosus does not predict future persistence in extremely preterm infants. *Acta Paediatr.* (2019) 108:1590–6. doi: 10.1111/apa.14752
33. Clyman RI, Kaempf J, Liebowitz M, Erdeve O, Bulbul A, Håkansson S, et al. PDA-TOLERATE trial investigators. Prolonged tracheal intubation and the association between patent ductus arteriosus and bronchopulmonary dysplasia: a secondary analysis of the PDA-TOLERATE trial. *J Pediatr.* (2020) 229:283–88.e2. doi: 10.1016/j.jpeds.2020.09.047
34. Okulu E, Erdeve O, Arslan Z, Demirel N, Kaya H, Gokce IK, et al. Turkish neonatal society INTERPDA study group. An observational, prospective, multicenter, registry-based cohort study comparing conservative and medical management for patent ductus arteriosus. *Front Pediatr.* (2020) 8:434. doi: 10.3389/fped.2020.00434
35. Chen YY, Wang HP, Chang JT, Chiou YH, Huang YF, Hsieh KS. Perinatal factors in patent ductus arteriosus in very low-birthweight infants. *Pediatr Int.* (2014) 56:72–6. doi: 10.1111/ped.12199
36. Sellmer A, Bjerre JV, Schmidt MR, McNamara PJ, Hjortdal VE, Høst B, et al. Morbidity and mortality in preterm neonates with patent ductus arteriosus on day 3. *Arch Dis Child Fetal Neonatal Ed.* (2013) 98:F505–10. doi: 10.1136/archdischild-2013-303816
37. Duan J, Kong X, Li Q, Hua S, Zhang S, Feng Z, et al. Association between hemoglobin levels in the first 3 days of life and bronchopulmonary dysplasia in preterm infants. *Am J Perinatol.* (2016) 33:998–1002. doi: 10.1055/s-0036-1583189

11

Initial Experience with Patent Ductus Arteriosus Ligation in Pre-Term Infants with Bidirectional Shunt Pattern

Ming-Chun Yang [1,2,3†], *Hsien-Kuan Liu* [1,3†], *Hsuan-Yin Wu* [3,4], *Shu-Leei Tey* [1,2], *Yung-Ning Yang* [1,2,3], *Chien-Yi Wu* [1,2] *and Jiunn-Ren Wu* [1*]

[1] *Department of Pediatrics, E-Da Hospital, Kaohsiung City, Taiwan,* [2] *School of Chinese Medicine for Post Baccalaureate, I-Shou University, Kaohsiung City, Taiwan,* [3] *School of Medicine for International Students, I-Shou University, Kaohsiung City, Taiwan,* [4] *Division of Cardiovascular Surgery, Department of Surgery, E-Da Hospital, Kaohsiung City, Taiwan*

Correspondence:
Jiunn-Ren Wu
jirewu@gmail.com

† These authors have contributed equally to this work and share first authorship

Background: Patent ductus arteriosus (PDA) with a bidirectional shunt reflects critical clinical conditions. The operability of PDA with a bidirectional shunt in pre-term infants is still not clearly clarified. This study aimed to investigate the feasibility and the outcomes of PDA ligation in pre-term infants with a bidirectional shunt PDA.

Methods: All pre-term infants receiving PDA ligation between 2013 and 2019 were enrolled in this prospective study. Patients were allocated into two groups based on the shunting direction of PDA, which were the left-to-right group (group A) and the bidirectional group (group B). Clinical characteristics and pre-op comorbidities were analyzed. Intraoperative complications, post-op neurological sequelae, necrotizing enterocolitis, survival, and mortality were compared between these two groups.

Results: Thirty-seven pre-term infants were enrolled (18 in group A, 19 in group B). The mean post-menstrual age at PDA surgery was 32.0 ± 1.3 and 32.8 ± 1.5 weeks, respectively. Before surgery, 44.4 and 89.5% (group A vs. B) of the patients were using invasive mechanical ventilator ($p < 0.01$). The requirement of high-frequency oscillatory ventilatory support was significantly higher in group B. PDA rupture-related bleeding during exposing PDA or ligating PDA occurred in four infants, and all were all in group B, including one with delayed hemothorax. Early surgical mortality within 30 days of surgery was higher in group B (0 vs. 21.1%, $p < 0.05$), but only one death could be attributed to the surgery, which was caused by a pain-induced pulmonary hypertension crisis. The 5-year survival was 100% in group A, and 73.7% in group B ($p < 0.05$).

Conclusion: We did not recommend routine PDA ligation in pre-term infants with a bidirectional shunt. However, a bidirectional shunt should not be an absolute contraindication if they fulfill indications of PDA closure. Unexpected intraoperative PDA rupture and delayed hemothorax in a bidirectional shunt PDA should be carefully monitored. Aggressive post-op pain control is also warranted to avoid pulmonary hypertension crisis. The post-op early mortality rate was higher in the bidirectional group, which could be inherent to their poor pre-operative lung condition. Only one death was directly related to the surgery.

Keywords: pre-term infant, pulmonary hypertension, patent ductus arteriosus ligation, outcomes, bidirectional shunt, contraindication, surgery

INTRODUCTION

The first cry of the newborn results in lung expansion and the pulmonary pressure begins to decline soon after birth. Patent ductus arteriosus (PDA) is the most common heart disease in pre-term infants (1). Functional closure of PDA occurs within 24–48 h after birth owing to increasing PaO_2 and decreasing circulatory vasodilators. Permanent anatomical closure occurs followed by the endothelial hyperplasia and fibrotic process (2, 3). Untreated hemodynamically significant PDA with a left-to-right shunt can result in increased pulmonary blood flow, heart failure, and pulmonary arterial (PA) hypertension (4–6), and can even progress to Eisenmenger syndrome.

Eisenmenger syndrome is an absolute contraindication for PDA closure in children and adults because the procedure could lead to pulmonary hypertension crisis, acute right ventricular failure, and even death. Pulmonary hypertension in pre-term infants is usually secondary to lung disease, mostly caused by respiratory distress syndrome and bronchopulmonary dysplasia (BPD), instead of PDA itself (7, 8). PDA with a bidirectional shunt reflects high PA pressure. Closure of hemodynamically significant PDA in pre-term infants with PA pressure lower than systemic blood pressure (left-to-right shunt) is reasonable, but PDA closure in very high PA pressure that is equal to systemic blood pressure (bidirectional shunt) is crucial because of the risk of acute right ventricular failure. However, the use of pulmonary vasodilator in pre-term infants with a bidirectional shunt will lead to a left-to-right ductal shunt and even pulmonary hemorrhage. This critical situation is more frequently encountered in extremely low-birth-weight pre-term infants. Surgical closure of hemodynamically significant PDA in pre-term infants with a bidirectional shunt remains a dilemma. Therefore, this study aimed to investigate the outcomes of hemodynamically significant PDA ligation in pre-term infants with a bidirectional shunt.

PATIENTS AND METHODS

Data of this case-control study was collected from in-patient and out-patient medical records. Ethical approval was given by the Institutional Review Board of Medical Ethics of E-DA Hospital (EMRP25106N), and all informed consents were approved by the participants' parents, with all patient information de-identified.

Abbreviations: LA/Ao ratio, left atrium-to-aorta ratio; HFOV, high frequency oscillatory ventilator; PA, pulmonary arterial; PASP, pulmonary arterial systolic pressure; PMA, post-menstrual age; PVL, periventricular leukomalacia.

Patients

Pre-term infants (gestational age < 37 weeks) admitted to our neonatal intensive care unit undergoing PDA ligation between April 2013 and March 2019 were enrolled in our study. Patients' gender, gestational age, birth bodyweight, and delivery method were all recorded. All echocardiography was performed by the same pediatric cardiologist (MC Yang), and echocardiographic assessment was repeated on the day of surgery. PDA size, left atrium-to-aorta ratio (LA/Ao ratio), transductal velocity, and pressure gradients (between the aorta and pulmonary artery) were recorded. Patients were divided into two groups according to the shunting directions of PDA. Group A was PDA with a continuous left-to-right shunt (**Figure 1A**), and group B was a bidirectional shunt (**Figures 1B–D**). The PA pressure measured in cardiac catheterization is regarded as the gold standard for the diagnosis of pulmonary hypertension. However, it is impractical for a pre-term infant to receive a cardiac catheterization procedure only for measuring PA pressure, and this forces pediatric cardiologists to rely on echocardiographic assessment. PDA blood flow is one of the methods to evaluate PA pressure (9). The shunting directions reflect the severity of pulmonary hypertension, and PA systolic pressure was estimated by echocardiographic transductal pressure gradient assessment comparing to simultaneous systemic blood pressure. In patients with left-to-right (or right-to-left) PDA shunt at the systolic phase, the PA systolic pressure equaled systolic blood pressure subtracted (or added) by transductal pressure gradient.

In our neonatal intensive care center, the strategy of respiratory support was to use nasal continuous positive airway pressure ventilation as much as possible to lower the incidence of lung injury (10). Pre-operative and post-operative neurosonography was checked by an experienced neonatologist (HK Liu). Intraventricular hemorrhage (IVH) grading was evaluated according to a standardized assessment. Briefly, grade 1 was the bleeding area confined to the germinal matrix plus up to 10% of the ventricle volume, grade 2 was germinal matrix hemorrhage and IVH between 10 and 50% of the lateral ventricle volume, grade 3 was germinal matrix hemorrhage and IVH more than 50% of the lateral ventricle volume, and grade 4 was periventricular hemorrhagic infarction (11). Mechanical ventilatory support, necrotizing enterocolitis (NEC), and BPD were all recorded. NEC was recorded if patients presented stage 2 or 3 NEC, which was defined according to modified Bell staging (12). The diagnosis of BPD was based on oxygen or ventilator requirements, while the timing of BPD assessment was based on gestational age. Patients who were <32 weeks of gestational age were evaluated at 36 weeks post-menstrual age or when discharged home, whichever came first. Patients who were ≥32 weeks of gestational age

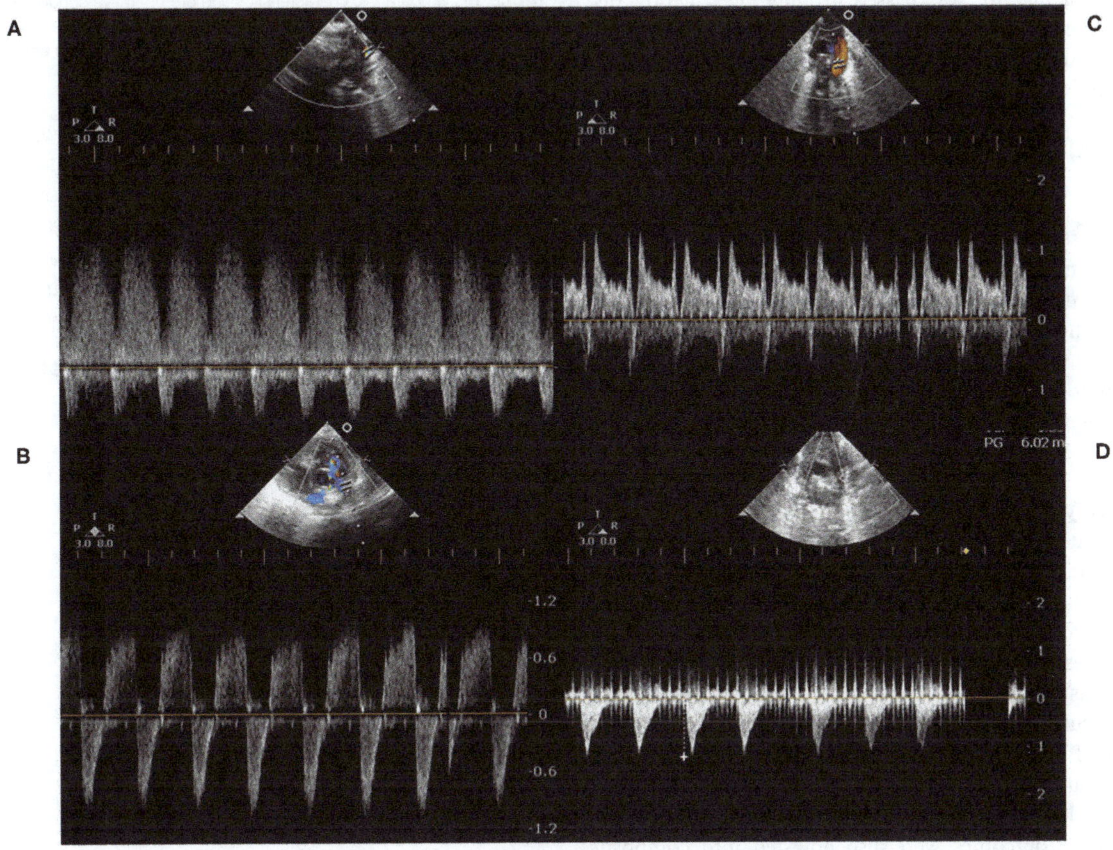

FIGURE 1 | (A) represented a continuous left-to-right shunt of a PDA, which was detected by pulse-wave Doppler. At the end-diastolic phase, there was a persistent left-to-right shunt; **(B,C)** represented a bidirectional shunt of a PDA. At the end-diastolic phase, the shunting directions were transient right-to-left; **(D)** represented a right-to-left shunt. There was rare left-to-right shunt either at the systolic or diastolic phase.

were evaluated at 28 days of age or when discharged home, depending on which came first (13). The definition of acute kidney injury was based on Kidney Diseases: Improving Global Outcomes consensus (14). Acute kidney injury was defined if serum creatinine rose $\geq$0.3 mg/dL within 48 h or serum creatinine $\geq$1.5–1.9 times of the lowest prior serum creatinine within 7 days.

Surgical Indications and Procedures

PDA ligations were performed by the same experienced cardiovascular surgeon (HY Wu). There were echocardiographic and clinical indications of hemodynamically significant PDA. Hemodynamically significant PDA was considered in patients fulfilling echocardiographic criteria, which were PDA diameter/bodyweight >1.3, antegrade PA diastolic flow, LA/Ao ratio $\geq$1.4, left ventricular enlargement, and retrograde diastolic flow in the descending aorta (15). Clinical criteria of hemodynamically significant PDA included PDA-related pulmonary hemorrhage, acute kidney injury, the need to upgrade ventilatory support, or difficulty in weaning a high-setting mechanical ventilator after excluding other etiologies. Fluid restriction to 90–100 cc/kg per day was applied if the PDA met the criteria of hemodynamically significant PDA. Once the PDA remained hemodynamically significant after fluid restriction, or fluid restriction resulted in significant electrolyte imbalance, oral ibuprofen or oral acetaminophen treatment was administered if enteral feeding had been successfully established. During the study period, intravenous ibuprofen was not commercially available in Taiwan because of small marketing requirements, which limited our use of ibuprofen in candidates. Surgical indications of PDA ligation were hemodynamically significant PDA plus one of the following (1) pre-term infants who could not tolerate enteral trophic feeding so that oral ibuprofen/acetaminophen could not be given; (2) infants who failed to respond to oral ibuprofen/acetaminophen treatment; (3) infants who were contraindicated to receive oral ibuprofen (active pulmonary hemorrhage, severe IVH, thrombocytopenia <100,000/uL, NEC, urine output <0.5 ml/kg/h, serum creatinine >1.7 mg/dL).

Surgical PDA ligation was performed via left posterolateral thoracotomy in the intensive care unit. The incision was carried out in the left third or fourth intercostal space at the right decubitus position. The ductus and the recurrent laryngeal nerve were exposed with the aid of a dissector. After PDA was exposed, a ligature was passed around PDA, gently tied town, and then a metal clip was placed for additional security. Body temperature, heart rate, and blood pressure were closely monitored and recorded right before the surgery and within 24 h after PDA ligation. Continuous intravenous morphine infusion (0.01 mg/kg/h) was given as a pain control protocol until 48 h after surgery.

Primary Outcome

Primary outcomes referred to complications occurring at or soon after surgery, including PDA rupture-related bleeding during the surgery, desaturation or unstable saturation during the surgical procedure that required temporary interruption of surgery, post-op pneumothorax, post-op hemothorax, vocal cord paralysis, phrenic nerve palsy, and immediate surgical mortality on the day of surgery.

Secondary Outcome

Secondary outcomes were complications within 30 days of the surgery, including neurological sequelae, NEC, and early mortality (16). BPD severity and 5-year survival were also included in secondary outcomes.

IVH progression was defined in patients whose IVH grading increment was equal to or more than 2 grades. Progression to periventricular leukomalacia (PVL) was defined in patients who had no PVL before PDA ligation, yet evolved into PVL after surgery at follow-up. Because early mortality might deter infants from developing post-op PVL, post-op NEC or BPD, these secondary outcomes were also adjusted into composite outcomes, including "early mortality or progression to PVL," "early mortality or post-op NEC," and "early mortality or BPD" to avoid comorbidity bias caused by early mortality.

STATISTICAL ANALYSIS

Data were analyzed by SPSS version 22 statistical software. Continuous variables were presented as mean ± standard deviation (SD). Independent Student's t-test was applied for comparison of mean values of the two groups, and the Mann-Whitney U-test was used to compared means if the data were not normally distributed. Pearson's chi-square test and Fisher's exact test were used to compare categorical variables, while the Kaplan-Meier model was applied to analyze survival, and the log-rank test was used to compare survival between the two groups. Statistical significance was defined as a p-value < 0.05.

RESULTS

Thirty-seven patients were enrolled in this study, including 18 in group A, and 19 in group B. The demographic characteristics and pre-op conditions are shown in **Table 1**. The mean age at surgery was 20.4 and 13.2 days old (3.1–37.7 vs. 1.7–24.9, 95% confidence interval). Respiratory distress was more severe in group B. In group A, nine infants had failure of non-invasive ventilatory support (including failure of nasal continuous positive airway pressure support in six infants, and failure of nasal intermittent positive airway pressure support in three infants) caused by hemodynamically significant PDA. The need to upgrade the setting of the original invasive mechanical ventilator was 50% (9/18) in group A, and 89.5% (17/19) in group B. One out of 18 infants (5.6%) in group A required high-frequency oscillatory ventilator, whereas 8 of 19 infants (42.1%) in group B required high frequency oscillatory ventilatory support ($p < 0.05$). Of those under invasive ventilatory support, the oxygen index was significantly higher in group B (4.7 ± 2.2 vs. 9.3 ± 2.7, $p < 0.05$). Two infants (2/37) in group B used inhaled nitric oxide to maintain adequate oxygenation, and one (1/37) of them also took sildenafil.

TABLE 1 | Demographic characteristics and pre-operative conditions.

	L-to-R shunt	Bidirectional shunt	*P*-value
Number	18	19	
Gestational age (week-old)	29.1 ± 0.8	30.9 ± 1.2	0.22
Birth body weight (gram)	1329 ± 201	1452 ± 187	0.66
Vaginal delivery	10 (55.6%)	5 (26.3%)	0.09
Male	9 (50%)	11 (57.9%)	0.63
Antenatal corticosteroid	7 (38.9%)	3 (15.8%)	0.11
Age at surgery (day-old)	20.4 ± 8.2	13.2 ± 5.5	0.22
Age at surgery (PMA, week-old)	32.0 ± 1.3	32.8 ± 1.5	0.68
Body weight at surgery (gram)	1544 ± 264	1585 ± 216	0.90
Pre-op complications			
Severe IVH	2 (11.1%)	4 (21.1%)	0.66
Periventricular leukomalacia	1 (5.6%)	1 (5.3%)	1.00
Meconium ileus	1 (5.6%)	0 (0%)	0.47
NEC	1 (5.6%)	0 (0%)	0.47
Pulmonary hemorrhage	5 (27.8%)	9 (47.4%)	0.31
Acute kidney injury	10 (55.6%)	11 (57.9%)	0.67
Pre-op ventilatory support			
Non-invasive ventilator or no support	9 (50%)	2 (10.5%)	<0.01*
Invasive ventilator	9 (50%)	17 (89.5%)	<0.01*
Conventional ventilator	8 (44.4%)	9 (47.4%)	0.09
HFOV	1 (5.6%)	8 (42.1%)	0.012*
Inhaled nitric oxide	0	2 (10.5%)	
Oxygen index	4.7 ± 2.2	9.3 ± 2.7	0.02*
LA/Ao ratio	1.73 ± 0.07	1.73 ± 0.08	0.97
PDA size/BW (mm/kg)	2.1 ± 0.2	2.4 ± 0.2	0.33
Cardiothoracic ratio on radiograph	0.60 ± 0.05	0.65 ± 0.08	0.74
Serum creatinine before PDA closure (mg/dL)	1.1 ± 0.6	1.4 ± 1.0	0.21
Prior ibuprofen/acetaminophen treatment	7 (38.9%)	3 (15.8%)	0.11

*HFOV, high frequency oscillatory ventilator; IVH, grade 3 or 4 intraventricular hemorrhage; LA/Ao ratio, left atrium-to-aorta ratio; NEC, stage 2 or 3 necrotizing enterocolitis; PMA, post-menstrual age; * represented statistically significant, $p < 0.05$.*

The LA/Ao ratio, PDA size indexed by body weight at surgery (PDA size/BW), and the cardiothoracic ratios on chest radiograph were similar between the two groups. There

TABLE 2 | Perioperative vital signs of the patients receiving PDA ligation.

	L-to-R shunt $n = 18$	Bidirectional shunt $n = 19$	*P*-value
Pre-op body temperature (°C)	36.7 ± 0.1	36.4 ± 0.2	0.23
Pre-op heart rate (bpm)	162 ± 2	165 ± 3	0.58
Tachycardia > 160 bpm	12	13	0.91
Use of dopamine	5	12	0.03*
Pre-op blood pressure (mmHg)			
Systolic blood pressure	64 ± 3	63 ± 3	0.91
Diastolic blood pressure	36 ± 2	35 ± 3	0.80
Mean blood pressure	45 ± 2	42 ± 2	0.83
Estimated PASP (mmHg)	41 ± 2	58 ± 3	<0.001*
Post-op body temperature (°C)	36.6 ± 0.1	36.6 ± 0.1	0.74
Post-op heart rate (bpm)	165 ± 3	166 ± 4	0.75
Post-op blood pressure (mmHg)			
Systolic blood pressure	66 ± 4	67 ± 5	0.88
Diastolic blood pressure	42 ± 3	44 ± 4	1.00
Mean blood pressure	50 ± 3	50 ± 4	0.95

*Bpm, beats per minute; PASP, pulmonary arterial systolic pressure; *represented statistically significant, p < 0.05.*

TABLE 3 | Primary outcome–immediate complications after PDA ligation.

	L-to-R shunt $n = 18$	Bidirectional shunt $n = 19$	*P*-value
PDA bleeding during surgery	0 (0%)	4 (21.1%)	0.04*
Intraoperative desaturation	1 (5.9%)	3 (15.8%)	0.32
Pneumothorax	1 (5.9%)	2 (10.5%)	0.62
Hemothorax	0 (0%)	1 (5.3%)	0.34
Vocal cord paralysis	1 (5.9%)	0 (0%)	0.28
Phrenic nerve palsy	2 (11.8%)	0 (0%)	0.12
Immediate surgical mortality	0 (0%)	0 (0%)	NS

*NS, non-significant; *represented statistically significant, p < 0.05.*

TABLE 4 | Secondary outcomes–late adverse outcomes after PDA ligation.

	L to R shunt $n = 18$	Bidirectional shunt $n = 19$	*P*-value
Neurological complications			
Post-op severe IVH	6 (33.3%)	5 (26.3%)	0.72
IVH progression	4 (22.2%)	1 (5.3%)	0.15
Post-op PVL	6 (33.3%)	4 (21.1%)	0.46
Progression to PVL	6 (33.3%)	1 (5.3%)	0.04*
Hydrocephalus	2 (11.1%)	3 (15.8%)	0.63
Post-op NEC	0	2 (10.5%)	0.16
Bronchopulmonary dysplasia			
Overall	16 (88.9%)	9 (47.4%)	0.054
Mild	3 (16.7%)	0	0.10
Moderate	1 (5.6%)	0	0.36
Severe	12 (66.6%)	9 (47.4%)	0.71
Early mortality	0	4 (21.1%)	0.04*
Overall Mortality	0	5 (26.3%)	0.02*
Composite outcomes			
Early mortality or progression to PVL	6 (33.3%)	7 (36.8%)	0.82
Early mortality or post-op NEC	0	5 (26.3%)	0.02*
Early mortality or BPD	16 (88.9%)	13 (68.4%)	0.13
Death after PDA ligation (days)	NA	29 ± 19	NA

*BPD, Bronchopulmonary dysplasia; IVH, intraventricular hemorrhage; NEC, Necrotizing enterocolitis; PVL, Periventricular leukomalacia; NA, not applicable; *represented statistically significant, p < 0.05.*

was no significant difference in serum creatinine level or incidence of acute kidney injury before surgery. The use of oral ibuprofen treatment was limited because seven patients developed acute kidney injury with serum creatinine >1.7 mg/dL, 17 patients were restricted from enteral feeding due to shock status requiring dopamine infusion, 14 patients developed active pulmonary hemorrhage, and one patient had NEC. Only ten infants received oral ibuprofen/acetaminophen before surgery.

Primary Outcomes

Perioperative vital signs are shown in **Table 2**. Infants in group B had a higher incidence of shock requiring dopamine infusion prior to the surgery ($p < 0.05$). However, under continuous dopamine infusion before surgical ligation, the systolic, diastolic, and mean blood pressure levels were similar between the two groups. Group B had higher estimated PA systolic pressure compared to group A (58 ± 3 vs. 41 ± 2 mmHg, $p < 0.001$) on the day of surgery. Milrinone, as a medical treatment of PDA in whom had congestive heart failure and reduced left ventricular contractility, was administered in five infants before surgery. After PDA ligation, there was no infant experiencing post-ligation syndrome, so adding of inotropes was not required.

The overall intraoperative and immediate post-operative complications are listed in **Table 3**. These complications included PDA rupture-related PDA bleeding (10.8%), intra-op desaturation (10.8%), post-op pneumothorax (8.1%), delayed post-op hemothorax (2.7%), vocal cord paralysis (2.7%), and phrenic nerve palsy (5.4%).

PDA rupture-related bleeding during exposing PDA or ligating PDA occurred in four infants in group B, whereas no infant experienced PDA rupture in group A ($p < 0.05$). Intra-op desaturation requiring temporary interruption of surgery occurred in four infants (1 in group A, and 3 in group B). Although it was non-significantly different, intra-op desaturation occurred more frequently in group B. One infant in group B received emergent chest tube insertion on the day of surgery because of delayed hemothorax, which was considered to be caused by PDA rupture-related bleeding. Her condition stabilized

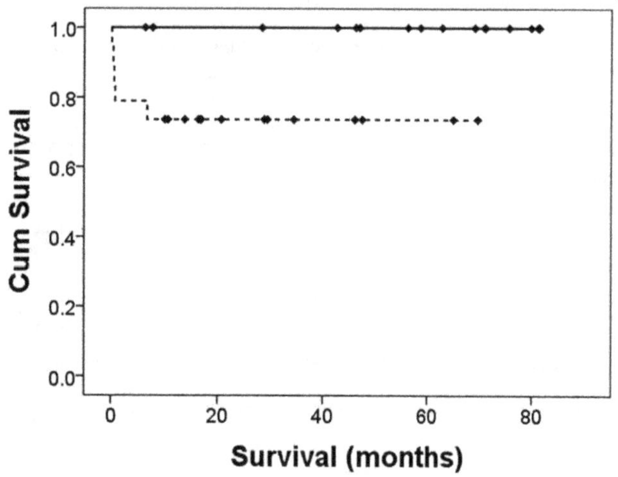

FIGURE 2 | Cumulative survival after PDA ligation. The solid line is the left-to-right group. The dotted line is the bidirectional group. The Log-rank test revealed a significant difference in survival, $p = 0.02$.

soon after the intervention. There was no immediate surgical mortality on the day of surgery in both groups.

Secondary Outcomes

As shown in **Table 4**, after PDA ligation, there were more infants in group A developing progression to PVL (33.3% in group A vs. 5.3% in group B, $p < 0.05$). Two infants developed NEC after surgery, and both of them were in group B. The overall incidence of BPD was 88.9% in group A, and 47.4% in group B ($p = 0.054$). Of the different severity of BPD, the incidence was similar between the two groups. Early mortality occurred only in group B (four infants, 21.1%). The causes of death were sepsis in two infants, stage 3 NEC in one infant, and pulmonary hypertensive crisis in one infant, with this infant expiring on the next day of surgery. Among the composite outcomes, only "early mortality or NEC" was significantly different (0% in group A vs. 26.3% in group B, $p < 0.05$). Although the overall mortality was higher in group B than that in group A (26.3 vs. 0%, $p < 0.05$), only one death could be attributed to PDA ligation. As shown in **Figure 2**, the 5-year survival was higher in group A (100 vs. 73.7%, $p = 0.02$).

DISCUSSION

This is a novel study of PDA closure in pre-term infants exploring the relationship between the shunting directions of PDA and surgical outcomes in the literature. There are several unique important findings in this study. Pre-term infants with a bidirectional shunt PDA were prone to have higher PA pressures, unstable blood pressures, and inherent worse respiratory conditions requiring more invasive mechanical ventilatory support. PDA rupture-related bleeding during the surgical procedure was a major challenge for both medical staff and patients, especially while exposing or ligating the PDA. Although there was no significant difference, intra-op desaturation occurred more frequently in the bidirectional group. Unexpected vascular bleeding and unstable oxygen saturation complicated the surgical procedure. Even after the procedure, delayed hemothorax several hours after PDA ligation still occurred and required emergent chest tube insertion in one infant. Among the composite outcomes of early mortality and post-op comorbidities, only NEC was more frequent in group B. NEC was a major concern that complicated clinical care after PDA surgery in group B. In most patients with bidirectional shunt pattern, PDA ligation was feasible. Only one death died of pulmonary hypertensive crisis could be attributed to PDA surgery. However, early mortality of 21.1% was observed.

The operability of PDA in PA pressure reaching systemic blood pressure is generally not feasible in children and adults. Eisenmenger syndrome remains an absolute contraindication of PDA closure in children and adults (17). The major concerns are post-op pulmonary hypertensive crisis and acute right heart failure because of irreversible pulmonary arterial hypertension (18–23). Nevertheless, pulmonary arterial smooth muscle cell hypertrophy and endothelial cell proliferation are believed to be the main pathophysiology in irreversible pulmonary hypertension, but it rarely happens before 1 year of age (24, 25).

Early PDA treatment within 7 days of birth is generally not recommended because of possible spontaneous closure in the first week, and early treatment is associated with higher mortality and higher BPD rate (26). In this cohort, six infants (two in group A, four in group B) underwent PDA ligation within 7 days old. Among these six infants, four infants had pulmonary hemorrhage, one infant developed PDA-related shock, and one infant had both pulmonary hemorrhage and shock. Emergent surgical ligation was performed in three infants because of refractory shock and persistent pulmonary hemorrhage. Another three infants with pulmonary hemorrhage also underwent surgical ligation after the failure of controlling PDA with fluid restriction.

In our study, most of the infants with bidirectional shunt were mainly left-to-right shunt (**Figures 1B,C**), but two infants were bidirectional with a mainly right-to-left shunt (**Figure 1D**). In pre-term infants, the PA pressures were dynamic and influenced by the lung condition. The persistent left-to-right shunt PDA (**Figure 1A**) or bidirectional pattern with mainly left-to-right shunt PDA (**Figures 1B,C**) ultimately contributed to pulmonary blood overflow and pulmonary edema. The pulmonary blood overflow further led to pulmonary hemorrhage at an unexpected timing. The occurrence would be abrupt within hours, especially in extremely low birth weight infants. Once pulmonary hemorrhage occurred, the PA pressure would suddenly elevate to the systemic level, which in turn caused right-to-left shunt. Medical management of pulmonary hemorrhage eventually stabilized the edema or hemorrhage, and the PA pressure would return to a lower level. However, the PDA became left-to-right shunt again afterward. This entered an endless vicious cycle, so that interruption of the cycle by ligating PDA provided benefit to these pre-term infants because no one could predict when would be the next episode of pulmonary hemorrhage. This was also the rationale why we needed to perform PDA ligation in an infant with a bidirectional shunt.

Because of the preserved reversibility of pulmonary hypertension, PDA ligation was performed in two particular pre-term infants with a mainly right-to-left shunt. Both of these infants were treated with high-frequency oscillatory ventilator, and were also the only two infants receiving inhaled nitric oxide during PDA ligation. One of these, whose birth body weight was 845 gram, had grade 4 RDS and severe persistent pulmonary hypertension of the newborn that was refractory to intratracheal surfactant administration, experiencing repeated pulmonary hemorrhage due to a transient left-to-right shunt and pulmonary overflow while inhaling 10 ppm nitric oxide. Pulmonary hemorrhage further aggravated pulmonary hypertension and led to the reappearance of a right-to-left shunt. Emergent PDA ligation was performed to interrupt the endless vicious cycle in this infant at the age of 2 days. He was weaned off the invasive mechanical ventilator successfully under intensive respiratory care and other medical treatments when he was 13 days old, and was discharged at corrected age of 52 days.

The other infant, whose birth bodyweight was 500 grams, was born at gestational age 27 weeks. He also received PDA ligation in the status of a right-to-left shunt. In the beginning, PDA was not hemodynamically significant, so it was treated conservatively. His pulmonary condition had never been well, so a high ventilator setting with intermittent administration of inhaled nitric oxide had been applied for 3 months. Weaning of invasive ventilator was not achievable in the first 3 months of life. Echocardiography at corrected age of 6 days revealed a 2.5 mm right-to-left shunt PDA. After titrating up nitric oxide, PDA became a bidirectional shunt on echocardiography. This response indicated the reversibility of pulmonary vasoreactivity. Because high mechanical ventilator setting and inhaled nitric oxide were unable to be weaned off successfully in the past 3 months, we decided to carry out PDA ligation and then use inhaled nitric oxide continuously to treat his severe pulmonary hypertension. PDA ligation was performed at the corrected age of 8 days. The PDA was edematous and fragile. PDA rupture happened intraoperatively, otherwise the whole surgical procedure was smooth. Afterwards, the patient was successfully weaned from an invasive mechanical ventilator 37 days after the operation, by the time he was at the corrected age of 44 days. Inhaled nitric oxide was shifted to oral sildenafil for the treatment of pulmonary hypertension. Although this patient had severe BPD, he needed oxygen hood with low oxygen fraction only. Our limited experience demonstrates the feasibility of PDA closure in pre-term infants with severe pulmonary hypertension, even though PA pressure was higher than systemic blood pressure.

There was an infant in group B who died from a pulmonary hypertensive crisis on the next day of PDA ligation. This infant's condition was stable initially after surgery, but he developed circulatory shock and desaturation 6 h later. Despite inhaled nitric oxide being administered, the patient still had acute right ventricular failure and shock. In this case, routine morphine was administered continuously after surgery, but the dosage was not increased while he had the severe pulmonary hypertensive crisis. On reflection, the pain-induced pulmonary hypertensive crisis was a major problem leading to death, and from this case, it was determined that management of pain control should be more aggressive in infants with very high PA pressure after PDA surgery.

There was a higher incidence of intra-operative PDA bleeding and post-op hemothorax in group B. Two of the four infants in group B with PDA bleeding received inhaled nitric oxide during surgery. The postulated hypothesis was that the intraductal blood pressure was very high because the PA pressure was approaching systemic blood pressure, which led to engorgement and fragility of the PDA. Once touching the vessel while exposing or ligating the PDA, a rupture occurred easily and resulted in bleeding. Inhaled nitric oxide also contributed to the bleeding because the exposure of nitric oxide might lead to a certain degree of coagulopathy (27). Transcatheter PDA closure in pre-term infants has become an available intervention and several trials presented promising outcomes (28, 29). The hemodynamic study can be measured during the cardiac catheterization, which even allows a test occlusion before PDA closure in pre-term infants with a bidirectional shunt. Our study demonstrated the feasibility of PDA ligation in pre-term infants with a bidirectional shunt. Although intra-operative PDA bleeding and post-op hemothorax was a concern in surgery, transcatheter closure might be an alternative choice to overcome the bleeding-related complications.

LIMITATIONS

This was a prospective case-control study, but the allocation of patients and the timing of surgery were not randomized. We allocated these patients into groups A or B according to their echocardiographic PDA blood flow findings on the day of surgery. The pre-op respiratory condition was worse in group B, and this might have influenced the post-operative outcomes. Due to the small marketing requirement of intravenous ibuprofen in Taiwan, the intravenous form had not been available until 2019. This resulted in few candidates receiving intravenous ibuprofen in our cohort. Hence, the experience of ibuprofen treatment may be quite different from other countries. Owing to the background, we had more infants undergoing surgical ligation, even in the status of a bidirectional shunt.

Approximately one-fourth of infants with moderate to severe BPD developed pulmonary hypertension later in their life (30). In our cohort, 22 infants developed moderate to severe BPD (13 in group A, nine in group B). Although group B had higher estimated PA pressure during the surgery, the development of BPD-related pulmonary hypertension was not evaluated.

There were only 37 pre-term infants enrolled in this study, so statistical calculations might not have reached significance because of the relatively small number of patients. No studies have focused on outcomes of PDA with a bidirectional shunt in pre-term infants. This can be regarded as an initial experience for similar subjects, and the conclusions would be more confidently regarded as valid if more patients could be enrolled in future research.

CONCLUSIONS

This is a novel study exploring outcomes of PDA ligation in pre-term infants with a bidirectional shunt. Post-op echocardiography revealed favorable left ventricular and right ventricular systolic function and no signs of acute right ventricular failure in our study, except for one patient expiring from a pulmonary hypertensive crisis. The relatively high mortality rate in group B could be attributed to poor pre-op conditions, including higher oxygen index and unstable blood pressure requiring dopamine infusion. Post-ligation outcomes proved the feasibility of PDA closure in critical pre-term infants with severe pulmonary hypertension and even with a bidirectional shunt. Composite outcomes showed neurological sequelae and the incidence of BPD did not differ between the two groups. According to this result, we did not recommend routine PDA ligation in pre-term infants with a bidirectional shunt. However, a bidirectional shunt should not be an absolute contraindication if pre-term infants fulfill indications of PDA closure. Surgeons need to be extremely careful while dissecting the tissue, exposing and ligating the PDA. Even though surgical ligation might be successfully performed, watchful monitoring for delayed hemothorax is still warranted. Post-operative pain control should be very aggressive if there are any signs of a pulmonary hypertension crisis.

ETHICS STATEMENT

The studies involving human participants were reviewed and approved by Institutional Review Board of Medical Ethics of E-DA Hospital. Written informed consent to participate in this study was provided by the participants' legal guardian/next of kin.

AUTHOR CONTRIBUTIONS

The ideas and protocol of this study were designed by M-CY. Medical records were obtained by M-CY, H-KL, H-YW, S-LT, Y-NY, and C-YW. M-CY and H-KL completed the manuscript and worked for the statistical analysis. J-RW revised the article. All authors contributed to the article and approved the submitted version.

REFERENCES

1. Lu CW, Wu MH. Patent ductus arteriosus: when does it become a significant lesion for full-term newborns? *Pediatr Neonatol.* (2010) 51:141–2. doi: 10.1016/S1875-9572(10)60026-5
2. Schneider DJ, Moore JW. Patent ductus arteriosus. *Circulation.* (2006) 114:1873–82. doi: 10.1161/CIRCULATIONAHA.105.592063
3. Wu JR, Yeh JL, Liou SF, Dai ZK, Wu BN, Hsu JH. Gamma-secretase inhibitor prevents proliferation and migration of ductus arteriosus smooth muscle cells through the Notch3-HES1/2/5 pathway. *Int J Biol Sci.* (2016) 12:1063–73. doi: 10.7150/ijbs.16430
4. Simonneau G, Montani D, Celermajer D, Denton C, Gatzoulis MA, Krowka M, et al. Haemodynamic definitions and updated clinical classification of pulmonary hypertension. *Eur Respir J.* (2019) 53:1801913. doi: 10.1183/13993003.01913-2018
5. Hansmann G, Koestenberger M, Alastalo TP, Apitz C, Austin ED, Bonnet D, et al. 2019 updated consensus statement on the diagnosis and treatment of pediatric pulmonary hypertension: the European pediatric pulmonary vascular disease network (EPPVDN), endorsed by AEPC, ESPR and ISHLT. *J Heart Lung Transplant.* (2019) 38:879–901. doi: 10.1016/j.healun.2019.06.022
6. Roth TS, Aboulhosn JA. Pulmonary hypertension and congenital heart disease. *Cardiol Clin.* (2016) 34:391–400. doi: 10.1016/j.ccl.2016.04.002
7. Yeh TF. Persistent pulmonary hypertension in preterm infants with respiratory distress syndrome. *Pediatr Pulmonol.* (2001) 23:103–6. doi: 10.1002/ppul.1950322341
8. Baker CD, Abman SH, Mourani PM. Pulmonary hypertension in preterm infants with bronchopulmonary dysplasia. *Pediatr Allergy Immunol Pulmonol.* (2014) 27:8–16. doi: 10.1089/ped.2013.0323
9. O'Connor MG, Cornfield DN, Austin ED. Pulmonary hypertension in the premature infant: a challenging comorbidity in a vulnerable population. *Curr Opin Pediatr.* (2016) 28:324–30. doi: 10.1097/MOP.0000000000000355
10. Sahni R, Schiaratura M, Polin RA. Strategies for the prevention of continuous positive airway pressure failure. *Semin Fetal Neonatal Med.* (2016) 21:196–203. doi: 10.1016/j.siny.2016.02.008
11. Inder TE, Perlman JM, Volpe JJ. Preterm Intraventricular Hemorrhage/Posthemorrhagic hydrocephalus. In: Volpe JJ, editor. *Volpe's Neurology of the Newborn.* 6th ed. Philadelphia, PA: Elsevier (2018). p.637. doi: 10.1016/B978-0-323-42876-7.00024-7
12. Neu J. Necrotizing enterocolitis: the search for a unifying pathogenic theory leading to prevention. *Pediatr Clin North Am.* (1996) 43:409. doi: 10.1016/S0031-3955(05)70413-2
13. Jobe AH, Bancalari E. Bronchopulmonary dysplasia. *Am J Respir Crit Care Med.* (2001) 163:1723–9. doi: 10.1164/ajrccm.163.7.2011060
14. Nada A, Bonachea EM, Askenazi DJ. Acute kidney injury in the fetus and neonate. *Semin Fetal Neonatal Med.* (2017) 22:90–7. doi: 10.1016/j.siny.2016.12.001
15. Sehgal A, McNamara PJ. Does echocardiography facilitate determination of hemodynamic significance attributable to the ductus arteriosus? *Eur J Pediatr.* (2009) 168:907–14. doi: 10.1007/s00431-009-0983-3
16. Jacobs JP, Mayer JE Jr, Mavroudis C, O'Brien SM, Austin EH III, Pasquali SK, et al. The society of thoracic surgeons congenital heart surgery database: 2017 update on outcomes and quality. *Ann Thorac Surg.* (2017) 103:699–709. doi: 10.1016/j.athoracsur.2017.01.004
17. Tharakan J, Venkateshwaran S. Large patent ductus arteriosus: to close or not to close. *Ann Pediatr Cardiol.* (2012) 5:141–4. doi: 10.4103/0974-2069.99615
18. Wang JK, Wu MH, Hwang JJ, Chiang FT, Lin MT, Lue HC. Transcatheter closure of moderate to large patent ductus arteriosus with the Amplatzer duct occluder. *Catheter Cardiovasc Interv.* (2007) 69:572–8. doi: 10.1002/ccd.20701
19. Bhalgat PS, Pinto R, Dalvi BV. Transcatheter closure of large patent ductus arteriosus with severe pulmonary arterial hypertension: short and intermediate-term results. *Ann Pediatr Cardiol.* (2012) 5:135–40. doi: 10.4103/0974-2069.99614
20. D'Alto M, Mahadevan VS. Pulmonary arterial hypertension associated with congenital heart disease. *Eur Respir Rev.* (2012) 21:328–37. doi: 10.1183/09059180.00004712
21. Niu MC, Mallory GB, Justino H, Ruiz FE, Petit CJ. Treatment of severe pulmonary hypertension in the setting of the large patent ductus arteriosus. *Pediatrics.* (2013) 131:e1643–9. doi: 10.1542/peds.2011-1417
22. Kalavrouziotis G, Kourtesis A, Paphitis C, Azariades P. Closure of a large patent ductus arteriosus in children and adults with pulmonary hypertension. *Hellenic J Cardiol.* (2010) 51:15–8.
23. Carmosino MJ, Friesen RH, Doran A, Ivy DD. Perioperative complications in children with pulmonary hypertension undergoing noncardiac surgery or cardiac catheterization. *Anesth Analg.* (2007) 104:521–7. doi: 10.1213/01.ane.0000255732.16057.1c

24. Adatia I, Kothari SS, Feinstein JA. Pulmonary hypertension associated with congenital heart disease: pulmonary vascular disease: the global perspective. *Chest.* (2010) 137:52S–61S. doi: 10.1378/chest.09-2861
25. Sakao S, Tatsumi K, Voelkel NF. Reversible or irreversible remodeling in pulmonary arterial hypertension. *Am J Respir Cell Mol Biol.* (2010) 43:629–34. doi: 10.1165/rcmb.2009-0389TR
26. Okulu E, Erdeve O, Arslan Z, Demirel N, Kaya H, Gokce IK, et al. An observational, prospective, multicenter, registry-based cohort study comparing conservative and medical management for patent ductus arteriosus. *Front Pediatr.* (2020) 8:434. doi: 10.3389/fped.2020.00434
27. Gries A, Bode C, Peter K, Herr A, Böhrer H, Motsch J, et al. Inhaled nitric oxide inhibits human platelet aggregation, P-selectin expression, and fibrinogen binding *in vitro* and *in vivo* *Circulation.* (1998) 97:1481–7. doi: 10.1161/01.CIR.97.15.1481
28. Vali P, Lakshminrusimha S, Pelech A, Underwood M, Ing F. Patent ductus arteriosus in preterm infants: is early transcatheter closure a paradigm shift? *J Perinatol.* (2019) 39:1449–61. doi: 10.1038/s41372-019-0506-7
29. Almeida-Jones M, Tang NY, Reddy A, Zahn E. Overview of transcatheter patent ductus arteriosus closure in preterm infants. *Congenit Heart Dis.* (2019) 14:60–4. doi: 10.1111/chd.12712
30. Hansmann G, Sallmon H, Roehr CC, Kourembanas S, Austin ED, Koestenberger M. Pulmonary hypertension in bronchopulmonary dysplasia. *Pediatr Res.* (2020). doi: 10.1038/s41390-020-0993-4. [Epub ahead of print].

12

Predictive Model of Early Spontaneous Ductus Arteriosus Closure Based on Neonatologist Performed Echocardiography in Preterm Infants

María Carmen Bravo [1], Rebeca Sánchez [1], Ana Isabel Blanco [1], Itsaso Losantos [2] and Adelina Pellicer [1]*

[1] *Department of Neonatology, La Paz University Hospital, Madrid, Spain,* [2] *Division of Statistics, La Paz University Hospital, Madrid, Spain*

Correspondence:
María Carmen Bravo
mcarmen.bravo@salud.madrid.org

Background: Patent ductus arteriosus (PDA) treatment remains controversial. Modeling on the predictive capacity of early spontaneous PDA closure would help in decision-making.

Aim: To design a predictive model of early spontaneous PDA closure.

Methods: As part of a trial to assess efficacy and safety of two ibuprofen treatment schemes for PDA, infants below 29 weeks' gestation were scanned between 18 and 72 h of birth, and serially if indicated. PDA treatment was decided based on echocardiography signs of lung overflow or systemic hypoperfusion and clinical criteria. A PDA score that included the echocardiographic parameters significantly associated with treatment prescription was retrospectively applied. Perinatal variables and screening score were included in a backwards elimination model to predict early spontaneous closure.

Results: Among 87 eligible infants (27 weeks' gestation; age at screening 45 h), 21 received ibuprofen at 69 h of life [screening score = 7 (IQR = 5–8.5); score at treatment = 9 (IQR = 8–9)], while 42 infants had conservative management, [screening score = 1 (IQR = 0–4)]. Twenty four infants were excluded (ibuprofen contraindication, declined consent or incomplete echocardiography). Screening score showed an AUC = 0.93 to predict early spontaneous PDA closure, [cut-off value = 4.5 (sensitivity = 0.90, specificity = 0.86)]. The predictive model for early spontaneous PDA closure followed the equation: Log (p/1-p) = −28.41 + 1.23* gestational age −0.87* PDA screening score.

Conclusions: A predictive model of early spontaneous PDA closure that includes gestational age and the screening PDA score is proposed to help clinicians in the decision- making for PDA treatment. In addition, this model could be used in future intervention trials aimed to prevent PDA related morbidities to improve the eligibility criteria.

Keywords: ductus arteriosus, echocardiography, preterm infant, ibuprofen, NPE

INTRODUCTION

The patent ductus arteriosus (PDA) is associated with several morbidities including intraventricular hemorrhage (IVH), necrotizing enterocolitis (NEC), bronchopulmonary dysplasia (BPD), and death as a result of pulmonary over-circulation and systemic hypoperfusion (1–6). Different management strategies have been studied in the last years, such as prophylactic treatment, early targeted treatment, treatment of a clinically symptomatic PDA, and the conservative approach of "watchful waiting" (7–12). The reported spontaneous closure rate reaches 73% at 2 months of postnatal age in extremely low gestational age neonates who survive beyond the neonatal period (11). Yet, none of these approaches have shown a reduction in the prevalence of PDA-related morbidities. This lack of benefit may be due to the fact that some infants with borderline ductal shunts (non-significant) were included in the treatment group in these trials (9). In addition, in case of active treatment is decided, there is not consensus on "how early" should treatment be started, as severe co-morbidities like IVH or pulmonary hemorrhage occur very early after birth and would be only prevented by prophylactic or very early targeted treatment (before 12 h form birth) (9, 13). Moreover, pharmacological efficacy of the cyclooxygenase inhibitors is inversely related to postnatal age at treatment administration (14).

Serial neonatologist performed echocardiography (NPE) facilitate identification of a hemodynamically significant PDA (hsPDA), and may also inform on the likelihood of spontaneous PDA closure. We hypothesized that an early predictive NPE model for spontaneous PDA closure beyond the first day of life will avoid overtreatment of babies with closing PDA patterns.

This retrospective study, that combines systematic serial NPE and prospective clinical data recordings, aims to build up a model to classify two populations of preterm infants early in the clinical course: those with a closing PDA pattern that will not be subsidiary of an active PDA treatment, from those with hsPDA and pathophysiologically related (lung hyperperfusion or systemic hypoperfusion) co-morbidities, therefore beneficiaries of an active early PDA treatment.

METHOD

Infants with <29 completed weeks of gestation underwent echocardiographic assessment between 18 and 72 h of birth, as part of the routine care at NICU, in the foregoing discussion named as screening NPE. Those with NPE criteria of hsPDA were considered eligible for a multicentre randomized controlled trial to compare the efficacy and safety of two different intravenous ibuprofen treatment schemes (15-min bolus infusion vs. 24-h continuous infusion). Pharmacological PDA closure at this stage was always indicated by the attending physician based on echocardiography data and the infant's clinical condition. Serial scans were performed until PDA closure was confirmed or hospital discharge, whatever came first.

A hsPDA was defined by NPE if PDA showed a diameter larger than 1.5 mm and echocardiographic signs indicating pulmonary overflow, systemic hypoperfusion, or both were present, following the latest recommendations of the European Special Interest Group "Neonatologist Performed Echocardiography" (15). Infants were excluded in the case ibuprofen treatment was contraindicated or had no informed consent signed. If an open duct was not judged as hsPDA, or even in the case of pulmonary overflow or systemic hypoperfusion the attending physician decided a "watchful waiting," serial scans were undertaken to confirm PDA closure or need for treatment prescription.

Infants who received ibuprofen for PDA closure at any time during the neonatal period formed the ibuprofen treatment (IB-T) group, and those who did not received any pharmacological treatment to close PDA formed the conservative management (CM) group.

The study protocol was approved by the Ethics Committee for Human Studies at La Paz University Hospital and the Spanish Medicines Agency at the National Ministry of Health (Eudract Code: 2016-002974-11 and ClinicalTrials.gov code: NCT04282941).

NPE Studies

An Aplio 500 ultrasound scanner (Toshiba Medical Systems B.V, Netherlands) with a multifrequency phased array transducer 7–10 Mhz was used. Structural normality of the heart was established on the initial scan and standardized criteria for PDA hemodynamic significance were followed (15–18).

Transductal diameter was measured from a high left-sided parasternal "ductal" view to obtain a clear 2D image of the ductus arteriosus. The probe was placed in a true sagittal plane to the left of the sternum with the marker pointing toward the head to obtain the ductal view. The ductal diameter was measured at the site of maximum constriction (shortest diameter) at the pulmonary end, using color Doppler imaging, increasing the gain until background noise was suppressed, and expressed in mm. Ductal maximum and minimum velocity (Vmax/Vmin) ratio, was measured applying pulsed-wave Doppler (PWD) at the pulmonary end of the ductal view. Antegrade left pulmonary artery (LPA) diastolic flow, was visualized from a high parasternal short axis view using color Doppler. End-diastolic velocity was measured by PWD in the LPA tracing the Doppler signal and expressed in cm/s. Left atrial/aortic ratio was measured from the parasternal long axis view using M-mode at end-diastole, positioning the probe perpendicular to the aorta at the level of the aortic valve. To calculate the left ventricular output (LVO), aortic root diameter was measured at the hinges of the aortic valve leaflets, from the long axis parasternal view. The velocity time integral (VTI) of the ascending aorta was obtained by PWD from the apical 5-chamber view, aligning the probe to become parallel to flow direction, without angle of correction. Three consecutive Doppler wave forms were averaged and used to estimate the VTI. LVO (mL/kg/min) was derived from the equation: $[(\text{aortic diameter}^2/4) * \pi * \text{VTI} * \text{heart rate}]/\text{weight}$. Superior vena cava

---

Abbreviations: PDA, patent ductus arteriosus; IVH, intraventricular hemorrhage; NEC, necrotizing enterocolitis; BPD, bronchopulmonary dysplasia; NPE, neonatologist performed echocardiographic studies; hsPDA, hemodynamically significant PDA; PWD, pulsed-wave Doppler; LPA, left pulmonary artery; LVO, left ventricular output; VTI, velocity time integral; SVC, superior vena cava.

(SVC) diameter was calculated from the parasternal long axis view with the ultrasound beam in a true sagittal plane and angled to the right of the ascending aorta. Maximum and minimum diameters of three to five consecutive cardiac cycles, obtained by M-mode at the point the SVC starts to open into the right atrium, were averaged. The VTI of the SVC was measured from a subcostal window and the angle of insonation was minimized by maneuvering the transducer inferiorly to allow visualization of the maximal amount of flow within the SVC before entry into the right atrium. The pulsed Doppler recording was made at the junction of the SVC and the right atrium. The averaged VTI from 5 to 10 consecutive cardiac cycles was obtained. SVC flow (mL/kg/min) was derived from the equation: [(mean SVC diameter^2/4) $* \pi *$ VTI $*$ heart rate] / weight. Then, the LVO/SVC flow was calculated.

E wave/A wave ratio was obtained from a four-chamber view with the probe positioned on the apex of the heart with the marker facing the left side. The probe was tilted to the right shoulder and the pulsed Doppler range gate was set slightly below the mitral valve annulus.

NPE were always performed by the same study team (MCB, RS, and AIB) for whom inter and intra-observer variability study was conducted ahead to the trial start on a sample of 57 scans. The intraclass correlation coefficient ranged between 0.88 and 0.98 ($p < 0.001$) for all the variables that were explored.

Statistical Analysis

The data were analyzed using the SAS version 9.4 (SAS Institute Inc. 2013). The quantitative perinatal data and echocardiographic variables were expressed as median and interquartile range (IQR), and the qualitative data as count and percentage (%). IB-T group and CM group were compared using the Mann-Whitney U or Kruskal-Wallis-test and Fisher's exact or χ^2-test for quantitative and qualitative variables, respectively.

A multiple regression analysis was performed to evaluate the association between perinatal and NPE variables with ibuprofen treatment. Different combinations of the NPE variables were used to calculate the best PDA score to categorize PDA disease and to predict early spontaneous PDA closure, adapted from that proposed by Sehgal et al. (19) for ductal disease severity staging. A receiver operating characteristics curve was constructed to assess the ability of PDA score at screening NPE to predict early spontaneous PDA closure.

The best model for PDA score was retrospectively calculated at screening NPE and at the time of treatment administration. In addition, a backwards elimination method was applied to create the best predictive model of early spontaneous PDA closure, based on the probability of the Wald statistic. A full (saturated) model including all the perinatal variables statistically associated with spontaneous closure (positive and negative associations) from the multiple regression model was created. Then, at each step the analysis gradually eliminates variables from the regression model to find a reduced model that best explains the data.

All the statistical analyses were considered bilateral, and values of $p < 0.05$ were considered significant.

RESULTS

From July 2018 to April 2020, 87 infants of 27 (25.6–27.8) weeks of gestation were eligible for the study (**Figure 1**). Of them, 85 underwent screening NPE assessment at a median postnatal age of 45 (24–49) h. Informed consent was declined in one infant, and an additional infant was not included due to incomplete data on screening NPE. Twenty one infants who were identified as having hsPDA by NPE received ibuprofen treatment (IB-T group) at a median postnatal age of 69 (52–158) h, while 42 infants who did not show echocardiographic signs of hsPDA were not treated and formed the CM group. Among the former, treatment was indicated in 7 infants as a result of the screening NPE, while in the remaining 14, a second NPE was needed for decision-making.

Twenty two additional infants underwent screening NPE but were not considered eligible for the intervention trial due to persistent pulmonary hypertension ($n = 9$) or other clinical conditions ($n = 13$). This precluded to have a complete systematic approach by NPE in this subset of infants and accordingly are not included in this retrospective analysis. Details of the study population chart flow are depicted on **Figure 1**.

Infants in the IB-T group had lower gestational age ($p < 0.001$), birth weight ($p = 0.003$), and 5-min Apgar ($p = 0.04$), showed higher rates of advanced resuscitation at birth ($p = 0.03$), and had larger transductal diameter ($p < 0.001$), higher ductal Vmax/Vmin ratio ($p < 0.001$) and higher LPA diastolic velocity ($p < 0.001$). In addition, reverse descending aorta diastolic flow was more prevalent at screening NPE in infants in the IB-T group than in those of the CM group ($p < 0.001$).

The predictive capacity of screening NPE for early spontaneous PDA closure was analyzed by different models of PDA score. This analysis yielded that the best model of PDA score included only the echocardiographic variables statistically associated with the CM group (**Tables 1, 2**). It showed an AUC = 0.93 (95% CI 0.88–0.99), with PDA score cut-off value <4.5 with a sensitivity of 0.90 (95% CI 0.71–0.97), specificity of 0.86 (95% CI 0.72–0.93), positive predictive value of 0.76 (95% CI 0.59–0.87), and negative predictive value of 0.95 (95% CI 0.83–0.98) (**Figure 2**).

Median screening PDA score was 7 (IQR: 5–8.5) and 1 (IQR: 0–4) for the IB-T group and the CM group, respectively ($p < 0.001$). Median PDA score at the time ibuprofen treatment was administered was 9 (IQR: 8–9) (**Tables 3, 4**).

The backward stepwise regression analysis showed that the best predictive model to estimate the likelihood of early spontaneous PDA closure included the gestational age [OR = 3.44 (95% CI 1.33–8.87)] and the screening PDA score [OR = 0.42 (95% CI 0.25–0.71)], according to the following equation,

$$\text{Log}(p/1\text{-}p) = -28.41 + 1.23^{*} \text{ gestational age } -0.87^{*} \text{ PDA score at screening NPE.}$$

Where, p is the probability of early spontaneous closure. Thus, for each unit increase in the PDA score at screening or in gestational age (in weeks), the likelihood of early spontaneous PDA closure decreases 58% or increases by 3.4 times, respectively.

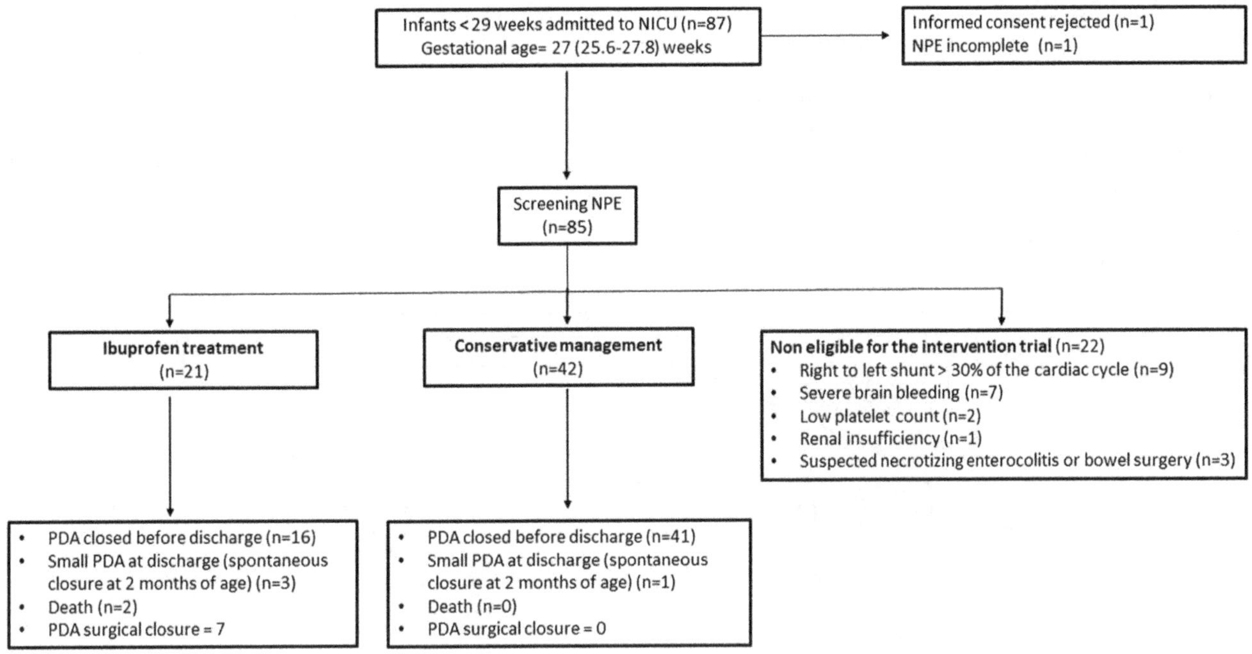

FIGURE 1 | Patient flowchart.

TABLE 1 | Proposed predicted models of early spontaneous PDA closure.

Predicted model	AUC (95% CI)	Cut-off value	Sensitivity (95% CI)	Specificity (95% CI)	PPV (95% CI)	NPV (95% CI)
Model 1	0.89 (0.82–0.97)	6.5	0.86 (0.65–0.95)	0.78 (0.64–0.88)	0.67 (0.52–0.78)	0.92 (0.79–0.97)
Model 2	0.89 (0.82–0.97)	6.5	0.80 (0.60–0.92)	0.80 (0.66–0.90)	0.68 (0.52–0.80)	0.89 (0.77–0.95)
Model 3	0.90 (0.83–0.97)	4.5	0.90 (0.71–0.97)	0.74 (0.59–0.85)	0.63 (0.50–0.74)	0.94 (0.80–0.98)
Model 4	0.89 (0.81–0.97)	6.5	0.86 (0.65–0.95)	0.81 (0.67–0.90)	0.69 (0.54–0.81)	0.92 (0.79–0.97)
Model 5	0.93 (0.88–0.99)	4.5	0.90 (0.71–0.97)	0.86 (0.72–0.93)	0.76 (0.59–0.87)	0.95 (0.83–0.98)

Model 1 includes all the echocardiographic variables (transductal diameter, ductal velocity Vmax/Vmin ratio, antegrade LPA diastolic flow, Left atrial: aortic ratio, LVO/SVC flow ratio, E wave/A wave ratio and reverse descending aorta diastolic velocity). Model 2 includes all the echocardiographic variables but E/A ratio. Model 3 includes all the echocardiographic variables but left atrial/aortic ratio. Model 4 includes all the echocardiographic variables but LVO/SVC flow. Model 5 includes only the echocardiographic variables significantly associated with conservative management (transductal diameter, ductal velocity Vmax/Vmin ratio, antegrade LPA diastolic flow and reverse descending aorta diastolic velocity).

Transductal diameter (mm): <1.5 = score 1; 1.5–3 = score 2; >3 = score 3; Ductal velocity Vmax/Vmin ratio (m/s): <1.5 = score 1; 1.5–2 = score 2; >2 = score 3. Antegrade LPA diastolic flow (cm/s): <30 = score 1; 30–50 = score 2; >50 = score 3; Left atrial: aortic ratio: <1.4:1 = score 0; 1.4–1.6:1 = score 2; >1.6:1 = score 3; LVO/SVC flow ratio: <4 = score 0; ≥4 = score 3; E wave/A wave ratio: <1 = score 0; 1–1.5 = score 2; >1.5 = score 3.

AUC, area under the curve; CI, confidence interval; PPV, positive predictive value; NPV, negative predictive value.

DISCUSSION

The results of this analysis support screening PDA score at the second day of life in very preterm infants as a valuable tool to discriminate between two different groups of patients: those with a PDA pattern with high probability of early spontaneous closure during the first 2 weeks of life, and those who will develop unequivocal signs of hemodynamic significance related to a patent duct. In the backward stepwise regression analysis, only the gestational age improved the predictive capacity of the model. This is particularly relevant at extreme gestational ages as, according to our data, the likelihood of early spontaneous PDA closure at 24 weeks of gestation and PDA screening score of 5 would be around 4%, while at 29 weeks and the same score, it would reach 94%. Thus, the strength of PDA score is especially remarkable for intermediate gestational age groups, such as 26 weeks of gestation, where a score of 3 or 6 modifies dramatically the likelihood for early spontaneous closure, ranging from 72% to 16%, respectively. These findings highlight the importance of early personalized management of PDA instead of considering PDA as an all or none phenomenon. This personalized approach is essential to avoid overtreatment in infants with high chances of early spontaneous closure, and will focus on babies with high NPE screening scores that

TABLE 2 | Ductal disease stage* (Model 5).

	Modality/position of sample gate	Score 0	Score 1	Score 2	Score 3
Transductal diameter, mm	Color Doppler, high left-sided parasternal	0	<1.5	1.5–3	>3
Ductal velocity Vmax/Vmin ratio, m/s	PWD at pulmonary end of duct view	0	<1.5	1.5–2	>2
Antegrade LPA diastolic flow, cm/s	PWD within left pulmonary artery	0	<30	30–50	>50
Descending aorta diastolic velocity	PWD within descending aorta. High parasternal	Forward	Absent	Reverse	

*adapted from Sehgal et al. (19): Maximum score = 11. Minimum score = 0.
LPA, left pulmonary artery; PWD, pulse wave Doppler.

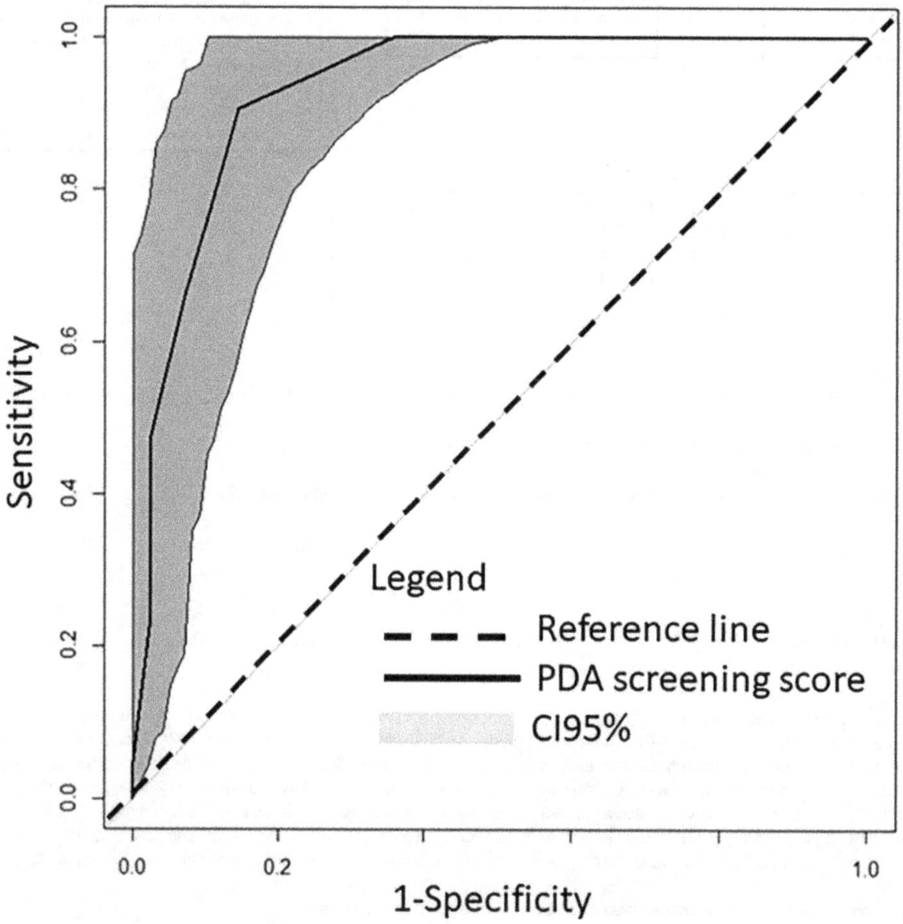

FIGURE 2 | Receiver operating characteristics curve of the ability of screening PDA score to differentiate between PDA ibuprofen treatment group and early PDA spontaneous closure (conservative management group).

would be beneficiaries of early pharmacological prescription for PDA closure.

Early identification of this specific group may offer two main advantages. First, it has been reported that the efficacy of ibuprofen is inversely related to postnatal age at the time treatment is started; thus, the earlier the treatment the higher the likelihood of closure (14). Second, this predictive model also recognizes a subgroup of infants potentially most vulnerable to develop PDA-related morbidities, as a consequence of being exposed to a large blood shunting from the systemic to the pulmonary circulation. This population should be the focus of preventive strategies to minimize the hidden impact of PDA blood flow shifting from specific territories, either from the perspective of clinical management but also for research purposes.

Although, prolonged ductal patency may be associated with a variety of adverse outcomes (1–6), the pathophysiological mechanistic approach involving PDA hemodynamic changes has not been established yet. In addition, although some trials on early pharmacological therapy have shown a reduction in the

TABLE 3 | Clinical data of the study population.

	Conservative management ($n = 42$)	Ibuprofen treatment ($n = 21$)	p-value
Gestational age (weeks), median (IQR)	27.8 (26.7–28.4)	26 (24.6–26.6)	<0.001
Birth weight (g), median (IQR)	1056 (858–1056)	850 (660–957)	0.003
Maternal age (years), median (IQR)	33 (30–35.7)	31 (26.5–34)	0.2
5-min Apgar score <5, (IQR)	8 (6–8)	6 (4.5–8)	0.04
Cord pH, median (IQR)	7.30 (7.25–7.36)	7.34 (7.31–7.34)	0.02
Premature rupture of membranes >24 h, n (%)	13 (31)	2 (9)	0.07
Advanced resuscitation, n (%)*	15 (36)	14 (67)	0.03
Chorioamnionitis, n (%)[†]	18 (62)	14 (70)	0.7
Antenatal steroids, n (%)[z]	29 (70)	14 (67)	0.7
Multiple, n (%)	18 (43)	6 (29)	0.4
Male sex, n (%)	19 (45)	13 (62)	0.3
Surfactant therapy, n (%)	25 (60)	16 (76)	0.3
Postnatal age at screening NPE, median (IQR)	47.5 (24–48)	45 (24–56)	0.7
Platelet count (× 10^3/ml) at screening NPE, median (IQR)	215 (134.5–282.5)	241 (161–305)	0.2
Hemoglobin (g/dL) at screening NPE, median (IQR)	14.4 (12.6–15.7)	13.9 (12.8–15.3)	0.6
Postnatal age at PDA closure (days), median (IQR)	5 (2–15)	19 (9–34)	<0.001

*intubation in the delivery room with or without assisted circulation.
[†]histological placental studies ($n = 29$, conservative management; $n = 20$, ibuprofen treatment).
[z]full course.

TABLE 4 | Neonatologist Performed Echocardiography (NPE) variables.

	Screening NPE			NPE at treatment	
	Conservative management ($n = 42$)	Ibuprofen treatment ($n = 21$)	p-value		p-value*
Transductal diameter, mm (median, IQR)	0 (0–1.5)	2 (1.7–2.6)	<0.001	2 (2.3–2.9)	0.01
Ductal velocity Vmax/Vmin ratio, m/s (median, IQR)	0 (0–1.4)	1.5 (1.2–2.2)	<0.001	2 (1.6–2.3)	0.02
Antegrade LPA diastolic flow, cm/s (median, IQR)	0.1 (0.08–0.18)	0.32 (0.17–0.38)	<0.001	0.36 (0.3–0.45)	0.006
Left atrial: aortic ratio (median, IQR)	1.6 (1.2–1.8)	1.7 (1.4–2)	0.3	1.9 (1.6–2.1)	0.01
LVO/SVC flow ratio (median, IQR)	2.2 (1.5–2.6)	2.4 (1.8–3.5)	0.07	3.7 (2.9–4.8)	0.02
E wave/A wave ratio (median, IQR)	0.75 (0.7–1)	0.8 (0.7–0.84)	0.8	0.8 (0.7–1)	0.08
Reverse descending aorta diastolic velocity, n (%)	2 (5)	11 (52)	<0.001	19 (90)	0.01
PDA Score (median, IQR)	1 (0–4)	7 (5–8.5)	<0.001	9 (8–9)	0.002

*screening vs. treatment.

short-term morbidities, such as pulmonary hemorrhage or severe IVH (9, 13), data on the long-term outcomes did not show benefits in the treatment group (7). The lack of long-term benefits in intervention trials on PDA closure could be explained by misclassification of the eligible population, as infants with PDA were selected for intervention independently of their individual PDA patterns, either if closing patterns were present or not.

We propose the early PDA score defined in this study as a tool for better selection of candidates for intervention in future trials on PDA treatment strategies. This early and objective score identified the population of low birth weight infants who received treatment for PDA closure, corresponding to one third of those who were systematically observed. Recent literature is aligned with our data, as spontaneous permanent closure of PDA by the end of the first week of life is reported in one third of the extremely low birth weight infants (16), and two thirds of them close their PDA by 2 months of life (20). These data have divided the scientific community in two currents with respect to PDA (treat or not treat) (7, 9, 11).

It is of note that active treatment with ibuprofen started at 69 h of birth in our study, although IB-T group screening NPE score was 7 at 42 h. The 27 h delay in ibuprofen treatment could have had a negative effect on treatment response, as the metabolism of ibuprofen has been shown to mature early in life (17).

Previous research focus on the management of PDA according to its capacity to cause harm (18, 19, 21). NPE offers information regarding hemodynamic PDA-related changes and allows the characterization of shunt volume over the lungs as well as the blood steal at the post-ductal circulation (15). Based on this information, different scores at random postnatal ages have been proposed (18, 19, 21) that have shown a relationship between shunt severity (higher PDA score) and IVH, NEC, BPD, or death (19, 21). In this retrospective study, screening NPE conducted on day 2 of birth only included in the PDA score the variables which predicted spontaneous early closure of PDA. Other parameters traditionally used to guide PDA treatment, such as left atrial to aortic ratio, LVO/SVC flow or E wave/A wave ratio, were excluded. These NPE variables may help to PDA disease staging but do not seem to be as useful for early in life treatment decision-making.

As opposite to previous reports (21), we decided not to use tissue Doppler imaging-derived variables to be included in our model because it was intended to define a more generalisable tool, easy to use by a wider population of neonatologists. Our score includes variables that define PDA size and flow (transductal diameter and ductal velocity), lung over-circulation (antegrade LPA diastolic flow), and systemic shunt effect (descending aorta diastolic velocity) according to the latest recommendations of the European Special Interest Group "Neonatologist Performed Echocardiography" (15). Neither platelet count nor the hemoglobin level (22) were found to be associated with PDA closing pattern in this study, so those were not included in the predictive model.

The main limitation of this study is its retrospective design so these results should be validated prospectively in a larger population. A greater predisposition of the neonatologist to treat infants with a lower gestational age and those with echocardiography-derived parameters indicating larger shunts is a matter of fact. As there was not a previously defined cut-off value to guide clinicians on when to start PDA treatment, only NPE variables statistically associated with treatment were included in the score that was retrospectively applied.

The strength, however, is to provide a tool to help clinicians in PDA decision making, by early identification of hsPDA that do not show closing patters, rather than to explore the association between PDA and morbidities. Future research will clarify whether prevention of PDA-related morbidities is feasible by effective early identification and treatment of hsPDA without closing patterns.

In conclusion, a predictive model of early spontaneous PDA closure that includes gestational age and the screening PDA score is proposed. This model may help clinicians in the decision-making process of PDA treatment but these results should be validated prospectively in a larger population. In addition, this model could be used to classify study groups for future intervention trials on ductal treatment that aim to prevent PDA related morbidities.

ETHICS STATEMENT

The studies involving human participants were reviewed and approved by Ethics Committee for Human Studies at La Paz University Hospital. Written informed consent to participate in this study was provided by the participants' legal guardian/next of kin.

AUTHOR CONTRIBUTIONS

MB conceptualized and designed the study, performed some of the echocardiographic scans, drafted the initial manuscript, collected the information from the medical charts, performed the initial analyses, and approved the final manuscript as submitted. RS performed some of the echocardiographic scans, collected the information from the medical charts, and approved the final manuscript as submitted. AB performed some of the echocardiographic scans, collected the information from the medical charts, and approved the final manuscript as submitted. IL performed the statistical analysis, reviewed the manuscript, and approved the final manuscript as submitted. AP conceptualized and designed the study, drafted the initial manuscript, and approved the final manuscript as submitted. All authors contributed to the article and approved the submitted version.

ACKNOWLEDGMENTS

We acknowledge the SAMID (Salud Materno Infantil y Desarrollo). Network (RD08/0072/0018 and RD12/0026/0004) of the Instituto de Salud Carlos III for their scientific support.

REFERENCES

1. Weber SC, Weiss K, Bührer C, Hansmann G, Koehne P, Sallmon H. Natural history of patent ductus arteriosus in very low birth weight infants after discharge. *J Pediatr.* (2015) 167:1149–15. doi: 10.1016/j.jpeds.2015.06.032
2. Osborn DA, Evans N, Kluckow M. Hemodynamic and antecedent risk factors of early and late periventricular/intraventricular hemorrhage in premature infants. *Pediatrics.* (2003) 112:33–9. doi: 10.1542/peds.112.1.33
3. Clyman RI The role of patent ductus arteriosus and its treatments in the development of bronchopulmonary dysplasia. *Semin Perinatol.* (2013) 37:102–7. doi: 10.1053/j.semperi.2013.01.006
4. Noori S, McCoy M, Friedlich P, Bright B, Gottipati V, Seri I, et al. Failure of ductus arteriosus closure is associated with increased mortality in preterm infants. *Pediatrics.* (2009) 123:e138–44. doi: 10.1542/peds.2008-2418
5. Schena F, Francescato G, Cappelleri A, Picciolli I, Mayer A, Mosca F, et al. Association between hemodynamically significant patent ductus arteriosus and bronchopulmonary dysplasia. *J Pediatr.* (2015) 16:1488–92. doi: 10.1016/j.jpeds.2015.03.012
6. Härkin P, Marttila R, Pokka T, Saarela T, Hallman M. Morbidities associated with patent ductus arteriosus in preterm infants. Nationwide cohort study. *J Matern Fetal Neonatal Med.* (2018) 31:2576–83. doi: 10.1080/14767058.2017.1347921
7. Schmidt B, Davis P, Moddemann D, Ohlsson A, Roberts RS, Saigal S, et al. Long-term effects of indomethacin prophylaxis in extremely-low-birth-weight infants. *N Engl J Med.* (2001) 344:1966–72. doi: 10.1056/NEJM200106283442602
8. Mosalli R, Alfaleh K. Prophylactic surgical ligation of patent ductus arteriosus for prevention of mortality and morbidity in extremely low birth weight infants. *Cochrane Database Syst Rev.* (2008) 1:CD006181. doi: 10.1002/14651858.CD006181.pub2
9. Kluckow M, Jeffery M, Gill A, Evans N. A randomised placebo-controlled trial of early treatment of the patent ductus arteriosus. *Arch Dis Child Fetal Neonatal Ed.* (2014) 99:F99–104. doi: 10.1136/archdischild-2013-304695
10. Malviya MN, Ohlsson A, Shah SS. Surgical versus medical treatment with cyclooxygenase inhibitors for symptomatic patent ductus arteriosus in preterm infants. *Cochrane Database Syst. Rev.* (2013)

2013:CD003951. doi: 10.1002/14651858.CD003951.pub3

11. Rolland A, Shankar-Aguilera S, Diomande D, Zupan-Simunek V, Boileau, P. Natural evolution of patent ductus arteriosus in the extremely preterm infant. *Arch Dis Child Fetal Neonatal Ed.* (2015) 100:F55–8. doi: 10.1136/archdischild-2014-306339
12. Benitz WE. Learning to live with patency of the ductus arteriosus in preterm infants. *J Perinatol.* (2011) 31(Suppl. 1):S42–8. doi: 10.1038/jp.2010.175
13. Fowlie PW, Davis PG, McGuire W. Prophylactic intravenous indomethacin for preventing mortality and morbidity in preterm infants. *Cochrane Database Syst Rev.* (2010) 2010:CD000174. doi: 10.1002/14651858.CD000174.pub2
14. Aranda JV, Clyman R, Cox B, Van Overmeire B, Wozniak P, Sosenko I, et al. A randomized, double-blind, placebo- controlled trial on intravenous ibuprofen L-lysine for the early closure of nonsymptomatic patent ductus arteriosus within 72 hours of birth in extremely low-birth-weight infants. *Am J Perinatol.* (2009) 26:235–46. doi: 10.1055/s-0028-1103515
15. van Laere D, van Overmeire B, Gupta S, El-Khuffash A, Savoia M, McNamara PJ, et al. Application of neonatologist performed Echocardiography in the assessment of a patent ductus arteriosus, on behalf of the European special interest group 'Neonatologist Performed Echocardiography' (NPE). *Pediatr Res.* (2018) 84:S46–56. doi: 10.1038/s41390-018-0077-x
16. Koch J, Hensley G, Roy L, Brown S, Ramaciotti C, Rosenfeld CR. Prevalence of spontaneous closure of the ductus arteriosus in neonates at a birth weight of 1000 grams or less. *Pediatrics.* (2006) 117:1113–21. doi: 10.1542/peds.2005-1528
17. Flint RB, ter Heine R, Spaans E, Burger DM, de Klerk JCA, Allegaert K, et al. Simulation-based suggestions to improve ibuprofen dosing for patent ductus arteriosus in preterm newborns. *Eur J Clin Pharmacol.* (2018) 74:1585–91. doi: 10.1007/s00228-018-2529-y
18. McNamara PJ, Sehgal A. Towards rational management of the patent ductus arteriosus: the need for disease staging. *Arch Dis Child Fetal Neonatal.* (2007) 92:F424–7. doi: 10.1136/adc.2007.118117
19. Sehgal A, Eldho P, Menahem S. Functional echocardiography in staging for ductal disease severity role in predicting outcomes. *Eur J Pediatr.* (2013) 172:179–84. doi: 10.1007/s00431-012-1851-0
20. Clyman RI, Liebowitz M, Kaempf J, Erdeve O, Bulbul A, Håkansson S, et al. PDA-TOLERATE trial: an exploratory randomized controlled trial of treatment of moderate-to-large patent ductus arteriosus at 1 week of age. *J Pediatr.* (2019) 205:41-8.e6. doi: 10.1016/j.jpeds.2018.09.012
21. El-Khuffash A, James AT, Corcoran JD, Dicker P, Franklin O, Elsayed YN, et al. A patent ductus arteriosus severity score predicts chronic lung disease or death before discharge. *J Pediatr.* (2015) 167:1354–61. doi: 10.1016/j.jpeds.2015.09.028
22. Dani C, Poggi C, Fontanelli G. Relationship between platelet count and volume and spontaneous and pharmacological closure of ductus arteriosus in preterm infants. *Am J Perinatol.* (2013) 30:359–64. doi: 10.1055/s-0032-1324702

13

Platelet Counts and Patent Ductus Arteriosus in Preterm Infants

*Gema González-Luis [1], Stefano Ghiradello [2], Pilar Bas-Suárez [3], Giacomo Cavallaro [2], Fabio Mosca [2], Ronald I Clyman [4] and Eduardo Villamor [5]**

[1] Department of Neonatology, Complejo Hospitalario Universitario Insular Materno-Infantil (CHUIMI) de Canarias, Las Palmas de Gran Canaria, Spain, [2] Neonatal Intensive Care Unit, Department of Clinical Sciences and Community Health, Fondazione IRCCS Cà Granda Ospedale Maggiore Policlinico, Università degli Studi di Milano, Milan, Italy, [3] Department of Pediatrics, Hospital Vithas Santa Catalina, Las Palmas de Gran Canaria, Spain, [4] Cardiovascular Research Institute, Department of Pediatrics, University of California, San Francisco, San Francisco, CA, United States, [5] Department of Pediatrics, Maastricht University Medical Center (MUMC+), School for Oncology and Developmental Biology (GROW), Maastricht, Netherlands

***Correspondence:**
Eduardo Villamor
e.villamor@mumc.nl

Background: A meta-analysis published in 2015 showed a significant association between low platelet counts in the first day(s) of life and risk of patent ductus arteriosus (PDA). The meta-analysis pooled data from 11 studies cohorts (3,479 preterm infants).

Objective: To update the meta-analysis by adding new studies on the topic and including other platelet parameters different from platelet counts.

Methods: PubMed/Medline and Embase databases were searched. Random-effects risk ratios (RR) and differences in means (DM) and 95% confidence intervals (CI) were calculated.

Results: We included 31 studies (7,638 infants). Meta-analysis showed that the risk of developing any PDA was significantly associated with platelet counts $<150 \times 10^9$/L (11 studies, RR 1.58, 95% CI 1.28 to 1.95), and $<100 \times 10^9$/L (7 studies, RR 1.61, 95% CI 1.14 to 2.28), but not $<50 \times 10^9$/L (4 studies, RR 1.34, 95% CI 0.77 to 2.32). Risk of developing hemodynamically significant PDA (hsPDA) was significantly associated with platelet counts $<150 \times 10^9$/L (12 studies, RR 1.33, 95% CI 1.09 to 1.63), and $<100 \times 10^9$/L (7 studies, RR 1.39, 95% CI 1.06 to 1.82), but not $<50 \times 10^9$/L (6 studies, RR 1.24, 95% CI 0.86 to 1.79). Infants with hsPDA had significantly lower mean platelet counts (19 studies, DM 22.0×10^9, 95% CI 14.9 to 29.1) and platelet mass (11 studies, DM 214.4, 95% CI 131.2 to 297.5) and significantly higher platelet distribution width (PDW, 9 studies, DM −0.53, 95% CI −1.01 to −0.05) than infants without hsPDA. Meta-analysis could not demonstrate significant differences in mean platelet volume (MPV).

Conclusion: Compared to the previous analysis, this updated meta-analysis included 21 additional studies that provide stronger evidence of the association between low platelet counts and PDA/hsPDA. Other platelet parameters such as platelet mass and PDW are also associated with hsPDA risk. However, the low number of platelets may be an epiphenomenon associated with the maturity and clinical stability of preterm infants rather than a contributing factor in the pathogenesis of PDA.

Keywords: ductus arteriosus, platelets, meta-analysis, platelet distribution width, thrombocytopenia

INTRODUCTION

Failure of ductus arteriosus (DA) closure in preterm infants is a conundrum that neonatologists have faced for decades and whose pathophysiological and clinical implications are far from being solved (1–10). In 2010, Echtler et al. made a significant contribution to the understanding of DA pathobiology when they showed that normal number and function of platelets were key factors for mice DA closure (11). They also reported an association between low platelet counts in the first day of life and risk of developing patent DA (PDA) in a cohort of 123 infants born at 24 to 30 weeks of gestation (11). The publication of these results prompted numerous groups of neonatologists to analyze the potential association between the number of platelets at birth and the presence of PDA in their populations (12–18).

In 2015, we conducted a systematic review and meta-analysis on the topic of platelet counts in the first days of life and PDA (19). The meta-analysis pooled data from 11 study cohorts (3,479 preterm infants) and showed a significant association between PDA and platelet counts $<150 \times 10^9$/L as well as platelet counts $<100 \times 10^9$/L. However, the results were largely limited by the low robustness of the association and the high degree of statistical heterogeneity among studies. The evidence was therefore highly susceptible to being modified as more researchers published new data. The objective of the present study was to update our previous meta-analysis. Since our original report, we have located 20 additional studies that we have included in a new meta-analysis. Several studies included information about other platelet factors in addition to platelet counts. These factors have been also included in our updated meta-analysis.

METHODS

The methodology employed in this updated systematic review and meta-analysis is similar to that previously described in our 2015 report (19).

Search

We set up a monthly electronic alert from PubMed for new articles containing the most relevant search terms of our previous meta-analysis (last update June 2020). In addition, a new search was conducted in Pubmed and Embase on April 15, 2020 and we searched the Science Citation Index and Google Scholar for articles citing our previous meta-analysis as well as the articles that were included in it.

Inclusion Criteria and Study Selection

Two investigators (G G-L, and EV) independently evaluated studies for inclusion and any disagreements were resolved by discussion. Studies were included for analysis if satisfying all following criteria: (1) full text was available in English, Spanish, Italian, Dutch, French, German, Portuguese, Galician, or Catalan; (2) a prospective or retrospective cohort study or case-control design was used; (3) primary data were reported in a manner that could be used to measure the association between PDA and platelet counts or other platelet parameters; and (4) the study population was comprised of preterm infants. As in our previous meta-analysis the studies were divided according to the way they considered small ductal shunts (19). Studies comparing closed DA vs. small plus large PDA, were classified as reporting on "any PDA." Studies comparing closed DA and/or small PDA vs. large PDA, were classified as reporting on "hemodynamically significant PDA" (hsPDA).

Data Extraction and Assessment of Study Quality

Two investigators (GG-L, EV) independently extracted data on study design, demographics, rate of PDA and/or hsPDA, platelet counts, and other quantitative or qualitative platelet factors. A second group of investigators (SC, GC) checked the data extraction for completeness and accuracy. In cases in which necessary data were missing from the studies, additional information was requested from the authors. Methodological quality was assessed using the Newcastle-Ottawa Scale (NOS) for cohort or case-control studies (20).

Statistical Analysis

Studies were combined and analyzed using COMPREHENSIVE META-ANALYSIS V 3.0 software (Biostat Inc., Englewood, NJ, USA). For dichotomous outcomes, the risk ratio (RR) with 95% confidence interval (CI) was calculated from the data provided in the studies. For continuous outcomes, the difference in means (DM) with 95% CI was calculated. When studies reported continuous variables as median and range or interquartile range, we requested the mean and standard deviation from the authors or, alternatively, we estimated them using the method of Wan et al. (21). Due to anticipated heterogeneity, summary statistics were calculated with a random-effects model. This model accounts for variability between studies as well as within studies. To identify any study that may have exerted a disproportionate influence on the summary effect, we deleted studies one at a time. Heterogeneity was assessed with the Q statistic and quantified using the I^2 statistic. Publication bias was assessed only for the analyses including at least 10 studies. We used the Egger's regression test and visual analysis of funnel plots to assess publication bias. Meta-regression, using random effects (method of moments estimator), was performed to explore the following sources of heterogeneity in the association between platelet counts and PDA/hSPDA: cohort mean or median gestational age (GA) and birth weight (BW), percent males, rate of PDA/hsPDA, thrombocytopenia rate, and number of infants included in the study. Meta-regression was performed only for the analyses including at least 10 studies. A probability value of <0.05 (0.10 for heterogeneity) was considered statistically significant.

RESULTS

Included Studies

The new search identified 20 articles (22–41) that were added to the 11 already included in our previous meta-analysis (19). The PRISMA flow diagram of the search process is shown in **Supplementary Figure 1**. The 31 studies yielded a population of 7,638 preterm infants. The main characteristics of the studies are shown in **Table 1**. All the studies were cohort studies and

TABLE 1 | Characteristics of the studies included in the meta-analysis.

Study	Year	n	Country	GA cohort (weeks)	BW cohort (g)	% males	Day PDA assessment	%PDA	%hsPDA	Range PL assessment (days)	% PL < 150	% PL < 100
Echtler (11)	2010	123	Germany	28.0	1036	48.8	3–5	70.7	23.6	1	15.4	0.0
Fujioka (14)	2011	118	Japan	27.9	1059	57.6	3–5	29.7	23.7[a]	1	16.1	6.8[a]
Shah (15)	2011	497	USA, Canada	25.8	825	52.6	3	34.0	NR	3	27.2[a]	8.7[a]
Dwarakanath[b] (42)	2011	148	USA	26.0	733	50.0	NR	60.8	45.9[c]	3	41.2	NR
Dizdar (12)	2012	361	Turkey	28.6	1054	46.5	3–5	NR	42.7	3	23.8	5.5[a]
Sallmon (16)	2012	1350	USA	28.3	1060	48.7	4–5	56.3	26.7	1	16.4	3.4
Dani (13)	2012	163	Italy	27.1	931	49.7	1–2	NR	82.8	1	32.5	19.6[a]
Brunner (43)	2013	322	Austria	29.0	1170	50.6	2–7	50.9	47.2	1	NR	2.8[d]
Bas-Suarez (18)	2014	194	Spain	27.9	1008	55.7	2–4	NR	54.6	2	11.3	6.7
Chen (17)	2014	77	Taiwan	29.5	1153	49.4	3–6	NR	44.2	1	NR	NR
Simon[e] (19)	2015	126	NL, Italy	28.4	1096	51.2	2–4	69.8	64.3	2	28.6	14.28
Engür (27)	2015	34	Turkey	29.8	1250	58.8	2	NR	32.3	2–5	NR	NR
Demir (25)	2016	235	Turkey	29.0	1549	54	3–5	NR	48.9	0–3	16.17	NR
Kulkarni (32)	2016	70	India	31.7	1197	51.4	3	28.6	17.4	1	50.0	24.3
Meinarde (33)	2016	88	Argentina	28.4	1112	50.0	3–7	NR	50.0	3	30.7	NR
Morawietz (34)	2016	368	Germany	28.0	1043	52.9	NR	64.1	36.9	NR	26.9	NR
Oliveira (38)	2016	328	Portugal	30.0	1231	48.8	1–3	30.2	NR	NR	19.5	NR
Olukman (35)	2016	824	Turkey	29.5	1193	45.9	3–4	NR	25.2	NR	NR	NR
Temel (22)	2017	97	Turkey	32.2	1809	48.5	3–5	NR	48.5	0–3	NR	NR
Kahvecioglu (29)	2018	60	Turkey	27.8	1024	45.0	3–4	NR	40.0	0–3	NR	NR
Bekmez (41)	2018	212	Turkey	29.0	1238	59.4	2–3	54.7	NR	2–3	NR	NR
Küçuk (31)	2018	75	Turkey	28.5	1180	56.0	0–3	NR	61.3	0–1	NR	NR
Akar (24)	2019	389	Turkey	29.5	1055	49.1	2–4	NR	45.7	0–1	NR	NR
Karabulut (30)	2019	148	Turkey	28.8	1092	45.9	1–3	NR	47.9	1–7	NR	NR
Kazanci (40)	2019	481	Turkey	28.0	1068	51.3	2–4	NR	35.1	1	NR	NR
Saldaña (39)	2019	250	Peru	NR	NR	51.6	NR	NR	34.8	NR	10.8	9.2
Demirel (26)	2020	100	Turkey	28.8	1238	NR	3–5	NR	50.0	1	NR	NR
Shekharappa (36)	2020	88	India	30.4	1335	46.6	NR	NR	82.9	NR	NR	NR
Ahmed (23)	2020	75	Egypt	31.7	NR	48.0	3	53.3	NR	2	NR	NR
Ghirardello (28)	2020	151	Italy	29.1	1098	44.4	1–3	NR	24.5	0	24.5	7.3
Kusuma (37)	2020	86	Indonesia	31.4	1535	47.7	NR	50	NR	NR	34.9	NR

[a]Data not reported in the original article but obtained after request to authors. [b]Abstract. [c]Based on numer of patients treated with COX inhibitors. [d]Patients with platelet count <50 × 10^9/L excluded. [e]Data published in the meta-analysis of Simon et al. as "CPS" group. GA, gestational age (mean or median); BW, birth weight total cohort (g, mean or median); PL, platelets (×10^9/L); NR, data not reported; PDA, patent ductus arteriosus; hsPDA, hemodynamically significant PDA. In the study of Shah et al. all the patients received prophylactic indomethacin. In the study of Echtler et al. a non-reported number of patients received prophylactic indomethacin.

only one (43) was prospective. Each study was allocated more than six NOS stars (**Supplementary Table 1**). The criteria used in each study for the definition of PDA and/or hsPDA are shown in **Supplementary Table 2**. From the included studies, 13 (11, 14–16, 19, 23, 32, 34, 37–39, 42, 43) reported on any PDA; that is, infants with a small PDA were included by the authors in the PDA group. Twenty-four studies (11–13, 16–19, 22–36, 41) compared infants with and without hsPDA; that is, infants with a small PDA were included by the authors in the non-PDA group. Six studies (11, 16, 19, 23, 32, 34) provided data on closed DA, small PDA and hsPDA. We included these studies in both analyses of any PDA and hsPDA. Twelve studies (22–27, 29–31, 35, 40, 41) reported data on mean platelet volume (MPV). Eleven studies (22–26, 29, 30, 35, 40, 41) reported data on platelet mass, and four studies (22, 26, 30, 41) reported data on plateletcrit. Since the plateletcrit is calculated with the formula platelet count ($10^4/\mu l$) × MPV (fL) × 10^{-3} (44) and the platelet mass is calculated with the formula platelet count (10^9/L) × MPV (fL) (45), plateletcrit values were converted into platelet mass values by multiplying by 10^4. Nine studies (22, 23, 25–27, 30, 35, 40, 41) reported data on platelet distribution width (PDW).

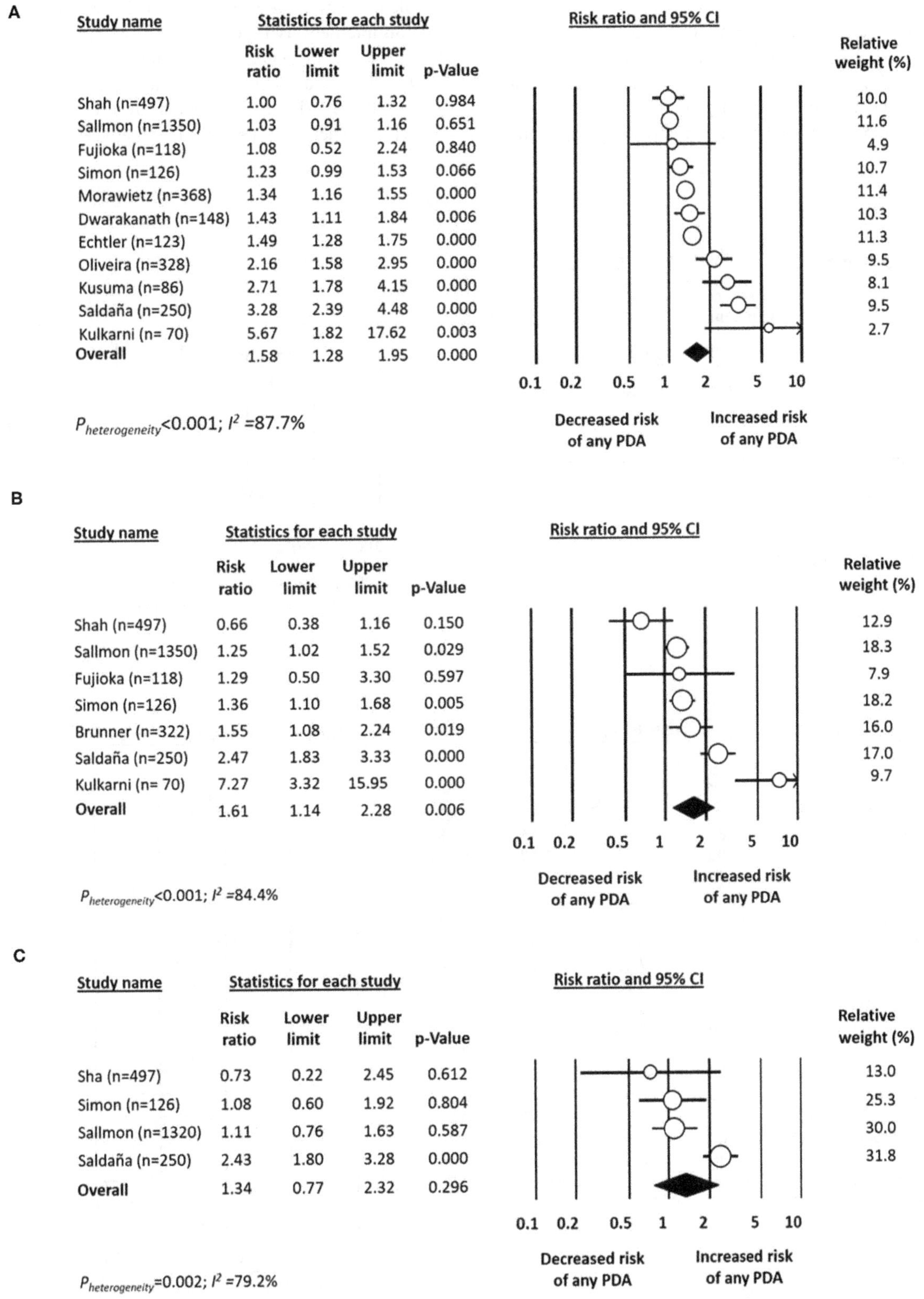

FIGURE 1 | Forest plot for studies examining the association between platelet counts below **(A)** 150 × 10^9/L, **(B)** 100 × 10^9/L, and **(C)** 50 × 10^9/L in the first day(s) of life on patent ductus arteriosus (PDA). Risk ratio >1 indicates increased risk of PDA.

Meta-Analysis

Any PDA

Data on rate of any PDA in infants with platelet counts above or below 150 × 10^9/L were available from 11 studies (11, 14–16, 19, 32, 34, 37–39, 42). There was a significant positive association between any PDA and platelet counts below 150 × 10^9/L (**Figure 1A**). The results of sensitivity analyses, excluding one study at a time, for this and all other analyses are shown in **Supplementary Table 3**. Neither visual inspection of the funnel plot (**Supplementary Figure 2A**) nor Egger's regression test (P = 0.066) revealed evidence of significant publication bias.

Data on rate of PDA in infants with platelet counts above or below 100 × 10^9/L were available from seven studies (14–16, 19, 32, 39, 43). There was a significant positive association between

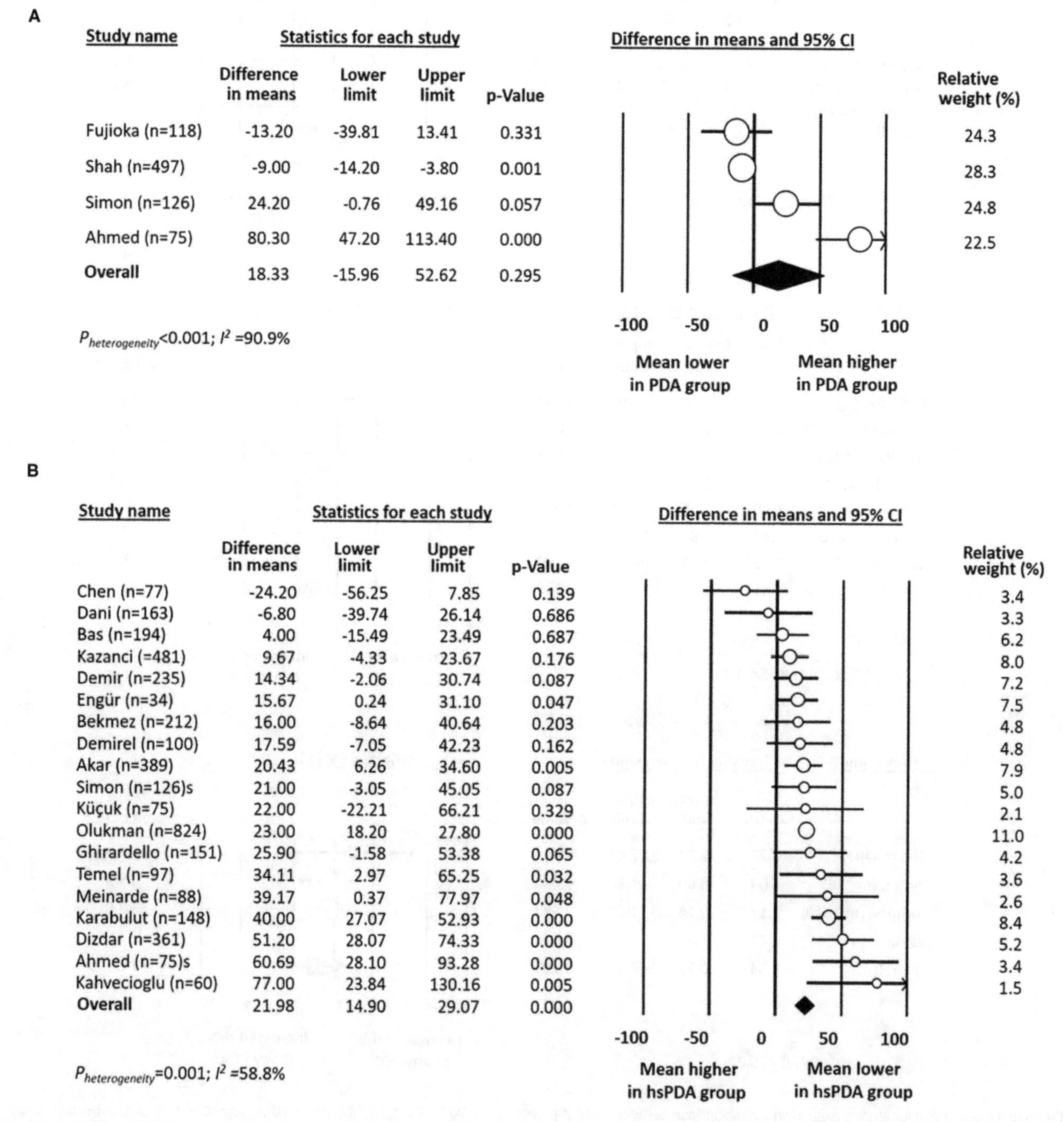

FIGURE 2 | Forest plot for studies examining the difference (PDA-no minus PDA-yes) in mean platelet count (×10^9/L) in the first day(s) of life in infants with and without any patent ductus arteriosus (PDA, **A**) and with and without hemodynamically significant patent ductus arteriosus (hsPDA, **B**).

any PDA and platelet counts below 100 × 10^9/L (**Figure 1B**). Data on rate of any PDA in infants with platelet counts above or below 50 × 10^9/L were available from four studies (15, 16, 19, 39). Meta-analysis could not detect a significant association between any PDA and platelet counts below 50 × 10^9/L (**Figure 1C**). Mean (SD) platelet counts in infants with and without any PDA were available from four studies (14, 15, 19, 23). Meta-analysis could not demonstrate a significant difference in mean platelet counts between the two groups (**Figure 2A**).

Hemodynamically Significant PDA

Data on rate of hsPDA in infants with platelet counts above or below 150 × 10^9/L were available from 12 studies (11–13, 16, 18, 19, 25, 28, 32–35). There was a significant positive association between hsPDA and platelet counts below 150 x 10^9/L (**Figure 3A**). Neither visual inspection of the funnel plot (**Supplementary Figure 2B**) nor Egger's regression test ($P = 0.130$) revealed evidence of significant publication bias.

Data on rate of hsPDA in infants with platelet counts above or below 100 × 10^9/L were available from seven studies (12, 13, 16, 18, 19, 28, 32). There was a significant positive association between any PDA and platelet counts below 100 x 10^9/L (**Figure 3B**). Data on rate of hsPDA in infants with platelet counts above or below 50 × 10^9/L were available from six studies (16, 18, 19, 25, 28, 36). Meta-analysis could not detect a significant association between any PDA and platelet counts below 50 × 10^9/L (**Figure 3C**).

Mean (SD) platelet counts in infants with and without hsPDA were available from 19 studies (12, 13, 17–19, 22–31, 33, 35, 40, 41). Platelet counts were significantly higher in the group without hsPDA (**Figure 2B**). Neither visual inspection of the funnel plot (**Supplementary Figure 2C**) nor Egger's regression test ($P = 0.941$) revealed evidence of significant publication bias.

Data on mean MPV in infants with and without any hsPDA were available from 12 studies (22–27, 29–31, 35, 40). Meta-analysis could not demonstrate a significant difference in MPV mean between the two groups (**Figure 4A**). Neither visual inspection of the funnel plot (**Supplementary Figure 2D**) nor Egger's regression test ($P = 0.678$) revealed evidence of significant publication bias.

Data on mean platelet mass in infants with and without any hsPDA were available from 11 studies (22–27, 29, 30, 35, 40, 41). Platelet mass was significantly higher in the group without hsPDA (**Figure 4B**). Neither visual inspection of the funnel plot (**Supplementary Figure 2E**) nor Egger's regression test ($P = 0.212$) revealed evidence of significant publication bias. Data on mean PDW in infants with and without any hsPDA were available from nine studies (22, 23, 25–27, 30, 35, 40, 41). Mean PDW was significantly lower in the hsPDA group (**Figure 4C**).

Meta-Regression Analyses

Potential sources of heterogeneity were assessed through random effects (method of moments) meta-regression analysis (46). Meta-regression was conducted only for the meta-analyses including 10 or more studies. The results of the meta-regression analyses are summarized in **Supplementary Table 4**. Meta-regression showed that the mean (or median) GA and BW of the cohort significantly correlated with the effect size of the association between any PDA and platelet counts <150 × 10^9/L (**Supplementary Table 4** and **Figure 2**). The GA of the cohort was associated with 22% (R^2 analog = 0.22) of the variance in the association between any PDA and platelet counts <150 × 10^9/L across studies. Each week that the GA of the cohort increased resulted in an increase in PDA log RR of 0.16 (the equivalent of going from a RR of 1.00 to a RR of 1.45). Similarly, the BW of the cohort was associated with 15% (R^2 analog = 0.15) of the variance in the association between any PDA and platelet counts <150 × 10^9/L across studies. Each increment of 100 g in the BW of the cohort resulted in an increase in PDA log RR of 0.11 (the equivalent of going from a RR of 1.00 to a RR of 1.29).

Meta-regression also showed that the rate of hsPDA of the cohort significantly correlated with the effect size of the association between any hsPDA and platelet counts <150 × 10^9/L (**Supplementary Table 4** and **Figure 2**). The hsPDA rate of the cohort was associated with 17% (R^2 analog = 0.17) of the variance in the association between hsPDA and platelet counts <150 × 10^9/L across studies. Each 10% decrease in hsPDA rate resulted in an increase in hsPDA log RR of 0.12 (the equivalent of going from a RR of 1.00 to a RR of 1.32).

DISCUSSION

This updated meta-analysis included 21 additional studies and doubled the number of infants, providing stronger evidence of the association between low platelet counts in the first day(s) of life and the risk of developing PDA or hsPDA. Besides low platelet counts, other platelet parameters such as platelet mass and PDW showed a significant association with hsPDA risk. Although the meta-analysis has gained in robustness with the increase in the number of studies and the inclusion of other platelet parameters, our results are still limited by the marked clinical and statistical heterogeneity among the different studies. In addition, the question that remains unanswered is to what extent the low number of platelets is an epiphenomenon associated with the maturity and clinical stability of preterm infants rather than a contributing factor in the pathogenesis of PDA (15).

As already discussed in the previous version of the meta-analysis, one of the main limitations for the study of the association between thrombocytopenia and PDA is the absence of uniform criteria to establish when these two entities have a clinical relevance (19). It has been argued that the definition of thrombocytopenia based on thresholds of 150 or even 100 × 10^9/L platelets is not clinically relevant for very preterm newborns (47, 48). In addition, neonatal thrombocytopenia and PDA share some potential etiopathogenic factors and this may confound the study of their potential association. The most frequent etiology of thrombocytopenia developing within the first days of life is intrauterine growth restriction (IUGR) and/or maternal hypertension (49, 50). This form of thrombocytopenia is rarely severe and platelet counts return to normal spontaneously in a short period of time (49, 50). The possible association between IUGR and PDA is controversial with studies reporting either a higher or lower risk of PDA in preterm

A

Study name	Risk ratio	Lower limit	Upper limit	p-Value	Relative weight (%)
Bas (n=194)	0.54	0.24	1.23	0.142	4.1
Dani (n=163)	0.94	0.80	1.10	0.426	11.5
Demir (n=235)	1.01	0.72	1.44	0.934	9.1
Sallmon (n=1350)	1.07	0.85	1.35	0.562	10.7
Simon (n=126)	1.12	0.85	1.46	0.425	10.2
Olukman (n=824)	1.26	0.98	1.63	0.073	10.4
Meinarde (n=88)	1.42	0.95	2.13	0.087	8.3
Ghirardello (n=151)	1.52	0.88	2.63	0.130	6.5
Morawietz (n=368)	1.53	1.18	1.99	0.002	10.3
Dizdar (n=361)	1.58	1.26	2.00	0.000	10.7
Echtler (n=123)	4.45	2.58	7.67	0.000	6.5
Kulkarni (=70)	5.00	1.18	21.19	0.029	1.7
Overall	1.33	1.09	1.63	0.006	

(Statistics for each study)

$P_{heterogeneity}$<0.001; I^2 =78.5%

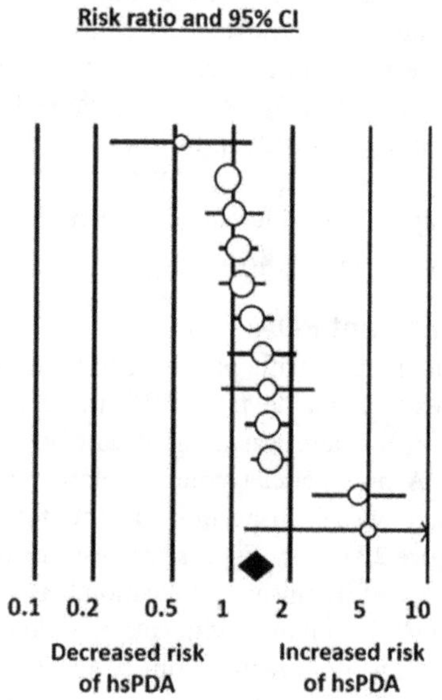

B

Study name	Risk ratio	Lower limit	Upper limit	p-Value	Relative weight (%)
Bas (n=194)	0.54	0.24	1.23	0.142	7.6
Sallmon (n=1350)	1.14	0.73	1.78	0.564	15.0
Dani (n=163)	1.17	1.03	1.32	0.013	24.2
Simon (n=126)	1.36	1.06	1.76	0.017	20.7
Dizdar (n=361)	1.70	1.24	2.32	0.001	18.9
Ghirardello (n=151)	1.82	0.90	3.69	0.098	9.3
Kulkarni (n=70)	9.35	2.85	30.65	0.000	4.3
Overall	1.39	1.06	1.82	0.018	

(Statistics for each study)

$P_{heterogeneity}$=0.002; I^2 =72.0%

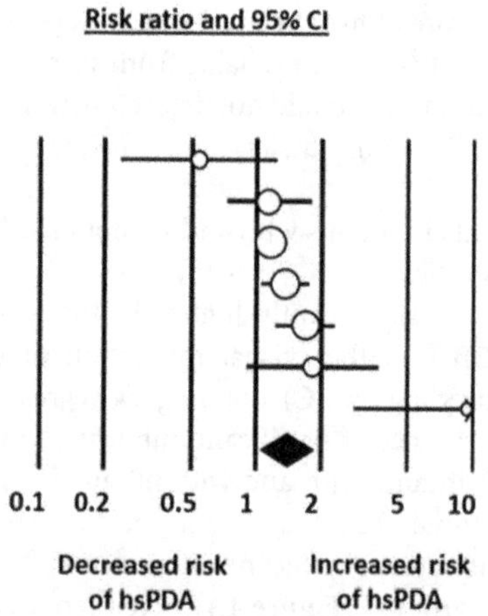

C

Study name	Risk ratio	Lower limit	Upper limit	p-Value	Relative weight (%)
Bas (n=194)	0.31	0.02	3.86	0.359	2.1
Sallmon (n=1350)	1.17	0.56	2.43	0.677	24.8
Simon (n=126)	1.17	0.66	2.10	0.591	39.3
Demir (n=235)	1.37	0.61	3.08	0.448	20.2
Shekarappa (n=88)	1.67	0.42	6.72	0.467	6.9
Ghirardello (n=151)	1.91	0.47	7.84	0.369	6.7
Overall	1.24	0.86	1.79	0.239	

(Statistics for each study)

$P_{heterogeneity}$=0.872; I^2 =0.0%

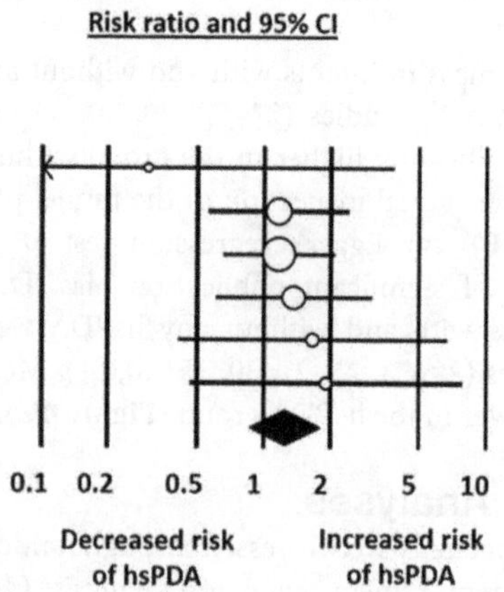

FIGURE 3 | Forest plot for studies examining the association between platelet counts **(A)** below 150 × 10^9/L, **(B)** below 100 × 10^9/L, and **(C)** below 50 × 10^9/L in the first day(s) of life on hemodynamically significant patent ductus arteriosus (hsPDA). Risk ratio >1 indicates increased risk of hsPDA.

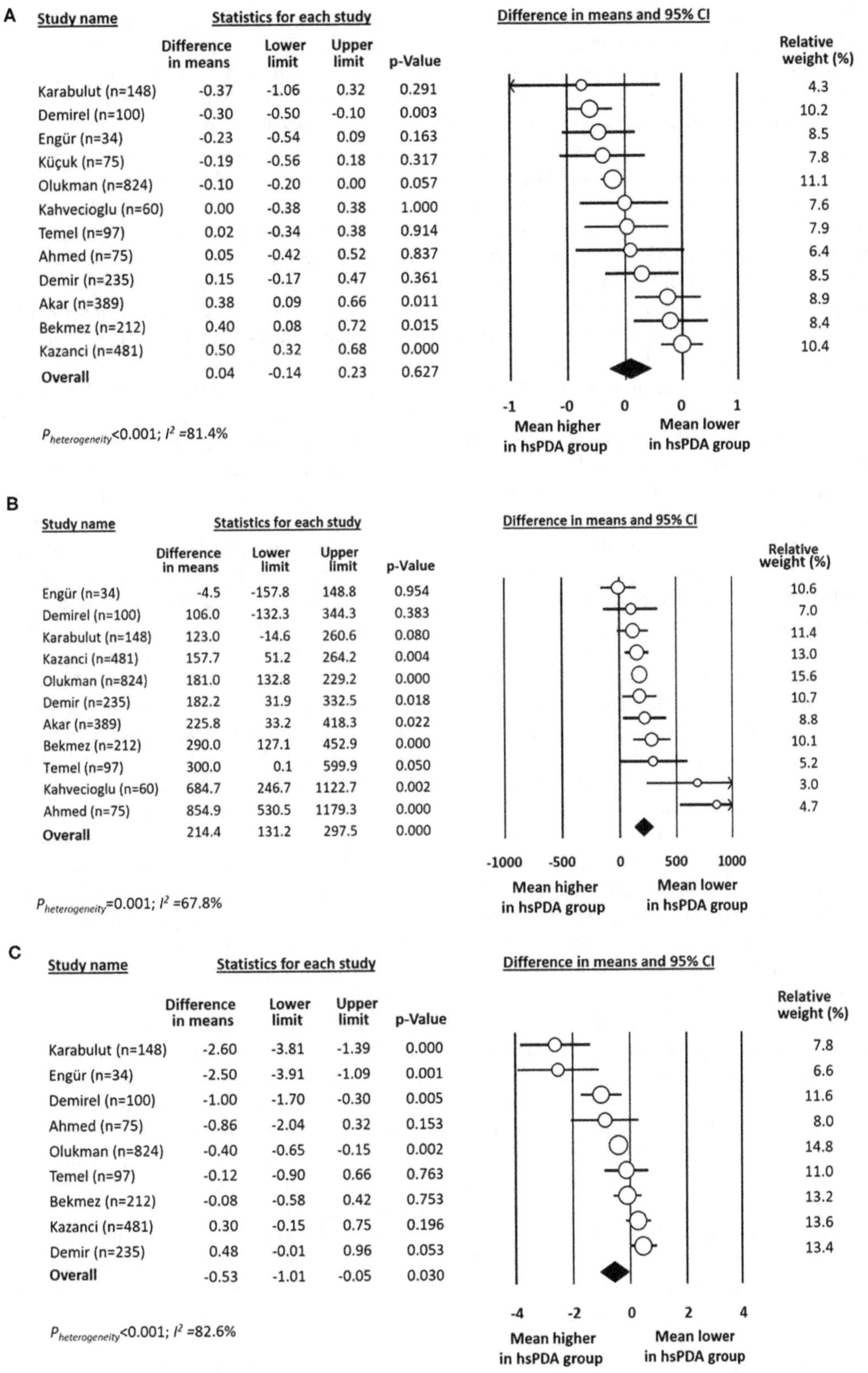

A

Study name	Difference in means	Lower limit	Upper limit	p-Value	Relative weight (%)
Karabulut (n=148)	-0.37	-1.06	0.32	0.291	4.3
Demirel (n=100)	-0.30	-0.50	-0.10	0.003	10.2
Engür (n=34)	-0.23	-0.54	0.09	0.163	8.5
Küçuk (n=75)	-0.19	-0.56	0.18	0.317	7.8
Olukman (n=824)	-0.10	-0.20	0.00	0.057	11.1
Kahvecioglu (n=60)	0.00	-0.38	0.38	1.000	7.6
Temel (n=97)	0.02	-0.34	0.38	0.914	7.9
Ahmed (n=75)	0.05	-0.42	0.52	0.837	6.4
Demir (n=235)	0.15	-0.17	0.47	0.361	8.5
Akar (n=389)	0.38	0.09	0.66	0.011	8.9
Bekmez (n=212)	0.40	0.08	0.72	0.015	8.4
Kazanci (n=481)	0.50	0.32	0.68	0.000	10.4
Overall	0.04	-0.14	0.23	0.627	

$P_{heterogeneity}$<0.001; I^2 =81.4%

B

Study name	Difference in means	Lower limit	Upper limit	p-Value	Relative weight (%)
Engür (n=34)	-4.5	-157.8	148.8	0.954	10.6
Demirel (n=100)	106.0	-132.3	344.3	0.383	7.0
Karabulut (n=148)	123.0	-14.6	260.6	0.080	11.4
Kazanci (n=481)	157.7	51.2	264.2	0.004	13.0
Olukman (n=824)	181.0	132.8	229.2	0.000	15.6
Demir (n=235)	182.2	31.9	332.5	0.018	10.7
Akar (n=389)	225.8	33.2	418.3	0.022	8.8
Bekmez (n=212)	290.0	127.1	452.9	0.000	10.1
Temel (n=97)	300.0	0.1	599.9	0.050	5.2
Kahvecioglu (n=60)	684.7	246.7	1122.7	0.002	3.0
Ahmed (n=75)	854.9	530.5	1179.3	0.000	4.7
Overall	214.4	131.2	297.5	0.000	

$P_{heterogeneity}$=0.001; I^2 =67.8%

C

Study name	Difference in means	Lower limit	Upper limit	p-Value	Relative weight (%)
Karabulut (n=148)	-2.60	-3.81	-1.39	0.000	7.8
Engür (n=34)	-2.50	-3.91	-1.09	0.001	6.6
Demirel (n=100)	-1.00	-1.70	-0.30	0.005	11.6
Ahmed (n=75)	-0.86	-2.04	0.32	0.153	8.0
Olukman (n=824)	-0.40	-0.65	-0.15	0.002	14.8
Temel (n=97)	-0.12	-0.90	0.66	0.763	11.0
Bekmez (n=212)	-0.08	-0.58	0.42	0.753	13.2
Kazanci (n=481)	0.30	-0.15	0.75	0.196	13.6
Demir (n=235)	0.48	-0.01	0.96	0.053	13.4
Overall	-0.53	-1.01	-0.05	0.030	

$P_{heterogeneity}$<0.001; I^2 =82.6%

FIGURE 4 | Forest plot for studies examining the difference (PDA-no minus PDA-yes) in **(A)** mean platelet volume (MPV), **(B)** platelet mass, and **(C)** platelet distribution width (PDW) in the first day(s) of life in infants with and without hemodynamically significant PDA (hsPDA).

infants with a history of IUGR (51). We analyzed this association in a recent meta-analysis (51). We observed a negative association between PDA and antenatal growth restriction (51). However, this association was only present in the meta-analysis pooling the studies that defined growth restriction as small for gestational age. The cohorts in which fetal growth assessment was conducted did not show a significant association with the risk of developing PDA (51). Therefore, the current evidence does not suggest that IUGR increases the incidence of PDA. Another pathological condition associated with both early-onset thrombocytopenia and PDA is perinatal infection (49, 50). Although individual studies and meta-analyses have shown an association between chorioamnionitis and PDA risk (52–54), this association was significantly biased by the lower GA of the group of infants exposed to chorioamnionitis (53). Nevertheless, neonatal sepsis is widely considered to be a major factor in the pathway leading from PDA to hsPDA (55).

Another important limitation of the previous (19) and present meta-analysis is the significant statistical heterogeneity observed in most of the analyses. We performed meta-regression analysis in order to investigate potential sources of heterogeneity. Meta-regression data suggest that the association between any PDA and platelet counts below 150×10^9/L correlated with the GA and BW of each cohort. That is, those studies that included children with higher GA and BW showed a stronger association between thrombocytopenia and PDA. However, this finding could not be confirmed in the other meta-regression analyses that we performed. The incidence of both PDA and hsPDA was highly variable across the different studies (see **Table 1**). This variability is probably a consequence of the lack of consensus on clinical or sonographic criteria to consider a ductal shunt as significant (1–10). Meta-regression showed that the association between hsPDA and low platelet counts ($<150 \times 10^9$/L) was stronger in the studies with a lower rate of hsPDA. Nevertheless, our meta-regression results should be interpreted with caution. The minimum number of studies recommended to perform a meta-regression analysis is 10 (46). Our analyses were conducted in most cases with 10–11 studies but a higher number would have been necessary to obtain more reliable results.

Several investigators proposed that it is not the number of platelets but other quantitative or qualitative platelet parameters that are associated with a greater risk of developing PDA. Since large platelets are more reactive than small platelets, an elevated platelet size (i.e., a high MPV) is considered a marker of platelet activation (56, 57). Elevated MPV has been associated with cardiovascular disease in adults (58) and several studies have analyzed the association between MPV and complications of prematurity such as bronchopulmonary dysplasia, sepsis, intraventricular hemorrhage, retinopathy of prematurity, or PDA (59–63). Nevertheless, our meta-analysis could not demonstrate an association between MPV and hsPDA (**Figure 4**). In contrast, the platelet mass was significantly lower in the group of infants with hsPDA. The platelet mass and the plateletcrit are calculations obtained by multiplying the MPV by the platelet count (44, 45). For example, a platelet count of 100×10^9/L and a MPV of 10 fL would equate to a platelet mass of 1,000 (45). Since in the mathematical formula the platelet count has a factor of hundreds while the MPV has a factor of tens, the former will have a weight 10 times greater than the latter in the final value of the platelet mass. Therefore, our findings regarding the association of platelet mass with hsPDA may be only a repetition of the findings on the association of platelet counts and risk of hsPDA.

As mentioned above, large platelets are considered to be metabolically and enzymatically more active than small platelets. PDW reflects the variability in the platelet size and its increase is considered as a sign of platelet activation (56, 57). According to the hypothesis of the role of platelets in DA closure, a higher degree of platelet activation, and therefore a higher PDW, would be expected in the infants without PDA. However, our meta-analysis shows that infants with hsPDA have higher PDW values than infants without the condition. The heterogeneity of this meta-analysis was very high and the included studies showed either increased or reduced PDW in the hsPDA group. In addition, high PDW and MPV have been proposed as useful markers to distinguish thrombocytopenia associated with sepsis from other etiologies (56). Thus again, the etiology of thrombocytopenia (i.e., sepsis vs. IUGR) may be the factor leading to the differences in results of the studies addressing the association between platelet parameters and PDA.

The hypothesis that the important risk factor for PDA is altered platelet function, not decreased platelet number, has also been investigated. Unfortunately, the low number of studies that included information on this topic did not allow us to pool them in a meta-analysis. Immature platelets may have different functional features when compared to mature platelets (64). Sallmon et al. investigated the immature platelet fraction in a cohort of infants with and without hsPDA (64). Although higher immature platelet fraction values were associated with hsPDA, logistic regression analysis revealed that only mature platelet counts on postnatal day 7 were independently associated with the condition (64). Ghirardello et al. investigated thromboelastographic, a technique for bedside hemostatic assessment, in preterm infants with and without hsPDA (28). They could not demonstrate significant differences in thromboelastographic profile in children having hsPDA, or in those who failed pharmacological treatment, compared to their respective controls (28). Engur et al. (27) and Ahmed et al. (23) reported significant lower levels of platelet derived growth factor in the first days of life in preterm infants developing hsPDA. Finally, Kahvecioglou et al. reported that a higher collagen-ADP duration was an independent risk factor for hsPDA. All these findings need to be confirmed in future studies.

It is still unclear which long-term benefits or harms are achieved by treating a PDA (1–9). The attitude of neonatologists toward PDA has progressively changed in the last years from advocating widespread treatment to close the PDA to a call for watchful observation (1–9). Although our meta-analysis focused on the effect of thrombocytopenia on "spontaneous" DA closure, we must take into account that rate of PDA closure may have been affected by the variations in the management of PDA among centers (8, 9). In a recent meta-analysis, Mitra et al. reported that low platelet counts were associated with higher odds of failure to PDA treatment with ibuprofen or indomethacin (65). Therefore, taking together the results of the meta-analysis of Mitra et al. and the present one, the evidence points to an association between low platelet counts and the presence of PDA as well as the lack of response to pharmacological treatment. Nevertheless, association does not mean causation.

Besides the observational studies on the association between platelet counts and PDA, the potential effect of platelet transfusion on DA closure has been investigated in two randomized controlled trials (RCTs). Andrew et al. compared two platelet count thresholds for prophylactic platelet transfusion (150×10^9/L vs. 50×10^9/L) (66). The incidence of either the primary outcome, intraventricular hemorrhage, or PDA, which was one of the secondary outcomes, was not significantly different between the two thresholds. (66). Very recently, Kumar et al. conducted a RCT with PDA as primary outcome and prophylactic transfusion thresholds of 100×10^9/L vs. 20×10^9/L platelets (67). This RCT could not demonstrate any positive effect of the higher threshold on DA closure. Interestingly, the group of infants in the higher threshold had a higher incidence of intraventricular hemorrhage (67). As reviewed by Fustolo-Gunnink et al., results from several studies suggest that platelet transfusions do not reduce bleeding risk of preterm infants, and even might increase it (68). Moreover, a recent RCT, which included 660 preterm infants (GA $<$ 34 weeks), reported a risk reduction of major bleeding and/or mortality in neonates assigned to a prophylactic platelet transfusion threshold of 25×10^9/L vs. a threshold of 50×10^9/L. These results have led to a revision of the criteria and guidelines for platelet transfusion in very preterm infants to be more restrictive (68–70). Altogether, the current evidence suggests that increasing platelet counts by transfusion to hypothetically accelerate DA closure may generate more harm than benefit.

In conclusion, the present updated meta-analysis provides stronger evidence of the association between low platelet counts in the first day(s) of life and risk of developing PDA and hsPDA. Identifying simple markers of platelet function may improve our diagnostic and therapeutic decisions in dealing with PDA or other neonatal conditions. However, due to the complexities involved with the pathogenesis of both neonatal thrombocytopenia and PDA, it is impossible to establish a cause-and-effect relationship between the two conditions. In fact, studies that have attempted to correct the thrombocytopenia through platelet transfusions have not only failed to alter the incidence of PDA, but also have even led to increased morbidity (67).

AUTHOR CONTRIBUTIONS

GG-L carried out the systematic search, selected studies for inclusion, extracted study data, contributed to statistical analyses, interpretation of results, and drafting of the manuscript. SG supervised study inclusion and data collection, contributed to interpretation of results, and reviewed and revised the manuscript. PB-S contributed to search and data collection, contributed to interpretation of results, and reviewed and revised the manuscript. GC supervised study inclusion and data collection, contributed to interpretation of results, and reviewed and revised the manuscript. FM and RC contributed to interpretation of results, and reviewed and revised the manuscript. EV conceptualized the study, carried out the systematic search, selected studies for inclusion, extracted study data, carried out the statistical analyses and interpretation of results, and drafted the manuscript. All authors contributed to the article and approved the submitted version.

ACKNOWLEDGMENTS

We thank I. Morioka, E. A. Dizdar, and C. Dani for kindly providing additional data and clarifications of their studies.

REFERENCES

1. Hundscheid T, Onland W, Van Overmeire B, Dijk P, van Kaam AH, Dijkman KP, et al. Early treatment versus expectative management of patent ductus arteriosus in preterm infants: a multicentre, randomised, non-inferiority trial in Europe (BeNeDuctus trial). *BMC Pediatrics*. (2018) 18:262. doi: 10.1186/s12887-018-1215-7
2. Smith A, EL-Khuffash AF. Defining "haemodynamic significance" of the patent ductus arteriosus: do we have all the answers? *Neonatology*. (2020) 117:1–8. doi: 10.1159/000506988
3. Mitra S, McNamara PJ. Patent ductus arteriosus—time for a definitive trial. *Clin Perinatol*. (2020) 47:617–39. doi: 10.1016/j.clp.2020.05.007
4. Reese J, Laughon MM. The patent ductus arteriosus problem: infants who still need treatment. *J Pediatr*. (2015) 167:954–6. doi: 10.1016/j.jpeds.2015.08.023
5. Clyman RI, Liebowitz M, Kaempf J, Erdeve O, Bulbul A, Håkansson S, et al. PDA-TOLERATE trial: an exploratory randomized controlled trial of treatment of moderate-to-large patent ductus arteriosus at 1 week of age. *J Pediatr*. (2019) 205:41–8. e6. doi: 10.1016/j.jpeds.2018.09.012
6. Sallmon H, Koehne P, Hansmann G. Recent advances in the treatment of preterm newborn infants with patent ductus arteriosus. *Clin Perinatol*. (2016) 43:113–29. doi: 10.1016/j.clp.2015.11.008
7. Clyman RI, Benitz WE. Transcatheter patent ductus arteriosus closure—will history repeat itself? *J Perinatol*. (2019) 39:1435–6. doi: 10.1038/s41372-019-0483-x
8. de Klerk J, Engbers A, van Beek F, Flint RB, Reiss I, Völler S, et al. Spontaneous closure of the ductus arteriosus in preterm infants: a systematic review. *Front Pediatr*. (2020) 8:541. doi: 10.3389/fped.2020.00541
9. Okulu E, Erdeve O, Arslan Z, Demirel N, Kaya H, Gokce IK, et al. An observational, prospective, multicenter, registry-based cohort study comparing conservative and medical management for patent ductus arteriosus. *Front Pediatr*. (2020) 8:434. doi: 10.3389/fped.2020.00434
10. Hamrick SE, Sallmon H, Rose AT, Porras D, Shelton EL, Reese J, et al. Patent ductus arteriosus of the preterm infant. *Pediatrics*. (2020) 146:e20201209. doi: 10.1542/peds.2020-1209
11. Echtler K, Stark K, Lorenz M, Kerstan S, Walch A, Jennen L, et al. Platelets contribute to postnatal occlusion of the ductus arteriosus. *Nat Med*. (2010) 16:75–82. doi: 10.1038/nm.2060
12. Dizdar AE, Ozdemir R, Nur Sari F, Yurttutan S, Gokmen T, Erdeve O, et al. Low platelet count is associated with ductus arteriosus patency in preterm newborns. *Early Hum Dev*. (2012) 88:813–6. doi: 10.1016/j.earlhumdev.2012.05.007
13. Dani C, Poggi C, Fontanelli G. Relationship between platelet count and volume and spontaneous and pharmacological closure of ductus arteriosus in preterm infants. *Am J Perinatol*. (2013) 30:359–64. doi: 10.1055/s-0032-1324702
14. Fujioka K, Morioka I, Miwa A, Morikawa S, Shibata A, Yokoyama N, et al. Does thrombocytopenia contribute to patent ductus arteriosus? *Nat Med*. (2011) 17:29–30. doi: 10.1038/nm0111-29

15. Shah NA, Hills NK, Waleh N, McCurnin D, Seidner S, Chemtob S, et al. Relationship between circulating platelet counts and ductus arteriosus patency after indomethacin treatment. *J Pediatr.* (2011) 158:919–23. e1–2. doi: 10.1016/j.jpeds.2010.11.018
16. Sallmon H, Weber SC, Huning B, Stein A, Horn PA, Metze BC, et al. Thrombocytopenia in the first 24 hours after birth and incidence of patent ductus arteriosus. *Pediatrics.* (2012) 130:e623–30. doi: 10.1542/peds.2012-0499
17. Chen YY, Wang HP, Chang JT, Chiou YH, Huang YF, Hsieh KS, et al. Perinatal factors in patent ductus arteriosus in very low-birthweight infants. *Pediatr Int.* (2014) 56:72–6. doi: 10.1111/ped.12199
18. Bas-Suarez MP, Gonzalez-Luis GE, Saavedra P, Villamor E. Platelet counts in the first seven days of life and patent ductus arteriosus in preterm very low-birth-weight infants. *Neonatology.* (2014) 106:188–94. doi: 10.1159/000362432
19. Simon SR, van Zogchel L, Bas-Suárez MP, Cavallaro G, Clyman RI, Villamor E. Platelet counts and patent ductus arteriosus in preterm infants: a systematic review and meta-analysis. *Neonatology.* (2015) 108:143–51. doi: 10.1159/000431281
20. Wells GA, Shea B, O'Connell D, Peterson J, Welch V, Losos M. *The Newcastle-Ottawa Scale (NOS) for Assessing the Quality of Nonrandomized Studies in Meta-Analyses.* (2019). Available online at: http://www.ohri.ca/programs/clinical_epidemiology/oxford.htm (accessed May 15, 2020).
21. Wan X, Wang W, Liu J, Tong T. Estimating the sample mean and standard deviation from the sample size, median, range and/or interquartile range. *BMC Med Res Methodol.* (2014) 14:135. doi: 10.1186/1471-2288-14-135
22. Temel M, Coskun M, Akbayram S, Demiryürek A. Association between neutrophil/lymphocyte ratio with ductus arteriosus patency in preterm newborns. *Bratisl Lek Listy.* (2017) 118:491–4. doi: 10.4149/BLL_2017_094
23. Ahmed EG, Samra NM, Amin SA, Borayek HA, Abdelrazek G. Platelets and platelet derived growth factor and ductus arteriosus in preterm neonates. *Prog Pediatr Cardiol.* (2020) 57:101226. doi: 10.1016/j.ppedcard.2020.101226
24. Akar S, Topcuoglu S, Tuten A, Ozalkaya E, Karatepe HO, Gokmen T, et al. Is the first postnatal platelet mass as an indicator of patent ductus arteriosus? *Arch Iran Med.* (2019) 22:687–91.
25. Demir N, Peker E, Ece I, Agengin K, Bulan KA, Tuncer O. Is platelet mass a more significant indicator than platelet count of closure of patent ductus arteriosus? *J Matern Fetal Neonatal Med.* (2016) 29:1915–8. doi: 10.3109/14767058.2015.1067296
26. Demirel G, Yilmaz A, Vatansever B, Tastekin A. Is high platelet distribution width in the first hours of life can predict hemodynamically significant patent ductus arteriosus in preterm newborns? *J Matern Fetal Neonatal Med.* (2020) 33:2049–53. doi: 10.1080/14767058.2018.1536743
27. Engür D, Kaynak-Türkmen M, Deveci M, Yenisey Ç. Platelets and platelet-derived growth factor in closure of the ductus arteriosus. *Turk J Pediatr.* (2015) 57:242–7.
28. Ghirardello S, Raffaeli G, Crippa BL, Gulden S, Amodeo I, Consonni D, et al. The thromboelastographic profile at birth in very preterm newborns with patent ductus arteriosus. *Neonatology.* (2020) 117:1–8. doi: 10.1159/000507553
29. Kahvecioglu D, Erdeve O, Akduman H, Ucar T, Alan S, Çakir U, et al. Influence of platelet count, platelet mass index, and platelet function on the spontaneous closure of ductus arteriosus in the prematurity. *Pediatr Neonatol.* (2018) 59:53–7. doi: 10.1016/j.pedneo.2017.01.006
30. Karabulut B, Arcagök BC, Simsek A. Utility of the platelet-to-lymphocyte ratio in diagnosing and predicting treatment success in preterm neonates with patent ductus arteriosus. *Fetal Pediatr Pathol.* (2019) 38:1–10. doi: 10.1080/15513815.2019.1686786
31. Küçük M, Bagci O, Igde M. The fate of patent ductus arteriosus is not affected by platelet count and mean platelet volume in premature infants< 32 gestational weeks. *Turkiye Klinikleri Cardiovascular Sciences.* (2018) 30:53–7. doi: 10.5336/cardiosci.2018-62380
32. Kulkarni VV, Dutta S, Sundaram V, Saini SS. Preterm thrombocytopenia and delay of ductus arteriosus closure. *Pediatrics.* (2016) 138:e20161627. doi: 10.1542/peds.2016-1627
33. Meinarde L, Hillman M, Rizzotti A, Basquiera AL, Tabares A, Cuestas E. C-reactive protein, platelets, and patent ductus arteriosus. *Platelets.* (2016) 27:821–3. doi: 10.1080/09537104.2016.1203398
34. Morawietz S. Korrelation eines hämodynamisch relevanten persistierenden Ductus arteriosus mit einer Thrombozytopenie in den ersten zehn Lebenstagen sowie die Auswirkungen einer Thrombozytopenie auf das Outcome einer Behandlung mit NSAID. Munich: Lmu (2016).
35. Olukman O, Ozdemir R, Karadeniz C, Calkavur S, Mese T, Vergin C. Is there a relationship between platelet parameters and patency of ductus arteriosus in preterm infants? *Blood Coagul Fibrinolysis.* (2017) 28:8–13. doi: 10.1097/MBC.0000000000000520
36. Shekharappa CB, Elizabeth EAB, Balachander B. Association of patent ductus arteriosus size with clinical features and short-term outcomes in preterm infants less than 34 weeks. *Indian J Child Health.* (2020) 7:105–8. doi: 10.32677/IJCH.2020.v07.i03.003
37. Kusuma AAMW, Gunawijaya E, Putra IGNS, Yantie NPVK, Kardana IM, Utama IMGDL, et al. Risk factors of patent ductus arteriosus in preterm. *Am J Pediatr.* (2020) 6:168–72. doi: 10.11648/j.ajp.20200602.29
38. Oliveira A, Soares P, Flor-de-Lima F, Neves ALs, Guimarães Hl. PDA management in VLBW infants: experience of a level III NICU. *J Pediatr Neonat Individ Med (JPNIM).* (2016) 5:e050227. doi: 10.7363/050227
39. Saldaña-Díaz CV, Roque-Quezada JCE, Saldaña-Montes SP, De-la-Cruz-Vargas J. Trombocitopenia como indicador predictivo de cierre deficitario de ductus arterioso en prematuros del Instituto Nacional Materno Perinatal. *Revista Peruana de Investigación Materno Perinatal.* (2019) 8:21–6. doi: 10.33421/inmp.2019150
40. Kazanci EG, Buyuktiryaki M, Unsal H, Tayman C. Useful platelet indices for the diagnosis and follow-up of patent ductus arteriosus. *Am J Perinatol.* (2019) 36:1521–7. doi: 10.1055/s-0039-1688821
41. Özer Bekmez B, Tayman C, Büyüktiryaki M, Çetinkaya AK, Çakir U, Derme T. A promising, novel index in the diagnosis and follow-up of patent ductus arteriosus: red cell distribution width-to-platelet ratio. *J Clin Lab Anal.* (2018) 32:e22616. doi: 10.1002/jcla.22616
42. Dwarakanath K, Dereddy N, Chabra D, Schabacker C, Calo J, Parton L. Spontaneous and pharmacological closure of PDAs in ELBW infants is influenced by thrombocyto-penia (abstract). *E-PAS 21.* (2011).
43. Brunner B, Hoeck M, Schermer E, Streif W, Kiechl-Kohlendorfer U. Patent ductus arteriosus, low platelets, cyclooxygenase inhibitors, and intraventricular hemorrhage in very low birth weight preterm infants. *J Pediatr.* (2013) 163:23–8. doi: 10.1016/j.jpeds.2012.12.035
44. Kanda H, Yamakuchi M, Mastumoto K, Mukaihara K, Shigehisa Y, Tachioka S, et al. Dynamic changes in platelets caused by shear stress in aortic valve stenosis. *Clin Hemorheol Microcirc.* (2020). doi: 10.3233/CH-200928. [Epub ahead of print].
45. Christensen RD. Platelet transfusion in the neonatal intensive care unit: benefits, risks, alternatives. *Neonatology.* (2011) 100:311–8. doi: 10.1159/000329925
46. Borenstein M, Hedges LV, Higgins JPT, Rothstein HR (editors). Meta-regression. In: *Introduction to Meta-Analysis.* Sussex: John Wiley & Sons (2009). p. 187–203.
47. Chakravorty S, Roberts I. How I manage neonatal thrombocytopenia. *Br J Haematol.* (2012) 156:155–62. doi: 10.1111/j.1365-2141.2011.08892.x
48. Sola-Visner M. Platelets in the neonatal period: developmental differences in platelet production, function, and hemostasis and the potential impact of therapies. *Hematology Am Soc Hematol Educ Program.* (2012) 2012:506–11. doi: 10.1182/asheducation.V2012.1.506.3798532
49. Beiner ME, Simchen MJ, Sivan E, Chetrit A, Kuint J, Schiff E. Risk factors for neonatal thrombocytopenia in preterm infants. *Am J Perinatol.* (2003) 20:049–54. doi: 10.1055/s-2003-37948
50. Roberts I, Murray NA, editors. Neonatal thrombocytopenia. *Seminars in Fetal And Neonatal Medicine.* Elsevier (2008).
51. Villamor-Martinez E, Kilani MA, Degraeuwe PL, Clyman RI, Villamor E. Intrauterine growth restriction and patent ductus arteriosus in very and extremely preterm infants: a systematic review and meta-analysis. *Front Endocrinol.* (2019) 10:58. doi: 10.3389/fendo.2019.00058
52. Park HW, Choi Y-S, Kim KS, Kim S-N. Chorioamnionitis and patent ductus arteriosus: a systematic review and meta-analysis. *PLoS ONE.* (2015) 10:e0138114. doi: 10.1371/journal.pone.0138114
53. Behbodi E, Villamor-Martínez E, Degraeuwe PL, Villamor E. Chorioamnionitis appears not to be a risk factor for patent ductus arteriosus in preterm infants: a systematic review and meta-analysis. *Sci Rep.* (2016) 6:37967. doi: 10.1038/srep37967

54. Green CA, Westreich D, Laughon MM, Stamilio DM, Strauss RA, Reese J, et al. Association of chorioamnionitis and patent ductus arteriosus in a national US cohort. *J Perinatol.* (2020). doi: 10.1038/s41372-020-00866-x. [Epub ahead of print].
55. Vucovich MM, Cotton RB, Shelton EL, Goettel JA, Ehinger NJ, Poole SD, et al. Aminoglycoside-mediated relaxation of the ductus arteriosus in sepsis-associated PDA. *Am J Physiol Heart Circ Physiol.* (2014) 307:H732–40. doi: 10.1152/ajpheart.00838.2013
56. Kim JY, Yoon J, Lim CS, Choi BM, Yoon S-Y. Clinical significance of platelet-associated hematological parameters as an early supplementary diagnostic tool for sepsis in thrombocytopenic very-low-birth-weight infants. *Platelets.* (2015) 26:620–6. doi: 10.3109/09537104.2014.963542
57. Kannar V, Deepthi A, Kumar MLH, Junjegowda K, Mariyappa N. Effect of gestational age, prematurity and birth asphyxia on platelet indices in neonates. *J Clin Neonatol.* (2014) 3:144. doi: 10.4103/2249-4847.140399
58. Chu S, Becker R, Berger P, Bhatt D, Eikelboom J, Konkle B, et al. Mean platelet volume as a predictor of cardiovascular risk: a systematic review and meta-analysis. *J Thromb Haemost.* (2010) 8:148–56. doi: 10.1111/j.1538-7836.2009.03584.x
59. Go H, Ohto H, Nollet KE, Takano S, Kashiwabara N, Chishiki M, et al. Using platelet parameters to anticipate morbidity and mortality among preterm neonates: a retrospective study. *Front Pediatr.* (2020) 8:90. doi: 10.3389/fped.2020.00090
60. Tao Y, Dong Y, Lu C-w, Yang W. Mean platelet volume in retinopathy of prematurity. *Graefes Arch Clin Exp Ophthalmol.* (2015) 253:2047–8. doi: 10.1007/s00417-015-3047-6
61. Dani C, Poggi C, Barp J, Berti E, Fontanelli G. Mean platelet volume and risk of bronchopulmonary dysplasia and intraventricular hemorrhage in extremely preterm infants. *Am J Perinatol.* (2011) 28:551–6. doi: 10.1055/s-0031-1274503
62. Grevsen AK, Hviid CV, Hansen AK, Hvas A-M, editors. The role of platelets in premature neonates with intraventricular hemorrhage: a systematic review and meta-analysis. Semin Thromb Hemost. (2020) 46:366–78. doi: 10.1055/s-0039-3402687
63. Wang J, Wang Z, Zhang M, Lou Z, Deng J, Li Q. Diagnostic value of mean platelet volume for neonatal sepsis: A systematic review and meta-analysis. *Medicine.* (2020) 99:e21649. doi: 10.1097/MD.0000000000021649
64. Sallmon H, Metze B, Koehne P, Opgen-Rhein B, Weiss K, Will JC, et al. Mature and immature platelets during the first week after birth and incidence of patent ductus arteriosus. *Cardiol Young.* (2020) 30:1–5. doi: 10.1017/S1047951120000943
65. Mitra S, Chan AK, Paes BA, Thrombosis, Group HiN. The association of platelets with failed patent ductus arteriosus closure after a primary course of indomethacin or ibuprofen: a systematic review and meta-analysis. *J Matern-Fetal Neonat Med.* (2017) 30:127–33. doi: 10.3109/14767058.2016.1163684
66. Andrew M, Vegh P, Caco C, Kirpalani H, Jefferies A, Ohlsson A, et al. A randomized, controlled trial of platelet transfusions in thrombocytopenic premature infants. *J Pediatr.* (1993) 123:285–91. doi: 10.1016/S0022-3476(05)81705-6
67. Kumar J, Dutta S, Sundaram V, Saini SS, Sharma RR, Varma N. Platelet transfusion for PDA closure in preterm infants: a randomized controlled trial. *Pediatrics.* (2019) 143:e20182565. doi: 10.1542/peds.2018-2565
68. Fustolo-Gunnink S, Huisman E, van der Bom J, van Hout F, Makineli S, Lopriore E, et al. Are thrombocytopenia and platelet transfusions associated with major bleeding in preterm neonates? A systematic review. *Blood Rev.* (2019) 36:1–9. doi: 10.1016/j.blre.2018.10.001
69. Fustolo-Gunnink SF, Fijnvandraat K, van Klaveren D, Stanworth SJ, Curley A, Onland W, et al. Preterm neonates benefit from low prophylactic platelet transfusion threshold despite varying risk of bleeding or death. *Blood.* (2019) 134:2354–60. doi: 10.1182/blood.2019000899
70. Lopriore E. Updates in red blood cell and platelet transfusions in preterm neonates. *Am J Perinatol.* (2019) 36(S 02):S37–40. doi: 10.1055/s-0039-1691775

14

Management of Patent Ductus Arteriosus in Premature Infants in 2020

Sarah Parkerson[1]*, Ranjit Philip*[2]*, Ajay Talati*[3] *and Shyam Sathanandam*[2*]

[1] Department of Pediatrics, University of Tennessee, Memphis, TN, United States, [2] Division of Pediatric Cardiology, University of Tennessee, Memphis, TN, United States, [3] Division of Neonatology, University of Tennessee, Memphis, TN, United States

***Correspondence:**
Shyam Sathanandam
ssathan2@uthsc.edu

The patent ductus arteriosus (PDA) is the most commonly found cardiac condition in neonates. While there have been several studies and thousands of publications on the topic, the decision to treat the PDA is still strongly debated among cardiologists, surgeons, and neonatologists. This is in part due to the shortage of long-term benefits with the interventions studied. Practice variations still exist within sub-specialties and centers. This article briefly summarizes the history, embryology and histology of the PDA. It also succinctly discusses the hemodynamic significance of a PDA which builds the framework to review all the available literature on PDA closure in premature infants, though not a paradigm shift just yet; it introduces transcatheter PDA closure (TCPC) as a possible armament to the clinician for this age-old problem.

Keywords: PDA, prematurity and low birth weight, transcatheter ductus closure, patent ductus arteriosus (patent arterial duct), surgical ligation of patent ductus arteriosus

INTRODUCTION

The patent ductus arteriosus (PDA) is the most common cardiac condition affecting neonates (1). While there has been several studies and thousands of publications on the topic, the decision to treat the PDA is still strongly debated among cardiologists, surgeons, and neonatologists (2–4).

Numerous studies have found an association with untreated PDAs and significant neonatal morbidities (5–7). When left untreated, the PDA and resulting left-to-right shunt can compromise systemic perfusion. Determining the volume of the shunt is a crucial step in deciding the course of action for premature infants with a PDA. Physicians use their clinical assessment, echocardiography, and indicators of systemic hypoperfusion or pulmonary over-circulation in order to quantify the shunt but this process has not been standardized (8, 9) and thus varies across institutions. While increased morbidity is associated with PDA, the management options have been linked to adverse outcomes (10–12); which leads to debate over whether or not to treat the PDA (2). Furthermore, if and when a PDA needs to be treated, how do we treat it? (13) This chapter intends to outline the current literature about the embryology, pathophysiology, and treatment approaches for the PDA in the premature infant in 2020.

HISTORY

The PDA was the first congenital heart lesion that was surgically repaired. This was performed by Dr. Robert Gross in 1938 (14). In the Second century, Galen was one of the first to describe a notion of blood traveling between the heart and the lungs. This concept was later developed into a complete anatomical and physiologic description of PDA many centuries later. In 1989, Krichenko et al. (15) angiographically classified the PDA based on the ductal lumen at the aortic and pulmonary ends. Closure of the PDA in a premature neonate with respiratory distress syndrome (RDS) was first detailed by Dr. ML Powell in 1963 (16). With the increasing survival of preterm neonates, the consequent increase in PDA closures in preterm infants and the special morphologic characteristics of the preterm ductus, the PDA was reclassified in 2016 to aid with the choice of device used for transcatheter device closure in this population (17).

EMBRYOLOGY

At the early embryonic stage, the ductus arteriosus (DA) is present on the right and left sides but the right atrophies between 37 and 40 days of embryonic gestation (18). The DA is created from the same embryonic structure that makes the pulmonary artery: the left 6th aortic arch. The DA attaches to the inner curve of the arch, distal to the left subclavian artery. There is a high resistance within the pulmonary vasculature (19) during development of the fetal lungs. Due to this degree of resistance, blood travels from the left pulmonary artery, through the DA, and into the descending aorta which preserves right ventricular function (20). If the DA were to close prematurely *in utero*, the right ventricular afterload increases and the fetus is at risk to develop right heart failure and fetal hydrops (21).

HISTOLOGY

Histologically, the walls of the DA are mainly muscular in contrast to the walls of the adjacent aorta and pulmonary artery, which are fibro-elastic (22). The DA is comprised of smooth muscle fibers which are arranged in longitudinal and spiral layers and surrounded by concentric layers of elastic tissue. The great arteries are composed primarily of elastic fibers arranged circumferentially. After birth, the medial smooth muscle fibers contract in response to the exposure to oxygen-rich ambient air (23). This leads to constriction of the lumen and shortening of the DA length which begins at the pulmonary end until there is functional closure between 24 and 48 h. The second stage of closure involves proliferation of the medial and intimal connective tissue and smooth muscle atrophy which leads to the conversion of a muscular vessel into a ligamentous non-contractile structure, the ligamentum arteriosum over the next 3 weeks (24). Vascular endothelial growth factor (VEGF) has been thought to be involved in DA closure. However, VEGF polymorphism rs2010963 status has not been shown to affect PDA incidence or successful treatment with cyclooxygenase inhibitors in preterm infants (25).

PHYSIOLOGY

The predominant cardiac output in fetal life bypasses the lungs via right to left shunting at the DA. This is possible due to the low systemic vascular resistance from the placenta and the high pulmonary vascular resistance in the lungs. Systemic vascular resistance is increased after birth when the cord is clamped (26). In addition, due to ventilation, the pulmonary vascular resistance is decreased and pulmonary blood flow is increased. This causes blood to shunt left to right through the DA. In term infants, predominant left to right shunting occurs within 10 min and is entirely left to right within 24 h of life (27).

PDA IN THE PREMATURE NEONATE

The incidence of PDA is inversely related to the gestational age. It remains open at 4 days of age in 10% of neonates born at 30–37 weeks, 80% of those between 25 and 28 weeks gestation and 90% born <24 weeks gestation (28–31). In these extremely premature infants, the PDA can persist for weeks, in comparison to infants born after 28 weeks in which the PDA is more likely to spontaneously close (32). Failure of closure of the DA in these infants is more commonly due to issues associated with prematurity rather than aberrations of the DA itself (33). The pressure gradient between the aorta and pulmonary artery (PA) as well as the size and resistance of the DA determine the hemodynamic effects of the PDA. The vessel's length, internal diameter, and intrinsic elastance properties define the resistance within the DA (34). Whereas, a small PDA may be left untreated without complications, a large PDA left open long-term can lead to pulmonary hypertension (19, 35). The role of platelet function in the spontaneous PDA closure in the preterm infant has been studied (36, 37). Lower counts of mature platelets are an independent predictor of a hsPDA (38).

The shunting of blood from left-to-right via the PDA causes pulmonary over-circulation and left-sided volume overload in the heart. This increase in pulmonary blood flow can affect the maturation of the pulmonary vasculature in a premature infant (33). It can result in pulmonary edema, reduced lung compliance, and ineffective gas exchange. This, in turn, leads to increased ventilator settings, which can cause parenchymal lung damage in the neonate (39). It has been suggested that PDA closure within the first 4 weeks of life may allow for faster weaning of oxygen and ventilatory support in extremely low birth weight (ELBW) infants (birth weight ≤1,000 g) (40); however, further investigation is needed.

With severe volume overload in the left heart, the end-diastolic pressure of the left atrium and ventricle can be elevated. The left ventricular myocardium undergoes remodeling to a larger and more spherical shape (41). The larger the left-to-right shunt, the more association with risk of necrotizing enterocolitis, intraventricular hemorrhage, acute kidney injury and death (7, 42, 43). Very low birth weight preterm infant survivors of pulmonary hemorrhage were associated with a PDA (79%) in comparison to their controls (55%) (44). Although, this mechanism is not completely understood. One widely accepted theory is that the shunting through the PDA results in lower systemic diastolic pressure and thus threatens end-organ perfusion. Others blame the morbidities of PDA on reperfusion injury suggesting that the left ventricle becomes more compliant overtime and thus increases its cardiac output. The reperfusion that occurs after a phase of hypoperfusion is thought to be the culprit of the end-organ damage in the premature neonate (45).

There is still widespread discordance about best management of a PDA and the timing in which to apply said management (4, 46, 47). A survey in 2018 found many disparities between neonatologists and cardiologists concerning the management of PDA in neonates (2). Most cardiologists believe that PDA closure alters the clinical outcomes in infants born <28 weeks' gestation, while almost half neonatologists surveyed disagree with this statement (2). There is currently not enough evidence to determine whether systemic complications associated with hemodynamically significant PDA in ELBW infants is due to the PDA or simply the result of prematurity (48).

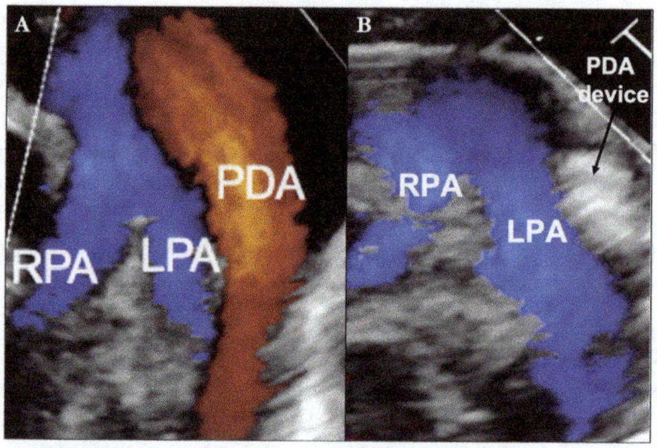

FIGURE 1 | (A) Transthoracic Echocardiogram (parasternal short axis image with color Doppler) demonstrating the relative size of the patent ductus arteriosus (PDA) in comparison to the left pulmonary artery (LPA) and right pulmonary artery (RPA). **(B)** Post-transcatheter PDA closure.

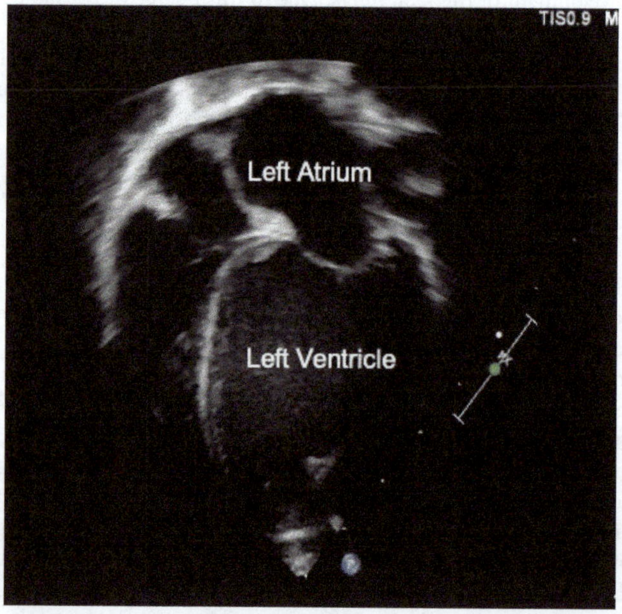

FIGURE 2 | Transthoracic Apical 4-chamber view showing left atrial and ventricular dilation suggestive of a hemodynamically significant PDA.

DEFINING A HEMODYNAMICALLY SIGNIFICANT PDA

There is a larger body of epidemiological data that reveals an association between a PDA and multiple morbidities including intraventricular hemorrhage (IVH), necrotizing enterocolitis (NEC), retinopathy of prematurity (ROP), and bronchopulmonary dysplasia (BPD) (5, 49, 50). However, significant differences have not been demonstrated in randomized trials of PDA closure. Prior to the twenty-first century, almost all PDAs were arbitrarily deemed hemodynamically significant and physicians aimed to close them soon after birth (51). That approach is no longer favored, and the majority of physicians prefer to watch and wait (46). The lack of quantifiable improvement in outcomes after PDA closure likely influenced this practice change. The outcomes without noticeable improvement after PDA closure include BPD, NEC, IVH, ROP, periventricular leukomalacia, long-term neurodevelopmental status, and death (52, 53).

Echocardiography has been examined in multiple studies as an objective measure of a hemodynamically significant PDA (hsPDA) (49, 54, 55). The echocardiographic parameters used in determining if a PDA is hemodynamically significant include the transductal diameter, evidence of left-sided volume overload, quantification of ductal shunting, and magnitude of pulmonary overcirculation (56). The transductal diameter and the flow pattern (low velocity flow) are used to quantify the shunt size as seen in **Figure 1A** (57). Indices of left-sided volume overload and pulmonary over-circulation are closely related and thus use many of the same indices for evaluation as seen in **Figure 2**. Albeit dated, one of the most used measurements to determine is a PDA is hemodynamically significant is the ratio of the left atrium diameter (LA) to the aortic root diameter (Ao) by M-mode echocardiography. If the LA:Ao ratio is >1.4, there is likely left-sided volume overload secondary to increased blood return from the lungs. Another important echocardiographic measurement includes reversal of flow in diastole in the abdominal aorta suggestive of a substantial shunt [i.e., evidence of systemic steal (**Figure 3**)]. Individually, these indices are not specific to a PDA but when presenting together in a premature infant with RDS, it is reasonable to believe there is a hemodynamically significant PDA present. Although there are numerous suggested protocols for assessment of a hsPDA (49, 50, 58–61), there is no validated protocol that confirms the echocardiographic information with real-time hemodynamic information from cardiac catheterization.

Echocardiography can also be useful as a predictive measure of whether a PDA will become hemodynamically significant. One study found that the ductal anatomy during the first 12 h of life, specifically a ductal length <5.2 mm, was predictive of a hsPDA by 72 h of life with a sensitivity of 83% and a specificity of 86% (62).

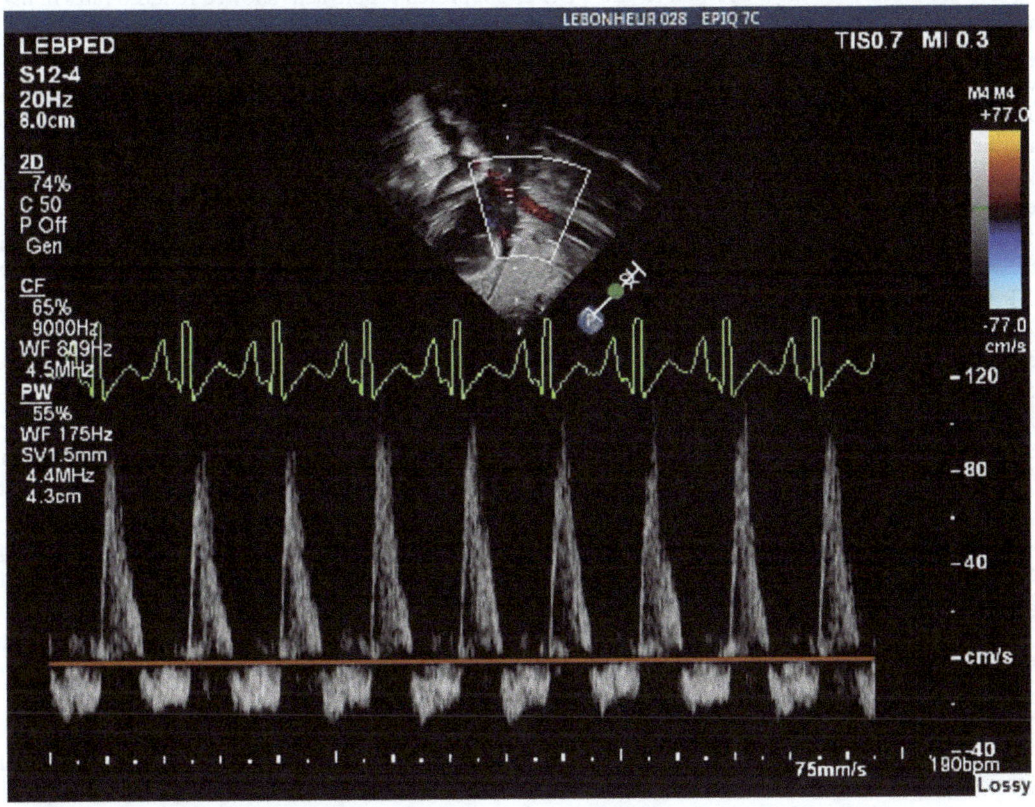

FIGURE 3 | Abdominal Aorta Doppler pattern showing diastolic flow reversal indicative of a hemodynamically significant PDA.

Multiple publications have investigated serum biochemical markers as indicators of a hsPDA both independently and with echocardiography. These markers include B-type natriuretic peptide (BNP), amino-terminal pro-B-type natriuretic peptide (NT-proBNP), and cardiac Troponin T (cTnT) (63, 64). There are also urinary markers such as Neutrophil gelatinase-associated lipocalin and heart-type fatty acid binding protein that have been used to predict ductal closure timing (65). While locally certified BNP or NT-proBNP assays can be useful to trend for appraisal of response to therapy, the variability of assays across institutions prevents universal assertions about their utilization (56). A study of premature neonates did find a correlation between the cTnT levels and the ductal diameter, LA:Ao ratio and descending aortic end-diastolic velocity (57). In addition, these biomarkers may help clinicians determine the effect of their treatments on infants' cardiac function. For example, one study found that even 2 weeks after treatment with oral ibuprofen, urinary NT-proBNP was still elevated, suggesting that there is still an effect on cardiac function even when the infant is clinically stable post-treatment (66).

Clinical judgment can be another useful resource in the decision to treat a PDA. One study found that presence or absence of certain clinical symptoms was appropriate for determining treatment of PDA and may prevent unnecessary medical treatments in this vulnerable population (67). Alone, echocardiographic indices and serum biochemical markers cannot reliably determine if a PDA is hemodynamically significant. However, when used in combination with clinical data, practitioners can make that determination on a case-by-case basis (9).

PROPHYLACTIC CLOSURE OF PDA

Though the presence of a moderate to large PDA has been associated with morbidity, as demonstrated in over 60 controlled trials, the lack of any decrease in morbidity and mortality with ductal closure has questioned the utility of prophylactic PDA closure in premature infants (68, 69). There are four possible explanations as described by McNamara for the lack of proven clinical benefit after ductal closure (70). First, the "hemodynamically significant" PDA has no true causal relationship with adverse outcomes. Second, the conclusions of many studies are unreliable due to the variable definition of "hemodynamically significant" and therefore results have been diluted by "hemodynamically non-significant" PDAs. Third, frequent cross-over between placebo and treatment groups may have obscured any visible benefits. Fourth, there is a causal relationship between the hsPDA and adverse outcomes but closure alone will not fully ameliorate the morbidities or mortalities. The multiple confounding factors that coexist may explain why the trials of prophylactic closure have shown only some reduction in various morbidities (52, 71).

Prophylactic medical closure of the PDA before the PDA becomes "hemodynamically significant" has been shown to reduce the incidence of severe IVH and the need for surgical ligation however it has not been shown to reduce BPD, NEC, or improve long-term neurodevelopmental outcomes (72). It is unclear why the decreased incidence of severe IVH has not translated into enhanced neurodevelopmental outcomes in the long-term. The Ment-trial in 1994 showed favorable neurodevelopment outcomes in 4.5 and 8-years old children who were treated with Indomethacin prophylaxis (73). However, the PDA-TOLERATE trial found medical treatment after the 1st week of life was not associated with reduced PDA ligations or PDAs present at discharge in infants born before 28 weeks gestation (74). In addition, the infants born between 26 and 28 weeks gestation had increased rates of late-onset sepsis and death when exposed to early medical treatment suggesting that early medical treatment is not without long-term negative effects (74). This has led many neonatologists to adopt a conservative approach, which compared to medical treatment, has resulted in similar rates of NEC, IVH, and ROP (75). In one study, premature infants who did not get treatment for their PDA had lower rates of mortality than the infants who received medical treatment (75). Spontaneous closure of PDAs and the need for rescue treatment for those in the conservative treatment group make it difficult to fully evaluate the morbidities associated with conservative treatment (76).

Prophylactic surgical ligation of PDA was a common practice before medical therapy was widely available. In 1989, Cassady published the first randomized controlled trial of prophylactic surgical ligation and found a significant reduction in rate of NEC but no reduction in mortality, severe IVH, BPD, or ROP (77). Due to the significant morbidities associated with surgical ligation, prophylactic surgical ligation is no longer an accepted practice (78, 79).

MEDICAL CLOSURE OF A HEMODYNAMICALLY SIGNIFICANT PDA

Both indomethacin and ibuprofen are accepted by the US Food and Drug Administration (FDA) for closing a PDA (80, 81). These drugs prevent the transition of arachidonic acid to prostaglandin by inhibiting the cyclooxygenase site of the prostaglandin synthase enzyme, thus causing constriction of the PDA. Ibuprofen can be as successful as indomethacin for closure of the PDA. In addition, ibuprofen offers a lower risk of NEC and acute kidney injury (82). The long-term benefits of using ibuprofen compared to indomethacin has not been extensively studied and thus the data is not currently available.

Ibuprofen is given in three doses 24 h apart. The standard dosing is 10 mg/kg for the first dose and half (5 mg/kg) for the second and third doses (83). However, new research has found a higher closure rate when the ibuprofen dose is doubled (54.8% closure compared to 30.6%) (84, 85). Mitra published a meta-analysis in 2018 which also observed a higher probability of PDA closure and no increase in adverse outcomes when the dose was doubled (86). Another RCT using early oral ibuprofen prophylaxis showed reduced rates of hsPDA albeit not statistically significant and with a high prevalence of adverse events (intestinal perforation and kidney injury) (87). This is further support by a study that found lower serum ibuprofen levels in premature infants whose hsPDA did not close after 3-dose treatment; specifically, the trough after the first dose was significantly lower compared to the group of infants whose hsPDA did close after 3-dose treatment (88).

The preferred route of ibuprofen administration has just been clarified by recent studies. A Cochrane review in 2015 observed that ibuprofen administered intravenously was less effective at PDA closure than ibuprofen administered orally (RR 0.37; 95% CI 0.23–0.61) (65). This was also seen in a large network meta-analysis (74). Pacifici suggested that the slower absorption and prolonged half-life with oral administration offered more time for the drug to interact with the PDA and thus made it more effective (89). However, a study of ELBW infants found that those infants who received oral ibuprofen for PDA closure had a higher rate of PDA reopening compared to those who received IV ibuprofen (90). In terms of safety, evidence supports that oral ibuprofen is as safe as IV ibuprofen in very low birth weight infants (91). Furthermore, one study observed that neurodevelopmental outcomes in premature infants who received oral ibuprofen vs. IV ibuprofen for PDA closure were not significantly different (92). Ibuprofen has been associated with higher risk of NEC, spontaneous intestinal perforation, and acute kidney injury (81) In addition, decreased blood flow to the kidneys, mesentery, and brain was revealed through near infrared spectroscopy (NIRS) and Doppler ultrasonography after indomethacin/ibuprofen was given for PDA closure (93–97). Consequently, withholding enteral feedings has become more popular when administering indomethacin/ibuprofen to premature infants in order to reduce the adverse gastrointestinal outcomes. However, some studies have investigated this and did not find a disparity in enteral feeding tolerance or harmful events involving the gastrointestinal tract when infants were given smaller volume enteral feeds during indomethacin/ibuprofen therapy (98, 99).

Recently, acetaminophen has been suggested as a substitute for indomethacin and ibuprofen. The US FDA has not approved the use of acetaminophen in neonates to close the PDA. The mechanism of acetaminophen is not completely known, but it is thought to inhibit the peroxidase section of the prostaglandin synthase enzyme causing narrowing of the PDA (100). Oral acetaminophen has not been extensively studied like the cyclooxygenase inhibitors, but was thought to be as successful as oral ibuprofen in closing a PDA (101). In addition, the incidence of renal insufficiency was reduced with oral acetaminophen administration compared to high dose oral ibuprofen (102). As seen with ibuprofen, one study found a lower serum acetaminophen level in premature infants whose PDA did not close after a 3-days course of acetaminophen (103). With potential for effective closure of the PDA and reduced adverse events (104), acetaminophen has become an appealing alternative to cyclooxygenase inhibitors (105), especially in infants with other morbidities easily aggravated by indomethacin/ibuprofen (106). However, a recent multicenter randomized control trial evaluating the effectiveness of IV acetaminophen over IV indomethacin in infants <32 weeks gestation with a birthweight ≤1,500 gms with a hemodynamically significant PDA by echocardiogram showed reduced effectiveness (5.9 vs. 55% closure rate) (107). In addition, a RCT evaluating the impacts of paracetamol compared to ibuprofen on neurodevelopment outcomes at 18–24 months corrected gestational age showed no significant difference (108). A single center trial of 12 infants evaluating the role of combined (paracetamol and ibuprofen) therapy to monotherapy-resistant hsPDA showed a 75% success rate (109). However, in a single center double-blinded randomized controlled pilot study, there was no benefit observed with adding IV paracetamol to IV ibuprofen for the treatment of hsPDA (110).

SURGICAL CLOSURE OF A HEMODYNAMICALLY SIGNIFICANT PDA

The first RCT evaluating surgical ligation vs. conservative "standard" medical care was done by Cotton and colleagues who tested ventilated VLBW neonates at 8–10 days of life. Albeit small, the study showed that routine early surgical ligations led to earlier extubations and a lower hospital bill (111). Unfortunately, surgical ligation has frequently been linked to increased morbidities including BPD, ROP, and long-term neurodevelopmental impairment (10, 112–116). The TIPP trial (trial of indomethacin prophylaxis in preterm infants) also corroborated that patients who underwent surgical ligation had more BPD, severe ROP, and 18–22 months neurosensory deficiency in comparison to patients who had medical therapy alone (72).

However, there are many confounding variables linked to surgical ligation that complicate the reasons for neurodevelopmental deficiency. It is unclear whether the outcomes are purely cause-and-effect or if surgery is an indication of clinical severity. With substantial adverse events depicted after surgical ligation (117–123) and the debate over whether a PDA even needs to be closed, most neonatologists err on the side of caution and defer surgical ligation even if medical management fails (2, 46).

PERCUTANEOUS CLOSURE OF HEMODYNAMICALLY SIGNIFICANT PDA

Transcatheter PDA closure (TCPC) has come to be the treatment of choice in adults and children (20). However, there is still hesitation with patient selection and timing of procedure due to opposing results on the safety of TCPC during infancy (124). The largest meta-analysis to date assessing infants undergoing percutaneous closure of their PDA was published by Backes in 2017. In 635 procedures within 38 studies, 92.2% were successful closures and the rate of adverse events was 23.3%, with only 10.1% being "clinically significant (125)." In 2016, Zahn evaluated TCPC in the extremely premature population, which included 24 infants with a mean weight of 1,249 grams. His successful closure rate was 88% and his adverse event rate was 12.5%. At follow up (median time of 11 months), all 24 patients were alive and did not have residual PDA, LPA stenosis, or aortic coarctation (126). At our institution, TCPC in premature infants had a significantly lower complication rate compared to surgical ligation (3.3 vs. 25.7%) (127, 128). We have currently performed TCPC on 108 infants weighing <1,000 grams at our institution. The complications in the 241 infants weighing between 500 and 2,000 grams at the time of the TCPC at our institute included: coarctation of the aorta (2), pericardial effusion needing drainage (2), tricuspid valve injury (1), one procedure related mortality early in the experience, device embolization and retrieval (1) and left pulmonary artery stenosis requiring device retrieval (1). In contrast, the surgical group ($n = 167$) had two procedure related mortalities, wound dehiscence (2), residual PDA requiring re-intervention (4), Pneumothorax (3), Sepsis/pneumonia (4), left ventricular wall motion abnormality needing digoxin at discharge (1), worsening respiratory status (2), and post-ligation syndrome (25).

While percutaneous PDA closure can be done at bedside using echocardiography and portable fluoroscopy, transporting the premature infant to the catheterization lab may be necessary. This transport requires thorough coordination since ELBW infants often require temperature and ventilatory regulation (129). In addition, there are some procedural alterations that can be made to better accommodate the premature infant during percutaneous PDA closure.

Since limb ischemia has been associated with accessing small diameter arteries in ELBW infants, the procedure is performed from a venous access only (130, 131). Femoral vessel nomograms allow for pre-procedure planning in certain settings but they may not include premature infants in the data set so it may be safest to avoid arterial access in premature infants (132). Reducing overall procedure time is especially important in premature infants and can be done by minimizing intracardiac catheter manipulation, contrast dosing, and unnecessary hemodynamic measurements (133, 134). Equally important is ensuring optimal device placement prior to device deployment (135). Without having arterial access, aortography is not possible so a transthoracic echocardiogram (TTE) should be used for evaluation of device placement as seen in **Figure 1B** (135). If a different device size is required due to inadequate placement or residual shunting, the initial device can be retrieved via catheter and a new device placed all within the same procedure setting (136). The risks associated with percutaneous PDA closure, while low even in ELBW infants, include device embolization, cardiac perforation, aortic coarctation, and LPA obstruction (125).

Currently, there are a number of PDA closure devices available for infants and children >5 kg. However, the DA morphology differs in ELBW infants in that it is long and tortuous (17) compared to older infants and children, which can compromise the effectiveness of these devices in ELBW infants (137). Recently, a new device was FDA approved for PDA closure in infants ≥ 700 g (138). The success rate with this new device was 95.5% (191/200) in all patients and 99% (99/100) in patients ≤ 2 kilograms. Of implanted patients, 99.4% reached the primary effectiveness endpoint. A primary safety endpoint event was reached in four patients (two transfusions, one hemolysis, and one aortic obstruction). No branch pulmonary artery obstructions were observed. Worsening of tricuspid regurgitation (TR) was found in five patients after the procedure. This study clearly showed safety and efficacy of TCPC even though it was restricted to 10 centers. It adds to the armament of the neonatologist in the early treatment of PDAs in premature infants and may encourage further investigation on the outcomes of early PDA closure in this population (138).

With growing experience, we have found that early PDA closure may afford better overall clinical outcomes in ELBW infants. In the past, early surgical ligation of the PDA did not demonstrate any benefit. However, unlike surgical ligation, TCPC involves no cutting or stitching to the infants' chest, there is no handling of the premature lungs and no inflammatory surge. Therefore, TCPC may be overall beneficial. It is similar to surgical ligation in that it affords immediate, definitive closure of the PDA unlike medical therapy, which is not 100% effective and requires a long time period to work. While TCPC is a technically feasible and safe therapeutic option, the lack of comparative trials and widespread operator experience, prevents it from being the current standard of care. Since ELBW infants who have undergone TCPC usually have multiple co-morbidities and are at high risk for hospital readmission during their 1st year of life, it is important to have a multidisciplinary follow-up visit after initial discharge to monitor their progress (139, 140). However, given the concerns of surgical ligation during infancy (52–55, 117–123), TCPC represents a potentially attractive alternative especially when medical therapy has failed.

POST-LIGATION SYNDROME

Substantial hemodynamic changes take place after ligation of PDA and they have only recently started being explored in a scientific manner. A sudden increase in afterload and a decrease in left ventricular (LV) preload occurs following ligation, putting the neonate at high risk for decreased cardiac output. In fact, decreased LV output has been reported in up to 50% of premature neonates after PDA ligation (141). This cardiac deterioration is termed post-ligation syndrome and can occur relatively quickly. Signs of a low cardiac output state include hypotension, increased metabolic acidosis and respiratory failure (142, 143). Studies have found a significantly lower incidence of post-ligation syndrome in ELBW infants who underwent transcatheter PDA closure compared to surgical ligation (144–146). Jain demonstrated that prophylactic milrinone administration reduced the incidence of post-ligation syndrome from 44 to 11% in high-risk patients (147). In addition, calcium chloride administration following transcatheter PDA closure can also reduce the incidence of post-ligation syndrome in ELBW infants (148).

CONCLUSION

Management of the PDA continues to be an elusive challenge for neonatologists and pediatric cardiologists despite it being the most common cardiac condition affecting premature neonates. After 50 years of scientific investigation yielding thousands of publications, there is still no agreement on the definition of a hemodynamically significant PDA and how best to treat it. However, many clinical lessons have been brought to light and cannot be ignored. We know that routine PDA closure soon after birth does not diminish the morbidities associated with a PDA. In addition, surgical ligation has been associated repeatedly with higher occurrence of BDP, ROP, and poorer neurodevelopmental outcomes. When medically treating the PDA, we have realized several medications which have had positive results, some with more adverse side effects than others. With the introduction of percutaneous PDA closure, we have the potential to be less invasive; however, as in most treatment modalities, the risks remain. Pharmacogenetics appears to be the next frontier as we contemplate the continued questions of who needs intervention for their hsPDA and how best to achieve this while minimizing the morbidity and mortality, specifically in premature infant population. With continued exploration, we continue to adapt our theories about the persistent ductus arteriosus and its effects.

AUTHOR CONTRIBUTIONS

All authors were involved in substantial contributions to the conception, design of the manuscript, drafting the article, and revising it critically for important intellectual content.

REFERENCES

1. Mitchell SC, Korones SB, Berendes HW. Congenital heart disease in 56,109 births: incidence and natural history. *Circulation.* (1971) 43:323–32. doi: 10.1161/01.CIR.43.3.323
2. Sathanandam S, Whiting S, Cunningham J, Zurakowski D, Apalodimas L, Waller BR, et al. Practice variation in the management of patent ductus arteriosus in extremely low birth weight infants in the United States: survey results among cardiologists and neonatologists. *Congenit Heart Dis.* (2019) 14:6–14. doi: 10.1111/chd.12729
3. Bose CL, Laughon M. Treatment to prevent patency of the ductus arteriosus: beneficial or harmful? *J Pediatr.* (2006) 148:713–4. doi: 10.1016/j.jpeds.2006.03.015
4. Benitz WE. Committee of the fetus and newborn. Patent ductus arteriosus in preterm infants. *Pediatrics.* (2016) 137:e20153730. doi: 10.1542/peds.2015-3730
5. Noori S, McCoy M, Friedlich P, Bright B, Gottipati V, Seri I, et al. Failure of ductus arteriosus closure is associated with increased mortality in preterm infants. *Pediatrics.* (2009) 123:e138– 44. doi: 10.1542/peds.2008-2418
6. Hamrick SE, Hansmann G. Patent ductus arteriosus of the pre- term infant. *Pediatrics.* (2010) 125:1020–30. doi: 10.1542/peds.2009-3506
7. Dollberg S, Lusky A, Reichman B. Patent ductus arteriosus, indomethacin and necrotizing enterocolitis in very low birth weight infants: a population-based study. *J Pediatr Gastroenterol Nutr.* (2005) 40:184–8. doi: 10.1097/00005176-200502000-00019
8. El-Khuffash A, Levy PT, Gorenflo M, Frantz ID. The definition of a hemodynamically significant ductus arteriosus. *Pediatr Res.* (2019) 85:740–1. doi: 10.1038/s41390-019-0342-7
9. Bischoff AR, Giesinger RE, Bell EF, McNamara PJ. Precision medicine in neonatal hemodynamics: need for prioritization of mechanism of illness and defining population of interest. *J Perinatol.* (2020) 40:1446–9. doi: 10.1038/s41372-020-0741-y

10. Clyman R, Cassady G, Kirklin JK, Collins M, Philips JB III. The role of patent ductus arteriosus ligation in bronchopulmonary dysplasia: reexamining a randomized controlled trial. *J Pediatr.* (2009) 154:873–6. doi: 10.1016/j.jpeds.2009.01.005
11. Sung SI, Chang YS, Chun JY, Yoon SA, Yoo HS, Ahn SY et al. Mandatory closure versus nonintervention for patent ductus arteriosus in very preterm infants. *J Pediatr.* (2016) 177:66–71. doi: 10.1016/j.jpeds.2016.06.046
12. El-Mashad AE, El-Mahdy H, El Amrousy D, Elgendy M. Comparative study of the efficacy and safety of paracetamol, ibuprofen, and indomethacin in closure of patent ductus arteriosus in preterm neonates. *Eur J Pediatr.* (2017) 176:233–40. doi: 10.1007/s00431-016-2830-7
13. Whiting S, Sathanandam S. Patent ductus arteriosus in extremely low birth weight infants - if, when and how to close it? In: Barría RM, editor. *Neonatal Intensive Care Unit.* Croatia: IntechOpen (2020). Available online at: https://www.intechopen.com/books/update-on-critical-issues-on-infant-and-neonatal-care/pda-closure-in-elbw-infants-if-when-and-how-to-do-it
14. Gross RE, Hubbard JP. Surgical ligation of a patent ductus arteriosus: a report of first successful case. *JAMA.* (1939) 112:729–31. doi: 10.1001/jama.1939.02800080049011
15. Krichenko A, Benson LN, Burrows P, Moes CA, McLaughlin P, Freedom RM. Angiographic classification of the isolated, persistently patent ductus arteriosus and implications for percutaneous catheter occlusion. *Am J Cardiol.* (1989) 63:877–80. doi: 10.1016/0002-9149(89)90064-7
16. Merritt TA, DiSessa TG, Feldman BH, Kirtkpatrick SE, Gluck L, Friedman WF. Closure of the patent ductus arteriosus with ligation and indomethacin: a consecutive experience. *J Pediatr.* (1978) 93:639–46. doi: 10.1016/S0022-3476(78)80909-3
17. Philip R, Waller BR 3rd, Agrawal V, Wright D, Arevalo A, Zurakowski D, et al. Morphologic characterization of the patent ductus arteriosus in the premature infant and the choice of transcatheter occlusion device. *Catheter Cardiovasc Interv.* (2016) 87:310–17. doi: 10.1002/ccd.26287
18. Congdon ED. Transformation of the aortic arch system during the development of the human embryo. *Contributions to Embryology.* (1922) 14:47–110.
19. Philip R, Johnson JN, Naik R, Kimura D, Boston U, Chilakala S, et al. Effect of patent ductus arteriosus on pulmonary vascular disease. *Congenit Heart Dis.* (2019) 14:37–41. doi: 10.1111/chd.12702
20. Schneider DJ, Moore JW. Patent ductus arteriosus. *Circulation.* (2006) 114:1873–82. doi: 10.1161/CIRCULATIONAHA.105.592063
21. Leal SD, Cavalle-Garrido T, Ryan G, Farine D, Helibut M, Smallhorn JF. Isolated ductal closure in utero diagnosed by fetal echocardiography. *Am J Perinatol.* (1997) 14:205–10. doi: 10.1055/s-2007-994128
22. Gittenberger-de Groot AC, Moulaert AJ, Harinck E, Becker AE. Histopathology of the ductus arteriosus after prostaglandin E1 administration in ductus dependent cardiac anomalies. *Br Heart J.* (1978) 40:215–20. doi: 10.1136/hrt.40.3.215
23. Reese J. Towards a greater understanding of the ductus arteriosus. *Semin Perinatol.* (2018) 42:199–202. doi: 10.1053/j.semperi.2018.05.001
24. Fay FS, Kooke PH. Guinea pig ductus arteriosus, II: irreversible closure after birth. *Am J Physiol.* (1972) 222:841– 9. doi: 10.1152/ajplegacy.1972.222.4.841
25. Sallmon H, Aydin T, Hort S, Kubinski A, Bode C, Klippstein T, et al. Vascular endothelial growth factor polymorphism rs2010963 status does not affect patent ductus arteriosus incidence or cyclooxygenase inhibitor treatment success in preterm infants. *Cardiol Young* (2019) 29:893–7. doi: 10.1017/S1047951119001033
26. Ovali F. Molecular and mechanical mechanisms regulating ductus arteriosus closure in preterm infants. *Front Pediatr.* (2020) 8:516. doi: 10.3389/fped.2020.00516
27. van Vonderen JJ, te Pas AB, Kolster-Bijdevaate C, van Lith JM, Blom NA, Hooper SB, et al. Non-invasive measurements of ductus arteriosus flow directly after birth. *Arch Dis Child Fetal Nenatal Ed.* (2014) 99:F408–12. doi: 10.1136/archdischild-2014-306033
28. Clyman RI, Couto J, Murphy GM. Patent ductus arteriosus: are current neonatal treatment options better or worse than no treatment at all?. *Semin Perinatol.* (2012) 36:123–9. doi: 10.1053/j.semperi.2011.09.022
29. Weinberg JG, Evans FJ, Burns KM, Pearson GD, Kaltman JR. Surgical ligation of patent ductus arteriosus in premature infants: trends and practice variation. *Cardiol Young.* (2016). 26:1107–14. doi: 10.1017/S1047951115001869
30. Heuchan AM, Clyman RI. Managing the patent ductus arteriosus: current treatment options. *Arch Dis Child Fetal Neonatal Ed.* (2014) 99:F431–6. doi: 10.1136/archdischild-2014-306176
31. Rolland A, Shankar-Aguilera S, Diomande D, Zupan-Simunek V, Boileau P. Natural evolution of patent ductus arteriosus in the extremely preterm infant. *Arch Dis Child Fetal Neonatal Ed.* (2015) 100:F55–8. doi: 10.1136/archdischild-2014-306339
32. Weber SC, Weiss K, Bührer C, Hansmann G, Koehne P, Sallmon H. Natural history of patent ductus arteriosus in very low birth weight infants after discharge. *J Pediatr.* (2015) 167:1149–51. doi: 10.1016/j.jpeds.2015.06.032
33. Kitterman JA, Edmunds LH Jr, Gregory GA, Heyman MA, Tooley WH, Rudolph AM. Patent ductus arteriosus in premature infants: incidence, relation to pulmonary disease and management. *N Engl J Med.* (1972) 287:473–7. doi: 10.1056/NEJM197209072871001
34. Tomita H, Fuse S, Hatakeyama K, Chiba S. Epinephrine-induced constriction of the persistent ductus arteriosus and its relation to distensibility. *Jpn Circ J.* (1998) 62:913–4. doi: 10.1253/jcj.62.913
35. Philip R, Towbin JA, Sathanandam S, Goldberg J, Yohannan T, Swaminathan N, et al. Effect of patent ductus arteriosus on the heart in preterm infants. *Congenit Heart Dis.* (2019) 14:33–6. doi: 10.1111/chd.12701
36. Kahvecioglu D, Erdeve O, Akduman H, Ucar T, Alan S, akir U, et al. Influence of platelet count, platelet mass index, and platelet function on the spontaneous closure of ductus arteriosus in the prematurity. *Pediatr Neonatol.* (2018) 59:53–7. doi: 10.1016/j.pedneo.2017.01.006
37. Alyamac Dizdar E, Ozdemir R, Sari FN, Yurttutan S, Gokmen T, Erdeve O, et al. Low platelet count is associated with ductus arteriosus patency in preterm newborns. *Early Hum Dev.* (2012) 88:813–6. doi: 10.1016/j.earlhumdev.2012.05.007
38. Sallmon H, Metze B, Koehne P, Opgen-Rhein B, Weiss K, Will JC, et al. Mature and immature platelets during the first week after birth and incidence of patent ductus arteriosus. *Cardiol Young.* (2020) 30:769–73. doi: 10.1017/S1047951120000943
39. Mirza H, Garcia J, McKinley G, Hubbard L, Sensing W, Schneider J, et al. Duration of significant patent ductus arteriosus and bronchopulmonary dysplasia in extremely preterm infants. *J Perinatol.* (2019) 39:1648–55. doi: 10.1038/s41372-019-0496-5
40. Philip R, Waller B, Chilakala S, Graham B, Stecchi N, Apalodimas L, et al. Hemodynamic and clinical consequences of early versus delayed closure of patent ductus arteriosus in extremely low birth weight infants. *J Perinatol.* (2020) doi: 10.1038/s41372-020-00772-2
41. deWaal K, Phad N, Collins N, Boyle A. Cardiac remodeling in preterm infants with prolonged exposure to a patent ductus arteriosus. *Congenit Heart Dis.* (2017) 12:364–72. doi: 10.1111/chd.12454
42. Brown ER. Increased risk of bronchopulmonary dysplasia in infants with patent ductus arteriosus. *J Pediatr.* (1979) 95:865–6. doi: 10.1016/S0022-3476(79)80454-0
43. Lipman B, Serwer GA, Brazy JE. Abnormal cerebral hemodynamics in preterm infants with patent ductus arteriosus. *Pediatrics.* (1982) 69:778–81.
44. Tomaszewska M, Stork E, Minich NM, Friedman H, Berlin S, Hack M. Pulmonary hemorrhage: clinical course and outcomes among very low-birth-weight infants. *Arch Pediatr Adolesc Med.* (1999)153:715–721. doi: 10.1001/archpedi.153.7.715
45. Deshpande P, Baczynski M, McNamara PJ, Jain A. Patent ductus arteriosus: the physiology of transition. *Semin Fetal Neonatal Med.* (2018) 23:225–31. doi: 10.1016/j.siny.2018.05.001
46. Benitz WE. Treatment of persistent patent ductus arteriosus in preterm infants: time to accept the null hypothesis? *J Perinatol.* (2010) 30:241–52. doi: 10.1038/jp.2010.3
47. Moodie DS, Sathanandam S, Qureshi AM. Proceedings of the International PDA symposium. *Congenit Heart Dis.* (2019) 14:5–5. doi: 10.1111/chd.12761
48. Thébaud B, Lacaze-Mazmonteil T. Patent ductus arteriosus in premature infants: a never-closing act. *Paediatr Child Health.* (2010) 15:267–70. doi: 10.1093/pch/15.5.267

49. McNamara PJ, Sehgal A. Towards rational management of the patent ductus arteriosus: the need for disease staging. *Arch Dis Child Fetal Neonatal Ed.* (2007) 92:F424–7. doi: 10.1136/adc.2007.118117
50. Chock VY, Punn R, Oza A, Benitz WE, Van Meurs KP, Whittemore AS, et al. Predictors of bronchopulmonary dysplasia or death in premature infants with a patent ductus arteriosus. *Pediatr Res.* (2014) 75:570–85. doi: 10.1038/pr.2013.253
51. Mahony L, Carnero V, Brett C, Heymann MA, Clyman RI. Prophylactic indomethacin therapy for patent ductus arteriosus in very-low-birth-weight infants. *N Engl J Med.* (1982) 306:506–10. doi: 10.1056/NEJM198203043060903
52. Kluckow M, Jeffery M, Gill A, Evans N. A randomized placebo-controlled trial of early treatment of the patent ductus arteriosus. *Arch Dis Child Fetal Neonatal Ed.* (2014) 99:F99–F104. doi: 10.1136/archdischild-2013-304695
53. Abdel-Hady H, Nasef N, Shabaan AE, Nour I. Patent ductus arteriosus in preterm infants: do we have the right answers? *BioMed Res Int.* (2013) 2013:676192. doi: 10.1155/2013/676192
54. Jain A, Shah PS. Diagnosis, evaluation, and management of patent ductus arteriosus in preterm neonates. *JAMA Pediatr.* (2015) 169:863–872. doi: 10.1001/jamapediatrics.2015.0987
55. Van Laere D, van Overmeire B, Gupta S, El-Khuffash A, Savoia M, McNamara PJ, et al. Application of neonatologist performed echocardiography in the assessment of a patent ductus arteriosus. *Pediatr Res.* (2018) 84:46–56. doi: 10.1038/s41390-018-0077-x
56. Paudel G, Joshi V. Echocardiography of the patent ductus arteriosus in premature infant. *Congenit Heart Dis.* (2019) 14:42–5. doi: 10.1111/chd.12703
57. Shepherd JL, Noori S. What is a hemodynamically significant PDA in preterm infants? *Congenit Heart Dis.* (2019) 14:21–6. doi: 10.1111/chd.12727
58. Sehgal A, Menahem S. Interparametric correlation between echocardiographic markers in preterm infants with patent ductus arteriosus. *Pediatr Cardiol.* (2013) 34:1212–7. doi: 10.1007/s00246-013-0640-5
59. Arlettaz R. Echocardiographic evaluation of patent ductus arteriosus in preterm infants. *Front Pediatr.* (2017) 5:147. doi: 10.3389/fped.2017.00147.eCollection 2017
60. Sehgal A, McNamara PJ. Does echocardiography facilitate determination of hemodynamic significance attributable to the ductus arteriosus? *Eur J Pediatr.* (2009) 168:907–14. doi: 10.1007/s00431-009-0983-3
61. El Hajjar M, Vaksmann G, Rakza T, Kongolo G, Storme L. Severity of the ductal shunt: a comparison of different markers. *Arch Dis Child Fetal Neonatal Ed.* (2005) 90:F419–22. doi: 10.1136/adc.2003.027698
62. Polat TB, Celik IH, Erdeve O. Early predictive echocardiographic features of hemodynamically significant patent ductus arteriosus in preterm VLBW infants. *Pediatr Int.* (2016) 58:589–94. doi: 10.1111/ped.12915
63. Kulkarni M, Gokulakrishnan G, Price J, Fernandes CJ, Leeflang M, Pammi M. Diagnosing significant PDA using natriuretic peptides in preterm neonates: a systematic review. *Pediatrics.* (2015) 135:e510–25. doi: 10.1542/peds.2014-1995
64. El-Khuffash AF, Molloy EJ. Influence of a patent ductus arteriosus on cardiac troponin T levels in preterm infants. *J Pediatr.* (2008) 153:350–3. doi: 10.1016/j.jpeds.2008.04.014
65. Slaughter JL, Cua CL, Notestine JL, Rivera BK, Marzec L, Hade EM, et al. Early prediction of spontaneous Patent Ductus Arteriosus (PDA) closure and PDA-associated outcomes: a prospective cohort investigation. *BMC Pediatr.* (2019) 19:333. doi: 10.1186/s12887-019-1708-z
66. Celik IH, Erdeve O, Demirel G, Canpolat FE, Dilmen U. Elevated urinary NT-proBNP after pharmacological closure of patent ductus arteriosus in very low birth weight infants. *Early Hum Dev.* (2013) 89:187–9. doi: 10.1016/j.earlhumdev.2012.09.020
67. Alan S, Karadeniz C, Okulu E, Kilic A, Erdeve O, Ucar T, et al. Management of patent ductus arteriosus in preterm infants: clinical judgment might be a fair option. *J Maternal-Fetal Neonatal Med.* (2013) 26:1850–4. doi: 10.3109/14767058.2013.801956
68. Clyman RI, Saha S, Jobe A, Oh W. Indomethacin prophylaxis for preterm infants: the impact of 2 multicentered randomized controlled trials on clinical practice. *J Pediatr.* (2007) 150:46–50. doi: 10.1016/j.jpeds.2006.09.001
69. Benitz WE, Bhombal S. The use of non-steroidal anti-inflammatory drugs for patent ductus arteriosus closure in preterm infants. *Semin Fetal Neonatal Med.* (2017) 22:302–7. doi: 10.1016/j.siny.2017.07.004
70. EL-Khuffash A,Weisz DE, McNamara PJ. Reflections of the changes in patent ductus arteriosus management during the last 10 years. *Arch Dis Child Fetal Neonatal Ed.* (2016) 101:F474–78. doi: 10.1136/archdischild-2014-306214
71. Fowlie PW, Davis PG, McGuire W. Prophylactic intravenous indomethacin for preventing mortality and morbidity in preterm infants. *Cochrane Database Syst Rev.* (2010) CD000174. doi: 10.1002/14651858.CD000174.pub2
72. Schmidt B, Asztalos EV, Roberts RS, Robertson CM, Sauve RS, Whitfield MF. Impact of bronchopulmonary dysplasia, brain injury, and severe retinopathy on the outcome of extremely low-birth-weight infants at 18 months: results from the trial of indomethacin prophylaxis in preterms. *JAMA.* (2003) 289:1124–9. doi: 10.1001/jama.289.9.1124
73. Ment LR, Vohr B, Allan W, Westerveld M, Sparrow SS, Schneider KC, et al. Outcome of children in the indomethacin intraventricular hemorrhage prevention trial. *Pediatrics.* (2000) 105:485–91. doi: 10.1542/peds.105.3.485
74. Clyman RI, Liebowitz M, Kaempf J, Erdeve O, Bulbul A, Håkansson S, et al. PDA-TOLERATE trial: an exploratory randomized controlled trial of treatment of moderate-to-large patent ductus arteriosus at 1 week of age. *J. Pediatr.* (2019) 205:41–8.e6. doi: 10.1016/j.jpeds.2018.09.012
75. Okulu E, Erdeve O, Arslan Z, Demirel N, Kaya H, Kursad I, et al. An Observational, prospective, multicenter, registry-based cohort study comparing conservative and medical management for patent ductus arteriosus. *Front Pediatr.* (2020) 8:434. doi: 10.3389/fped.2020.00434
76. Liebowitz M, Kaempf J, Erdeve O, Bulbul A, Håkansson S, Lindqvist J, et al. Comparative effectiveness of drugs used to constrict the patent ductus arteriosus: a secondary analysis of the PDA-TOLERATE trial (NCT01958320). *J Perinatol.* (2019) 39:599–607. doi: 10.1038/s41372-019-0347-4
77. Cassady G, Crouse DT, Kirklin JW, Strange MJ, Joiner CH, Godoy G, et al. A randomized, controlled trial of very early prophylactic ligation of the ductus arteriosus in babies who weighed 1000 g or less at birth. *N Engl J Med.* (1989) 320:1511–6. doi: 10.1056/NEJM198906083202302
78. Mikhail M, Lee W, Toews W, Synhorst DP, Hawes CR, Hernandez J, et al. Surgical and medical experience with 734 premature infants with patient ductus arteriosus. *J Thorac Cardiovasc Surg.* (1982) 83:349–57. doi: 10.1016/S0022-5223(19)37268-X
79. El-Khuffash AF, Jain A, McNamara PJ. Ligation of the patent ductus arteriosus in preterm infants: understanding the physiology. *J Pediatr.* (2013) 162:1100–6. doi: 10.1016/j.jpeds.2012.12.094
80. US Food and Drug Administration (FDA). *Sterile Indocin1 I.V. (Indomethacin for Injection). FDA Label.* (2009). (2014). Available online at: http://www.accessdata.fda.gov/drugsatfda_docs/label/2010/018878s027lbl.pdf (accessed November 6, 2014).
81. US Food and Drug Administration (FDA). *NeoProfen1 (ibuprofen lysine) Injection. NDA 21-903; Approval Letter.* April (2006). Available online at: http://www.accessdata.fda.gov/drugsatfda_docs/label/2006/021903lbl.pdf (accessed November 7, 2014).
82. Ohlsson A, Walia R, Shah SS. Ibuprofen for the treatment of patent ductus arteriosus in preterm or low birth weight (or both) infants. *Cochrane Database Syst Rev.* (2015) CD003481. doi: 10.1002/14651858.CD003481.pub6
83. van Overmeire B, Touw D, Schepens PJ, Kearns GL, van den Anker JN. Ibuprofen pharmacokinetics in preterm infants with patent ductus arteriosus. *Clin Pharmacol Ther.* (2001) 70:336–43. doi: 10.1067/mcp.2001.118453
84. Hirt D, van Overmeire B, Treluyer JM, Langhendries JP, Marguglio A, Eisinger MJ, et al. An optimized ibuprofen dosing scheme for preterm neonates with patent ductus arteriosus, based on a population pharmacokinetic and pharmacodynamic study. *Br J Clin Pharmacol.* (2008) 65:629–36. doi: 10.1111/j.1365-2125.2008.03118.x
85. Desfrere L, Zohar S, Morville P, Brunhes A, Chevret S, Pons G, Moriette G, Rey E, Treluyer JM. Dose-finding study of ibuprofen in patent ductus arteriosus using the continual reassessment method. *J Clin Pharm Ther.* (2005) 30:121–32. doi: 10.1111/j.1365-2710.2005.00630.x

86. Mitra, S, Florez ID, Tamayo ME. Association of placebo, indomethacin, ibuprofen, and acetaminophen with closure of hemodynamically significant patent ductus arteriosus in preterm infantsA systematic review and meta-analysis. *JAMA.* (2018) 319:1221–38. doi: 10.1001/jama.2018.1896
87. Kanmaz G, Erdeve O, Canpolat FE, Oguz SS, Uras N, Altug N, et al. Serum ibuprofen levels of extremely preterm infants treated prophylactically with oral ibuprofen to prevent patent ductus arteriosus. *Eur J Clin Pharmacol.* (2013) 69:1075201381. doi: 10.1007/s00228-012-1438-8
88. Yurttutan S, Oncel MY, Dilmen U, Erdeve O, Ozdemir R. The relationship between trough drug concentrations and ductal closure in preterm infants treated with three-dose-oral ibuprofen. *J Matern Fetal Neonatal Med.* (2013) 26:1306–10. doi: 10.3109/14767058.2013.784739
89. Pacifici GM. *Clinical Pharmacology of Ibuprofen in Preterm Infants: A Meta-Analysis of Published Data.* Available online at: http://www.gnresearch.org/doi/10.5935/MedicalExpress.2014.02.02 (accessed September 30, 2016).
90. Erdeve O, Yurttutan S, Altug N, Ozdemir R, Gokmen T, Dilmen U, et al. Oral versus intravenous ibuprofen for patent ductus arteriosus closure: a randomised controlled trial in extremely low birthweight infants. *Arch Dis Child Fetal Neonatal Ed.* (2012) 97:F279–83. doi: 10.1136/archdischild-2011-300532
91. Gokmen T, Erdeve O, Altug N, Oguz SS, Uras N, Dilmen U. Efficacy and safety of oral versus intravenous ibuprofen in very low birth weight preterm infants with patent ductus arteriosus. *J Pediatr.* (2011) 158:549–54.e1. doi: 10.1016/j.jpeds.2010.10.008
92. Eras Z, Gokmen T, Erdeve O, Ozyurt BM, Saridas B, Dilmen U. Impact of oral versus intravenous ibuprofen on neurodevelopmental outcome: a randomized controlled parallel study. *Am J Perinatol.* (2013) 30:857–62. doi: 10.1055/s-0033-1333667
93. Pezzati M, Vangi V, Biagiotti R, Bertini G, Cianciulli D, Rubaltelli FF. Effects of indomethacin and ibuprofen on mesenteric and renal blood flow in preterm infants with patent ductus arteriosus. *J Pediatr.* (1999) 135:733–8. doi: 10.1016/S0022-3476(99)70093-4
94. Patel J, Roberts I, Azzopardi D, Hamilton P, Edwards AD. Randomized double-blind controlled trial comparing the effects of ibuprofen with indomethacin on cerebral hemodynamics in preterm infants with patent ductus arteriosus. *Pediatr Res.* (2000) 47:36–42. doi: 10.1203/00006450-200001000-00009
95. Guzoglu N, Sari FN, Ozdemir R, Oguz SS, Uras N, Altug N, et al. Renal and mesenteric tissue oxygenation in preterm infants treated with oral ibuprofen. *J Matern Fetal Neonatal Med.* (2014) 27:197–203. doi: 10.3109/14767058.2013.811485
96. Van Bel F, Van Zwieten PH, Den Ouden LL. Contribution of color Doppler flow imaging to the evaluation of the effect of indomethacin on neonatal cerebral hemodynamics. *J Ultrasound Med.* (1990) 9:107–9. doi: 10.7863/jum.1990.9.2.107
97. Van Bel F, Van Zoeren D, Schipper J, Guit GL, Baan J. Effect of indomethacin on superior mesenteric artery blood flow velocity in preterm infants. *J Pediatr.* (1990) 116:965–70. doi: 10.1016/S0022-3476(05)80662-6
98. Clyman R, Wickremasinghe A, Jhaveri N, Hassinger DC, Attridge JT, Sanocka U, et al. Enteral feeding during indomethacin and ibuprofen treatment of a patent ductus arteriosus. *J Pediatr.* (2013) 163:406–11. doi: 10.1016/j.jpeds.2013.01.057
99. Yanowitz TD, Reese J, Gillam-Krakauer M, Cochran CM, Jegatheesan P, Lau J, et al. Superior mesenteric artery blood flow velocities following medical treatment of a patent ductus arteriosus. *J Pediatr.* (2014) 164:661–3. doi: 10.1016/j.jpeds.2013.11.002
100. Ferguson, JM. Pharmacotherapy for patent ductus arteriosus closure. *Congenit Heart Dis.* (2019) 14:52–6. doi: 10.1111/chd.12715
101. Oncel MY, Yurttutan S, Erdeve O, Uras N, Altug N, Oguz SS, et al. Oral paracetamol versus oral ibuprofen in the management of patent ductus arteriosus in preterm infants: a randomized controlled trial. *J Pediatr.* (2014) 164:510–4.e1. doi: 10.1016/j.jpeds.2013.11.008
102. Ohlsson A, Shah PS. Paracetamol (acetaminophen) for patent ductus arteriosus in preterm or low-birth-weight infants. *Cochrane Database Syst Rev.* (2015) CD010061. doi: 10.1002/14651858.CD010061.pub2
103. Yurttutan S, Oncel MY, Arayici S, Uras N, Altug N, Erdeve O, et al. A different first-choice drug in the medical management of patent ductus arteriosus: oral paracetamol. *J Matern Fetal Neonatal Med.* (2013) 26:825–7. doi: 10.3109/14767058.2012.755162
104. Oncel MY, Erdeve O. Oral medications regarding their safety and efficacy in the management of patent ductus arteriosus. *World J Clin Pediatr.* (2016). 5:75–81. doi: 10.5409/wjcp.v5.i1.75
105. Oncel MY, Erdeve O. Safety of therapeutics used in management of patent ductus arteriosus in preterm infants. *Curr Drug Saf.* (2015) 10:106–112. doi: 10.2174/1574886309999141030142847
106. Terrin G, Conte F, Oncel MY, Scipione A, McNamara PJ, Simons S, et al. Paracetamol for the treatment of patent ductus arteriosus in preterm neonates: a systematic review and meta-analysis. *Arch Dis Child Fetal Neonatal Ed.* (2016). 101:F127–36. doi: 10.1136/archdischild-2014-307312
107. Davidson JM, Ferguson J, Ivey E, Philip R, Weems MF, Talati AJ. A randomized trial of intravenous acetaminophen versus indomethacin for treatment of hemodynamically significant PDAs in VLBW infants. *J Perinatol.* (2020). doi: 10.1038/s41372-020-0694-1
108. Oncel MY, Eras Z, Uras N, Canpolat FE, Erdeve O, Oguz SS. Neurodevelopmental outcomes of preterm infants treated with oral paracetamol versus ibuprofen for patent ductus arteriosus. *Am J Perinatol.* (2017) 34:1185–9. doi: 10.1055/s-0037-1601564
109. Yurttutan S, Bozkaya A, Hüdayioglu F, Oncel MY. The effect of combined therapy for treatment of monotherapy-resistant PDA in preterm infants. *J Matern Fetal Neonatal Med.* (2019) 32:3662–5. doi: 10.1080/14767058.2018.1481043
110. Hochwald O, Mainzer G, Borenstein-Levin L, Jubran H, Dinur G, Zucker M, et al. Adding paracetamol to Ibuprofen for the treatment of patent ductus arteriosus in preterm infants: a double-blind, randomized, placebo-controlled pilot study. *Am J Perinatol.* (2018) 35:1319–25. doi: 10.1055/s-0038-1653946
111. Cotton RB, Stahlman MT, Bender HW, Graham TP, Catterton WZ, Kovar I. Randomized trial of early closure of symptomatic patent ductus arteriosus in small preterm infants. *J Pediatr.* (1978) 93:647–51.
112. Raval MV, Laughon MM, Bose CL, Phillips JD. Patent ductus arteriosus ligation in premature infants: who really benefits, and at what cost? *J Pediatr Surg.* (2007) 42:69–75. doi: 10.1016/j.jpedsurg.2006.09.040
113. Madan JC, Kendrick D, Hagadorn JI, Frantz ID 3rd. Patent ductus arteriosus therapy: impact on neonatal and 18-month outcome. *Pediatrics.* (2009) 123:674–81. doi: 10.1542/peds.2007-2781
114. Mirea L, Sankaran K, Seshia M, Ohlsson A, Allen AC, Aziz K, et al. Treatment of patent ductus arteriosus and neonatal mortality/morbidities: adjustment for treatment selection bias. *J Pediatr.* (2012) 161:689–94. doi: 10.1016/j.jpeds.2012.05.007
115. Janz-Robinson EM, Badawi N, Walker K, Bajuk B, Abdel-Latif ME. Neonatal intensive care units network. Neurodevelopmental outcomes of premature infants treated for patent ductus arteriosus: a population-based cohort study. *J Pediatr.* (2015) 167:1025–32.
116. Weisz DE, More K, McNamara PJ, Shah PS. PDA ligation and health outcomes: a meta-analysis. *Pediatrics.* (2014) 133:e1024–46. doi: 10.1542/peds.2013-3431
117. Benjamin JR, Smith PB, Cotten CM, Jaggers J, Goldstein RF, Malcolm WF. Long-term morbidities associated with vocal cord paralysis after surgical closure of a patent ductus arteriosus in extremely low birth weight infants. *J Perinatol.* (2010) 30:408–13. doi: 10.1038/jp.2009.124
118. Chen H, Weng G, Chen Z, Wang H, Xie Q, Bao J, et al. Comparison of posterolateral thoracotomy and video-assisted thoracoscopic clipping for the treatment of patent ductus arteriosus in neonates and infants. *Pediatr Cardiol.* (2011) 32:386–90. doi: 10.1007/s00246-010-9863-x
119. Clement WA, El-Hakim H, Phillipos EZ, Cote JJ. Unilateral vocal cord paralysis following patent ductus arteriosus ligation in extremely low-birth-weight in- fants. *Arch Otolaryngol Head Neck Surg.* (2008) 134:28–33. doi: 10.1001/archoto.2007.2
120. Hsu KH, Chiang MC, Lien R, Chu JJ, Chang YS, Chu SM, et al. Diaphragmatic paralysis among very low birth weight infants following ligation for patent ductus arteriosus. *Eur J Pediatr.* (2012) 171:1639–44. doi: 10.1007/s00431-012-1787-4
121. Mandhan P, Brown S, Kukkady A, Samarakkody U. Surgical closure of patent ductus arteriosus in preterm low birth weight infants. *Congenit Heart Dis.* (2009) 4:34–7. doi: 10.1111/j.1747-0803.2008.00241.x

122. Smith ME, King JD, Elsherif A, Muntz HR, Park AH, Kouretas PC. Should all newborns who undergo patent ductus arteriosus ligation be examined for vocal fold mobility? *Laryngoscope.* (2009) 119:1606–9. doi: 10.1002/lary.20148
123. Spanos WC, Brookes JT, Smith MC, Burkhart HM, Bell EF, Smith RJ. Unilateral vocal fold paralysis in premature infants after ligation of patent ductus arteriosus: vascular clip versus suture ligature. *Ann Otol Rhinol Laryngol.* (2009) 118:750–3. doi: 10.1177/000348940911801011
124. Baruteau AE, Hascoët S, Baruteau J, Boudjemline Y, Lambert V, Angel CY, et al. Transcatheter closure of patent ductus arteriosus: past, present and future. *Arch Cardiovasc Dis.* (2014) 107:122–32. doi: 10.1016/j.acvd.2014.01.008
125. Backes CH, Rivera BK, Bridge JA, Armstrong AK, Boe BA, Berman DP, et al. Percutaneous patent ductus arteriosus (PDA) closure during infancy: a meta-analysis. *Pediatrics.* (2017) 139:e20162927. doi: 10.1542/peds.2016-2927
126. Zahn EM, Peck D, Phillips A, Nevin P, Basaker K, Simmons C, et al. Transcatheter closure of patent ductus arteriosus in extremely premature newborns: early results and midterm follow-up. *JACC Cardiovasc Interv.* (2016) 9:2429–37. doi: 10.1016/j.jcin.2016.09.019
127. Sathanandam S, Balduf K, Chilakala S, Washington K, Allen K, Knott-Craig C, et al. Role of transcatheter patent ductus arteriosus closure in extremely low birth weight infants. *Catheter Cardiovasc Interv.* (2019) 93:89–6. doi: 10.1002/ccd.27808
128. Agrawal H, Parkerson S, Lighter D, Fowke J, Goedecke P, Towbin J, et al. Transcatheter closure of PDA compared to surgical ligation in premature neonates: clinical outcomes and cost comparison. *Catheter Cardiovasc Interv.* (2020) 95:1–229. doi: 10.12669/pjms.324.10048
129. Willis A, Pereiras L, Head T, Dupuis G, Sessums J, Corder G, et al. Transport of extremely low birth weight neonates for persistent ductus arteriosus closure in the catheterization lab. *Congenit Heart Dis.* (2019) 14:69–73. doi: 10.1111/chd.12706
130. Tadphale S, Yohannan T, Kauffmann T, Maller V, Agrawal V, Lloyd H, et al. Accessing femoral arteries less than 3 mm in diameter is associated with increased incidence of loss of pulse following cardiac catheterization in infants. *Pediatr Cardiol.* (2020) 41:1058–66. doi: 10.1007/s00246-020-02357-4
131. Alexander J, Yohannan T, Abutineh I, Agrawal V, Lloyd H, Zurakowski D, et al. Ultrasound-guided femoral arterial access in pediatric cardiac catheterizations: a prospective evaluation of the prevalence, risk factors, and mechanism for acute loss of arterial pulse. *Catheter Cardiovasc Interv.* (2016) 88:1098–107. doi: 10.1002/ccd.26702
132. Tadphale SD, Zurakowski D, Bird LE, Yohannan TM, Agrawal VK, Lloyd H, et al. Construction of femoral vessel nomograms for planning cardiac interventional procedures in children 0-4 years old. *Pediatr Cardiol.* (2020) 41:1135–44. doi: 10.1007/s00246-020-02363-6
133. Sathanandam S, Agrawal H, Chilakala S, Johnson J, Allen K, Knott-Craig C, et al. Can transcatheter PDA closure be performed in neonates ≤1,000 grams? The Memphis experience. *Congenit Heart Dis.* (2019) 14:79–84. doi: 10.1111/chd.12700
134. Sathanandam S, Justino H, Waller BR 3rd, Radke W, Qureshi A. Initial clinical experience with the medtronic micro vascular plug^{TM} in transcatheter occlusion of PDAs in extremely premature infants. *Catheter Cardiovasc Interv.* (2017) 89:1051–8. doi: 10.1002/ccd.26878
135. Johnson JN, Sathanandam S, Naik R, Philip R. Echocardiographic guidance for transcatheter patent ductus arteriosus closure in extremely low birth weight infants. *Congenit Heart Dis.* (2019) 14:74–8. doi: 10.1111/chd.12725
136. Sathanandam S, Gianinni A, Sefton E, Greer K, Stecchi N, Allen K, et al. Live broadcast of transcatheter PDA closure in a 700 grams ELBW infant during the international PDA symposium. *Congenit Heart Dis.* (2019) 14:85–9. doi: 10.1111/chd.12710
137. Agrawal H, Waller BR, Surendan S, Sathanandam S. New patent ductus arteriosus closure devices and techniques. *Interv Cardiol Clin.* (2019) 8:23–32. doi: 10.1016/j.iccl.2018.08.004
138. Sathanandam SK, Gutfinger D, O'Brien L, Forbes TJ, Gillespie MJ, Berman DP, et al. Amplatzer Piccolo Occluder clinical trial for percutaneous closure of the patent ductus arteriosus in patients ≥700 grams. *Catheter Cardiovasc Interv.* (2020) 96:1266–76. doi: 10.1002/ccd.28973
139. Apalodimas L, Waller BR, Philip R, Crawford J, Cunningham J, Sathanandam S. A comprehensive program for preterm infants with patent ductus arteriosus. *Congenit Heart Dis.* (2019) 14:90–4. doi: 10.1111/chd.12705
140. Sathanandam S, Apalodimas L, Weems M, Rush Waller B, Philip R. Establishing a Robust Transcatheter PDA Closure Program for Extremely Low Birth Weight Infants. *Congenital Cardiology Today – March (2018). Issue featured article. ISSN 1554-7787; ISSN 1554-0499.*
141. Kimball TR, Ralston MA, Khoury P, Crump RG, Cho FS, Reuter JH. Effect of ligation of patent ductus arteriosus on left ventricular performance and its determinants in premature neonates. *J Am Coll Cardiol.* (1996) 27:193–7. doi: 10.1016/0735-1097(95)00452-1
142. Ulrich TJB, Hansen TP, Reid KJ, Bingler MA, Olsen SL. Post-ligation cardiac syndrome is associated with increased morbidity in preterm infants. *J Perinatol.* (2018) 38:537–42. doi: 10.1038/s41372-018-0056-4
143. McNamara PJ, Stewart L, Shivananda SP, Stephens D, Sehgal A. Patent ductus arteriosus ligation is associated with impaired left ventricular systolic performance in premature infants weighing less than 1000 g. *J Thorac Cardiovasc Surg.* (2010) 140:150–7. doi: 10.1016/j.jtcvs.2010.01.011
144. Philip R, Waller B, Chilakala S, Apalodimas L, Sathanandam S. Comparison of low cardiac output syndrome after PDA ligation and transcatheter PDA closure in extremely low birth weight infants. *J Am Coll Cardiol.* (2019) 73(9 Suppl.):575. doi: 10.1016/S0735-1097(19)31183-0
145. Serrano RM, Madison M, Lorant D, Hoyer M, Alexy R. Comparison of 'post-patent ductus arteriosus ligation syndrome' in premature infants after surgical ligation vs. percutaneous closure. *J Perinatol.* (2020) 40:324–9. doi: 10.1038/s41372-019-0513-8
146. Harvey E, Philip R, Waller B, Johnson J, Cunningham J, Chilakala S, et al. Scoring system for post ligation cardiac syndrome and its utility after transcatheter and surgical patent ductus arteriosus ligation in extremely low birthweight infants. *Circulation.* (2019) 140:A14799. Available online at: https://www.ahajournals.org/doi/abs/10.1161/circ.140.suppl_1.14799?af=R
147. Jain A, Sahni M, El-Khuffash A, Khadawardi E, Sehgal A, McNamara PJ. Use of targeted neonatal echocardiography to prevent postoperative cardiorespiratory instability after patent ductus arteriosus ligation. *J Pediatr.* (2012) 160:584–9. doi: 10.1016/j.jpeds.2011.09.027
148. Tailor N, Philip R, Harvey E, Dupuis G, Waller B, Stecchi N, et al. Effect of intravenous calcium administration during transcatheter PDA closure in ELBW infants. *Catheter Cardiovasc Interv.* (2020) 95:1–229. doi: 10.1002/ccd.28864

15

Echocardiography-Guided Management of Preterms with Patent Ductus Arteriosus Influences the Outcome

Gianluca Terrin, Maria Di Chiara, Giovanni Boscarino, Paolo Versacci, Violante Di Donato, Antonella Giancotti, Elisabetta Pacelli, Francesca Faccioli, Elisa Onestà, Chiara Corso, Alessandra Ticchiarelli and Mario De Curtis*

Department of Maternal and Child Health, University of Rome La Sapienza, Rome, Italy

***Correspondence:**
Gianluca Terrin
gianluca.terrin@uniroma1.it

Introduction: Echocardiography (ECHO) with color flow Doppler is considered as the gold standard to identify a hemodynamic patent ductus arteriosus (hs-PDA). However, the optimal diagnostic and therapeutic management for newborns with hs-PDA is still controversial. We aimed to investigate two clinical strategies: (1) targeted treatment based on ECHO criteria and (2) treatment based on ECHO criteria in addition to clinical signs and symptoms.

Materials and Methods: This is a cohort study including all neonates consecutively admitted in the Neonatal Intensive Care Unit of University La Sapienza in Rome, with gestational age <32 weeks or body birth weight <1,500 g and with a diagnosis of hs-PDA as confirmed by ECHO evaluation performed within 72 h of life. We classified the babies in two cohorts: (A) pharmacological treatment immediately after ECHO screening and (B) pharmacological therapy for PDA was administered when the relevance of a hs-PDA was associated with clinical signs of hemodynamic instability.

Results: We considered as primary outcome newborns who survived without any morbidities (A: 48.1% vs. B: 22.2%, $p = 0.022$). In particular, we found that the rate of intraventricular hemorrhage stage ≥2 was increased in cohort B (A: 3.7% vs. B 24.4%, $p = 0.020$). A multivariate analysis showed that assignment to cohort A independently influences the primary outcome.

Conclusions: Adopting an hs-PDA management option based on ECHO-directed therapy regardless of symptoms may reduce the morbidity and improve the survival of very low birth weight infants.

Keywords: newborn, morbidity, intraventricular hemorrhage (IVH), very low birth weight (VLBW), survival

INTRODUCTION

Patent ductus arteriosus (PDA) is essential for fetal life (1). Normally, the ductus arteriosus closes within a few days after birth. In preterm infants, the ductus fails to close, leading to a left heart volume overload and systemic hypoperfusion (2). The persistence of a PDA may increase the risk of intraventricular hemorrhage (IVH), necrotizing enterocolitis (NEC), and chronic lung disease (CLD) (1, 3).

There is no consensus regarding the optimal diagnostic approach of PDA. The 2D echocardiography (ECHO) with color flow Doppler is the gold standard to identify hemodynamically significant PDA (hs-PDA) (4, 5). Nevertheless, it remains to be clarified if the assessment of a hs-PDA at the ECHO is enough to establish an indication for a pharmacological therapeutic intervention or if symptoms should guide the decision to start therapy. If hs-PDA defined only by echocardiographic criteria may not produce significant clinical effects, in many cases, symptoms appear to manifest when the effects of hemodynamic instability already occurred. Pharmacological intervention (i.e., ibuprofen, indomethacin, paracetamol), the first therapeutic option to close PDA in preterm newborns, is associated with the occurrence of severe side effects. Furthermore, clinical evidence demonstrating a reduction in morbidity and mortality in newborns treated for PDA is still scarce (2, 6–9). These findings, associated with spontaneous ductal closure in a number of preterm newborns, suggest an expectant management of PDA based on clinical observation without pharmacological therapy (10, 11). However, prospective studies reported a significantly higher rate of morbidities when a permissive tolerance of PDA strategy was adopted (12). All these considerations raised controversy regarding whom to treat and when to treat preterm infants with hs-PDA. If some infants might benefit from pharmacological therapy, the criteria for PDA treatment remain currently unclear. The American Academy of Pediatrics and Experts on PDA agree that further studies are advocated to evaluate the efficacy of different diagnostic and therapeutic management of newborns with PDA (13–16). Starting from these considerations, we aimed to compare, in a cohort study, two management options: (1) targeted treatment based on ECHO criteria and (2) treatment based on ECHO criteria in addition to clinical signs and symptoms.

MATERIALS AND METHODS

Study Population

All newborns consecutively admitted to the Neonatal Intensive Care Unit (NICU) of University La Sapienza of Rome from January 2016 to November 2019, with gestational age (GA) <32 weeks or body birth weight (BW) <1,500 g and with a diagnosis of hs-PDA as confirmed by echocardiographic evaluation performed within 72 h of life, were included. Infants with congenital malformations, inborn errors of metabolism, congenital infections, and hospital discharge or death within 72 h of life were excluded (17). A consensus definition for a clinical diagnosis of PDA is lacking (18). We performed a differential diagnosis process in order to exclude conditions that may have a clinical presentation that overlaps those of symptomatic hs-PDA, such as sepsis, pulmonary hemorrhage, and pneumothorax.

We defined PDA as hemodynamically significant in the presence of at least one of the following criteria: (1) PDA ≥1.5 mm, (2) unrestrictive pulsatile transductal flow, (3) left atrial-to-aortic root ratio ≥1.5, and (4) absent (end-) diastolic flow in descending aorta.

We classified the babies in two cohorts. Cohort A included newborns consecutively observed in the first 22 months of the study. After that period, the protocol regarding the management of newborns with hs-PDA was changed; thus, we enrolled newborns in cohort B.

In the first period of the study (cohort A), we started pharmacological treatment immediately after echocardiographic evaluation, while in the second period of the study (cohort B) the newborns received pharmacological therapy for PDA when the relevance of a hs-PDA, at echocardiographic evaluation, was associated with clinical signs of hemodynamic instability including acidosis, increased refill capillary time (evaluated three times consecutively), increased oxygen requirement, oliguria, and persistent hypotension (evaluated within 12 h).

Outcomes

We considered as primary outcome the rate of newborns who survived without any morbidities upon discharge from NICU. Morbidity was defined as the presence of at least one of the following conditions occurring after enrollment: NEC Bell stage ≥2, IVH stage ≥2 (observed after 72 h of life), retinopathy of prematurity stage ≥2, bronchopulmonary dysplasia (BPD), periventricular leukomalacia, prolonged mechanical ventilation (more than 7 days consecutively), and acute renal failure (1, 2, 14, 15, 19, 20). We considered as secondary outcome the rate of newborns with ductal closure within the first 2 weeks of life.

Data Collection

Medical staff who were blinded to the study aims evaluated the eligibility of newborns observed in NICU. Physicians who were not involved in the care of the newborns collected the informed consent and all data for statistical analysis. A third-party observer unaware of the study aims collected data on primary and secondary outcomes. A statistician blinded to the study performed data analysis.

Prenatal, perinatal, and postnatal data were prospectively recorded in separate data forms. All infants were monitored until discharge, transfer to other hospital, or death. Data GA, BW, gender, type of delivery, antenatal steroid administration, congenital disorders, and occurrence of all relevant obstetric information were collected (21–23). Apgar score at 5 min after birth, pH on cord blood, respiratory distress syndrome, occurrence of hypotension, feeding tolerance, and other gastrointestinal disorders were also prospectively recorded (22, 24, 25). Data on survival, morbidity, and duration of hospital stay were collected in a separate and codified data form. Diagnosis of the main neonatal morbidities was performed according to the standard criteria by physicians unaware of the study design and aims as previously described (26, 27). Nutritional management was performed as previously described (24, 26, 28). Hypotension was defined as any mean blood pressure value below the infant's postmenstrual age (29).

Therapeutic Protocol of Newborns With hs-PDA

The first-line therapy for all enrolled newborns was pharmacological treatment. Pharmacological treatment with ibuprofen was the first therapeutic choice for PDA treatment. We administered, as first cycle treatment, a dosing regimen of 10 mg/kg ibuprofen, followed by 5 mg/kg ibuprofen at 24 and 48 h later. In case of contraindications to ibuprofen, we administered a paracetamol dose of 20 mg/kg as first dose, followed by 7.5 mg/kg paracetamol every 6 h thereafter, for a total of 6 days. A second pharmacological cycle was performed in the occurrence of symptoms related to hs-PDA for the two study cohorts. We administered a therapeutic cycle of ibuprofen (10 mg/kg, followed by 5 mg/kg ibuprofen at 24 and 48 h later) or, in case of contraindications to it, a cycle of paracetamol (7.5 mg/kg, every 6 h thereafter, for a total of 6 days).

A third pharmacological cycle was performed still in newborns that showed a slight but not significant improvement of clinical conditions and/or ECHO findings. If clinical conditions remained unchanged or worsened after two pharmacological cycles of treatment, the newborns underwent surgery. After the third pharmacological cycle of treatment, if we observed a further improvement of clinical conditions and/or ECHO findings, we administered a fourth pharmacological cycle with indomethacin for a total of 5 days. In case of reopening of hs-PDA associated with signs of hemodynamic instability, we administered one more cycle of ibuprofen or, if there are contraindications to it, paracetamol at the same dosing regimen before the surgery.

Cranial Ultrasonography Examination

The transducer frequency was set at 7.5 MHz. Images were recorded in coronal and sagittal planes, according to standard procedure, as previously described (30). The anterior fontanel represented the acoustic window for the optimal visualization of the supratentorial structures, whereas the mastoid fontanel was used to evaluate the cerebellum. The cranial ultrasound (cUS) scans were performed in all preterm infants within the first 72 h (T0) at 7 days of life (T1) and at 28 days of life (T2) contemporarily by two physicians with high training in cUS (more than 200 cUS per year) and who were unaware of the study aims. The two sonographers performed each measure three times, and then they calculated the mean value and reported the results in a specific data form. Each measurement was confirmed after an agreement between the sonographers.

Ethics

The study was conducted in accordance with the World Medical Association Declaration of Helsinki for medical research involving human subjects. To conduct this research, we compared two historical cohorts of newborns using data collected during a study previously approved by the Ethical Committee (no. 5089). Data are available from the Department of Maternal and Child Health Policlinico Umberto I Hospital, La Sapienza University of Rome, Italy, Institutional Data Access for researchers who meet the criteria for access to confidential data.

Statistics

Statistical analysis was performed per protocol using Statistical Package for Social Science software (SPSS Inc, Chicago, IL, USA), version 22.0. We assessed statistical significance by the tests described below, considering that the level of significance for all statistical tests was two-sided with $p < 0.05$. We checked for normality using the Shapiro–Wilk test. The mean and 95% confidence interval summarized the continuous variables. We compared the cohorts using χ^2 test for categorical variables and t-test or Mann–Whitney for paired and unpaired variables.

We performed binary logistic regression analysis to evaluate whether gender (female or male), BW in model 1 (>1,500 or ≤1,500 g) or GA in model 2 (<29 or ≥29 weeks of PMA), prenatal steroid use (no or yes), alteration of Doppler velocimetry of uterine arteries (no or yes), respiratory distress syndrome (no or yes), and cohort assignment (A or B) influenced primary outcome.

RESULTS

The number of newborns that met the inclusion criteria was 106. We excluded 34 newborns because of major congenital malformations or inborn errors of metabolism or congenital infections (n = 11), death before 72 h of life (n = 13), and transfer to another hospital before 72 h of life (n = 10). Thus, the analysis of data was performed on 27 and 45 newborns enrolled in cohort A and cohort B, respectively. The baseline clinical characteristics of enrolled newborns were not different in the two study cohorts, as reported in **Table 1**. In **Table 2**, we reported the echocardiographic pattern of PDA observed in the two cohorts of the study.

The primary outcome (A: 48.1% vs. B: 22.2%, $p = 0.022$) of the study is reported in **Figure 1**. Among the morbidities observed in the study cohorts, the occurrence of IVH was higher in cohort B compared with that in cohort A (**Table 3**). The preterm newborns without hs-PDA, of the same study periods, were similar in baseline characteristics and outcomes (**Supplementary Table 1**). The mean length of hospitalization of patients in cohort A (96.5 days, 95% CI 69.7–123.4) was similar to those in cohort B (78.6 days, 95% CI 64.5–92.6, $p = 0.185$).

In **Table 4**, no difference in the rate of ductal closure, reopening, and need of surgical intervention was observed between the study cohorts. The rate of PDA closure before the first 2 weeks of life was similar in cohort A (44.4%) compared with that in cohort B (51.1%, p = 0.621). The mean age of definitive ductal closure was similar in cohort A (17.3 days, 95% CI 6.5–28.2) compared with that in cohort B (15.5 days, 95% CI 9.4–21.6, $p = 0.746$).

In **Table 5**, we report the modalities of treatment in the two cohorts of the study. The rate of newborns treated with specific drugs for PDA was similar between the two cohorts (A: 100% vs. B: 95.6%, $p = 0.387$).

A multivariate analysis showed that cohort A assignment independently reduces the risk of combined morbidity and mortality in our population (**Table 6**).

DISCUSSION

We demonstrated that an ECHO-guided therapy regardless of symptoms may increase the probability of survival without morbidity in very low birth weight infants. The reduction in morbidity observed in cohort A was associated with a significant

TABLE 1 | Baseline clinical characteristics of the study cohorts.

	Cohort A $n = 27$	Cohort B $n = 45$	*p*
Female	11 (40.7)	22 (48.9)	0.502
Gestational age, median weeks (IQR)	28 (4)	27 (2)	0.135
Birth weight, median g (IQR)	1,020 (500)	900 (480)	0.161
Twins	9 (33.3)	8 (17.8)	0.132
Cesarean section	23 (85.2)	35 (77.8)	0.214
Antenatal steroids[a]	16 (59.2)	27 (60)	0.586
Pregnancy-induced hypertension	8 (29.6)	12 (26.7)	0.444
Alteration of doppler velocimetry of uterine arteries	4 (14.8)	6 (13.3)	0.441
pH at birth, median (IQR)	7.25 (0.17)	7.26 (0.09)	0.187
Respiratory distress syndrome	21 (77.8)	39 (86.7)	0.254
FEF, median days (IQR)	21 (22)	25 (19)	0.926
Hypotension requiring inotropes	4 (14.8)	20 (44.4)	0.009
Temperature at 1st h of life, median °C (IQR)	36.1 (0.7)	36.1 (0.3)	0.289
Normoglycemia	8 (53.3)	15 (40.5)	0.400
APGAR score at 5 min of life, median (IQR)	7 (1)	7 (2)	0.815
Sepsis	6 (22.2)	10 (22.2)	0.620

[a]*Intramuscular steroid cycle in two doses of 12 mg over a 24-h period. Data are expressed as number (%) when not specified.*
FEF, full enteral feeding.

TABLE 2 | Echocardiographic pattern of patent ductus arteriosus at the time of diagnosis in the two study cohorts.

	Cohort A $n = 27$	Cohort B $n = 45$	*p*
Diameter ≥1.5 mm	21 (77.8)	33 (73.3)	0.673
Unrestrictive ductal flow (unidirectional left–right or pulsatile bidirectional)	26 (96.3)	44 (97.8)	0.634
Left atrium/aorta ratio ≥1.5	11 (40.7)	17 (37.8)	0.707
Absent or reverse flow in descending aorta	4 (14.8)	5 (11.1)	0.430

The diagnosis of hemodynamic significance of ductus arteriosus based on echocardiographic parameters. Data are expressed as number (%).

reduction in IVH. Current evidence suggests that many neonatal-related outcomes may depend on the management of PDA. Nevertheless, the literature review reports contradicting findings that mainly rely on the type of the designed study (31). Randomized controlled trials (RCTs) exploring the effects of a prophylactic treatment of PDA found that the occurrence of both death and long-term neurodevelopmental outcomes was not reduced. However, observational studies demonstrated the association between PDA exposure duration and long-term morbidities (14, 32, 33). In addition, retrospective studies found a relationship between symptomatic hs-PDA and morbidity combined with mortality (3).

A Cochrane review from 2010 demonstrated a significant reduction in morbidity associated with prophylactic administration of COX inhibitors in newborns with PDA (9). In contrast, a more recent Cochrane review showed that prophylactic treatment did not result in a reduction of morbidity (8). The concern about the possible exposure of newborns without hs-PDA to unnecessary treatments and the potential harm associated with ductal closure in subjects with elevated pulmonary pressure has raised doubts about the opportunity of the use of medical therapy for hs-PDA (19). In addition, recent evidence demonstrating an unchanged neonatal outcome after the implementation of a more conservative management plan lends support to the argument that PDA treatment should not be useful (6).

A recent retrospective study demonstrated that the rate of spontaneous closure before hospital discharge occurs in the majority of patients (33). However, the authors excluded the deceased infants from the analysis. Indeed out of 26 infants who died, 16 had a recorded cause of death that could be potentially related to PDA, including IVH, and 10 infants who died before 7 days of age had point-of-care ECHO done, and all of them had documented PDA. The authors concluded that the outcome of some deceased infants could have been influenced by the criteria used for treatment (33). Besides that, Okulu et al. in an observational, prospective, and multi-center study, compared the effects of conservative approach and early medical treatment options in newborns with GA <29 weeks. It was found that early treatment was associated with higher mortality and BPD/death. However, in this cohort study, each center used their individual preferences in the decision of PDA management (34).

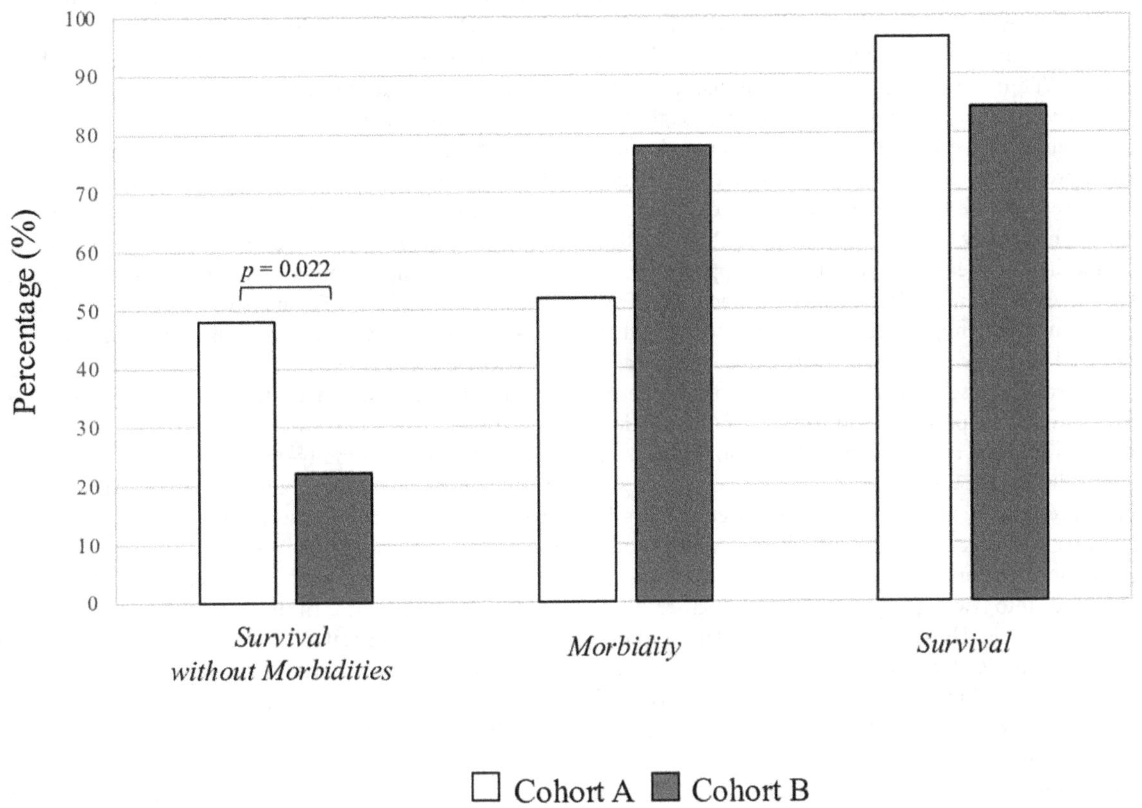

FIGURE 1 | Percentage of morbidity and survival in the two study Cohorts.

TABLE 3 | Morbidity in the two study cohorts.

	Cohort A $n = 27$	Cohort B $n = 45$	p
BPD	4 (14.8)	7 (15.6)	0.607
NEC	0 (0)	0 (0)	N/A
IVH	4 (14.8)	13 (28.9)	0.173
Stage ≥2	1 (3.7)	11 (24.4)	0.020
ROP	10 (37)	18 (40)	0.803
Stage ≥ 2	8 (29.6)	9 (20)	0.352
PLV	5 (18.5)	6 (13.3)	0.393
Prolonged invasive mechanical ventilation	4 (14.8)	14 (31.1)	0.122
Acute renal failure	0 (0)	2 (4.4)	0.387

BPD, bronchopulmonary dysplasia; NEC, necrotizing enterocolitis (Bell stage ≥2); IVH, intraventricular hemorrhage; ROP, retinopathy of prematurity; PLV, periventricular leukomalacia.
Data are expressed as number (%).

TABLE 4 | Clinical evolution of patent ductus arteriosus.

	Cohort A $n = 27$	Cohort B $n = 45$	p
Close after the first cycle of therapy	21 (77.8)	31 (68.9)	0.596
Definitive closure of PDA	23 (85.2)	39 (86.7)	0.561
Reopening of PDA	5 (18.5)	8 (17.8)	0.576
Surgical intervention	2 (7.4)	1 (2.2)	0.314

PDA, patency of the ductus arteriosus.
Data are expressed as number (%).

Thus, it is crucial to identify subjects on whom the advantages of medical treatments outweigh the risks of severe related side effects. To date, evidence regarding when to treat a hs-PDA in a preterm neonate is contrasting. Recent RCTs demonstrated that an early treatment, before the occurrence of symptoms, is safe and results in a lower incidence of late neonatal morbidity (35–37). The DETECT trial on early asymptomatic treatment showed a significant decrease in pulmonary hemorrhage rate in infants treated within the 1st h of life (35). In the PDA-TOLERATE trial enrolling <28-week newborns with a moderate-to-large PDA, the infants were randomized to receive either routine pharmacologic treatment or a conservative approach. The authors did not find any significant differences in terms of PDA closure and late neonatal morbidities. However, they showed that routine treatment, starting from 7 days of life, in infants with GA >26 weeks delayed full enteral feeding and increased the risk of morbidity and death. In this trial, the infants were not enrolled until the end of the 1st week, resulting in 14% of excluded newborns with PDA-related symptoms and

18% of infants not recruited owing to the physician's lack of equipoise (36). Liebowitz et al. starting from these findings, designed an observational study comparing newborns enrolled in the PDA-TOLERATE trial with those infants screened for PDA-TOLERATE who were excluded from the trial (even though they were potentially eligible) because the medical team wanted to use pharmacologic treatment. Interestingly, infants treated earlier within the 1st week of life had a significantly lower incidence of late neonatal morbidity and mortality despite their relative immaturity and their greater need of respiratory support (37).

Our results suggest that an ECHO-guided approach of a PDA, regardless of symptoms, might help to select newborns that should be treated in order to improve their clinical outcomes, hindering a potentially useless drug administration. Targeted treatment based on ECHO parameters may allow for the selection of preterm infants at a high risk of complications prior to the duct becoming clinically significant.

Our results are consistent with those of Rozé et al. This is a French national, prospective, population-based cohort study enrolling extremely preterm infants with GA < 29 weeks, who were placed into two groups based on whether they had undergone early ECHO screening or not. The authors reported that an early ECHO-guided treatment was associated with reduction in-hospital mortality and a reduced likelihood of pulmonary hemorrhage, even though they found no differences in late neonatal morbidity (38).

It has been demonstrated that hemodynamic instability is a major risk factor of several late neonatal complications such as IVH, BPD, and NEC (1, 4, 15, 20, 39). Although the accuracy of hs-PDA diagnosis increases with the presence of suggestive symptoms associated with ECHO findings, we hypothesize that waiting for the onset of symptoms may prolong the exposure to hemodynamic instability that, in turn, may increase the rate of morbidity and death. Accordingly, we found an increased morbidity when we decided to treat PDA only after the symptoms' appearance.

The differences in morbidity observed in our study rely mainly on IVH. A retrospective study reported an increased incidence of IVH in infants with persistent exposure to PDA (40). Besides that, it has been shown that medical prophylaxis within the 1st h of life results in a reduction in the incidence of IVH (41).

The literature review on the relation between PDA and IVH is controversial. A recent retrospective cohort study including infants born <29 weeks demonstrated a relation between the presence of hs-PDA and severe IVH. In particular, it was found that a hs-PDA requiring treatment was associated with a higher risk of IVH and that early treatment of hs-PDA was associated with a decreased severity of IVH (40). However, many of previous trials have included infants with PDA regardless of hemodynamic significance (42–44). Therefore, any beneficial effect of a protocol for PDA management may have been masked by the absence of clinical consequences of a physiologic PDA. In addition, the presence of confounders may have influenced the results of these studies. Kim et al. designed a cohort study including newborns with GA < 29 weeks to assess the relation between the size of PDA and cerebral hemodynamics within the 1st week of life (45). They indicated that cerebral hemodynamics was found to be stable regardless of the size of PDA in those premature infants. However, the authors did not report a specified protocol for ECHO, which was done at the direction of the attending neonatologist. Moreover, ECHO evaluation was not focused on the hemodynamic significance of the PDA. The strategy adopted in newborns in cohort A has produced a positive effect on the occurrence of IVH, probably by reducing the time of hemodynamic instability. Finally, we speculate that our selective approach may have reduced the possible consequences of hemodynamic instability, due to prolonged exposure to hs-PDA, on cerebral flow. Further studies are needed to establish the causality between the hemodynamic consequences of PDA and the occurrence of IVH.

Our findings should be taking into account several study limitations. The association between early ECHO evaluation and combined morbidity–mortality outcome may be related to the effects of chance (random error), bias, or confounding factors. The two cohorts were similar for conditions affecting morbidity and mortality. We verified that the effect on the main outcome of the study persisted even after correction for confounding variables. In keeping with the available evidence, we included antenatal and postnatal risk factors associated with IVH. Despite of everything, other confounding variables, unknown or not considered in our statistical analysis, may have influenced the study results. This is a small but not a randomized trial. To limit selection bias, physicians prescribing therapy for PDA were not blinded to the ECHO findings and the clinical condition of the baby. This made the study more feasible and affordable but may have compromised its external validity. However, physicians evaluating eligibility were blinded to the study aims and used objective inclusion criteria such as GA and BW. On the other hand, designing a double-blind clinical trial could have influenced the parents' consent of enrollment due to the increasingly strong association between significant PDA and important morbidities. A recent paper reported that the risk of lack of equipoise within physicians caring for infants with hs-PDA could be very high. Hence, it is not easy to design an RCT in newborns of critically ill conditions. The results of this study may encourage designing a specific RCT that could best address this topic. Researchers not involved in eligibility assessment and clinical practice, who were unaware of the cohort assignment to limit observer bias, collected the data for statistical analysis. The protocol for the collection, measurement, and interpretation of data was discussed and defined before starting the study. A statistician blinded to the study performed the analysis. We divided the two study cohorts on a temporal basis. The classification of the subjects on a temporal basis may represent a bias. However, the baseline features were similar between the study cohorts. We did not change the policies during the study period, but we cannot exclude the fact that unknown differences in clinical practice or changes in the medical staff composition may have influenced the outcomes of the study. We used previously described criteria for the definition of hs-PDA (1, 5, 19, 32, 46). Even if other parameters could be useful to define the hemodynamic significance of a PDA, information regarding ECHO findings on pulmonary overflow and systemic steal was not collected.

TABLE 5 | Pharmacological treatment in the two study cohorts.

	Cohort A $n = 27$	Cohort B $n = 45$	*p*
Need more than one cycle of therapy, number (%)	4 (14.8)	13 (28.9)	0.143
Number of cycles	1.3 (1.1–1.5)	1.5 (1.2–1.7)	0.277
Start of the first cycle of medical therapy, days	3.8 (2.7–4.9)	3.8 (3.0–4.5)	0.895
Duration of medical therapy, days	4.4 (3.4–5.3)	5.3 (4.3–6.3)	0.202
Paracetamol in the first cycle of medical therapy, number (%)	5 (18.5)	18 (40.0)	0.068
Ibuprofen in the first cycle of medical therapy, number (%)	22 (81.5)	25 (55.6)	0.068
No treatment, number (%)	0 (0.0)	2 (4.4)	0.068

Data are expressed as mean (95% CI) when not specified.

TABLE 6 | Binary logistic regression analysis to evaluate the influence of covariates on primary outcome.

Primary Outcome	B	p-value	OR	95.0% confidence interval	
				Lower limit	Upper limit
Model 1					
Birth weight	2.027	0.175	7.588	0.405	142.239
Twins	−0.497	0.519	0.608	0.134	2.758
Pregnancy-induced hypertension	−0.789	0.328	0.454	0.093	2.212
pH on cord blood	−1.176	0.239	0.309	0.044	2.185
Alteration of doppler velocimetry of uterine arteries	−0.149	0.877	0.862	0.130	5.699
Gender	−1.056	0.179	0.348	0.075	1.622
Antenatal corticosteroids[a]	0.324	0.661	1.383	0.324	5.896
Respiratory distress syndrome	0.868	0.336	2.383	0.406	14.000
Cohort	−1.825	0.024	0.161	0.033	0.784
Model 2					
Gestational age	−3.913	0.007	0.020	0.001	0.347
Twins	−1.276	0.155	0.279	0.048	1.621
Pregnancy-induced hypertension	−0.892	0.313	0.410	0.073	2.314
pH on cord blood	−1.297	0.258	0.273	0.029	2.603
Alteration of doppler velocimetry of uterine arteries	1.068	0.333	2.909	0.334	25.314
Gender	−1.579	0.083	0.206	0.035	1.227
Antenatal corticosteroids[a]	0.499	0.553	1.648	0.316	8.587
Respiratory distress syndrome	1.526	0.143	4.598	0.596	35.488
Cohort	−2.243	0.020	0.106	0.016	0.703

[a]*Intramuscular steroid cycle in two doses of 12 mg over a 24-h period.*

The ECHO data did not include more detailed parameters that could be useful for assessing the hemodynamic significance of a PDA. The ECHO findings collected in this study were limited to the definition of the hemodynamic significance of a PDA. Several of the criteria of hs-PDA are subject to considerable operator variability. Thus, different diagnostic criteria could lead to different conclusions. Our study was focused on short-term outcomes. Further research should investigate the relationship of different strategies to manage PDA closure on brain function and long-term neurodevelopmental outcomes. The small number of the newborns enrolled in the study and the differences in the number of subjects enrolled in the two cohorts limit the generalizability of the results.

In conclusion, an ECHO-based management of PDA regardless of symptoms is a safe and feasible approach useful to improve combined morbidity and mortality outcome in preterm newborns. The optimal protocol for the assessment and treatment of a newborn with hs-PDA should aim not only to an increased rate of PDA closure but also at a reduction in morbidity and mortality. Our results outline the importance of the early identification of newborns with hs-PDA trough ECHO-based protocol and may facilitate the design of a randomized trial on PDA management based on ECHO markers of PDA significance.

ETHICS STATEMENT

Ethical review and approval was not required for the study on human participants in accordance with the local legislation and institutional requirements. Written informed consent to participate in this study was provided by the participants' legal guardian/next of kin.

AUTHOR CONTRIBUTIONS

GT, MDi, GB, PV, and EP conceptualized and designed the study, organized the acquisition of data, reviewed, and revised both the analyses and the manuscript. GT, MDi, GB, PV, VDD, AG, EP, FF, EO, CC, AT, and MDe drafted the article and revised it critically for important intellectual content. All the authors approved the final manuscript to be published.

REFERENCES

1. Bhat R, Das UG. Management of patent ductus arteriosus in premature infants. *Indian J Pediatr.* (2015) 82:53–60. doi: 10.1007/s12098-014-1646-6
2. Benitz WE. Treatment of persistent patent ductus arteriosus in preterm infants: time to accept the null hypothesis? *J Perinatol.* (2010) 30:241–52. doi: 10.1038/jp.2010.3
3. Brown ER. Increased risk of bronchopulmonary dysplasia in infants with patent ductus arteriosus. *J Pediatr.* (1979) 95:865–6. doi: 10.1016/s0022-3476(79)80454-0
4. Wyllie JP, Gupta S. Prophylactic and early targeted treatment of patent ductus arteriosus. *Semin Fetal Neonatal Med.* (2018) 23:250–4. doi: 10.1016/j.siny.2018.03.005
5. Kindler A, Seipolt B, Heilmann A, Range U, Rüdiger M, Hofmann SR. Development of a diagnostic clinical score for hemodynamically significant patent ductus arteriosus. *Front Pediatr.* (2017) 5:280. doi: 10.3389/fped.2017.00280
6. El-Khuffash A, Weisz DE, McNamara PJ. Reflections of the changes in patent ductus arteriosus management during the last 10 years. *Arch Dis Child Fetal Neonatal Ed.* (2016) 101:F474–8. doi: 10.1136/archdischild-2014-306214
7. Terrin G, Conte F, Oncel MY, Scipione A, McNamara PJ, Simons S, et al. Paracetamol for the treatment of patent ductus arteriosus in preterm neonates: a systematic review and meta-analysis. *Arch Dis Child Fetal Neonatal Ed.* (2016) 101:F127–36. doi: 10.1136/archdischild-2014-307312
8. Ohlsson A, Walia R, Shah SS. Ibuprofen for the treatment of patent ductus arteriosus in preterm or low birth weight (or both) infants. *Cochrane Database Syst Rev.* (2015) 9:CD003481. doi: 10.1002/14651858.CD003481.pub6
9. Fowlie PW, Davis PG. Prophylactic intravenous indomethacin for preventing mortality and morbidity in preterm infants. *Cochrane Database of Syst Rev.* (2002) CD000174. doi: 10.1002/14651858.CD000174
10. Rolland A, Shankar-Aguilera S, Diomandé D, Zupan-Simunek V, Boileau P. Natural evolution of patent ductus arteriosus in the extremely preterm infant. *Arch Dis Child Fetal Neonatal Ed.* (2015) 100:F55–8. doi: 10.1136/archdischild-2014-306339
11. Sung SI, Chang YS, Chun JY, Yoon SA, Yoo HS, Ahn SY, et al. Mandatory closure versus nonintervention for patent ductus arteriosus in very preterm infants. *J Pediatr.* (2016) 177:66–71.e1. doi: 10.1016/j.jpeds.2016.06.046
12. Sathanandam S, Whiting S, Cunningham J, Zurakowski D, Apalodimas L, Waller BR, et al. Practice variation in the management of patent ductus arteriosus in extremely low birth weight infants in the United States: survey results among cardiologists and neonatologists. *Congenit Heart Dis.* (2019) 14:6–14. doi: 10.1111/chd.12729
13. El-Khuffash A, James AT, Corcoran JD, Dicker P, Franklin O, Elsayed YN, et al. A patent ductus arteriosus severity score predicts chronic lung disease or death before discharge. *J Pediatr.* (2015) 167:1354–61.e2. doi: 10.1016/j.jpeds.2015.09.028
14. Elsayed YN, Fraser D. Patent ductus arteriosus in preterm infants, part 1: understanding the pathophysiologic link between the patent ductus arteriosus and clinical complications. *Neonatal Netw.* (2017) 36:265–72. doi: 10.1891/0730-0832.36.5.265
15. Clyman RI. Patent ductus arteriosus, its treatments, and the risks of pulmonary morbidity. *Semin Perinatol.* (2018) 42:235–42. doi: 10.1053/j.semperi.2018.05.006
16. Slaughter JL, Cua CL, Notestine JL, Rivera BK, Marzec L, Hade EM, et al. Early prediction of spontaneous Patent Ductus Arteriosus (PDA) closure and PDA-associated outcomes: a prospective cohort investigation. *BMC Pediatr.* (2019) 19:333. doi: 10.1186/s12887-019-1708-z
17. Ferreira CR, van Karnebeek CDM. Inborn errors of metabolism. *Handb Clin Neurol.* 162:449–81. doi: 10.1016/B978-0-444-64029-1.00022-9
18. Gillam-Krakauer M, Reese J. Diagnosis and management of patent ductus arteriosus. *NeoReviews.* (2018) 19:e394–402. doi: 10.1542/neo.19-7-e394
19. McNamara PJ, Sehgal A. Towards rational management of the patent ductus arteriosus: the need for disease staging. *Arch Dis Child Fetal Neonatal Ed.* (2007) 92:F424–7. doi: 10.1136/adc.2007.118117
20. Alfaleh K, Smyth JA, Roberts RS, Solimano A, Asztalos EV, Schmidt B. Prevention and 18-month outcomes of serious pulmonary hemorrhage in extremely low birth weight infants: results from the trial of indomethacin prophylaxis in preterms. *Pediatrics.* (2008) 121:e233–8. doi: 10.1542/peds.2007-0028
21. Canani RB, Terrin G. Recent progress in congenital diarrheal disorders. *Curr Gastroenterol Rep.* (2011) 13:257–64. doi: 10.1007/s11894-011-0188-6
22. Passariello A, Terrin G, Baldassarre ME, de Curtis M, Paludetto R, Berni Canani R. Diarrhea in neonatal intensive care unit. *World J Gastroenterol.* (2010) 16:2664. doi: 10.3748/wjg.v16.i21.2664
23. Salvia G, Cascioli CF, Ciccimarra F, Terrin G, Cucchiara S. A case of protein-losing enteropathy caused by intestinal lymphangiectasia in a preterm infant. *Pediatrics.* (2001) 107:416–417. doi: 10.1542/peds.107.2.416
24. Terrin G, Passariello A, Canani RB, Manguso F, Paludetto R, Cascioli C. Minimal enteral feeding reduces the risk of sepsis in feed-intolerant very low birth weight newborns. *Acta Paediatr.* (2009) 98:31–5. doi: 10.1111/j.1651-2227.2008.00987.x
25. Lebreton E, Crenn-Hébert C, Menguy C, Howell EA, Gould JB, Dechartres A, et al. Composite neonatal morbidity indicators using hospital discharge data: a systematic review. *Paediatr Perinat Epidemiol.* (2020) 34:350–65. doi: 10.1111/ppe.12665
26. Terrin G, Coscia A, Boscarino G, Faccioli F, Di Chiara M, Greco C, et al. Long-term effects on growth of an energy-enhanced parenteral nutrition in preterm newborn: a quasi-experimental study. *PLoS ONE.* (2020) 15:e0235540. doi: 10.1371/journal.pone.0235540
27. Terrin G, Boscarino G, Di Chiara M, Iacobelli S, Faccioli F, Greco C, et al. Nutritional intake influences zinc levels in preterm newborns: an observational study. *Nutrients.* (2020) 12:529. doi: 10.3390/nu12020529
28. Berni Canani R, Passariello A, Buccigrossi V, Terrin G, Guarino A. The nutritional modulation of the evolving intestine. *J Clin Gastroenterol.* (2008) 42:S197–200. doi: 10.1097/MCG.0b013e31817da155
29. Cayabyab R, McLean CW, Seri I. Definition of hypotension and assessment of hemodynamics in the preterm neonate. *J Perinatol.* (2009) 29:S58–62. doi: 10.1038/jp.2009.29
30. Terrin G, De Nardo MC, Boscarino G, Di Chiara M, Cellitti R, Ciccarelli S, et al. Early protein intake influences neonatal brain measurements in preterms: an observational study. *Front Neurol.* (2020) 11:885. doi: 10.3389/fneur.2020.00885
31. Sallmon H, Koehne P, Hansmann G. Recent advances in the treatment of preterm newborn infants with patent ductus arteriosus. *Clin Perinatol.* (2016) 43:113–29. doi: 10.1016/j.clp.2015.11.008
32. Conrad C, Newberry D. Understanding the pathophysiology, implications, and treatment options of patent ductus arteriosus in the neonatal population. *Adv Neonatal Care.* (2019) 19:179–87. doi: 10.1097/ANC.0000000000000590
33. Semberova J, Sirc J, Miletin J, Kucera J, Berka I, Sebkova S, et al. Spontaneous closure of patent ductus arteriosus in infants $\leq$1500 g. *Pediatrics.* (2017) 140:e20164248. doi: 10.1542/peds.2016-4258
34. Okulu E, Erdeve O, Arslan Z, Demirel N, Kaya H, Gokce IK, et al. An observational, prospective, multicenter, registry-based cohort study comparing conservative and medical management for patent ductus arteriosus. *Front Pediatr.* (2020) 8:434. doi: 10.3389/fped.2020.00434
35. Kluckow M, Jeffery M, Gill A, Evans N. A randomised placebo-controlled trial of early treatment of the patent ductus arteriosus. *Arch Dis Child Fetal Neonatal Ed.* (2014) 99:F99–104. doi: 10.1136/archdischild-2013-304695
36. Clyman RI, Liebowitz M, Kaempf J, Erdeve O, Bulbul A, Håkansson S, et al. PDA-TOLERATE trial: an exploratory randomized controlled trial of treatment of moderate-to-large patent ductus arteriosus at 1 week of age. *J Pediatr.* (2019) 205:41–8.e6. doi: 10.1016/j.jpeds.2018.09.012

37. Liebowitz M, Katheria A, Sauberan J, Singh J, Nelson K, Hassinger DC, et al. Lack of equipoise in the PDA-TOLERATE trial: a comparison of eligible infants enrolled in the trial and those treated outside the trial. *J Pediatr.* (2019) 213:222–6.e2. doi: 10.1016/j.jpeds.2019.05.049
38. Rozé J-C, Cambonie G, Marchand-Martin L, Gournay V, Durrmeyer X, Durox M, et al. Association between early screening for patent ductus arteriosus and in-hospital mortality among extremely preterm infants. *JAMA.* (2015) 313:2441–8. doi: 10.1001/jama.2015.6734
39. Su B-H, Lin H-Y, Huang F-K, Tsai M-L, Huang Y-T. Circulatory management focusing on preventing intraventricular hemorrhage and pulmonary hemorrhage in preterm infants. *Pediatr Neonatol.* (2016) 57:453–62. doi: 10.1016/j.pedneo.2016.01.001
40. Khanafer-Larocque I, Soraisham A, Stritzke A, Al Awad E, Thomas S, Murthy P, et al. Intraventricular hemorrhage: risk factors and association with patent ductus arteriosus treatment in extremely preterm neonates. *Front Pediatr.* (2019) 7:408. doi: 10.3389/fped.2019.00408
41. Cooke L, Steer PA, Woodgate PG. Indomethacin for asymptomatic patent ductus arteriosus in preterm infants. *Cochrane Database Syst Rev.* (2003) CD003745. doi: 10.1002/14651858.CD003745
42. Sosenko IRS, Fajardo MF, Claure N, Bancalari E. Timing of patent ductus arteriosus treatment and respiratory outcome in premature infants: a double-blind randomized controlled trial. *J Pediatr.* (2012) 160:929–35.e1. doi: 10.1016/j.jpeds.2011.12.031
43. Mahony L, Carnero V, Brett C, Heymann MA, Clyman RI. Prophylactic indomethacin therapy for patent ductus arteriosus in very-low-birth-weight infants. *N Engl J Med.* (1982) 306:506–10. doi: 10.1056/NEJM198203043060903
44. van Overmeire B, van de Broek H, van Laer P, Weyler J, Vanhaesebrouck P. Early versus late indomethacin treatment for patent ductus arteriosus in premature infants with respiratory distress syndrome. *J Pediatr.* (2001) 138:205–11. doi: 10.1067/mpd.2001.110528
45. Kim ES, Kaiser JR, Rios DR, Bornemeier RA, Rhee CJ. Cerebral hemodynamics are not affected by the size of the patent ductus arteriosus. *Neonatology.* (2020) 117:182–8. doi: 10.1159/000506835
46. Keusters L, Purna J, Deshpande P, Mertens L, Shah P, McNamara PJ, et al. Clinical validity of systemic arterial steal among extremely preterm infants with persistent patent ductus arteriosus. *J Perinatol.* (2020). doi: 10.1038/s41372-020-0663-8. [Epub ahead of print].

16

Conservative Management of Patent Ductus Arteriosus in Preterm Infants—A Systematic Review and Meta-Analyses Assessing Differences in Outcome Measures Between Randomized Controlled Trials and Cohort Studies

Tim Hundscheid[1], Esther J. S. Jansen[1], Wes Onland[2], Elisabeth M. W. Kooi[3], Peter Andriessen[4,5] and Willem P. de Boode[1]*

[1] Division of Neonatology, Department of Paediatrics, Radboud Institute for Health Sciences, Amalia Children's Hospital, Radboud University Medical Centre, Nijmegen, Netherlands, [2] Department of Neonatology, Amsterdam University Medical Centers, VU University Medical Center, Emma Children's Hospital, University of Amsterdam, Amsterdam, Netherlands, [3] Division of Neonatology, University Medical Center Groningen, Beatrix Children's Hospital, University of Groningen, Groningen, Netherlands, [4] Department of Neonatology, Máxima Medical Center Veldhoven, Eindhoven, Netherlands, [5] Department of Applied Physics, School of Medical Physics and Engineering, Eindhoven University of Technology, Eindhoven, Netherlands

Correspondence:
Tim Hundscheid
tim.hundscheid@radboudumc.nl

Objective: This study aims to evaluate outcome after conservative management (no pharmacological/surgical intervention other than fluid restriction, diuretics, or ventilator adjustments) compared with active (pharmacological and/or surgical) treatment for patent ductus arteriosus (PDA) in preterm infants and analyze differences in outcome between randomized controlled trials (RCTs) and cohort studies.

Study Design: This is a systematic literature review using PubMed, EMBASE, and Cochrane library. RCTs and cohort studies comparing conservative management with active treatment were included. Meta-analysis was used to compare conservative management with any active (pharmacological and/or surgical), any pharmacological (non-prophylactic and prophylactic), and/or surgical treatment for mortality as primary and major neonatal morbidity as secondary outcome measure. Fixed-effect analysis was used, unless heterogeneity (I^2) was >50%. Outcome is presented as relative risk (RR) with 95% confidence interval.

Results: Twelve cohort studies and four RCTs were included, encompassing 41,804 and 720 patients, respectively. In cohort studies, conservative management for PDA was associated with a significantly higher risk for mortality (RR, 1.34 [1.12–1.62]) but a significantly lower risk for bronchopulmonary dysplasia (RR, 0.55 [0.46–0.65]), necrotizing enterocolitis (RR, 0.85 [0.77–0.93]), intraventricular hemorrhage (RR, 0.88 [0.83–0.95]), and retinopathy of prematurity (RR, 0.47 [0.28–0.79]) compared with any active PDA treatment. Meta-analysis of the RCTs revealed no significant differences in outcome between conservative management and active treatment.

Conclusion: No differences in mortality or morbidity for conservative management compared with active treatment regimens were observed in RCTs. Findings from cohort studies mainly highlight the lack of high-quality evidence for conservative management for PDA in preterm infants.

Keywords: PDA, ibuprofen, indomethacin, paracetamol, ligation, placebo, morbidity, mortality

INTRODUCTION

A patent ductus arteriosus (PDA) is very common in very low birth weight (VLBW) infants (<1,500 g) (1). It is associated with mortality and severe morbidity, such as bronchopulmonary dysplasia (BPD), necrotizing enterocolitis (NEC), intraventricular hemorrhage (IVH), and retinopathy of prematurity (ROP) (2).

Prophylactic treatment with indomethacin has been shown to reduce the incidence of symptomatic PDA, ligation, and severe IVH (3). Network meta-analysis of randomized controlled trials (RCTs) showed a significant effect on ductus arteriosus (DA) closure in pharmacologically treated children compared with placebo/no treatment (4). However, effective closure of the DA has not resulted in an improvement either in survival or major neonatal morbidity. When analyzing these RCTs, one has to be aware of the great heterogeneity in used definitions (and therefore inclusion criteria) for hemodynamically significant PDA (hsPDA) (5) and the remarkably high rate of open-label-treated patients in the control group (6). Ligation is an effective strategy to close the DA as well but has been associated with adverse outcome (7). Recent studies that adjusted for confounders prior to ligation, showed no association between ligation and adverse outcome (8, 9).

In the last decade, there has been a shift from aggressive pharmacological and/or surgical treatment toward a more conservative management (10). This change in policy can be justified by two arguments. First, since pharmacological treatment is not associated with an improvement in overall outcome (3, 4, 6, 11), fragile preterm infants are withheld from possible adverse effects of the pharmacological intervention. Second, there is a substantial rate of spontaneous closure of the DA (12, 13), even after failed pharmacological treatment (14). In summary, it is perceived that closure of the DA is delayed in preterm infants and treatment seems to only accelerate closure without improving outcome.

In this review and meta-analyses, we systematically reviewed the literature regarding mortality and morbidity associated with a conservative management for PDA in preterm and/or VLBW infants and compare most relevant outcome measures between RCTs and cohort studies.

METHODS

We performed a systematic literature review on 1 July 2020 in PubMed, EMBASE, and Cochrane library using the following search terms "preterm infant," "very low birth weight infant," "PDA," "conservative treatment," and "placebo" (**Table 1**). We excluded articles before 2000, as in this period antenatal corticosteroids and surfactant were not part of routine care. Reference lists of reviews and included articles were screened for additional studies. The Preferred Reporting Items for Systematic Reviews and Meta-Analyses (PRISMA) was followed (15). No review protocol was published.

Articles were included when it concerned (a) preterm infants <32 weeks' gestation or VLBW infants <1,500 g, with a PDA (irrespective of diagnostic criteria) in (b) a RCT or cohort study with (c) at least one study group managed conservatively (defined as <25% open-label pharmacological treatment with ibuprofen, indomethacin, or paracetamol and/or ligation/endovascular closure for RCTs and <25% active treatment during follow-up for cohort studies) as our aim is to compare active treatment with conservative management instead of "delayed" treatment and when (d) data about the primary outcome (mortality) or secondary outcome measures (BPD, NEC, IVH, and ROP) were available. Conservative management was defined as the absence of any pharmacological or surgical/endovascular intervention with the intention to actively close the DA other than fluid restriction, diuretics, and/or ventilator adjustments.

Articles were excluded if: (a) data about outcome measurements were not available per treatment regimen; (b) language was not English, German or Dutch; and (c) the paper was a conference abstract.

Two reviewers (TH and EJ) screened the title and abstract of the retrieved papers. Disagreements were resolved by a third reviewer (WdB). For eligible studies, corresponding authors were contacted for missing data from subgroups. Two reviewers (TH and EJ) assessed the risk of bias with the Cochrane Risk of Bias Tool for included RCTs (16) and the Newcastle-Ottawa Scale (NOS) for cohort studies (17). Disagreements were resolved by a third reviewer (WdB).

Data extraction regarding study design, study population, definition of (hs)PDA (not specified, clinical parameters only, echocardiographic parameters only, or both clinical and echocardiographic parameters), definition of conservative management (respiratory adjustments, fluid restriction and/or diuretics, or no pharmacological/surgical PDA treatment), percentage open-label active treatment (pharmacological and/or surgical) in the conservative management group, and outcome parameters (mortality, BPD, NEC, IVH, and ROP) from included studies were done by two reviewers (TH and EJ).

If available from the cohort studies, adjusted odds ratio (aOR) was also extracted and expressed as conservative management group compared with the active treatment regimen.

Conservative management was compared with five active treatment regimens, namely (1) any active treatment, defined as

TABLE 1 | Search strategy.

ID	Search	Hits
PubMed		
#1	Ductus arteriosus, patent [MeSH Terms]	8,951
#2	Patent ductus arteriosus [Title/Abstract]	8,328
#3	Patency of the ductus arteriosus [Title/Abstract]	198
#4	Persistent ductus arteriosus [Title/Abstract]	490
#5	hsPDA [Title/Abstract]	190
#6	PDA [Title/Abstract]	12,050
#7	#1 OR #2 OR #3 OR #4 OR #5 OR #6	21,577
#8	Infant, extremely premature [MeSH Terms]	2,477
#9	Preterm [Title/Abstract]	75,235
#10	VLBW [Title/Abstract]	33,696
#11	Very low birth weight infant [Title/Abstract]	485
#12	Extremely premature infant [Title/Abstract]	145
#13	Premature birth [Title/Abstract]	3,607
#14	Prematurity [Title/Abstract]	21,967
#15	Infant, low birth weight [MeSH Terms]	34,180
#16	#8 OR #9 OR #10 OR #11 OR #12 OR #13 OR #14	114,537
#17	Conservative treatment [MeSH Terms]	2,955
#18	Conservative [Title/Abstract]	105,930
#19	Expectative [Title/Abstract]	141
#20	Expectant [Title/Abstract]	5,866
#21	Placebo [Title/Abstract]	214,408
#22	Placebos [MeSH Terms]	34,946
#23	No treatment [Title/Abstract]	30,200
#24	#17 OR #18 OR #19 OR #20 OR #21 OR #22 OR #23	365,730
#25	#7 AND #16 AND #24	214
#26	#25 with filters: Publication date from 01 Jan 2000	175
EMBASE		
#1	Patent ductus arteriosus.ti. or patent ductus arteriosus.ab.	9,985
#2	PDA.ti. or PDA.ab.	16,176
#3	Patency of the ductus arteriosus.ti. or patency of the ductus arteriosus.ab.	276
#4	Persistent ductus arteriosus.ti. or persistent ductus arteriosus.ab.	558
#5	hsPDA.ti. or hsPDA.ab.	162
#6	#1 OR #2 OR #3 OR #4 OR #5	22,852
#7	Extremely preterm infant.ti. or extremely preterm infant.ab.	161
#8	Extremely premature infant.ti. or extremely premature infant.ab.	156
#9	Extreme preterm infant.ti. or extreme preterm infant.ab.	15
#10	Extreme premature infant.ti. or extreme premature infant.ab.	17
#11	Very low birth weight.ti. or very low birth weight.ab.	9,275
#12	VLBW.ti. or VLBW.ab.	5,016
#13	Prematurity.ti. or prematurity.ab.	28,702
#14	Premature birth.ti. or premature birth.ab.	4,534
#15	#7 OR #8 OR #9 OR #10 OR #11 OR #12 OR #13 OR #14	42,047
#16	Conservative treatment.ti. or conservative treatment.ab.	39,060
#17	Conservative.ti. or conservative.ab.	137,261

(Continued)

TABLE 1 | Continued

ID	Search	Hits
#18	Expectative.ti. or expectative.ab.	214
#19	No treatment.ti. or no treatment.ab.	44,953
#20	Placebo.ti. or placebo.ab.	307,386
#21	Expectant.ti. or expectant.ab.	7,805
#22	#16 OR #17 OR #18 OR #19 OR #20 OR #21	489,991
#23	#6 AND #15 AND #22	117
#24	Limit #23 to year = "2000–current"	93
Cochrane library		
#1	MeSH descriptor: [Ductus Arteriosus, Patent] explode all trees	285
#2	(Patent ductus arteriosus):ti,ab	750
#3	(PDA):ti,ab	959
#4	(Persistent ductus arteriosus):ti,ab	92
#5	(hsPDA):ti,ab	33
#6	(Patency of the ductus arteriosus):ti,ab	34
#7	(#6 OR #5 OR #4 OR #3 OR #2 OR #1)	1,403
#8	(Extremely preterm):ti,ab	564
#9	MeSH descriptor: [Infant, Extremely Premature] explode all trees	177
#10	MeSH descriptor: [Infant, Low Birth Weight] explode all trees	2,157
#11	(Preterm):ti,ab	13,188
#12	(VLBW):ti,ab	896
#13	(Very low birth weight infants):ti,ab	1,680
#14	(Infant, Extremely Premature):ti,ab	103
#15	(Premature birth):ti,ab	2,672
#16	(Prematurity):ti,ab	2,349
#17	#9 OR #10 OR #11 OR #12 OR #13 OR #14 OR #15 OR #16	17,085
#18	MeSH descriptor: [Conservative Treatment] explode all trees	119
#19	(Conservative):ti,ab	8,311
#20	(Expectative):ti,ab	90
#21	(Expectant):ti,ab	1,097
#22	(Placebo):ti,ab	293,798
#23	(No treatment):ti,ab	262,232
#24	MeSH descriptor: [Placebos] explode all trees	23,914
#25	#18 OR #19 OR #20 OR #21 OR #22 OR #23 OR #24	489,460
#26	#7 AND #17 AND #25	339
#27	#26 with Cochrane Library publication date between Jan 2000 and 1 Jul 2020	282

treatment with either ibuprofen, indomethacin, or paracetamol and/or ligation/endovascular closure; (2) any pharmacological treatment, defined as treatment with ibuprofen, indomethacin, and/or paracetamol, both prophylactic and non-prophylactic; (3) non-prophylactic pharmacological treatment, defined as treatment with ibuprofen, indomethacin, and/or paracetamol beyond a postnatal age of 24 h; (4) prophylactic pharmacological treatment, defined as treatment with ibuprofen, indomethacin, or paracetamol within a postnatal age of 24 h irrespective of PDA status; and (5) ligation/endovascular closure, defined as ligation/endovascular closure without preceding pharmacological treatment.

Some studies included a subgroup without a PDA. Those subgroups were excluded from the initial analysis, but in a subgroup analysis, we included those low-risk patients in the conservative treatment group to investigate their modulating effect on outcome measures. Furthermore, our main inclusion criterium for PDA was irrespective of diagnostic criteria used. In a subgroup analysis, we will only include studies with an echocardiographically confirmed PDA >1.5 mm in both subgroups.

Outcome measures were entered in Review Manager Software for meta-analysis (Revman version 5.3 Copenhagen: The Nordic Cochrane Center, The Cochrane Collaboration, 2014). Meta-analysis was performed for RCTs and cohort studies separately per defined treatment regimen. We used random effect if the heterogeneity (I^2) was >50% (18) and fixed effect in case of a lower heterogeneity. Effects are presented as risk ratio (RR) and risk difference (RD) with 95% confidence interval (95% CI).

The methodological quality of the studies' outcome parameters was examined with the GRADE method (19). We assessed imprecision as serious if the total number of events was <300 or if the width of the CI of the RR was >0.25. We used the GRADE-pro GDT 2016 software (GRADEpro Guideline Development Tool [Software], McMaster University, 2015) to create a "summary of findings" table to report the quality of evidence. The GRADE approach results in an assessment of the evidence in one of four grades of evidence: high, moderate, low, or very low certainty.

RESULTS

Our search revealed 388 unique articles, of which four RCTs (20–23) and 12 cohort studies (7, 24–34) could be included in the meta-analyses. **Figure 1** depicts the PRISMA flow diagram showing the retrieval process of the included articles (15). Due to our inclusion criterium of strict conservative management, we had to exclude many RCTs (n = 18) because of >25% open-label active treatment and cohort studies (n = 13) because of >25% active treatment during follow-up in the conservative management arm.

Study Characteristics

A total of 63,254 patients were analyzed, of which 720 patients from RCTs and 41,804 from cohort studies were included in the initial meta-analyses. The remaining (n = 20,730) were classified as a subgroup without a PDA in four cohort studies and did not receive any (prophylactic) treatment (26, 29) and were therefore excluded from the initial analyses.

In **Table 2**, the characteristics of the included RCTs and cohort studies are shown. The used definitions for a (hs)PDA varied extensively between studies. Patient characteristics are presented in **Table 3**.

Three RCTs were placebo controlled (20, 22, 23), while for one RCT, the control arm was not specified (21). In the cohort studies, the definition of conservative management ranged from no treatment at all to a regimen with fluid restriction, diuretics, and/or adaptation in ventilator settings or the absence of any pharmacological/surgical treatment.

Mortality was heterogeneously defined, since four studies excluded early neonatal deaths within 24–72 postnatal hours (7, 30, 32, 34). The outcome parameter BPD was defined according to the international criteria at 36 weeks postmenstrual age in 12 papers (7, 20, 22, 26–34). NEC was defined according to the Bell stadium in nine studies (7, 20, 22, 23, 26, 27, 30, 31, 34). Thirteen studies defined IVH as grade III or higher (7, 20–23, 25–32, 34), ROP was defined as stage 3 or higher in five studies (7, 22, 26, 28, 34). No study described endovascular closure.

Risk of Bias

The quality of the included RCTs was high, given the low risk of bias (**Table 4**). The quality of the cohort studies was classified as moderate (**Table 5**).

Meta-Analysis

Meta-Analysis Outcome Measures Randomized Controlled Trials

Meta-analysis of the four included RCTs did not show significant differences for mortality or morbidity in any of the predefined groups, as is shown in **Table 6** (**Supplementary Material 1**). The quality of the evidence was graded as moderate to low (**Supplementary Material 2**).

Meta-Analysis Outcome Measures Cohort Studies

Meta-analysis of the cohort studies revealed that conservative management was associated with a higher risk for mortality compared with any active treatment (RR, 1.34 [1.12–1.62]; RD, 0.03 [0.01–0.06]), any pharmacological treatment (RR, 1.46 [1.14–1.85]; RD, 0.05 [0.01–0.08]), and non-prophylactic pharmacological treatment (RR, 1.54 [1.13–2.09]; RD, 0.04 [0.00–0.07]) (**Table 6**; **Supplementary Material 3**). The quality of the evidence was graded as very low (**Supplementary Material 4**).

Conservative management was associated with a lower risk for BPD and ROP compared with both each separate active treatment regimen and any active treatment. The risk for NEC was significantly lower for conservative management in comparison with any active treatment (RR, 0.85 [0.77–0.93]; RD, −0.01 [−0.02 to −0.01]), prophylactic pharmacological treatment (RR, 0.77 [0.67–0.88]; RD, −0.02 [−0.03 to −0.01]), and ligation (RR, 0.49 [0.35–0.68]; RD, −0.07 [−0.12 to −0.02]). Conservative management was associated with a lower risk for IVH compared with any active treatment (RR, 0.88 [0.83–0.95]; RD, −0.02 [−0.03 to 0.01]) and ligation (RR, 0.65 [0.48–0.88]; RD, −0.09 [−0.15 to −0.03]) (**Table 6**; **Supplementary Material 3**). The quality of the evidence was graded as very low (**Supplementary Material 4**).

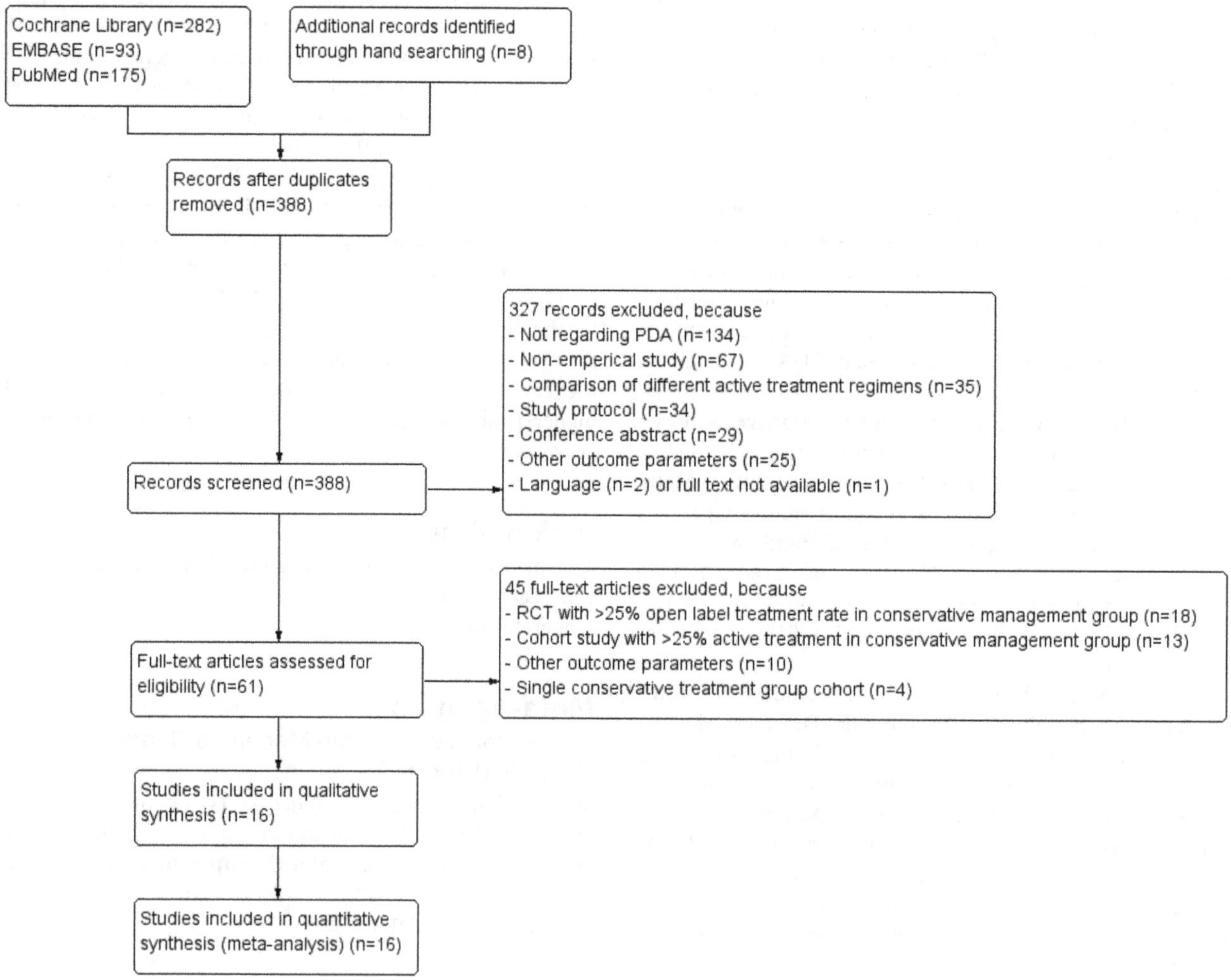

FIGURE 1 | Preferred Reporting Items for Systematic Reviews and Meta-Analysis (PRISMA) flow diagram of systematic literature review (15).

Meta-Analysis Outcome Measures Cohort Studies Including Patients Without a PDA

Subgroup baseline characteristics and outcome measures were available for patients without a PDA in three studies ($n = 20,497$) (26–28). In this subgroup, analysis outcome of those patients was added to the conservative management group (**Table 7**). The higher risk for mortality lost significance in almost all subgroups, while the lower risk for morbidity was even more pronounced (**Table 8, Supplementary Material 5**).

Meta-Analysis Outcome Measures Cohort Studies With Echocardiographic Defined PDA

We performed a subgroup meta-analysis on the two cohort studies that used echocardiographic definitions ($n = 316$) (29, 34). Outcome measurements, as presented in **Table 9**, showed a significant lower risk for BPD in the conservative treated group compared with the available subgroups any treatment and any/non-prophylactic pharmacological treatment. Mortality and other morbidity outcomes showed no difference.

Adjusted Outcome

Adjusted Outcome Measures From Cohort Studies

Eight cohort studies calculated aOR for baseline characteristics between conservative management and either pharmacological therapy, ligation, or pharmacological therapy followed by ligation (7, 26, 28, 30, 31, 33–35). **Table 10** shows a statistically significant higher risk for mortality and an overall lower risk for morbidity, especially BPD, in the conservatively managed group.

Adjusted Composite Outcome Measures From Cohort Studies

Studies that calculated an adjusted composite outcome, mainly involving mortality and/or BPD, observed lower aOR after conservative management in comparison with pharmacological treatment (30), to ligation alone (7, 30, 34), and pharmacological therapy and/or ligation (7, 30) (**Table 11**). One study defined composite outcome as survival without death or BPD and found no difference between conservative treatment and pharmacological treatment (aOR, 1.72 [0.92–3.23]) (31).

TABLE 2 | Study characteristics of included studies.

	References	Period	Design	Treatment strategies	Main inclusion criteria	Main exclusion criteria	Infants (*n*)	Conservative management	Used drug(s) (dosage if available)	(hs)PDA diagnosis	hsPDA definition
RCTs	Härkin et al. (20)	2013 2015	Double-blind Monocenter	CONS (placebo) vs. PPT	GA <32 weeks	CM, lethal disease, PPHN	48	Placebo (0.45% saline)	Paracetamol (once 20 mg/kg; 24 × 7.5 mg/kg every 6 h)	CLIN + ECHO	CLIN: increased respiratory support, decreased blood pressure, increased pulse pressure, pulmonary congestion, cardiomegaly, hepatomegaly, murmur, hyperdynamic precordium, bounding pulses ECHO: LA/Ao >1.4, PDA diameter/LPA >1.5, large LtR shunt
	Kumar Nair et al. (21)	1998 2001	Non-blinded Monocentre	CONS vs. PPT	BW 750–1,250 g, absence of IVH prior to inclusion	GA <26 weeks, AS[5] <5, CM, sepsis, contraindication for PPT	115	Not defined	INDO (3 × 0.1 mg/kg/day) start 6–12 h PNA	CLIN + ECHO	CLIN: hemorrhagic pulmonary edema, cardiomegaly on chest X-ray or failure of weaning from ventilatory support ECHO: not defined
	Sung et al. (22)	2014 2019	Double-blinded Monocenter	CONS (placebo) vs. PT	GA 23–30-weeks with respiratory support and PDA at PNA 6–14 days	CHD, life threatening CM, predominant RtL shunt, IVH ≥3, contraindication for PT	142	Placebo (0.9% saline)	IBU p.o. (10–5–5 mg/kg)	ECHO	ECHO: diameter >1.5 mm with predominant LtR shunt
	Van Overmeire et al. (23)	1999 2001	Double-blind Multicenter	CONS (placebo) vs. PPT	GA 24–30 weeks within 6 h PNA	Major CM, IVH > grade I, AS[5] <5, sepsis, hypotension, contraindication for PPT	415	Placebo	IBU (10–5–5 mg/kg)	Not defined	Not defined
Cohort studies	Alexander et al. (24)	1996 2005	Retrospective (chart review) Monocentre	CONS vs. PT or LIG or LIG after PT	BW <1,000 g with ECHO of PDA documented	Not defined	298	No PT and/or LIG	INDO (3 × 0.2 mg/kg every 12 h)	ECHO	Not defined
	Bourgoin et al. (25)	2003 2011	Prospective Multicenter	CONS for (non-hs)PDA vs. PT or LIG for hsPDA	Discharged alive	Dead <2 years, CM, lost to follow-up	857	No PT and/or LIG	IBU (10–5–5 mg/kg)	ECHO	PDA diameter >1.5 mm; LA/Ao >1.5; pulsatile flow in the DA; retrograde/absent diastolic flow in the cerebral anterior artery or in the descending thoracic aorta.
	Härkin et al. (26)	2005 2013	Retrospective (FMBR database) Multicentre	CONS vs. PT and/or LIG or no PDA	GA <32 weeks	Mortality <7 days PNA, severe CM	3,668	No PT and/or LIG	INDO or IBU	CLIN + ECHO	CLIN: murmur, hyperdynamic precordium, bounding pulses, increased need for respiratory support and increased pulse pressure ECHO: not defined
	Heuchan et al. (27)	2005 2009	Retrospective Monocentre	CONS vs. LIG or no PDA	Echocardiogram performed at PNA 6–48 h	CHD	25	No PT and/or LIG	None (primary LIG)	CLIN + ECHO	CLIN: murmur, hypotension, pulmonary hemorrhage, renal impairment ECHO: color Doppler diameter

(Continued)

TABLE 2 | Continued

References	Period	Design	Treatment strategies	Main inclusion criteria	Main exclusion criteria	Infants (*n*)	Conservative management	Used drug(s) (dosage if available)	(hs)PDA diagnosis	hsPDA definition
Laughon et al. (28)	1997 2004	Retrospective Multicenter	CONS vs. PPT or STG or LIG or no PDA	GA 23–30-weeks	Not defined	34,602	No PT and/or LIG	INDO	Not defined	Not defined
Letshwiti et al. (29)	2004 2011	Retrospective Monocenter	CONS vs. PT (subdivided in ETG and STG) or no PDA	BW <1,500 g	Not defined	371	PEEP ≥5 cmH_2O, FR (130–150 ml/kg/day)	IBU (10–5–5 mg/kg)	ECHO	PDA diameter >2 mm; LA/Ao >1.5; evidence of reduced splanchnic Doppler flow
Lokku et al. (30)	2006 2012	Retrospective (CNN database) Multicentre	CONS vs. PT and/or LIG	GA 23–32-weeks with CLIN and/or ECHO of PDA	Dead <72 h PNA, severe CM, ≥triplet, missing data regarding date of birth or sex	5,824	No PT and/or LIG	INDO	CLIN ± ECHO	CLIN: systolic murmur, bounding pulses, wide pulse pressure ECHO: not defined
Mirea et al. (7)	2004 2008	Retrospective (CNN database) Multicenter	CONS vs. PT and/or LIG	GA ≤32 weeks with CLIN and/or ECHO of PDA	Dead <72 h PNA, CHD	3,556	FR and/or diuretics	INDO	CLIN ±- ECHO	Not defined
Mohamed et al. (31)	2001 2014 2014	Retrospective (database) Monocentre	CONS vs. PT	BW <1,500 g	Not defined	643	Standard respiratory setting, no FR	INDO [2001–2006] IBU [2006–2014]	CLIN + ECHO	CLIN: cardiac murmur, pulsating pericardium, wide peripheral pulses, increasing metabolic acidosis (base excess <-8 mEq/L) ECHO: moderate to severe PDA
Sadeck et al. (32)	2010 2011	Retrospective (BNRN database) Multicentre	CONS vs. PT and/or LIG	BW <1,000 g, GA <33 weeks with ECHO of PDA	Died or transferred <3 days PNA, congenital infections, CM	494	No PT and/or LIG	INDO/IBU	Not defined	Not defined
Slaughter et al. (33)	2006 2013	Retrospective (PHIS database) Multicentre	CONS vs. PT	GA <28 weeks	Hospitalized <3 days, admitted >24 h PNA, no recorded discharge status	12,018	No PT and/or LIG	INDO/IBU	Not defined	Not defined
Sung et al. (34)	2009 2014	Retrospective (database) Monocentre	CONS vs. PT and/or LIG	GA 23–26-weeks	Died <48 h, CHD, PDA <2 mm or off ventilator	178	FR and diuretics if indicated	INDO (3 × 0.2 mg/kg every 12 h)	CLIN + ECHO	CLIN: deterioration in respiratory condition, cardiac murmur, hyperactive precordium, hypotension and widened pulse pressure ECHO: PDA diameter ≥2 mm with predominant LtR shunt

AS^5, Apgar score at 5 min postpartum; BNRN, Brazilian Neonatal Research Network; BW, birth weight; CHD, congenital heart disease; CM, congenital malformation and/or chromosomal abnormality and/or genetic syndrome; CNN, Canadian Neonatal Network; CLIN, clinical diagnosis; CONS, conservative management; d, days; DA, ductus arteriosus; ECHO, echocardiographic parameters; ETG, early treatment group; FMBR, Finnish Medical Birth Register; FR, fluid restriction; GA, gestational age; IBU, ibuprofen; INDO, indomethacin; IVH, intraventricular hemorrhage; LA/Ao, left atrium to aortic root ratio; LIG, ligation; LPA, left pulmonary artery; LtR, left to right; (hs)PDA, (hemodynamically significant) patent ductus arteriosus; PEEP, positive end expiratory pressure; PHIS, Pediatric Health Information System; PNA, postnatal age; PPHN, persistent pulmonary hypertension of a newborn; PT, pharmacological treatment; PPT, prophylactic pharmacological treatment; RCTs, randomized controlled trials; RtL, right to left; STG, standard treatment group.

TABLE 3 | Patient characteristics of included studies.

		Patient characteristics															
		Conservative management				Prophylactic pharmacological treatment			Pharmacological treatment			Ligation closure			Pharmacotherapy and/or ligation closure		
	References	**Infants (male/N)**	**GA (weeks)**	**BW (grams)**	**Open-label treatment**	**Infants (male/N)**	**GA (weeks)**	**BW (g)**	**Infants (male/N)**	**GA (weeks)**	**BW (g)**	**Infants (male/N)**	**GA (weeks)**	**BW (g)**	**Infants (male/N)**	**GA (weeks)**	**BW (g)**
RCTs	Härkin et al. (20)	14/25	28.3 ± 2.06	1,120 ± 340	12.0%	13/23	28.4 ± 2.36	1,220 ± 430	–	–	–	–	–	–	–	–	–
	Kumar Nair et al. (21)	NA/59	27.9 ± 1.4	995 ± 83.6	NA	NA/56	27.8 ± 1.2	989.5 ± 93.5	–	–	–	–	–	–	–	–	–
	Sung et al. (22)	41/72	26.7 ± 2.0	915 ± 243	0%	–	–	–	28/70	26.8 ± 2.1	893 ± 256	–	–	–	–	–	–
	Van Overmeire et al. (23)	NA/210	28.1 ± 1.6	1,065 ± 324	24.8%	NA/205	28.1 ± 1.7	1,048 ± 315	–	–	–	–	–	–	–	–	–
Cohort studies	Alexander et al. (24)	NA/54	25.7 ± 1.9	729.6 ± 169.6	0%	–	–	–	?/198	**26.1 ± 1.9**	**739 ± 140.5**	?/46	**24.8 ± 1.5**	**678.7 ± 153.5**	–	–	–
	Bourgoin et al. (25)	254/505	NA	977 ± 212	0%	–	–	–	134/248	NA	**911 ± 191**	40/104	NA	**833 ± 225**	–	–	–
	Härkin et al. (26)	98/182	28.82 ± 2.41	1,225 ± 402	0%	–	–	–	395/770	**26.3 ± 1.2**	**1,115 ± 336**	66/112	**25.6 ± 1.4**	**834 ± 297**	134/250	**25.5 ± 1.3**	**846 ± 278**
	Heuchan et al. (27)	4/7	27 [25–28]	1,046 [680–1,440]	0%	–	–	–	–	–	–	8/11	26 [24–27]	780 [613–1,240]	–	–	–
	Laughon et al. (28)	2,201/ 3,886	27 [26–29]	970 [750–1,220]	0%	3,293/ 6,189	**26 [25–28]**	873 [703–1075]	3,021/ 5,690	27 [25–29]	**960 [760–1,205]**	388/701	**25 [24–27]**	**730 [624–895]**	–	–	–
	Letshwiti et al. (29)[§]	16/34	27.4 ± 2.7	1,010 ± 250	14.7%	–	–	–	**15/52**	27.9 ± 2.0	1,040 ± 270	–	–	–	–	–	–
									26/52	27.5 ± 1.9	1,010 ± 280						
	Lokku et al. (30)[†]	811/ 1,486	28.2 ± 2.3	NA	0%	–	–	–	1,754/ 3,226	**27.1 ± 2.1**	NA	165/280	**26.0 ± 2.2**	NA	423/832	**25.6 ± 1.7**	NA
			28.2 ± 2.4	NA						**26.6 ± 2.0**	NA		**26.0 ± 1.8**	NA		**25.3 ± 1.6**	NA
	Mirea et al. (7)	321/577	28.3 ± 2.3	NA	0%	–	–	–	1,062/ 2,026	**27.0 ± 2.1**	NA	185/327	**26.0 ± 2.3**	NA	325/626	**25.5 ± 1.7**	NA
	Mohamed et al. (31)	122/228	28.0 ± 3.4	1,016 ± 340	0%	–	–	–	216/415	27.7 ± 2.9	988 ± 311	–	–	–	–	–	–
	Sadeck et al. (32)	91/187	27.6 ± 2.2	772 ± 142.3	0%	–	–	–	90/205	27.4 ± 1.9	**804 ± 121.6**	48/102	**26.6 ± 1.8**	781 ± 118.5	–	–	–
	Slaughter et al. (33)	4,302/ 8,130	NA	NA	0%	–	–	–	2,068/ 3,888	NA	NA	–	–	–	–	–	–
	Sung et al. (34)	54/97	24.5 ± 1.0	718 ± 137	0%	–	–	–	–	–	–	35/81	24.6 ± 1.1	728 ± 134	–	–	–

Data presented as number, percentage, mean ± standard deviation or median [interquartile range]. Statistical difference between other groups in same study are bold.

ETG; early treatment group, GA; gestational age, N; total infants, NA; not available, PDA; patent ductus arteriosus, RCTs; randomized controlled trials, STG; symptomatic treatment group.

[§]Pharmacological treatment in study subdivided between early treatment and symptomatic treatment.

[†]Cohort subdivided in cohort 2006–2008 and 2009–2012. BW; birth weight.

DISCUSSION

In this systematic review, we reviewed the available literature of the last two decades regarding a conservative management for a PDA in preterm infants. Meta-analysis of the included RCTs showed no differences in outcome for the conservative management group compared with active treatment groups. This is in line with a recent network meta-analysis that demonstrated no differences in severe neonatal morbidities between pharmacological treatment and no (active) treatment (4). This meta-analysis also included RCTs with an overall high rate of open-label active treatment in the conservative management (no treatment/placebo) group. However, our meta-analysis only including strict conservative management regimens RCTs, also showed no differences in mortality and/or morbidity in the small number of patients included.

Contrarily, meta-analysis of the cohort studies suggest an association with a significant higher risk for mortality in the conservative management group compared with most active treatment groups. Our meta-analysis hereby adds to the available evidence indicating an association between PDA and mortality (2); however, causality remains unproven. Remarkably, a significant lower risk for severe neonatal morbidities was found in our meta-analysis of the cohort studies in the conservative management group compared with various active treatment regimens.

The risk of bias of the included cohort studies was classified as moderate. The main risk of bias was treatment selection bias or confounding by indication, since patients could be managed conservatively due to contraindications for ibuprofen/indomethacin or because of a non-hsPDA. The lower incidence of neonatal morbidity might be due to survival bias, as patients who died cannot develop BPD. Furthermore, patients at the highest risk to develop (severe) morbidities are more likely to die. This might be enhanced by the exclusion of early neonatal death in four cohort studies (7, 30, 32, 34). Many cohort studies were derived from databases (7, 26, 30–34), which are at risk of poor diagnostic precision. These biases might explain the observed higher risk for mortality on the one hand, and the lower risk for morbidity on the other hand for conservatively managed patients compared with active treatment regimens.

Our subgroup analysis including patients without a PDA ("best-case scenario") further suggests treatment selection bias, as patients with the highest *a priori* risk for mortality were possibly not treated for their PDA while low-risk patients might have been excluded from retrospective cohort studies. The higher risk for mortality lost significance, while the lower risk for morbidity was even more pronounced. This supports

TABLE 4 | Risk of bias assessment of included randomized controlled trials according to the cochrane risk of bias tool (16).

	Härkin et al. (20)	Kumar Nair et al. (21)	Sung et al. (22)	Van Overmeire et al. (23)
Adequate sequence generation	+	+	+	+
Allocation concealment	+	+	+	+
Performance bias	+	−	+	+
Detection bias	+	?	+	+
Attrition bias	+	+	+	+
Reporting bias	+	+	+	+
Other bias	?	?	?	?

TABLE 5 | Risk of bias assessment of included cohort studies according to Newcastle–Ottawa scale (NOS) (17).

References	Selection				Comparability	Outcome		
	A	B	C	D	E	F	G	H
Alexander et al. (24)	*	*	*	*	**	*	–	*
Bourgoin et al. (25)	*	*	*	*	**	*	*	*
Härkin et al. (26)	*	*	*	*	**	*	*	*
Heuchan et al. (27)	*	*	*	*	–	*	–	*
Laughon et al. (28)	–	*	*	*	**	*	–	*
Letshwiti et al. (29)	*	*	*	*	–	*	–	*
Lokku et al. (30)	*	*	*	*	*	*	–	*
Mirea et al. (7)	*	*	*	*	**	*	*	*
Mohamed et al. (31)	*	*	*	*	**	*	*	*
Sadeck et al. (32)	*	*	*	*	–	*	–	*
Slaughter et al. (33)	*	*	*	*	*	*	*	*
Sung et al. (34)	*	*	*	*	**	*	–	*

A; representatives of the exposed cohort, B; selection of non-exposed cohort, C; ascertainment of exposure, D; demonstration that outcome of interest was not present at start of study, E; comparability of cohorts on the basis of the design or analysis, F; assessment of outcome, G; was follow-up long enough for outcomes to occur, H; adequacy of follow-up of cohorts.

Maximum score for each item is one star (*), except for comparability for which two stars (**) can be scored, and if not scored positive presented as "–".

TABLE 6 | Outcome measurements after meta-analysis.

Comparison	(Sub)group	Mortality	BPD (any definition)	NEC (any stage)	IVH (any grade)	ROP (any stage)
Conservative management vs. any active treatment	RCTs	1.09§ (0.73–1.61)	0.80 (0.55–1.17)	1.17§ (0.65–2.13)	1.00§ (0.71–1.40)	0.85§ (0.45–1.60)
		0.01 (−0.04 to 0.06)	*−0.06 (−0.16 to 0.04)*	*0.01 (−0.02 to 0.04)*	*0.00 (−0.04 to 0.05)*	*−0.03 (−0.13 to 0.08)*
		[4; 720]	[4; 709]	[4; 720]	[4; 720]	[2; 190]
	Cohort studies	**1.34 (1.12–1.62)**	**0.55 (0.46–0.65)**	**0.85§ (0.77–0.93)**	**0.88§ (0.83–0.95)**	**0.47 (0.28–0.79)**
		0.03 (0.01–0.06)	***−0.18 (−0.24 to −0.12)***	***−0.01 (−0.02 to −0.01)***	***−0.02 (−0.03 to −0.01)***	***−0.06 (0.10 to −0.02)***
		[11; 40,916]	**[11; 39,993]**	**[9; 28,004]**	**[10; 28,504]**	**[8; 26,608]**
Conservative management vs. any pharmacological treatment	RCTs	1.09§ (0.73–1.61)	0.80 (0.55–1.17)	1.17§ (0.65–2.13)	1.00§ (0.71–1.40)	0.85§ (0.45–1.60)
		0.01 (−0.04 to 0.06)	*−0.06 (−0.16 to 0.04)*	*0.01 (−0.02 to 0.04)*	*0.00 (−0.04 to 0.05)*	*−0.03 (−0.13 to 0.08)*
		[4; 720]	[4; 709]	[4; 720]	[4; 720]	[2; 190]
	Cohort studies	**1.46 (1.14–1.85)**	**0.63 (0.51–0.78)**	1.06 (0.78–1.46)	0.95§ (0.89–1.02)	**0.57 (0.40–0.82)**
		0.05 (0.01–0.08)	***−0.12 (−0.17 to −0.06)***	*0.01 (−0.02 to 0.03)*	*−0.01 (−0.02 to 0.00)*	***−0.04 (−0.06 to −0.02)***
		[7; 24,729]	**[7; 24,104]**	[6; 23,965]	[7; 24,446]	**[5; 22,892]**
Conservative management vs. nonprophylactic pharmacological treatment	RCTs	0.97§ (0.33–2.87)	0.89§ (0.60–1.32)	0.42§ (0.11–1.55)	1.94§ (0.37–10.28)	0.91§ (0.47–1.74)
		0.00 (−0.09 to 0.09)	*−0.05 (−0.22 to 0.12)*	*−0.06 (−0.14 to 0.03)*	*0.03 (−0.04 to 0.09)*	*−0.02 (−0.15 to 0.11)*
		[1; 142]	[1; 131]	[1; 142]	[1; 142]	[1; 142]
	Cohort studies	**1.54 (1.13–2.09)**	**0.60 (0.48–0.76)**	1.01 (0.81–1.26)	0.97§ (0.90–1.04)	**0.57 (0.37–0.87)**
		0.04 (0.00–0.07)	***−0.13 (−0.18 to −0.07)***	*0.00 (−0.02 to 0.01)*	*0.00 (−0.02 to 0.01)*	***−0.04 (−0.06 to −0.01)***
		[6; 18,148]	**[6; 17,779]**	[5; 17,640]	[6; 18,141]	**[4; 16,567]**
Conservative management vs. prophylactic pharmacological treatment	RCTs	1.11§ (0.72–1.69)	0.66 (0.25–1.76)	1.63§ (0.81–3.31)	0.96§ (0.68–1.35)	0.31§ (0.01–7.20)
		0.01 (−0.04 to 0.07)	*−0.06 (−0.19 to 0.07)*	*0.03 (−0.01 to 0.07)*	*−0.01 (−0.06 to 0.05)*	*−0.04 (−0.15 to 0.07)*
		[3; 578]	[3; 578]	[3; 578]	[3; 578]	[1; 48]
	Cohort studies	0.92§ (0.83–1.01)	**0.82§ (0.78–0.87)**	**0.77§ (0.67–0.88)**	0.91§ (0.81–1.01)	**0.66§ (0.59–0.75)**
		−0.01 (−0.03 to 0.00)	***−0.07 (−0.09 to −0.05)***	***−0.02 (−0.03 to −0.01)***	*−0.01 (−0.03 to 0.00)*	***−0.05 (−0.06 to −0.03)***
		[1; 10,075]	**[1; 9,580]**	**[1; 9,580]**	[1; 9,580]	**[1; 9,580]**
Conservative management vs. ligation	RCTs	NA	NA	NA	NA	NA
	Cohort studies	1.25 (0.76–2.05)	**0.36 (0.27–0.47)**	**0.49 (0.35–0.68)**	**0.65 (0.48–0.88)**	**0.23 (0.18–0.31)**
		0.07 (−0.02 to 0.16)	***−0.36 (−0.47 to −0.26)***	***−0.07 (−0.12 to −0.02)***	***−0.09 (−0.15 to −0.03)***	***−0.17 (−0.28 to −0.07)***
		[7; 7,867]	**[7; 8,021]**	**[6; 7,535]**	**[7; 8,020]**	**[6; 7,146]**

Data presented as risk ratio (95% confidence interval) and risk difference (95% confidence interval) after random effect unless otherwise specified, [number of studies; number of patients]. BPD; bronchopulmonary dysplasia, IVH; intraventricular hemorrhage, NA; not available, NEC; necrotizing enterocolitis, RCTs; randomized controlled trials, ROP; retinopathy of prematurity.
§Fixed effect. Significant differences are depicted in bold fonts. To show difference between risk ratio with 95% confidence interval in non-italic font, risk difference with 95% confidence interval in italic and number of studies/patients within brackets.

TABLE 7 | Patient characteristics of cohort studies with subgroup without patent ductus arteriosus.

	Patient characteristics					
	Conservative management			No or asymptomatic PDA		
References	Infants (male/*N*)	GA (weeks)	BW (grams)	Infants (male/N)	GA (weeks)	BW (g)
Härkin et al. (26)	98/182	28.82 ± 2.41	1,225 ± 402	1,398/2,536†	**29.7 ± 1.9**	**1,340 ± 371**
Heuchan et al. (27)	4/7	27 [25–28]	1,046 [680–1,440]	3/7	26 [24–28]	912 [500–1,440]
Laughon et al. (28)	2,201/3,886	27 [26–29]	970 [750–1,220]	9,796/18,136	**29 [27–30]**	**1,170 [895–1,400]**

Data presented as number, mean ± standard deviation or median [interquartile range]. Statistical difference between other treatment groups in same study are in bold.
BW; birth weight, GA; gestational age, N; total infants, PDA; patent ductus arteriosus.
†Including 182 patients with PDA that were conservatively managed and analyzed separately.

TABLE 8 | Outcome measurements after meta-analysis of cohort studies including patient without patent ductus arteriosus.

Comparison	Mortality	BPD (any definition)	NEC (any stage)	IVH (any grade)	ROP (any stage)
Conservative management vs. any active treatment	1.14 (0.91–1.43) *0.02 (−0.01 to 0.04)* [11; 61,372]	**0.47** **(0.38–0.57)** ***−0.20 (−0.26 to −0.14)*** **[11; 57,400]**	**0.78** **(0.61–0.99)** ***−0.02 (−0.04 to 0.00)*** **[9; 45,831]**	**0.71** **(0.50–0.99)** ***−0.04 (−0.07 to −0.01)*** **[10; 46,266]**	**0.34** **(0.27–0.43)** ***−0.07 (−0.10 to −0.03)*** **[8; 44,371]**
Conservative management vs. any pharmacological treatment	1.20 (0.94–1.54) *0.02 (−0.01 to 0.04)* [7; 45,178]	**0.51** **(0.42–0.61)** ***−0.15 (−0.20 to −0.10)*** **[7; 41,504]**	0.92 (0.63–1.35) *0.00 (−0.03 to 0.02)* [6; 41,785]	0.77 (0.53–1.12) *−0.02 (−0.05 to 0.01)* [7; 42,221]	**0.39** **(0.33–0.46)** ***−0.05 (−0.09 to −0.01)*** **[5; 40,648]**
Conservative management vs. non-prophylactic pharmacological treatment	1.20 (0.97–1.49) *0.01 (−0.01 to 0.04)* [6; 38,597]	**0.47** **(0.39–0.57)** ***−0.16 (−0.22 to −0.10)*** **[6; 35,179]**	0.83 (0.60–1.15) *−0.01 (−0.04 to 0.01)* [5; 35.460]	0.72 (0.50–1.05) *−0.03 (−0.06 to 0.00)* [6; 35,896]	**0.42** **(0.33–0.53)** ***−0.05 (−0.09 to −0.02)*** **[4; 32,138]**
Conservative management vs. prophylactic pharmacological treatment	**0.74** **(0.69–0.79)** ***−0.04 (−0.05 to −0.03)*** **[1; 28,211]**	0.54 (0.51–0.56) *−0.19 (−0.20 to −0.17)* [1; 25,151]	**0.59** **(0.53–0.65)** ***−0.04 (−0.05 to −0.03)*** **[1; 25,151]**	**0.44** **(0.40–0.48)** ***−0.07 (−0.08 to −0.07)*** **[1; 25,151]**	0.35 (0.32–0.39) *−0.09 (−0.10 to −0.08)* [1; 25,151]
Conservative management vs. ligation	0.96 (0.49–1.87) *0.05 (−0.05 to 0.14)* [7; 28,323]	**0.30** **(0.20–0.43)** ***−0.39 (−0.49 to −0.28)*** **[7; 25,428]**	**0.40** **(0.28–0.57)** ***−0.09 (−0.14 to −0.03)*** **[6; 25,410]**	**0.49** **(0.25–0.94)** ***−0.11 (−0.20 to −0.03)*** **[7; 25,782]**	**0.16** **(0.14–0.18)** ***−0.18 (−0.30 to −0.06)*** **[6; 24,909]**

Data presented as risk ratio (95% confidence interval) and risk difference (95% confidence interval) after random effect, [number of studies; number of patients]. Significant differences are depicted in bold fonts.

BPD; bronchopulmonary dysplasia, IVH; intraventricular hemorrhage, NEC; necrotizing enterocolitis, RCTs; randomized controlled trials, ROP; retinopathy of prematurity. To show difference between risk ratio with 95% confidence interval in non-italic font, risk difference with 95% confidence interval in italic and number of studies/patients within brackets.

TABLE 9 | Outcome measurements after meta-analysis of cohort studies including echocardiographic defined patent ductus arteriosus.

Comparison	Mortality	BPD (any definition)	NEC (any stage)	IVH (any grade)	ROP (any stage)
Conservative management versus any active treatment	0.79 (0.35–1.78) *−0.02 (−0.08 to 0.04)* [2; 316]	**0.43 (0.32 to 0.58)** ***−0.38 (−0.49 to −0.27)*** **[2; 287]**	0.94 (0.47 to 1.88) *−0.01 (−0.08 to 0.06)* [2; 316]	0.66 (0.36 to 1.22) *−0.06 (−0.14 to 0.02)* [2; 316]	1.17 (0.39 to 3.54) *0.01 (−0.06 to 0.08)* [1; 178]
Conservative management versus any pharmacological treatment/non -prophylactic pharmacological treatment	0.61 (0.07 to 5.06) *−0.02 (−0.09 to 0.05)* [1; 138]	**0.38 (0.18 to 0.80)** ***−0.30 (−0.47 to −0.14)*** **[1; 132]**	0.76 (0.17 to 3.43) *−0.02 (−0.11 to 0.08)* [1; 138]	0.66 (0.20 to 2.14) *−0.05 (−0.16 to 0.07)* [1; 138]	NA

Data presented as risk ratio (95% confidence interval) and risk difference (95% confidence interval) after fixed effect, [number of studies; number of patients]. Significant differences are depicted in bold fonts. BPD, bronchopulmonary dysplasia; IVH, intraventricular haemorrhage; NA, not available; NEC, necrotizing enterocolitis; RCTs, randomised controlled trials; ROP, retinopathy of prematurity.

To show difference between risk ratio with 95% confidence interval in non-italic font, risk difference with 95% confidence interval in italic and number of studies/patients within brackets.

our hypothesis that the decreased risk for morbidity might be due to the inclusion of relatively well children in the conservative treatment group. Furthermore, treated patients were systematically younger and/or smaller than conservatively treated patients. We also included a subgroup analysis of patients with an echocardiographic confirmed PDA ("worst-case scenario") in an attempt to exclude preterm infants with a small PDA that did not necessitated treatment as it would close spontaneously. In this subgroup, only the risk for BPD was significantly lower for the conservative management group. This might be due to the clinicians' tendency to treat a PDA, even with the same echocardiographic PDA characteristics, in case of ventilator dependency which in itself is a risk factor for BPD (36).

The higher risk for mortality and lower risk for morbidity in conservatively managed infants remained significant in three cohort studies after adjustment for baseline characteristics (26, 28, 34). Only one study observed a significantly lower risk for mortality for conservatively managed infants, without a difference in risk for morbidity. This might be due to differences in neonatal practice overall, since they compared a first epoch

TABLE 10 | Adjusted odds ratio for outcome parameters in non-randomized cohort studies.

Comparison	References	Adjusted for	Mortality	BPD	NEC	IVH	ROP
Conservative management vs. pharmacological treatment	Härkin et al. (26)	GA, SGA, RDS, delivery hospital, and ACS	**2.0 (1.1–3.3)**	**0.5 (0.3–0.9)**	0.8 (0.6–1.1)	0.9 (0.6–1.4)	0.9 (0.4–2.0)
	Laughon et al. (28)	BW, GA, inborn status, and ACS	**1.7 (1.4–2.0)**	**0.7 (0.6–0.8)**	NS	NS	**0.7 (0.6–0.8)**
	Mohamed et al. (31)	GA, BW, sex, and maternal conditions	**0.51 (0.25–0.99)**	0.71 (0.28–1.80)	0.84 (0.46–1.53)	1.31 (0.61–2.81)	1.31 (0.51–3.38)
Conservative management vs. ligation	Härkin et al. (26)	GA, SGA, RDS, delivery hospital, and ACS	1.0 (0.6–2.0)	**0.3 (0.1–0.5)**	**0.5 (0.3–0.8)**	**0.2 (0.1–0.4)**	1.7 (0.3–10.0)
	Sung et al. (34)	GA, BW, SGA, sex, AS^5, and ACS	0.8§ (0.3–2.2)	**0.4§ (0.2–0.8)**	–	–	–
Conservative management vs. pharmacological treatment and/or ligation	Härkin et al. (26)	GA, SGA, RDS, delivery hospital, and ACS	**3.3 (1.4–5.0)**	**0.2 (0.1–0.3)**	0.7 (0.4–1.1)	0.8 (0.5–1.3)	0.7 (0.3–1.7)

Data presented as adjusted odds ratio (95% confidence interval) after multivariable logistic regression unless otherwise specified. Significant differences are bold.
§ Propensity score adjusted.
ACS; antenatal corticosteroids, AS^5; Apgar score at 5 min postpartum, BPD; bronchopulmonary dysplasia, BW; birth weight, CS; Cesarean section, GA; gestational age, IVH; intraventricular hemorrhage, NEC; necrotizing enterocolitis, NS; not significant, RDS; respiratory distress syndrome, ROP; retinopathy of prematurity, SGA; small for gestational age.

characterized by active pharmacological treatment (2001–2009) with a second epoch with predominantly a conservative management (2010–2014) (31). The composite outcome, heterogeneously defined as mortality and/or morbidity, was significantly lower in the conservatively managed group (7, 30, 34).

Adjustment for baseline perinatal characteristics does not completely reduce treatment selection bias in the cohort studies, since they cannot correct for all relevant clinical conditions after birth and potential unmeasured confounders. These confounders might have influenced the clinician's decision whether or not to treat a PDA in an infant. The importance of these confounders might be crucial, since in analogy the association between ligation and morbidity lost significance only after the adjustment for postnatal, preligation covariates like sepsis, cardiovascular drug support, NEC, and severe IVH (9).

We could not replicate the finding that prophylactic treatment significantly reduces the risk of IVH (3). This might be due to our exclusion criteria, since most trials regarding prophylactic indomethacin were conducted before 2000 and/or had >25% open-label active treatment in the placebo group (37). In the only included cohort comparing conservative management to prophylactic treatment, although conservatively treated infants were significantly less mature, there was no difference in IVH in both the adjusted and unadjusted analysis (28).

This systematic literature review highlights the main pitfalls of the available evidence regarding PDA treatment in preterm and/or VLBW infants. Eligible RCTs are scarce, due to our strict inclusion criteria. Consequentially, most included studies were retrospective cohort studies with the accompanying heterogeneity and higher risk of bias. Heterogeneity occurred due to different diagnostic approaches and variety in used definition of (hs)PDA. Conservative management in the included studies was predominantly classified as no treatment with indomethacin, ibuprofen, acetaminophen, and/or ligation. If specifically defined, it was highly variable from watchful waiting to the use of diuretics and/or fluid restriction and/or ventilator adjustments.

With the currently available literature regarding conservative PDA management, one might conclude that it appears safe to wait for delayed spontaneous closure based on RCT data. However, cohort studies suggest that conservative management is associated with a higher risk for mortality, but a lower risk for morbidity, albeit with a very low level of evidence. Therefore, a conservative management cannot be generalized to all preterm infants with a PDA and considered evidence-based practice at this moment.

Instead of dichotomizing a PDA as present or not, one should consider the PDA as a spectrum in which the amount of shunt volume across the PDA is thought to be associated with adverse outcome. To asses shunt volume (neonatologist performed), echocardiography could play an important role (38). Additional objective measurements indicative of transductal left-to-right shunt volume, rather than DA diameter alone, could better indicate hemodynamic significance, for example, the PDA severity score (39).

The high amount of active treatment in cohort studies and open-label treatment in RCTs suggests that in case of PDA associated morbidities clinicians might try to rule

TABLE 11 | Adjusted odds ratio for composite outcome in cohort studies.

References	Adjusted for	Cohort	Composite outcome according to comparison		
			Conservative management vs. pharmacological treatment	**Conservative management vs. ligation**	**Conservative management vs. pharmacological treatment and/or ligation**
Lokku et al. (30)†	GA, SGA, sex, SNAP II score >20, outborn, maternal hypertension, and ACS	2006–2008 2009–2012	1.05 (0.79–1.41) **0.61 (0.51–0.74)**	**0.53 (0.31–0.93)** **0.24 (0.13–0.43)**	**0.36 (0.23–0.56)** **0.27 (0.19–0.38)**
Mirea et al. (7)†	GA, SGA, sex, SNAP II >20, year of birth, site, inborn/outborn,		0.91 (0.72–1.16)	**0.56 (0.37–0.87)**	**0.43 (0.30–0.60)**
	maternal hypertension, gestational		0.99§ (0.76–1.28)	**0.52§ (0.29–0.93)**	**0.45§ (0.29–0.70)**
	diabetes, chorioamnionitis, and ACS		0.99§§ (0.72–1.35)	**0.59§§ (0.42–0.82)**	**0.80§§ (0.66–0.97)**
Sung et al. (34)††	GA, BW, SGA, AS5, sex, and ACS		–	**0.5§ (0.2–0.9)**	–

Data presented as adjusted odds ratio (95% confidence interval) after multivariable logistic regression unless otherwise specified. Significant differences are bold.
ACS; antenatal corticosteroids, AS5; Apgar score at 5 min postpartum, BW; birth weight, GA; gestational age, SGA; small for gestational age, SNAP II; Score for Neonatal Acute Physiology, version II.
§ Propensity score adjusted.
§§ Propensity score matched.
† Composite outcome defined as mortality or any severe morbidity (IVH grade ≥3, or periventricular leukomalacia, ROP stage ≥3, BPD defined as oxygen need at 36 weeks postmenstrual age and NEC stages ≥2).
†† Composite outcome defined as mortality or BPD.

out a putative causal role of a PDA and therefor initiate active treatment in an attempt to achieve PDA closure. As included cohort studies mainly stratified patients regarding their final PDA treatment ("as treated"), instead of the initial management to which RCTs randomize ("intention to treat"), our meta-analysis could not correct for treatment selection bias, which is one of the main limitations.

The tendency of clinicians to actively close the DA in case of associated findings, hence absence of clinical equipoise, remains one of the main limitations in RCTs. In the PDA TOLERATE trial (40), 48% of the patients allocated to conservative management received open-label active treatment, referred to as "rescue" treatment (40). For future RCTs, we would suggest defining "open-label treatment" criteria as "rescue treatment" insinuates treatment is superior to conservative management in preterm infants with a PDA for which evidence is lacking. Together with the different types of bias in both RCTs and cohort studies rescue treatment contributes to the everlasting conundrum on PDA management.

In conclusion, we found no differences in outcome in the included RCTs. Our meta-analysis highlights the lack of high-quality evidence for conservative management for PDA in preterm infants.

The current trend toward conservative management cannot be justified based on these scarce, mainly retrospective and very heterogeneous cohort studies. Further cohort studies will not be able to provide a final and conclusive answer to the question whether we should consider a PDA in preterm infants as an epiphenomenon which can be managed conservatively or as an important causal factor or contributing factor to adverse outcome in preterm infants. High-quality RCTs with a conservative management group with a limited—preferably without—open-label treatment rate are needed to elucidate the conundrum whether or not to treat a PDA in extremely preterm infants.

AUTHOR CONTRIBUTIONS

TH, EJ, and WB initiated the idea for this systematic review and meta-analysis. TH, WB, and WO contributed to the design of the study. Data acquisition and analysis were done by TH and EJ. WO, EK, PA, and WB revised the article critically for important intellectual content. All authors approved the final version.

ACKNOWLEDGMENTS

We would like to thank Dr. R. Donders, biostatistician for his input on the statistical analysis plan of this systematic review and meta-analysis.

REFERENCES

1. Lee JA, Kim MJ, Oh S, Choi BM. Current status of therapeutic strategies for patent ductus arteriosus in very-low-birth-weight infants in Korea. *J Korean Med Sci.* (2015) 30(Suppl. 1):S59–66. doi: 10.3346/jkms.2015.30.S1.S59
2. Brooks JM, Travadi JN, Patole SK, Doherty DA, Simmer K. Is surgical ligation of patent ductus arteriosus necessary? The Western Australian experience of conservative management. *Arch Dis Child Fetal Neonatal Ed.* (2005) 90:F235–9. doi: 10.1136/adc.2004.057638
3. Fowlie PW, Davis PG, McGuire W. Prophylactic intravenous indomethacin for preventing mortality and morbidity in preterm infants. *Cochrane Database Syst Rev.* (2010) 2010:CD000174. doi: 10.1002/14651858.CD000174.pub2
4. Mitra S, Florez ID, Tamayo ME, Mbuagbaw L, Vanniyasingam T, Veroniki AA, et al. Association of placebo, indomethacin, ibuprofen, and acetaminophen with closure of hemodynamically significant patent ductus arteriosus in preterm infants: a systematic review and meta-analysis. *JAMA.* (2018) 319:1221–38. doi: 10.1001/jama.2018.1896
5. Zonnenberg I, de Waal K. The definition of a haemodynamic significant duct in randomized controlled trials: a systematic literature review. *Acta Paediatr* (2012) 101:247–51. doi: 10.1111/j.1651-2227.2011.02468.x
6. Hundscheid T, Onland W, van Overmeire B, Dijk P, van Kaam A, Dijkman KP, et al. Early treatment versus expectative management of patent ductus arteriosus in preterm infants: a multicentre, randomised, non-inferiority trial in Europe (BeNeDuctus trial). *BMC Pediatr.* (2018) 18:262. doi: 10.1186/s12887-018-1215-7
7. Mirea L, Sankaran K, Seshia M, Ohlsson A, Allen AC, Aziz K, et al. Treatment of patent ductus arteriosus and neonatal mortality/morbidities: adjustment for treatment selection bias. *J Pediatr.* (2012) 161:689–94.e1. doi: 10.1016/j.jpeds.2012.05.007
8. Weisz DE, Mirea L, Resende MHF, Ly L, Church PT, Kelly E, et al. Outcomes of surgical ligation after unsuccessful pharmacotherapy for patent ductus arteriosus in neonates born extremely preterm. *J Pediatr.* (2018) 195:292–6 e3. doi: 10.1016/j.jpeds.2017.11.029
9. Weisz DE, Mirea L, Rosenberg E, Jang M, Ly L, Church PT, et al. Association of patent ductus arteriosus ligation with death or neurodevelopmental impairment among extremely preterm infants. *JAMA Pediatr.* (2017) 171:443–9. doi: 10.1001/jamapediatrics.2016.5143
10. Ngo S, Profit J, Gould JB, Lee HC. Trends in patent ductus arteriosus diagnosis and management for very low birth weight infants. *Pediatrics.* (2017) 139:e20162390. doi: 10.1542/peds.2016-2390
11. Farooqui MA, Elsayed Y, Jeyaraman MM, Dingwall O, Tagin M, Zarychanski R, et al. Pre-symptomatic targeted treatment of patent ductus arteriosus in preterm newborns: a systematic review and meta-analysis. *J Neonatal Perinatal Med.* (2018) 12:1–7. doi: 10.3233/NPM-17130
12. Sung SI, Chang YS, Kim J, Choi JH, Ahn SY, Park WS. Natural evolution of ductus arteriosus with noninterventional conservative management in extremely preterm infants born at 23–28 weeks of gestation. *PLoS ONE.* (2019) 14:e0212256. doi: 10.1371/journal.pone.0212256
13. Semberova J, Sirc J, Miletin J, Kucera J, Berka I, Sebkova S, et al. Spontaneous closure of patent ductus arteriosus in infants $\leq$ 1500 g. *Pediatrics.* (2017) 140:e20164258. doi: 10.1542/peds.2016-4258
14. Weber SC, Weiss K, Buhrer C, Hansmann G, Koehne P, Sallmon H. Natural history of patent ductus arteriosus in very low birth weight infants after discharge. *J Pediatr.* (2015) 167:1149–51. doi: 10.1016/j.jpeds.2015.06.032
15. Moher D, Liberati A, Tetzlaff J, Altman DG, Group P. Preferred reporting items for systematic reviews and meta-analyses: the PRISMA statement. *J Clin Epidemiol.* (2009) 62:1006–12. doi: 10.1016/j.jclinepi.2009.06.005
16. Higgins JP, Altman DG, Gotzsche PC, Juni P, Moher D, Oxman AD, et al. The cochrane collaboration's tool for assessing risk of bias in randomised trials. *BMJ.* (2011) 343:d5928. doi: 10.1136/bmj.d5928
17. Wells GA, Shea B, O'Connell D, Peterson J, Welch V, Losos M. *The Newcastle-Ottawa Scale (NOS) for Assessing the Quality of Nonrandomized Studies in Meta-Analyses.* (2000). Available online at: http://www.ohri.ca/programs/clinical_epidemiology/oxford.htm (accessed June 1, 2020).
18. Serghiou S, Goodman SN. Random-effects meta-analysis: summarizing evidence with caveats. *JAMA.* (2019) 321:301–2. doi: 10.1001/jama.2018.19684
19. GRADE. *Handbook for Grading Quality of Evidence and Strength of Recommendations: The GRADE Working Group.* (2013). Available online at: guidelinedevelopment.org/handbook (accessed June 1, 2020).
20. Harkin P, Harma A, Aikio O, Valkama M, Leskinen M, Saarela T, et al. Paracetamol accelerates closure of the ductus arteriosus after premature birth: a randomized trial. *J Pediatr.* (2016) 177:72–7 e2. doi: 10.1016/j.jpeds.2016.04.066
21. Kumar Nair PA, Pai MG, Gazal HA, Da Costa DE, Al Khusaiby SM. Indomethacin prophylaxis for intraventricular hemorrhage in very low birth weight babies. *Indian Pediatr.* (2004) 41:551–8.
22. Sung SI, Lee MH, Ahn SY, Chang YS, Park WS. Effect of nonintervention vs oral ibuprofen in patent ductus arteriosus in preterm infants: a randomized clinical trial. *JAMA Pediatr.* (2020) 174:755–63. doi: 10.1001/jamapediatrics.2020.1447
23. Van Overmeire B, Allegaert K, Casaer A, Debauche C, Decaluwe W, Jespers A, et al. Prophylactic ibuprofen in premature infants: a multicentre, randomised, double-blind, placebo-controlled trial. *Lancet.* (2004) 364:1945–9. doi: 10.1016/S0140-6736(04)17477-1
24. Alexander F, Chiu L, Kroh M, Hammel J, Moore J. Analysis of outcome in 298 extremely low-birth-weight infants with patent ductus arteriosus. *J Pediatr Surg.* (2009) 44:112–7. disscusion 7. doi: 10.1016/j.jpedsurg.2008.10.019
25. Bourgoin L, Cipierre C, Hauet Q, Basset H, Gournay V, Roze JC, et al. Neurodevelopmental outcome at 2 years of age according to patent ductus arteriosus management in very preterm infants. *Neonatology.* (2016) 109:139–46. doi: 10.1159/000442278
26. Harkin P, Marttila R, Pokka T, Saarela T, Hallman M. Morbidities associated with patent ductus arteriosus in preterm infants. Nationwide cohort study. *J Matern Fetal Neonatal Med.* (2018) 31:2576–83. doi: 10.1080/14767058.2017.1347921
27. Heuchan AM, Young D. Early colour doppler duct diameter and symptomatic patent ductus arteriosus in a cyclo-oxygenase inhibitor naive population. *Acta Paediatr, Int J Paediatr.* (2013) 102:254–7. doi: 10.1111/apa.12103
28. Laughon M, Bose C, Clark R. Treatment strategies to prevent or close a patent ductus arteriosus in preterm infants and outcomes. *J Perinatol.* (2007) 27:164–70. doi: 10.1038/sj.jp.7211662
29. Letshwiti JB, Semberova J, Pichova K, Dempsey EM, Franklin OM, Miletin J. A conservative treatment of patent ductus arteriosus in very low birth weight infants. *Early Hum Dev.* (2017) 104:45–9. doi: 10.1016/j.earlhumdev.2016.12.008
30. Lokku A, Mirea L, Lee SK, Shah PS. Trends and outcomes of patent ductus arteriosus treatment in very preterm infants in Canada. *Am J Perinatol.* (2017) 34:441–50. doi: 10.1055/s-0036-1593351
31. Mohamed MA, El-Dib M, Alqahtani S, Alyami K, Ibrahim AN, Aly H. Patent ductus arteriosus in premature infants: to treat or not to treat? *J Perinatol.* (2017) 37:652–7. doi: 10.1038/jp.2017.4
32. Sadeck LS, Leone CR, Procianoy RS, Guinsburg R, Marba ST, Martinez FE, et al. Effects of therapeutic approach on the neonatal evolution of very low birth weight infants with patent ductus arteriosus. *J Pediatr.* (2014) 90:616–23. doi: 10.1016/j.jped.2014.04.010
33. Slaughter JL, Reagan PB, Newman TB, Klebanoff MA. Comparative effectiveness of nonsteroidal anti-inflammatory drug treatment vs no treatment for patent ductus arteriosus in preterm infants. *JAMA Pediatr.* (2017) 171:e164354. doi: 10.1001/jamapediatrics.2016.4354
34. Sung SI, Chang YS, Chun JY, Yoon SA, Yoo HS, Ahn SY, et al. Mandatory closure versus nonintervention for patent ductus arteriosus in very preterm infants. *J Pediatr.* (2016) 177:66–71 e1. doi: 10.1016/j.jpeds.2016.06.046
35. Isayama T, Mirea L, Mori R, Kusuda S, Fujimura M, Lee SK, et al. Patent ductus arteriosus management and outcomes in Japan and Canada: comparison of proactive and selective approaches. *Am J Perinatol.* (2015) 32:1087–94. doi: 10.1055/s-0035-1548727
36. Clyman RI, Hills NK. The effect of prolonged tracheal intubation on the association between patent ductus arteriosus and bronchopulmonary dysplasia (grades 2 and 3). *J Perinatol.* (2020) 40:1358–65. doi: 10.1038/s41372-020-0718-x
37. Schmidt B, Davis P, Moddemann D, Ohlsson A, Roberts RS, Saigal S, et al. Long-term effects of indomethacin prophylaxis in extremely-low-birth-weight infants. *N Engl J Med.* (2001) 344:1966–72. doi: 10.1056/NEJM2001062834 42602

38. van Laere D, van Overmeire B, Gupta S, El-Khuffash A, Savoia M, McNamara PJ, et al. Application of NPE in the assessment of a patent ductus arteriosus. *Pediatr Res.* (2018) 84(Suppl. 1):46–56. doi: 10.1038/s41390-018-0077-x
39. El-Khuffash A, James AT, Corcoran JD, Dicker P, Franklin O, Elsayed YN, et al. A patent ductus arteriosus severity score predicts chronic lung disease or death before discharge. *J Pediatr.* (2015) 167:1354–61.e2. doi: 10.1016/j.jpeds.2015.09.028
40. Clyman RI, Liebowitz M, Kaempf J, Erdeve O, Bulbul A, Hakansson S, et al. PDA-TOLERATE trial: an exploratory randomized controlled trial of treatment of moderate-to-large patent ductus arteriosus at 1 week of age. *J Pediatr.* (2018) *205:41–8.e6*. doi: 10.1016/j.jpeds.2018.09.012

17

Factors Associated with Benefit of Treatment of Patent Ductus Arteriosus in Preterm Infants

Esther J. S. Jansen [1], Tim Hundscheid [1], Wes Onland [2], Elisabeth M. W. Kooi [3], Peter Andriessen [4,5] and Willem P. de Boode [1]*

[1] Radboud University Medical Center Nijmegen, Radboud Institute for Health Sciences, Amalia Children's Hospital, Nijmegen, Netherlands, [2] Emma Children's Hospital, Amsterdam University Medical Centers, VU University Medical Center, University of Amsterdam, Amsterdam, Netherlands, [3] University Medical Center Groningen, Beatrix Children's Hospital, University of Groningen, Groningen, Netherlands, [4] Máxima Medical Center, Veldhoven, Netherlands, [5] Department of Applied Physics, School of Medical Physics and Engineering, Eindhoven University of Technology, Eindhoven, Netherlands

***Correspondence:**
Esther J. S. Jansen
esther.jansen@radboudumc.nl

Context: There is an ongoing debate on the optimal management of patent ductus arteriosus (PDA) in preterm infants. Identifying subgroup of infants who would benefit from pharmacological treatment might help.

Objective: To investigate the modulating effect of the differences in methodological quality, the rate of open-label treatment, and patient characteristics on relevant outcome measures in randomized controlled trials (RCTs).

Data Sources: Electronic database search between 1950 and May 2020.

Study Selection: RCTs that assessed pharmacological treatment compared to placebo/no treatment.

Data Extraction: Data is extracted following the PRISMA guidelines. Outcome measures were failure to ductal closure, surgical ligation, incidence of necrotizing enterocolitis, bronchopulmonary dysplasia, sepsis, periventricular leukomalacia, intraventricular hemorrhage (IVH) grade ≥3, retinopathy of prematurity and mortality.

Results: Forty-seven studies were eligible. The incidence of IVH grade ≥3 was lower in the treated infants compared to the placebo/no treatment (RR 0.77, 95% CI 0.64–0.94) and in the subgroups of infants with either a gestational age <28 weeks (RR 0.77, 95% CI 0.61–0.98), a birth weight <1,000 g (RR 0.77, 95% CI 0.61–0.97), or if untargeted treatment with indomethacin was started <24 h after birth (RR 0.70, 95% CI 0.54–0.90).

Limitations: Statistical heterogeneity caused by missing data and variable definitions of outcome parameters.

Conclusions: Although the quality of evidence is low, this meta-analysis suggests that pharmacological treatment of PDA reduces severe IVH in extremely preterm, extremely low birth weight infants or if treatment with indomethacin was started <24 h after birth. No other beneficial effects of pharmacological treatment were found.

Keywords: ductus botalli, patent ductus arteriosis, premature (babies), ibuprofen, indometacin, acetaminophen

INTRODUCTION

Patent ductus arteriosus (PDA) is common in preterm and very low birth weight infants (1). Persistence is associated with a higher risk of morbidities, including bronchopulmonary dysplasia (BPD), necrotizing enterocolitis (NEC), and intraventricular hemorrhage (IVH), and mortality (2). Nevertheless, pharmacological treatment or surgical closure of PDA is not without adverse effects (3, 4). After many decades of clinical research, the question remains open if, when, and how PDA should be treated in preterm infants (5). Globally, there has been a shift from early pharmacological treatment toward a more expectant management policy (6). A uniform definition of a hemodynamic significant PDA does not exist, nor is there clear evidence in favor of or against many of the approaches to treating PDA (7–9). Since 1976 we know that pharmacological treatment is an effective way of ductal closure (10). A recent meta-analysis, however, showed that neither short-term nor long-term outcomes seem to differ between treated and untreated patients (11). This sparked an ongoing debate on the optimal approach to treating PDA, which ranges from expectant management to aggressive treatment with a variety of cyclooxygenase inhibitors or acetaminophen with varying doses and at different intervals (5). Although the results of randomized controlled trails (RCTs) on PDA treatment have been reviewed extensively, only a small number of reviews stratified the results according to infant characteristics, methodological quality (11, 12), timing of treatment (12), or to the definitions of a hemodynamic significant PDA (9).

To the best of our knowledge this is the first comprehensive systematic review of RCTs to investigate the modulating effect of the methodological quality, the rate of open-label treatment in the placebo/no treatment groups, and several patient characteristics on the benefits, or adverse effects, of pharmacological treatment of PDA in preterm infants. We aim to identify specific subgroups of preterm infants at high risk of adverse outcomes, who would benefit from active closure of PDA.

METHODS

Our study is performed in accordance with the Preferred Reporting Items for Systematic Reviews and Meta-Analyses (PRISMA) guidelines (13).

Search Strategy

We searched the following databases: PubMed, the Ovid Embase, and the Cochrane Library. We searched for papers published between 1950 up to and including April 2020. By using the Boolean operators AND and OR, we used all possible combinations of the following search terms: infant, newborn, neonate, preterm, premature, ductus, arteriosus, Botalli. We also used the Mesh terms "Infant, premature," "Ductus Arteriosus, Patent," and "Ductus Arteriosus" in the PubMed database. The complete search strategy can be found in **Supplement 1.** Subsequently, we assessed the publications cited by the selected studies for relevant material eligible for possible additional inclusion.

Study Selection

Three authors (EJ, TH, and WdB) independently screened the publications identified in our initial search for eligibility on the basis of their titles and abstracts. Where disagreement arose, the full text was assessed and then discussed in order to reach consensus. We selected studies with a RCT design and written in either English, Dutch, or German. Generally speaking, we included all studies that assessed pharmacological treatment with either ibuprofen, indomethacin, or acetaminophen vs. placebo/no treatment. We excluded animal studies, studies on antenatal treatment, studies that included patients with a post term age of more than 1 month, and studies concerning patients with a congenital heart defect.

Data Extraction

Two authors (EJ and TH) performed data extraction. The data we extracted from the selected studies were general study parameters, demographic parameters pertaining to the participants, treatment regime(s), and outcomes. We collected the parameters study design, total number of patients, mean gestational age (GA), birth weight (BW), postnatal age (PNA) at the start of treatment, and the rate of open-label treatment in the placebo/no treatment group. The following outcome parameters were collected (if reported in the studies) and analyzed: mortality, failure to close the DA, the need for surgical ligation, the incidence of NEC (any definition), BPD (any definition), sepsis, periventricular leukomalacia (PVL), IVH grade ≥ 3, retinopathy of prematurity (ROP), oliguria, other respiratory morbidity (e.g., pneumothorax), other gastrointestinal morbidity [e.g., spontaneous intestinal perforation (SIP)], and long-term neurodevelopmental impairment. In case of missing data, we tried to contact the corresponding authors of the studies in question and requested them to kindly provide these data.

Statistical Analysis

As ibuprofen, indomethacin, and acetaminophen are comparable regarding their effectiveness in DA closure (11, 14), but their side effect profiles may differ (11, 14), we performed two analyses. In the first analysis we combined all studies reporting either of these three drugs in comparison with placebo/no treatment. In a second analysis we divided the studies according to which drug was used. Subgroups were made, related to known risk factors (GA, BW) and other factors influencing efficacy of treatment, such as PNA. Moreover, the consequences of open label treatment percentage in the control group were analyzed since this is an important methodologic flaw in the RCTs. The following strata were analyzed: BW in five subgroups: <1,000 g, 1,000–1,250 g, 1,251–1,500 g, >1,500 g, and data unknown; GA in four subgroups: <28 weeks, 28–33 weeks, >33 weeks, and data unknown; PNA at the start of treatment in four subgroups: <24 h, 24–72 h, >72 h, and data unknown. Studies with start of treatment <24 h PNA were divided into untargeted (start treatment irrespective whether the ductus is open or closed) and targeted (start treatment only after clinically and/or echocardiographically confirmation of a PDA) treatment. The rate of open-label treatment in the placebo/no treatment arm was expressed as a percentage and divided into four groups:

<25%, 25–50%, >50%, and data unknown. For statistical analysis we used Review Manager (RevMan version 5.3 Copenhagen: The Nordic Cochrane Center, The Cochrane Collaboration, 2014). The risk ratio (RR) and risk difference (RD) with a 95% confidence interval (CI) were calculated with the Mantel-Haenszel method. We calculated the number needed to treat (NNT) with a 95% CI for each different outcome in case of statistical significance. We used random-effect meta-analysis if the heterogeneity (I^2) was >50% (15) and fixed-effect in case of low heterogeneity.

Risk of Bias

We critically examined the methodological quality of the selected studies and the risk of bias in accordance with the Cochrane guidelines (16). The quality parameters included the type of analysis, random sequence generation, allocation concealment, blinding of participants and personnel, and blinding of outcome assessment. Two authors (EJ and TH) assessed the risk of bias assessment. When disagreement arose, a third author (WdB) assessed the studies in order to reach consensus. The risk of bias was calculated (low risk: 1 point, unclear risk: 2 points, and high risk: 3 points) and the cumulative score was divided into three subgroups: low (7–9 points in total), intermediate (10–12 points), and high (13–21 points). We examined the methodological quality of the studies' outcome parameters with the GRADE method (17). We assessed imprecision as serious if the total number of events was <300 or if the width of the CI of the RR was >0.25. We used the GRADE-pro GDT 2016

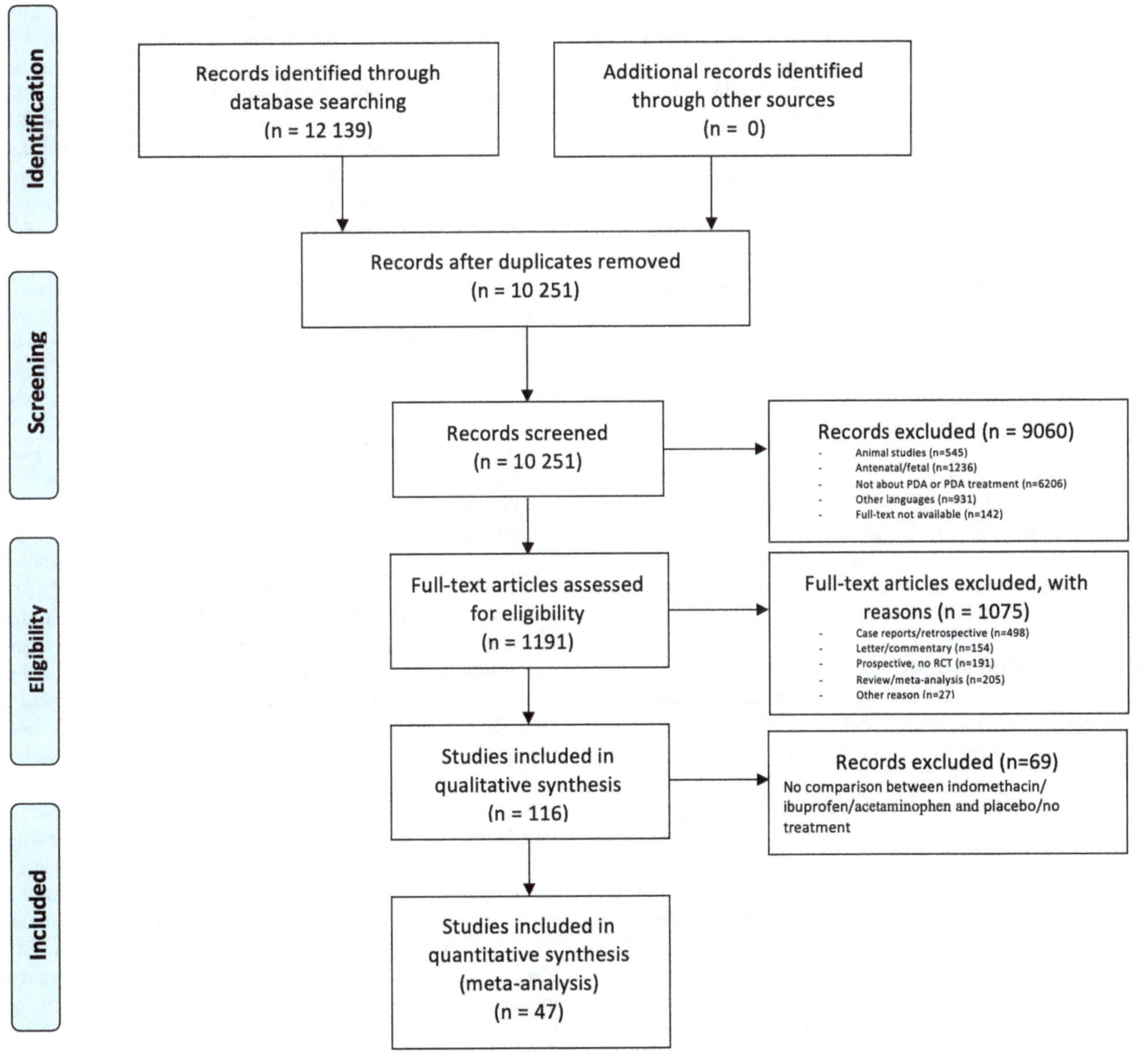

FIGURE 1 | PRISMA flow diagram.

software [GRADEpro Guideline Development Tool (Software) McMaster University, 2015] to create a "summary of findings" table to report the quality of evidence. The GRADE approach results in an assessment of the quality of a body of evidence in one of four grades: high, moderate, low, or very low.

RESULTS

Study Selection

Out of the 12,139 articles we identified 10,251 as unique in our initial search. After selection (see **Figure 1**) a final 47 papers were eligible, comprising a total of 5,242 infants (18–64).

Study Characteristics and Risk of Bias

The relevant characteristics of the 47 papers are described in **Table 1** (18–64). Thirty-two (68%) of the studies analyzed the effect of indomethacin (18–44, 46, 47, 55, 60, 61), 12 (26%) studied the effect of ibuprofen (45, 48–54, 56–59), two (4%) studied acetaminophen (62, 64), and one (2%) studied the effect of either indomethacin, ibuprofen, or acetaminophen (63). Thirteen papers (28%) included preterm infants with a mean GA < 28 weeks (42, 44, 46–48, 50, 53, 55–58, 61, 63), and 30 (64%) included infants with a mean GA between 28 and 32 weeks (18, 20–24, 26–30, 32–41, 43, 45, 47, 49, 51, 52, 59, 60, 62, 64). Seventeen papers (36%) included preterm infants with a mean BW < 1,000 g (33, 35, 39, 41–46, 48, 50, 53, 55, 56, 58, 61, 63), and 19 (40%) included infants weighing between 1,000 and 1,250 g (20, 22–24, 27–30, 34, 36–38, 40, 47, 49, 52, 57, 62, 64). Most studies (62%) investigated treatment that was started within 24 h' PNA (26, 29, 30, 32, 34, 35, 37–53, 55, 58, 60–62, 64). More than two third of the studies reported the rate of open-label treatment, namely 25–50% in 16 (34%) (20, 22, 31, 32, 36, 37, 42, 46, 48, 50, 52, 53, 58, 60, 61, 63), and >50% in 15 (32%) studies (18, 19, 23–25, 27, 33, 34, 40, 43, 45, 47, 51, 55, 56). The median rate of the open-label treatment was 44.5% (range 0–85%). Twenty-one studies (45%) were classified as having a low risk of bias (18, 21–23, 25, 27, 29, 31, 33, 37, 38, 42, 43, 46, 47, 49, 50, 53, 56, 61, 62). Six papers (13%) were assessed as having a high risk of bias (19, 26, 34, 39, 40, 63).

Outcome Measures

Despite our efforts to contact the corresponding authors and our request to provide missing data, not all data on GA, BW and rate of open-label treatment could be retrieved. Data on GA (19, 25, 31) and/or BW (25, 31, 60) were unavailable in four trials (453 and 499 infants for GA and BW, respectively). The rate of open-label treatment was unavailable for nine trials (21, 26, 28, 30, 39, 44, 57, 59, 64).

RR of outcomes, stratified by the patient characteristics, the quality of the studies, and the rate of open-label treatment in the placebo/no treatment group are described in **Table 2**. The meta-analyses revealed that in comparison to placebo/no treatment, the administration of indomethacin, ibuprofen, or acetaminophen resulted in a significantly reduced risk of failed ductal closure (RR 0.40, 95% CI 0.33–0.48; RD −0.32, 95% CI −0.38, −0.27; NNT 3.4, 95% CI 3.1–3.7) or risk of surgical ligation (RR 0.61, 95% CI 0.49–0.76; RD −0.04, 95% CI −0.06, −0.02; NNT 22.8, 95% CI 15.8–40.7), irrespective of the used drug. This result was similar for the subcategories based on mean BW, GA, and PNA at the start of treatment. The quality of evidence was graded as very low or very low to low, respectively (**Supplement 2**).

We found no difference for BPD, NEC, sepsis, PVL, ROP or mortality between the intervention and control group overall, or in any of the subgroups (**Table 2**), irrespective of the used drug. In most studies BPD was defined as supplemental oxygen requirement at 28 days' PNA or at 36 weeks' postmenstrual age (PMA). Seven RCTs used radiographic criteria (19, 22, 26, 31, 33, 35, 36). Four RCTs did not state their definition of BPD clearly (32, 43, 51, 52). Neither the overall meta-analyses nor the subgroup analyses of the 28 days' PNA and 36 weeks' PMA definition of BPD revealed any differences between the placebo/no treatment and the pharmacological treatment group.

Twenty-eight out of 47 studies started the treatment <24 h PNA. Of these 28 studies, five started treatment only after clinically and/or echocardiographically confirmation of a PDA (targeted treatment) (26, 47, 51, 52, 61). All the other RCTs started irrespective whether the ductus was open or closed within the first 24 h after birth (untargeted treatment).

Compared to the no treatment group, the infants allocated to the pharmacological treatment group had a lower risk of IVH grade ≥3 (RR 0.76, 95% CI 0.62–0.93; RD −0.03, 95% CI −0.05, −0.01; NNT 34, 95% CI 18.9–136.6). This reduced risk of IVH grade ≥3 was also observed in the subgroups GA <28 weeks (RR 0.77, 95% CI 0.61–0.98; RD −0.03, 95% CI −0.06, −0.00; NNT 30.3, 95% CI 16.1–262.9), BW <1,000 g (RR 0.77, 95% CI 0.61–0.97; RD −0.03, 95% CI −0.06, −0.00; NNT 30.2, 95% CI 16.4–199.9), or if treatment was given untargeted <24 h' PNA (RR 0.70; 95% CI 0.57–0.87; RD −0.04, 95% CI −0.06, −0.02; NNT 26, 95% CI 15.7–64.1).

We found a significant reduction in severe IVH only when untargeted treatment with indomethacin was used < 24 h PNA compared to no treatment (RR 0.70, 95% CI 0.54–0.90; RD −0.04, 95% CI −0.07, −0.01). Forest plots for the risk of IVH grade ≥3 are depicted for the different subgroups in **Figure 2**. Furthermore, the incidence of IVH grade ≥3 in the treatment group was significantly lower in the low and intermediate risk of bias groups and if the rate of open-label treatment was 25–50%. The quality of evidence was graded as very low to low (**Supplement 2**).

Subgroup analyses of the other outcome measurements proved impossible on account of the scarcity of available data. Five RCTs described data on oliguria (37, 40–42, 62). Five studies described the incidence of pneumothorax (30, 32, 37–39), six studies pulmonary hemorrhage (37, 42, 46, 60, 61, 63), and one study reported pulmonary hypertension as outcome measure (60). Five studies described the incidence of gastrointestinal bleeding (24, 27, 32, 40, 61), while two studies reported the incidence of SIP (46, 61). Only three RCTs described the long-term data on neurodevelopmental outcomes regarding motor delay, cognitive delay, the incidence of deafness and blindness, and neurodevelopmental impairment in general (44, 46, 64).

TABLE 1 | Treatment, patient and, study characteristics of the RCTs included.

References	Patients (n)	Treatment characteristics			Patient characteristics		Study characteristics								
		Intervention	Control	Start at PNA	GA (w)	BW (g)	Open-label treatment	1	2	3	4	5	6	7	Risk of bias
Nestrud et al. (18)	23	Indomethacin	Placebo	> 72 h	28–32	1,251–1,500	> 50%	+	+	+	?	+	+	?	Low
Merritt et al. (19)	24	Indomethacin	No treatment	24–72 h	unknown	1,251–1,500	> 50%	–	–	–	?	–	+	?	High
Neu et al. (20)	21	Indomethacin	Placebo	> 72 h	28–32	1,000–1,250	25–50%	?	+	+	+	–	+	?	Intermediate
Yanagi et al. (21)	17	Indomethacin	Placebo	> 72 h	28–32	1,251–1,500	unknown	+	+	+	?	+	+	?	Low
Yeh et al. (22)	55	Indomethacin	Placebo	> 72 h	28–32	1,000–1,250	25–50%	+	?	+	+	+	+	?	Low
Mahony et al. (23)	47	Indomethacin	Placebo	> 72 h	28–32	1,000–1,250	> 50%	+	+	+	+	+	+	?	Low
Mullett et al. (24)	47	Indomethacin	Placebo	> 72 h	28–32	1,000–1,250	> 50%	?	+	+	?	+	–	?	Intermediate
Gersony et al. (25)	405	Indomethacin	Placebo	> 72 h	unknown	unknown	> 50%	+	+	+	?	+	+	?	Low
Kaapa et al. (26)	27	Indomethacin	No treatment	<24 h T	28–32	>1,500	unknown	+	?	–	?	?	+	?	High
Rudd et al. (27)	30	Indomethacin	Placebo	> 72 h	28–32	1,000–1,250	> 50%	+	+	+	+	+	+	?	Low
Yeh et al. (28)	47	Indomethacin	Placebo	> 72 h	28–32	1,000–1,250	unknown	+	?	+	?	?	+	?	Intermediate
Mahony et al. (29)	104	Indomethacin	Placebo	< 24 h UT	28–32	1,000–1,250	< 25%	+	+	+	+	?	+	?	Low
Ment et al. (30)	48	Indomethacin	Placebo	< 24 h UT	28–32	1,000–1,250	unknown	–	?	+	+	?	+	?	Intermediate
Hammerman et al. (31)	24	Indomethacin	Placebo	> 72 h	unknown	unknown	25–50%	+	+	+	+	?	+	?	Low
Rennie et al. (32)	50	Indomethacin	Placebo	< 24 h UT	28–32	1,251–1,500	25–50%	?	?	+	+	?	?	?	Intermediate
Hammerman et al. (33)	24	Indomethacin	Placebo	> 72 h	28–32	<1,000	> 50%	+	+	+	+	+	+	?	Low
Krueger et al. (34)	32	Indomethacin	No treatment	< 24 h UT	28–32	1,000–1,250	> 50%	?	?	–	?	?	+	?	High
Vincer et al. (35)	30	Indomethacin	Placebo	< 24 h UT	28–32	<1,000	< 25%	?	–	+	?	+	+	?	Intermediate
Weesner et al. (36)	26	Indomethacin	Placebo	24–72 h	28–32	1,000–1,250	25–50%	+	?	+	+	?	+	?	Intermediate
Bandstra et al. (37)	199	Indomethacin	Placebo	< 24 h UT	28–32	1,000–1,250	25–50%	+	+	+	+	+	+	?	Low
Hanigan et al. (38)	111	Indomethacin	Placebo	< 24 h UT	28–32	1,000–1,250	< 25%	+	+	+	+	?	+	?	Low
Ment et al. (39)	36	Indomethacin	Placebo	< 24 h UT	28–32	<1,000	unknown	–	?	+	+	–	+	?	High
Lai et al. (40)	32	Indomethacin	Placebo	< 24 h UT	28–32	1,000–1,250	> 50%	–	–	?	?	?	+	?	High
Ment et al. (41)	431	Indomethacin	Placebo	< 24 h UT	28–32	<1,000	< 25%	+	+	?	+	–	+	?	Intermediate
Couser et al. (42)	90	Indomethacin	Placebo	< 24 h UT	< 28	<1,000	25–50%	+	?	+	+	+	+	?	Low
Supapannachart et al. (43)	30	Indomethacin	Placebo	< 24 h UT	28–32	<1,000	> 50%	+	+	+	?	+	+	?	Low
Couser et al. (44)	90	Indomethacin	Placebo	< 24 h UT	< 28	<1,000	unknown	+	?	+	+	–	+	?	Intermediate
De Carolis et al. (45)	46	Ibuprofen	No treatment	< 24 h UT	28–32	<1,000	> 50%	+	–	–	+	+	+	?	Intermediate
Schmidt et al. (46)	1,202	Indomethacin	Placebo	< 24 h UT	< 28	<1,000	25–50%	+	+	+	+	?	+	?	Low
Osborn et al. (47)	70	Indomethacin	Placebo	< 24 h T	< 28	1,000–1,250	> 50%	?	+	+	+	+	+	?	Low
Gournay et al. (48)	131	Ibuprofen	Placebo	< 24 h UT	< 28	<1,000	25–50%	+	+	+	+	–	+	–	Intermediate
van Overmeire et al. (49)	415	Ibuprofen	Placebo	< 24 h UT	28–32	1,000–1,250	< 25%	+	+	+	+	+	+	?	Low
Dani et al. (50)	155	Ibuprofen	Placebo	< 24 h UT	< 28	<1,000	25–50%	+	+	+	+	?	+	?	Low
Sangtawesin et al. (51)	42	Ibuprofen	Placebo	< 24 h T	28–32	1,251–1,500	> 50%	?	?	+	+	+	+	?	Intermediate
Sangtawesin et al. (52)	62	Ibuprofen	Placebo	< 24 h T	28–32	1,000–1,250	25–50%	?	?	+	+	+	+	?	Intermediate
Aranda et al. (53)	136	Ibuprofen	Placebo	24–72 h	< 28	<1,000	25–50%	+	+	+	+	+	+	?	Low
Amoozgar et al. (54)	51	Ibuprofen	Placebo	> 72 h	> 33	>1,500	< 25%	?	?	?	?	+	+	?	Intermediate
Maruyama et al. (55)	19	Indomethacin	Placebo	< 24 h UT	< 28	<1,000	> 50%	+	+	?	?	+	+	?	Intermediate
Sosenko et al. (56)	105	Ibuprofen	Placebo	24–72 h	< 28	<1,000	> 50%	+	+	+	+	+	+	?	Low
Bagnoli et al. (57)	134	Ibuprofen	Placebo	> 72 h	< 28	1,000–1,250	Unknown	?	?	?	?	+	+	?	Intermediate
Kanmaz et al. (58)	46	Ibuprofen	No treatment	< 24 h UT	< 28	<1,000	25–50%	+	+	–	+	–	+	?	Intermediate
Ding et al. (59)	72	Ibuprofen	Placebo	Unknown	28–32	1,251–1,500	Unknown	?	?	?	+	+	+	?	Intermediate
Jannatdoust et al. (60)	70	Indomethacin	No treatment	< 24 h UT	28–32	Unknown	25–50%	+	+	–	?	?	+	?	Intermediate
Kluckow et al. (61)	92	Indomethacin	Placebo	< 24 h T	< 28	<1,000	25–50%	+	+	+	+	+	+	–	Low
Harkin et al. (62)	48	Acetaminophen	Placebo	< 24 h UT	28–32	1,000–1,250	< 25%	+	+	+	+	+	+	?	Low
Clyman et al. (63)	202	Any	No treatment	> 72 h	< 28	<1,000	25–50%	+	?	–	?	+	+	–	High
Juujarvi et al. (64)	44	Acetaminophen	Placebo	< 24 h UT	28–32	1,000–1,250	Unknown	+	+	+	+	?	?	?	Intermediate

BW, birth weight; GA, gestational age; h, hour; n, number; NA, not available; PNA, postnatal age; any, indomethacin/ibuprofen/acetaminophen; T, targeted treatment, UT, untargeted treatment; risk of bias numbers stand for (1) random sequence generation (selection bias); (2) allocation concealment (selection bias); (3) blinding of participants and personnel (performance bias); (4) blinding of outcome assessment (detection bias); (5) incomplete outcome data (attrition bias); (6) selective reporting (reporting bias), and; (7) other bias.

TABLE 2 | Risk ratio of outcomes, stratified by the patient characteristics, the quality of the studies, and the rate of open-label treatment in the placebo/no treatment group.

	Failed closure PDA	Need for ligation	NEC	BPD	Sepsis	PVL	IVH (Grade ≥ 3)	ROP	Mortality
Whole population	**0.40 [0.33–0.48] 40; 4,291**	**0.61 [0.49–0.76] 24; 3,289**	1.10 [0.89–1.37] 29; 3,686	0.97 [0.85–1.10] 26; 3,005	1.02 [0.82–1.25] 13; 1,205	0.93 [0.65–1.33] 11; 1,619	**0.76 [0.62–0.93] 19; 3,071**	0.99 [0.86–1.15] 19; 1,489	1.02 [0.89–1.17] 37; 3,987
BW < 1,000 g	**0.48 [0.37–0.63] 13; 2,045**	**0.61 [0.46–0.80] 11; 2,102**	1.07 [0.84–1.37] 14; 2,330	0.94 [0.79–1.12] 13; 1,983	1.09 [0.84–1.41] 7; 720	0.84 [0.55–1.28] 8; 951	**0.77 [0.61–0.97] 12; 2,251**	1.18 [0.95–1.47] 9; 864	1.08 [0.91–1.28] 15; 2,368
BW 1,000–1,250 g	**0.37 [0.27–0.51] 18; 1,516**	**0.60 [0.41–0.89] 10; 1,088**	1.21 [0.74–1.97] 13; 1,291	1.07 [0.90–1.26] 8; 857	0.89 [0.61–1.29] 6; 485	1.22 [0.60–2.48] 3; 668	0.78 [0.54–1.13] 6; 851	0.82 [0.67–1.00] 9; 585	0.98 [0.75–1.28] 15; 1,413
BW 1,251–1,500 g	**0.32 [0.16–0.65] 5; 204**	1.08 [0.08–15.46] 2; 75	1.27 [0.54–3.01] 1; 41	0.67 [0.10–4.53] 3; 114	-	-	-	1.36 [0.25–7.27] 1; 40	0.65 [0.33–1.28] 5; 155
BW > 1,500 g	0.15 [0.02–1.09] 1;27	-	-	0.54 [0.06–5.26] 1; 27	-	-	-	-	0.27 [0.03–2.11] 1; 27
BW unknown	**0.28 [0.18–0.44] 3; 499**	0.56 [0.13–2.33] 1; 24	0.70 [0.07–6.70] 1; 24	1.05 [0.78–1.41] 1; 24	-	-	0.69 [0.12–3.85] 1; 69	-	1.40 [0.55–3.57] 1; 24
GA < 28 w	**0.63 [0.47–0.84] 9; 2,039**	**0.67 [0.52–0.87] 9; 2,130**	1.20 [0.94–1.54] 12; 2,367	0.92 [0.74–1.15] 9; 1,858	1.15 [0.89–1.49] 5; 644	0.90 [0.59–1.37] 8; 959	**0.77 [0.61–0.98] 9; 2,008**	1.17 [0.94–1.46] 7; 809	1.05 [0.88–1.25] 12; 2,369
GA 28–32 w	**0.34 [0.28–0.41] 29; 1,823**	**0.45 [0.29–0.71] 13; 1,110**	0.86 [0.56–1.34] 16; 1,295	1.06 [0.92–1.21] 15; 1,100	0.83 [0.58–1.18] 8; 561	1.02 [0.50–2.04] 3; 660	0.77 [0.55–1.09] 10; 1,063	0.86 [0.71–1.04] 12; 680	0.97 [0.76–1.24] 23; 1,570
GA > 33 w	-	-	-	-	-	-	-	-	-
GA unknown	**0.31 [0.22–0.42] 2; 429**	0.66 [0.19–2.28] 2; 49	0.70 [0.07–6.70] 1; 24	0.57 [0.08–4.09] 2; 47	-	-	-	-	0.88 [0.38–2.04] 2; 48
PNA < 24 h (targeted)	0.59 [0.25–1.35] 3; 159	0.22 [0.01–4.41] 1; 92	1.56 [0.45–5.42] 3; 224	0.68 [0.42–1.09] 3; 177	0.85 [0.48–1.49] 1; 92	1.70 [0.54–5.37] 2; 146	-	0.46 [0.16–1.32] 2; 150	0.76 [0.41–1.42] 3; 189
PNA <24 h (untargeted)	**0.39 [0.32–0.48] 21; 2,916**	**0.53 [0.39–0.72] 13; 2,502**	1.04 [0.79–1.36] 17; 2,677	0.96 [0.75–1.22] 14; 2,235	0.95 [0.69–1.32] 8; 704	0.82 [0.50–1.33] 6; 1,036	**0.70 [0.57–0.87] 16; 2,630**	1.02 [0.85–1.21] 9; 706	1.04 [0.88–1.21] 20; 2,872
PNA 24–72 h	**0.12 [0.02–0.63] 2; 68**	0.78 [0.35–1.76] 2; 130	1.26 [0.71–2.22] 3; 276	0.93 [0.61–1.43] 5; 288	-	0.58 [0.18–1.83] 2; 235	0.92 [0.50–1.70] 2;239	1.20 [0.90–1.61] 4; 294	0.77 [0.42–1.42] 5; 289
PNA > 72 h	**0.41 [0.30–0.57] 13;1,076**	0.75 [0.52–1.07] 8; 565	1.33 [0.87–2.04] 7; 907	[0.86–1.19] 4; 305	1.15 [0.84–1.58] 4; 409	1.20 [0.57–2.51] 1; 202	1.63 [0.82–3.24] 1; 202	0.78 [0.48–1.27] 4; 339	1.21 [0.81–1.81] 9; 637
PNA unknown	0.13 [0.02–1.00] 1; 72	-	-	-	-	-	-	-	-
Low risk of bias	**0.39 [0.30–0.50] 18; 3,049**	**0.55 [0.42–0.71] 13; 2,548**	1.04 [0.80–1.35] 15; 2,767	0.97 [0.83–1.14] 13; 2,284	0.92 [0.73–1.18] 10; 925	0.85 [0.53–1.36] 8; 1,240	**0.79 [0.63–0.98] 9; 2,393**	[0.86–1.17] 11; 1,029	1.03 [0.88–1.21] 19; 2,940
Intermediate risk of bias	**0.37 [0.26–0.53] 17; 927**	0.74 [0.46–1.20] 8; 483	1.61 [0.98–2.64] 11; 655	1.03 [0.74–1.44] 8; 408	[0.07–15.04] 1; 46	0.90 [0.36–2.22] 2; 177	**0.55 [0.32–0.96] 7; 410**	0.83 [0.48–1.42] 6; 226	0.98 [0.70–1.38] 12; 694
High risk of bias	**0.42 [0.19–0.97] 5; 315**	0.90 [0.45–1.82] 3; 258	0.84 [0.47–1.53] 3; 264	0.88 [0.68–1.13] 5; 313	1.40 [0.89–2.21] 2; 234	1.20 [0.57–2.51] 1; 202	1.02 [0.57–1.82] 3; 268	1.12 [0.68–1.86] 2; 234	1.05 [0.62–1.77] 6; 353
Open-label treatment < 25%	**0.38 [0.29–0.50] 6; 762**	**0.39 [0.15–0.97] 3; 549**	0.65 [0.31–1.33] 5; 658	1.09 [0.90–1.31] 3; 493	0.97 [0.47–1.99] 2; 152	2.05 [0.71–5.89] 1; 415	1.06 [0.63–1.78] 4; 635	0.93 [0.45–1.93] 3; 164	1.14 [0.81–1.62] 6; 769
Open-label treatment 25–50%	**0.40 [0.31–0.52] 14; 2,323**	**0.52 [0.39–0.70] 11; 2,226**	1.09 [0.85–1.39] 12; 2,379	0.94 [0.78–1.13] 14; 2,160	1.07 [0.82–1.39] 6; 793	0.72 [0.47–1.11] 7; 999	**0.76 [0.61–0.95] 9; 2,152**	[0.87–1.17] 10; 1,036	1.05 [0.89–1.24] 14; 2,457
Open-label treatment > 50%	**0.40 [0.25–0.62] 13; 843**	**0.63 [0.40–0.99] 8; 361**	1.24 [0.68–2.28] 10; 467	0.98 [0.76–1.26] 8; 325	0.90 [0.61–1.34] 5; 260	1.63 [0.58–4.53] 3; 205	0.57 [0.25–1.30] 4; 200	1.17 [0.64–2.15] 4; 212	0.86 [0.55–1.33] 12; 499
Open-label treatment unknown	**0.37 [0.21–0.66] 7; 363**	1.89 [0.91–3.93] 1; 134	[0.07–15.08] 1; 48	0.54 [0.06–5.26] 1; 27	-	-	0.26 [0.05–1.48] 2; 84	0.32 [0.07–1.42] 1; 47	0.41 [0.15-1.13] 5; 262

Risk ratio with 95% confidence interval. Number of studies and infants. RR < 1 favors treatment; RR > 1 favors placebo/no treatment. In bold the statistically significant differences. BW, birth weight; GA, gestational age; PNA, postnatal age; PDA, patent ductus arteriosus; NEC, necrotizing enterocolitis; BPD, bronchopulmonary dysplasia; PVL, periventricular leukomalacia; IVH, intraventricular hemorrhage; ROP, retinopathy of prematurity. w, weeks; h, hours. - means not estimable.

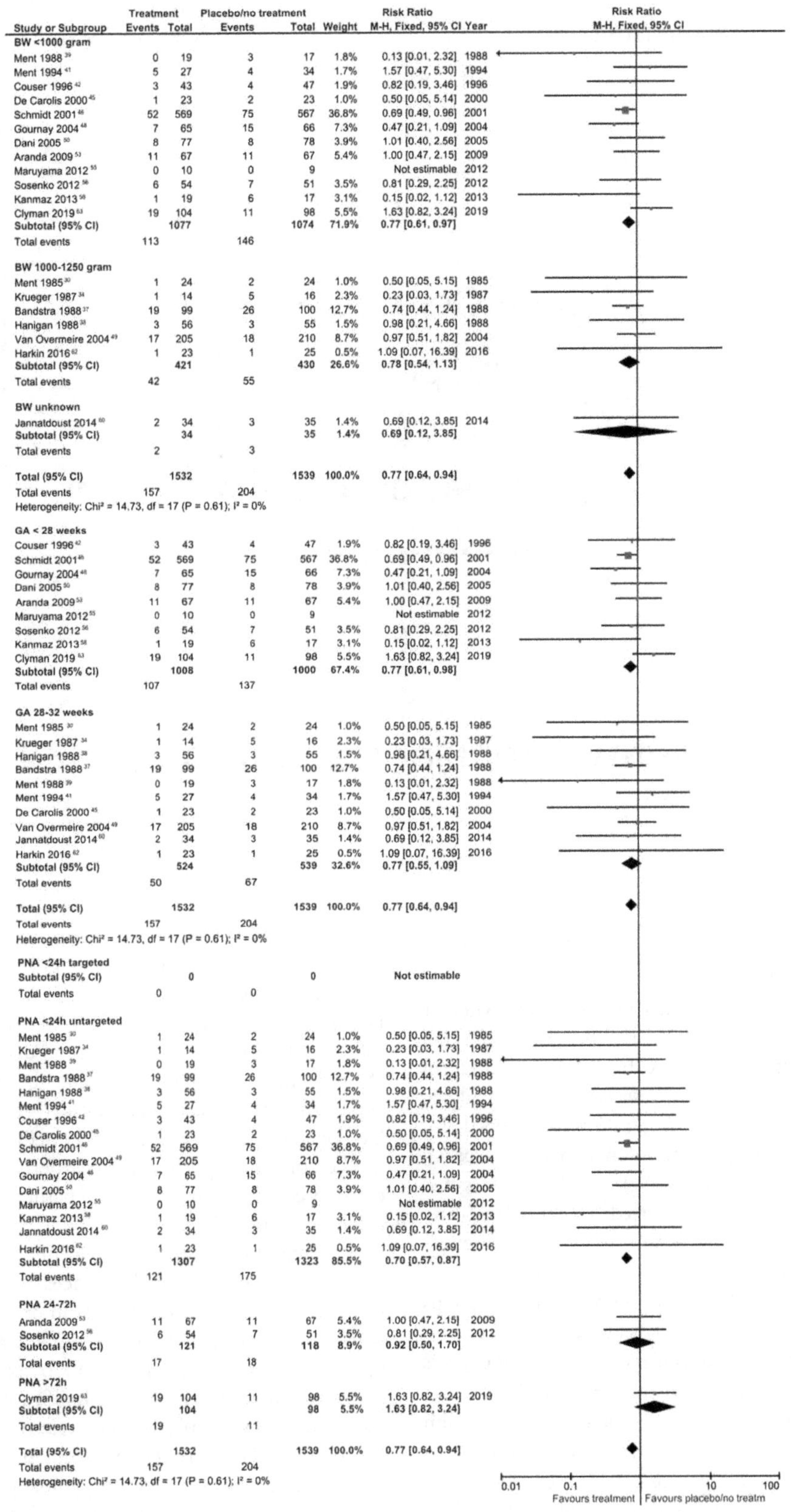

FIGURE 2 | Forest plots regarding the risk for intraventricular hemorrhage grade ≥ 3. BW, birth weight; GA, gestational age; PNA, postnatal age.

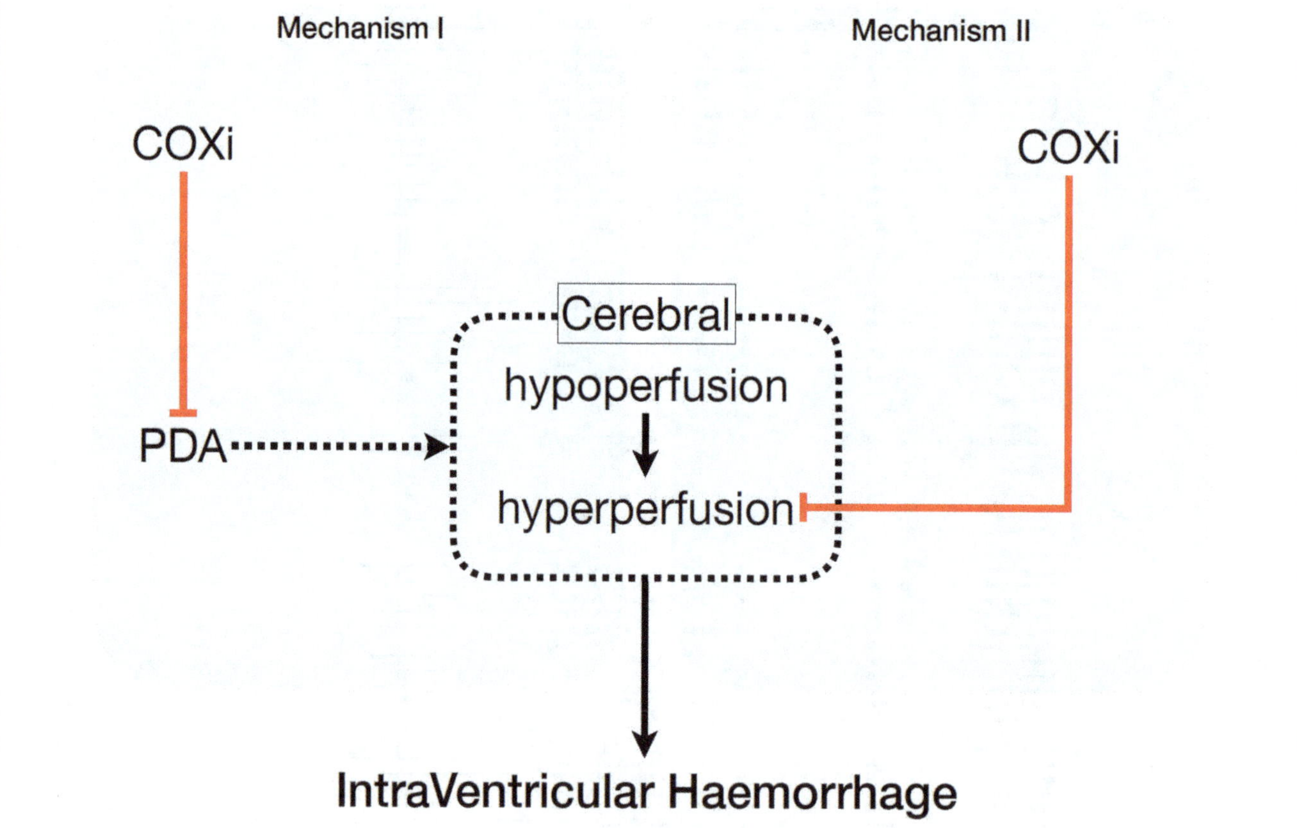

FIGURE 3 | Potential pathophysiological mechanisms of pharmacologic cyclo-oxygenase inhibition on intraventricular hemorrhage. COXi, cyclo-oxygenase; PDA, patent ductus arteriosus.

DISCUSSION

Summary of Evidence

The aim of this systematic review was to investigate whether patient characteristics or study characteristics modulate the beneficial or adverse effects of PDA treatment in preterm infants. The main finding of this review was that pharmacologic treatment of PDA is associated with a significantly reduced risk of IVH grade ≥3 in extremely preterm infants (GA <28 weeks), extremely low BW infants (BW <1,000 g), or when untargeted treatment with indomethacin was started <24 h after birth. Moreover, this review revealed no relevant significant differences for the outcome measures NEC, BPD, mortality, sepsis, PVL, and ROP between intervention and control groups in the subgroups BW, GA, risk of bias, and rate of open-label treatment.

Our findings regarding the reduced risk of IVH grade ≥3 is in line with a previous review comprising 2,588 newborns <37 weeks' gestation, which showed that untargeted administration of indomethacin is associated with a decreased risk of IVH (65). In our meta-analysis a total of 2,937 preterm infants were assessed for IVH grade ≥3 and stratified by BW, GA, and PNA. Out of the infants allocated to the treatment group 10% had IVH grade ≥3 compared to 13% of the infants in the placebo/no treatment group. Dividing the included studies who treated the infants <24 h after birth into untargeted treatment or targeted treatment, we found only reduction of severe IVH in the former group if indomethacin was used. The hypothesis is that this reduction of severe IVH is probably not a direct effect of ductal closure itself and therefore limiting cerebral perfusion disturbances, but mediated by prevention of hyperperfusion by a direct drug-induced cerebrovascular vasoconstriction (see **Figure 3**). This effect has been demonstrated for indomethacin and might prevent the cerebral hypoperfusion-hyperperfusion sequence, which is considered to be an important pathophysiological mechanism associated with IVH (66–69).

Subdividing the studies according to which drug was used, we found no significant differences in the incidences of NEC, BPD, ROP or mortality, which is in line with recently published papers (11, 14). In contrast to our meta-analysis, these papers used any grade of IVH instead of severe IVH as outcome parameter and observed no significant differences in any of the used drugs vs. placebo/no treatment. Our review selected studies published between 1985 and 2019, whereas currently, as opposed to the previous century, most preterm infants will have received corticosteroids antenatally and surfactants postnatally, if required. We know that this approach reduces the risk of an IVH (70). Including only those studies published in the last 25 years, the significant reduction of severe IVH is still observed in the youngest, smallest and untargeted treated infants.

Although untargeted treatment constitutes the only convincing evidence for active closure of PDA, it is currently seldom provided (1). It might, however, be argued that any evidence-based reduction in the risk of IVH grade ≥3 is beneficial to the infant, but sufficient evidence is lacking. In a 2015 meta-analysis about neurodevelopmental impairment after a severe IVH, only observational cohort studies were identified and on the whole the risk of bias was high (71). Moreover, there is also little evidence of improved long-term developmental outcome and mortality after prophylactic treatment (44, 45, 65).

In addition, we stratified by rate of open-label treatment, something that to our knowledge has not been done before. The median rate of the open-label treatment in the studies was 44.5% (calculated from 38 out of 47 studies). Since we reviewed the raw data in our meta-analysis to determine the morbidity and mortality of the different subgroups, we could not analyze whether the original studies performed intention to treat or per protocol analysis. We hypothesized that the potential effects of active treatment of a PDA would be attenuated in RCTs with a high proportion of open label treatment in the control/placebo arm. However, this was not observed. Failure of DA closure and the need for surgical ligation were significantly lower in the treatment group independent of the rate of open-label treatment. To our surprise, however, this subgroup analysis, which stratified the studies according to a high rate vs. a lower rate of open-label treatment in the control group, showed no difference in morbidity and mortality. We found no significant reduction of major clinical outcomes, not even in the subgroup of RCTs with low open-label treatment rates in the no treatment group of patients. This raises the question whether a PDA should be considered as an epiphenomenon as was suggested by recent cohort studies using restrictive treatment policies (72, 73). This should, however, be supported or refuted by well-powered high-quality RCTs targeting the high-risk population (<28 weeks' GA and/or BW <1,000 g) with low-rate open-label treatment of the placebo/no treatment group.

Limitations

The first limitation of this meta-analysis are the missing data in the RCTs. Unfortunately, even though we tried to reduce selection bias by contacting the corresponding authors, not all missing data could be retrieved. As a consequence, we could not include all studies in our subgroup stratification.

Secondly, a meta-analysis has to deal with heterogeneity of the included RCTs. The high statistical heterogeneity in this meta-analysis is comparable with a previously published meta-analyses (74). Heterogeneity leads to lower quality of evidence (5, 75). In an attempt to reduce clinical heterogeneity, we stratified the results in several subgroups and subdivided treatment started <24 h after birth in untargeted treatment and targeted treatment. Moreover, the definitions of outcome measures in the included RCTs in a meta-analysis vary. In the current meta-analysis, the outcomes BPD and NEC were not uniformly defined in the selected studies. The possible reason is the large spread in publication years; criteria for short-term morbidities have changed over the years. Nevertheless, neither the overall meta-analyses nor the subgroup analyses of the different BPD definitions revealed any differences. The heterogeneity of studies analyzing NEC was low. Unfortunately, subgroup analyses could not be performed for the outcome measures pneumothorax, pulmonary hemorrhage, pulmonary hypertension, gastro-intestinal bleeding, SIP, and oliguria, because of the scarcity of available data. Last, another important factor that could be a major factor contributing to heterogeneity is the classification of hemodynamic significance of the PDA. Zonnenberg et al. showed that there is substantial variability in the definition of a significant PDA in clinical trials (9). In the 47 included RCTs the used definition of a PDA varied much, ranging from clinical, radiographic and echocardiographic parameters.

Future research is required with unambiguously definitions of outcome measures and larger groups of preterm infants. There is a need for well-powered high-quality RCTs with low-rate open-label treatment of the placebo/no treatment group. In addition, more research is needed to investigate which mechanisms might be responsible for the reduction of IVH grade ≥3 in the youngest, the smallest, or in the preterm infants that are treated untargeted with indomethacin within the first 24 h of life.

Conclusions

In this systematic review, in which we investigated the modulating effects of patient characteristics and study characteristics by performing subgroup meta-analyses, the degree of heterogeneity among the included studies and variability in study quality is high. Therefore, the quality of evidence following GRADE assessment is low. Pharmacological treatment of a PDA in extremely preterm infants with either a GA <28 weeks, a BW <1,000 g, or if untargeted treatment with indomethacin is given <24 h PNA is associated with a significantly lower risk of developing IVH grade ≥3. We found no differences in the incidence of other morbidities or in mortality when we stratified the subgroups by BW, GA, and PNA at start of treatment. Important data on long-term consequences of neurodevelopmental impairment are lacking for these studies. More high-quality and low-rate open-label treatment studies are needed to unravel the effects of pharmacological PDA treatment on short-term and long-term morbidity and to elucidate underlying pathophysiologic mechanisms.

AUTHOR CONTRIBUTIONS

EJ conceptualized and designed the study, collected the data, drafted the initial manuscript, and analyzed and interpreted the data. TH collected, analyzed and interpreted the data, and reviewed and revised the manuscript. WO, EK, and PA analyzed and interpreted the data, critically reviewed the manuscript, and provided administrative, technical, or material support. WB coordinated and supervised data collection, analyzed data, and critically reviewed the manuscript for important intellectual content. All authors approved the final manuscript as submitted and agree to be accountable for all aspects of the work.

REFERENCES

1. Lee JA, Kim MJ, Oh S, Choi BM. Current status of therapeutic strategies for patent ductus arteriosus in very-low-birth-weight infants in Korea. *J Korean Med Sci.* (2015) 30(Suppl. 1):S59–66. doi: 10.3346/jkms.2015.30.S1.S59
2. Sellmer A, Bjerre JV, Schmidt MR, McNamara PJ, Hjortdal VE, Host B, et al. Morbidity and mortality in preterm neonates with patent ductus arteriosus on day 3. *Arch Dis Child Fetal Neonatal Ed.* (2013) 98:F505–10. doi: 10.1136/archdischild-2013-303816
3. Heuchan AM, Clyman RI. Managing the patent ductus arteriosus: current treatment options. *Arch Dis Child Fetal Neonatal Ed.* (2014) 99:F431–6. doi: 10.1136/archdischild-2014-306176
4. Bourgoin L, Cipierre C, Hauet Q, Basset H, Gournay V, Roze JC, et al. Neurodevelopmental outcome at 2 years of age according to patent ductus arteriosus management in very preterm infants. *Neonatology.* (2016) 109:139–46. doi: 10.1159/000442278
5. Sankar MN, Bhombal S, Benitz WE. PDA: to treat or not to treat. *Congenit Heart Dis.* (2019) 14:46–51. doi: 10.1111/chd.12708
6. Ngo S, Profit J, Gould JB, Lee HC. Trends in patent ductus arteriosus diagnosis and management for very low birth weight infants. *Pediatrics.* (2017) 139:e20162390. doi: 10.1542/peds.2016-2390
7. Bose CL, Laughon MM. Patent ductus arteriosus: lack of evidence for common treatments. *Arch Dis Child Fetal Neonatal Ed.* (2007) 92:F498–502. doi: 10.1136/adc.2005.092734
8. Clyman RI, Couto J, Murphy GM. Patent ductus arteriosus: are current neonatal treatment options better or worse than no treatment at all? *Semin Perinatol.* (2012) 36:123–9. doi: 10.1053/j.semperi.2011.09.022
9. Zonnenberg I, de Waal K. The definition of a haemodynamic significant duct in randomized controlled trials: a systematic literature review. *Acta Paediatr.* (2012) 101:247–51. doi: 10.1111/j.1651-2227.2011.02468.x
10. Friedman WF, Hirschklau MJ, Printz MP, Pitlick PT, Kirkpatrick SE. Pharmacologic closure of patent ductus arteriosus in the premature infant. *N Engl J Med.* (1976) 295:526–9. doi: 10.1056/NEJM197609022951003
11. Mitra S, Florez ID, Tamayo ME, Mbuagbaw L, Vanniyasingam T, Veroniki AA, et al. Association of placebo, indomethacin, ibuprofen, and acetaminophen with closure of hemodynamically significant patent ductus arteriosus in preterm infants: a systematic review and meta-analysis. *JAMA.* (2018) 319:1221–38. doi: 10.1001/jama.2018.1896
12. Benitz WE. Treatment of persistent patent ductus arteriosus in preterm infants: time to accept the null hypothesis? *J Perinatol.* (2010) 30:241–52. doi: 10.1038/jp.2010.3
13. Moher D, Liberati A, Tetzlaff J, Altman DG. Preferred reporting items for systematic reviews and meta-analyses: the PRISMA statement. *PLoS Med.* (2009) 6:e1000097. doi: 10.1371/journal.pmed.1000097
14. El-Mashad AE, El-Mahdy H, El Amrousy D, Elgendy M. Comparative study of the efficacy and safety of paracetamol, ibuprofen, and indomethacin in closure of patent ductus arteriosus in preterm neonates. *Eur J Pediatr.* (2017) 176:233–40. doi: 10.1007/s00431-016-2830-7
15. Serghiou S, Goodman SN. Random-effects meta-analysis: summarizing evidence with caveats. *JAMA.* (2019) 321:301–2. doi: 10.1001/jama.2018.19684
16. Higgins JP, Altman DG, Gotzsche PC, Juni P, Moher D, Oxman AD, et al. The Cochrane Collaboration's tool for assessing risk of bias in randomised trials. *BMJ.* (2011) 343:d5928. doi: 10.1136/bmj.d5928
17. GRADE handbook for grading quality of evidence and strength of recommendations. In: Schünemann H, Brozek J, Guyatt G, Oxman A, ed.: *The GRADE Working Group* (2013_: guidelinedevelopment.org/handbook (accessed August 7, 2019).
18. Nestrud RM, Hill DE, Arrington RW, Beard AG, Dungan WT, Lau PY, et al. Indomethacin treatment in patent ductus arteriosus. A double-blind study utilizing indomethacin plasma levels. *Dev Pharmacol Ther.* (1980) 1:125–36. doi: 10.1159/000455530
19. Merritt TA, Harris JP, Roghmann K, Wood B, Campanella V, Alexson C, et al. Early closure of the patent ductus arteriosus in very low-birth-weight infants: a controlled trial. *J Pediatr.* (1981) 99:281–6. doi: 10.1016/S0022-3476(81)80479-9
20. Neu J, Ariagno RL, Johnson JD, Pitlick PT, Cohen RS, Beets CL, et al. A double blind study of the effects of oral indomethacin in preterm infants with patent ductus arteriosus who failed medical management. *Pediatric Pharmacol.* (1981) 1:245–9.
21. Yanagi RM, Wilson A, Newfeld EA, Aziz KU, Hunt CE. Indomethacin treatment for symptomatic patent ductus arteriosus: a double-blind control study. *Pediatrics.* (1981) 67:647–52.
22. Yeh TF, Luken JA, Thalji A, Raval D, Carr I, Pildes RS. Intravenous indomethacin therapy in premature infants with persistent ductus arteriosus–a double-blind controlled study. *J Pediatr.* (1981) 98:137–45. doi: 10.1016/S0022-3476(81)80560-4
23. Mahony L, Carnero V, Brett C, Heymann MA, Clyman RI. Prophylactic indomethacin therapy for patent ductus arteriosus in very-low-birth-weight infants. *N Engl J Med.* (1982) 306:506–10. doi: 10.1056/NEJM198203043060903
24. Mullett MD, Croghan TW, Myerberg DZ, Krall JM, Neal WA. Indomethacin for closure of patent ductus arteriosus in prematures. *Clin Pediatr.* (1982) 21:217–20. doi: 10.1177/000992288202100404
25. Gersony WM, Peckham GJ, Ellison RC, Miettinen OS, Nadas AS. Effects of indomethacin in premature infants with patent ductus arteriosus: results of a national collaborative study. *J Pediatr.* (1983) 102:895–906. doi: 10.1016/S0022-3476(83)80022-5
26. Kaapa P, Lanning P, Koivisto M. Early closure of patent ductus arteriosus with indomethacin in preterm infants with idiopathic respiratory distress syndrome. *Acta Paediatrica Scand.* (1983) 72:179–84. doi: 10.1111/j.1651-2227.1983.tb09693.x
27. Rudd P, Montanez P, Hallidie-Smith K, Silverman M. Indomethacin treatment for patent ductus arteriosus in very low birthweight infants: double blind trial. *Arch Dis Child.* (1983) 58:267–70. doi: 10.1136/adc.58.4.267
28. Yeh TF, Raval D, Pyati S, Pildes RS. Retinopathy of prematurity (ROP) and indomethacin therapy in premature infants with patent ductus arteriosus (PDA). *Prostaglandins.* (1983) 25:385–91. doi: 10.1016/0090-6980(83)90041-2
29. Mahony L, Caldwell RL, Girod DA, Hurwitz RA, Jansen RD, Lemons JA, et al. Indomethacin therapy on the first day of life in infants with very low birth weight. *J Pediatr.* (1985) 106:801–5. doi: 10.1016/S0022-3476(85)80361-9
30. Ment LR, Duncan CC, Ehrenkranz RA, Kleinman CS, Pitt BR, Taylor KJ, et al. Randomized indomethacin trial for prevention of intraventricular hemorrhage in very low birth weight infants. *J Pediatr.* (1985) 107:937–43. doi: 10.1016/S0022-3476(85)80197-9
31. Hammerman C, Strates E, Valaitis S. The silent ductus: its precursors and its aftermath. *Pediatr Cardiol.* (1986) 7:121–7. doi: 10.1007/BF02424985
32. Rennie JM, Doyle J, Cooke RW. Early administration of indomethacin to preterm infants. *Arch Dis Child.* (1986) 61:233–8. doi: 10.1136/adc.61.3.233
33. Hammerman C, Strates E, Komar K, Bui K. Failure of prophylactic indomethacin to improve the outcome of the very low birth weight infant. *Dev Pharmacol Ther.* (1987) 10:393–404. doi: 10.1159/0004 57771
34. Krueger E, Mellander M, Bratton D, Cotton R. Prevention of symptomatic patent ductus arteriosus with a single dose of indomethacin. *J Pediatr.* (1987) 111:749–54. doi: 10.1016/S0022-3476(87)80262-7
35. Vincer M, Allen A, Evans J, Nwaesei C, Stinson D, Rees E, et al. Early intravenous indomethacin prolongs respiratory support in very low birth weight infants. *Acta Paediatrica Scand.* (1987) 76:894–7. doi: 10.1111/j.1651-2227.1987.tb17260.x
36. Weesner KM, Dillard RG, Boyle RJ, Block SM. Prophylactic treatment of asymptomatic patent ductus arteriosus in premature infants with respiratory distress syndrome. *Southern Med J.* (1987) 80:706–8. doi: 10.1097/00007611-198706000-00010
37. Bandstra ES, Montalvo BM, Goldberg RN, Pacheco I, Ferrer PL, Flynn J, et al. Prophylactic indomethacin for prevention of intraventricular hemorrhage in premature infants. *Pediatrics.* (1988) 82:533–42.
38. Hanigan WC, Kennedy G, Roemisch F, Anderson R, Cusack T, Powers W. Administration of indomethacin for the prevention of periventricular-intraventricular hemorrhage in high-risk neonates. *J Pediatr.* (1988) 112:941–7. doi: 10.1016/S0022-3476(88)80224-5
39. Ment LR, Duncan CC, Ehrenkranz RA, Kleinman CS, Taylor KJ, Scott DT, et al. Randomized low-dose indomethacin trial for prevention of intraventricular hemorrhage in very low birth weight neonates. *J Pediatr.* (1988) 112:948–55. doi: 10.1016/S0022-3476(88)80225-7
40. Lai TH, Soong WJ, Hwang B. Indomethacin for the prevention of symptomatic patent ductus arteriosus in very low birth weight infants. *Zhonghua Min Guo Xiao Er Ke Yi Xue Hui Za Zhi.* (1990) 31:17–23.
41. Ment LR, Oh W, Ehrenkranz RA, Philip AG, Vohr B, Allan W, et al. Low-dose

indomethacin and prevention of intraventricular hemorrhage: a multicenter randomized trial. *Pediatrics.* (1994) 93:543–50.

42. Couser RJ, Ferrara TB, Wright GB, Cabalka AK, Schilling CG, Hoekstra RE, et al. Prophylactic indomethacin therapy in the first twenty-four hours of life for the prevention of patent ductus arteriosus in preterm infants treated prophylactically with surfactant in the delivery room. *J Pediatr.* (1996) 128(5 Pt 1):631–7. doi: 10.1016/S0022-3476(96)80127-2
43. Supapannachart S, Khowsathit P, Patchakapati B. Indomethacin prophylaxis for patent ductus arteriosus (PDA) in infants with a birth weight of less than 1250 grams. *J Med Assoc Thai.* (1999) 82(Suppl. 1):S87–92.
44. Couser RJ, Hoekstra RE, Ferrara TB, Wright GB, Cabalka AK, Connett JE. Neurodevelopmental follow-up at 36 months' corrected age of preterm infants treated with prophylactic indomethacin. *Arch Pediatr Adolesc Med.* (2000) 154:598–602. doi: 10.1001/archpedi.154.6.598
45. De Carolis MP, Romagnoli C, Polimeni V, Piersigilli F, Zecca E, Papacci P, et al. Prophylactic ibuprofen therapy of patent ductus arteriosus in preterm infants. *Eur J Pediatr.* (2000) 159:364–8. doi: 10.1007/s004310051288
46. Schmidt B, Davis P, Moddemann D, Ohlsson A, Roberts RS, Saigal S, et al. Long-term effects of indomethacin prophylaxis in extremely-low-birth-weight infants. *N Engl J Med.* (2001) 344:1966–72. doi: 10.1056/NEJM200106283442602
47. Osborn DA, Evans N, Kluckow M. Effect of early targeted indomethacin on the ductus arteriosus and blood flow to the upper body and brain in the preterm infant. *Arch Dis Child Fetal Neonatal Ed.* (2003) 88:F477–82. doi: 10.1136/fn.88.6.F477
48. Gournay V, Roze JC, Kuster A, Daoud P, Cambonie G, Hascoet JM, et al. Prophylactic ibuprofen versus placebo in very premature infants: a randomised, double-blind, placebo-controlled trial. *Lancet.* (2004) 364:1939–44. doi: 10.1016/S0140-6736(04)17476-X
49. Van Overmeire B, Allegaert K, Casaer A, Debauche C, Decaluwe W, Jespers A, et al. Prophylactic ibuprofen in premature infants: a multicentre, randomised, double-blind, placebo-controlled trial. *Lancet.* (2004) 364:1945–9. doi: 10.1016/S0140-6736(04)17477-1
50. Dani C, Bertini G, Pezzati M, Poggi C, Guerrini P, Martano C, et al. Prophylactic ibuprofen for the prevention of intraventricular hemorrhage among preterm infants: a multicenter, randomized study. *Pediatrics.* (2005) 115:1529–35. doi: 10.1542/peds.2004-1178
51. Sangtawesin V, Sangtawesin C, Raksasinborisut C, Sathirakul K, Kanjanapattanakul W, Khorana M, et al. Oral ibuprofen prophylaxis for symptomatic patent ductus arteriosus of prematurity. *J Med Assoc Thai.* (2006) 89:314–21.
52. Sangtawesin C, Sangtawesin V, Lertsutthiwong W, Kanjanapattanakul W, Khorana M, Ayudhaya JK. Prophylaxis of symptomatic patent ductus arteriosus with oral ibuprofen in very low birth weight infants. *J Med Assoc Thai.* (2008) 91(Suppl. 3):S28–34.
53. Aranda JV, Clyman R, Cox B, Van Overmeire B, Wozniak P, Sosenko I, et al. A randomized, double-blind, placebo-controlled trial on intravenous ibuprofen L-lysine for the early closure of nonsymptomatic patent ductus arteriosus within 72 hours of birth in extremely low-birth-weight infants. *Am J Perinatol.* (2009) 26:235–45. doi: 10.1055/s-0028-1103515
54. Amoozgar H, Ghodstehrani M, Pishva N. Oral ibuprofen and ductus arteriosus closure in full-term neonates: a prospective case-control study. *Pediatr Cardiol.* (2010) 31:40–3. doi: 10.1007/s00246-009-9542-y
55. Maruyama K, Fujiu T. Effects of prophylactic indomethacin on renal and intestinal blood flows in premature infants. *Pediatr Int.* (2012) 54:480–5. doi: 10.1111/j.1442-200X.2012.03583.x
56. Sosenko IR, Fajardo MF, Claure N, Bancalari E. Timing of patent ductus arteriosus treatment and respiratory outcome in premature infants: a double-blind randomized controlled trial. *J Pediatr.* (2012) 160:929–35.e921. doi: 10.1016/j.jpeds.2011.12.031
57. Bagnoli F, Rossetti A, Messina G, Mori A, Casucci M, Tomasini B. Treatment of patent ductus arteriosus (PDA) using ibuprofen: renal side-effects in VLBW and ELBW newborns. *J Matern Fetal Neonatal Med.* (2013) 26:423–9. doi: 10.3109/14767058.2012.733775
58. Kanmaz G, Erdeve O, Canpolat FE, Oguz SS, Uras N, Altug N, et al. Serum ibuprofen levels of extremely preterm infants treated prophylactically with oral ibuprofen to prevent patent ductus arteriosus. *Eur J Clin Pharmacol.* (2013) 69:1075–81. doi: 10.1007/s00228-012-1438-8
59. Ding YJ, Han B, Yang B, Zhu M. NT-proBNP plays an important role in the effect of ibuprofen on preterm infants with patent ductus arteriosus. *Eur Rev Med Pharmacol Sci.* (2014) 18:2596–8.
60. Jannatdoust A, Samadi M, Yeganehdoust S, Heydarzadeh M, Alikhah H, Piri R, et al. Effects of intravenous indomethacin on reduction of symptomatic patent ductus arteriosus cases and decreasing the need for prolonged mechanical ventilation. *J Cardiovasc Thorac Res.* (2014) 6:257–9. doi: 10.15171/jcvtr.2014.022
61. Kluckow M, Jeffery M, Gill A, Evans N. A randomised placebo-controlled trial of early treatment of the patent ductus arteriosus. *Arch Dis Child Fetal Neonatal Ed.* (2014) 99:F99–104. doi: 10.1136/archdischild-2013-304695
62. Harkin P, Harma A, Aikio O, Valkama M, Leskinen M, Saarela T, et al. Paracetamol accelerates closure of the ductus arteriosus after premature birth: a randomized trial. *J Pediatr.* (2016) 177:72–7 e72. doi: 10.1016/j.jpeds.2016.04.066
63. Clyman RI, Liebowitz M, Kaempf J, Erdeve O, Bulbul A, Hakansson S, et al. PDA-TOLERATE trial: an exploratory randomized controlled trial of treatment of moderate-to-large patent ductus arteriosus at 1 week of age. *J Pediatr.* (2019) 205:41–8 e46. doi: 10.1016/j.jpeds.2018.09.012
64. Juujarvi S, Kallankari H, Patsi P, Leskinen M, Saarela T, Hallman M, et al. Follow-up study of the early, randomised paracetamol trial to preterm infants, found no adverse reactions at the two-years corrected age. *Acta Paediatr.* (2019) 108:452–8. doi: 10.1111/apa.14614
65. Fowlie PW, Davis PG, McGuire W. Prophylactic intravenous indomethacin for preventing mortality and morbidity in preterm infants. *Cochrane Database Syst Rev.* (2010) 2010:CD000174. doi: 10.1002/14651858.CD000174.pub2
66. Keating P, Verhagen E, van Hoften J, ter Horst H, Bos AF. Effect of indomethacin infused over 30 minutes on cerebral fractional tissue oxygen extraction in preterm newborns with a patent ductus arteriosus. *Neonatology.* (2010) 98:232–7. doi: 10.1159/000283946
67. Patel J, Roberts I, Azzopardi D, Hamilton P, Edwards AD. Randomized double-blind controlled trial comparing the effects of ibuprofen with indomethacin on cerebral hemodynamics in preterm infants with patent ductus arteriosus. *Pediatr Res.* (2000) 47:36–42. doi: 10.1203/00006450-200001000-00009
68. Khanafer-Larocque I, Soraisham A, Stritzke A, Al Awad E, Thomas S, Murthy P, et al. Intraventricular hemorrhage: risk factors and association with patent ductus arteriosus treatment in extremely preterm neonates. *Front Pediatr.* (2019) 7:408. doi: 10.3389/fped.2019.00408
69. Nelin TD, Pena E, Giacomazzi T, Lee S, Logan JW, Moallem M, et al. Outcomes following indomethacin prophylaxis in extremely preterm infants in an all-referral NICU. *J Perinatol.* (2017) 37:932–7. doi: 10.1038/jp.2017.71
70. Roberts D, Brown J, Medley N, Dalziel SR. Antenatal corticosteroids for accelerating fetal lung maturation for women at risk of preterm birth. *Cochrane Database Syst Rev.* (2017) 3:Cd004454. doi: 10.1002/14651858.CD004454.pub3
71. Mukerji A, Shah V, Shah PS. Periventricular/intraventricular hemorrhage and neurodevelopmental outcomes: a meta-analysis. *Pediatrics.* (2015) 136:1132–43. doi: 10.1542/peds.2015-0944
72. Harkin P, Marttila R, Pokka T, Saarela T, Hallman M. Morbidities associated with patent ductus arteriosus in preterm infants. Nationwide cohort study. *J Maternal-Fetal Neonatal Med.* (2018) 31:2576–83. doi: 10.1080/14767058.2017.1347921
73. Mohamed MA, El-Dib M, Alqahtani S, Alyami K, Ibrahim AN, Aly H. Patent ductus arteriosus in premature infants: to treat or not to treat? *J Perinatol.* (2017) 37:652–7. doi: 10.1038/jp.2017.4
74. Ohlsson A, Walia R, Shah SS. Ibuprofen for the treatment of patent ductus arteriosus in preterm or low birth weight (or both) infants. *Cochrane Database Syst Rev.* (2018) 9:Cd003481. doi: 10.1002/14651858.CD003481.pub7
75. Jansen EJS, Dijkman KP, van Lingen RA, de Vries WB, Vijlbrief DC, de Boode WP, et al. Using benchmarking to identify inter-centre differences in persistent ductus arteriosus treatment: can we improve outcome? *Cardiol Young.* (2017) 27:1488–96. doi: 10.1017/S104795111700052X

18

Transcatheter Closure of Patent Ductus Arteriosus in Infants with Weight Under 1,500 Grams

Alain Fraisse [1,2], *Carles Bautista-Rodriguez* [1,2], *Margarita Burmester* [2,3], *Mary Lane* [1,2] and *Yogen Singh* [4,5]*

[1] *Pediatric Cardiology Services, Royal Brompton Hospital, London, United Kingdom,* [2] *National Heart and Lung Institute, Imperial College London, London, United Kingdom,* [3] *Pediatric Cardiac Intensive Care Unit, Royal Brompton Hospital, London, United Kingdom,* [4] *Department of Pediatrics—Pediatric Cardiology and Neonatal Medicine, Cambridge University Hospitals NHS Foundation Trust, Cambridge, United Kingdom,* [5] *University of Cambridge School of Clinical Medicine, Cambridge, United Kingdom*

***Correspondence:**
Yogen Singh
yogen.singh@nhs.net

Persistent patent ductus arteriosus (PDA) is very common in preterm infants, especially in extremely preterm infants. Despite significant advances in management of these vulnerable infants, there has been no consensus on management of PDA—when should we treat, who should we treat, how should we treat and in fact there is no agreement on how we should define a hemodynamically significant PDA. Medical management with non-steroidal anti-inflammatory drugs (NSAIDs) remains the first line of therapy with moderate success rate in closing the PDA. Paracetamol has been reported to be a safe and equally effective medical therapy for closure of PDA. However, additional studies on its long-term safety and efficacy in extremely low birth weight infants are needed before paracetamol can be recommended as standard treatment for a PDA in preterm infants. Surgical ligation of PDA is not without an increased risk of mortality and co-morbidities. Recently, there has been a significant interest in percutaneous transcatheter closure of PDA in preterm infants, including extremely low birth weight infants. Transcatheter PDA closure in preterm ELBW infants is technically feasible with high PDA occlusion success rates and acceptable complication rates as compared to surgical ligation. Many centers have reported promising early- and mid-term follow-up results. However, they need to be further tested in the prospective well-designed studies and randomized controlled trials comparing the results and outcomes of this technique with current treatment strategies including medical treatment before they can be used as the new standard of care for PDA closure in extremely low birth weight infants.

Keywords: patent ductus arteriosus, prematurity, transcatheter closure, patent ductus arteriosus (PDA), extremely preterm infants, percutaneous closure

INDICATIONS AND CONVENTIONAL TREATMENT OF A HEMODYNAMIC SIGNIFICANT PDA IN EXTREMELY LOW BIRTH WEIGHT INFANTS

A persistent patent ductus arteriosus (PDA), defined as failure of the ductus to close within 72 h postnatally, is very common in extremely low birth weight infants and seen in around 50% of infants born under 28 weeks of gestation and / or birth weight <1,000 g (1). Preterm infants under 1,500 g are categorized as very low birth weight infants and those under 1,000 g are considered as extremely low birth weight (ELBW) infants (1, 2). The pathophysiology and echocardiographic diagnosis have been covered in the different articles of Frontier's Research topic on "management of PDA in preterm infants" and this article is primarily focused at advances in management *via* transcatheter closure of PDA in preterm infants weighing under 1,500 g. This article is not focused at whether we should treat or not treat PDA but on the feasibility of closing PDA in ELBW infants via transcatheter route when required as an alternative to surgical ligation.

The left to right shunt across a persistent PDA may lead to pulmonary over-circulation and left heart volume-overload (2). Delayed closure of a hemodynamically significant PDA has been reported to be associated with increased risk of bronchopulmonary dysplasia (BPD) / chronic respiratory disease (CLD), prolonged assisted ventilation, necrotizing enterocolitis (NEC), pulmonary hemorrhage, intraventricular hemorrhage (IVH), renal impairment and increased risk of mortality (2–10). This association led to numerous (more than 60) randomized controlled trials (RCTs) trying to prove that the treatment of PDA would be beneficial. However, these trials have failed to demonstrate any improvement in the long term outcomes such as death or BPD / CLD (11). Some trials have reported short term benefits such as early prophylactic use of indomethacin reported reduction of IVH and acute pulmonary hemorrhage and prophylactic surgical ligation reported reduction in NEC (12–14). There are no other proven benefits shown in terms of improvement in long-term outcomes (such as death or BPD) and there are some adverse outcomes [e.g., increased incidence of chronic lung disease was reported in infants treated with ibuprofen (11)].

Despite the reported association between persistent PDA, increased risk of mortality and significant co-morbidities, the treatment strategy remains controversial which could be because of proven benefits from treating the PDA in ELBW infants (11, 15, 16). There is no agreed consensus on management of PDA in preterm infants and there are numerous trials on-going at the moment testing different treatment approaches to placebo or no treatment.

Treatments with non-steroidal anti-inflammatory drugs (NSAIDs) or paracetamol have been used to promote closure when a PDA was found to be hemodynamically significant. NSAIDs, cyclo-oxygenase inhibitors, have moderate success rate in closing the PDA and they may have adverse effects in some infants or even may be contraindicated in presence of certain conditions such as NEC or intestinal perforation and significant renal impairment (17, 18). Medical treatment fails in 20–40% of the cases (19, 20). Following a recent systemic review (2020) by Ohlsson et al., concluded that paracetamol appears to be a promising alternative to indomethacin and ibuprofen for the closure of a PDA with possibly fewer adverse effects. A possible association between prenatal paracetamol and the development of autism or autism spectrum disorder in childhood and language delay in girls has been reported (21). Therefore, additional studies on its long-term safety and efficacy in ELBW infants are needed before paracetamol can be recommended as standard first line treatment for closure of PDA in preterm infants (21).

Surgical ligation of the PDA is often the alternative to failed pharmacological treatment and it is usually performed through left thoracotomy. It is not without the increased risk of mortality and significant morbidities in this vulnerable group of infants. Thirty days mortality rate has been reported around 5–8% (22, 23). Surgical ligation been reported to be associated to post-ligation cardiac syndrome (PLCS), phrenic nerve and vocal cord palsy, pneumothorax, bleeding, and infection (24–26). The post-operative course of preterm infants undergoing surgical ligation of PDA is often complicated by PLCS and despite targeted milrinone prophylaxis, some infants continue to experience hemodynamic instability and postoperative respiratory deterioration (27–30). Studies have also that it may also worsen long-term outcomes, including increasing the risk for bronchopulmonary dysplasia, retinopathy of prematurity and neurosensory impairment, however, controversies remain whether these are related to surgical ligation or prolonged exposure of preterm infants to PDA itself or associated co-morbidities (31–33).

Conservative management approach, consisting of fluid restriction, diuretics and positive end-expiratory pressure, is also being practiced in many neonatal units because of the lack of proven long-term benefits from PDA closure in this population (34–37). Many studies have concluded that conservative management approach is a reasonable option as compared to pharmacologic or surgical treatment (35–41) while some studies have questioned about the safety of this approach because of increased mortality and morbidity (8, 9, 15). Results from RCTs and well-designed prospective studies are awaited to establish risks and benefits of the conservative management approach.

In absence of proven long term benefits from treating PDAs and lack of superiority of one approach to another, currently there is no universal consensus on how best PDA should be managed in preterm infants. However, there is consensus among the neonatal community that well-designed prospective randomized controlled trials of different modalities against placebo are needed, and there are more than 10 large randomized trials of different approaches on-going worldwide (42). This would be interesting to see the results of these trials in the coming years.

Recently there has been an increased interest in transcutaneous closure of PDA, whether this approach can be used as an alternative to surgical ligation or even to medical treatment in the ELBW infants. We describe the background, current evidence and feasibility of this approach in closure of PDA in infants under 1,500 g.

TRANSCATHETER CLOSURE OF PDA IN EXTREMELY PRETERM INFANTS: BACKGROUND

In the most recent years, several cohort studies reported preliminary experience with transcatheter technique, using various devices for PDA closure in premature infants (43–55). Comparison with surgical ligation revealed a positive impact on post procedure pulmonary outcome (49, 50). The procedure has been well-described in preterm infants, including extremely low birth weight (ELBW) infants as small as 640 g (50). Following the results of an ongoing prospective trial using the ADO II AS, this device received FDA and CE approval for transcatheter closure of PDA in premature babies weighting more than 700 g and over 3 days old (51). This has been renamed as Amplatzer Piccolo Occluder® (APO). More recently, a retrospective comparison between surgery and transcatheter closure by Regan et al. reported an increased mechanical ventilation duration during the NICU stay after surgery as compared to infants undergoing transcatheter closure. Additionally, hospital stay could potentially be shorter in cases where transcatheter closure was performed in the 1st month of life (52).

PATIENT SELECTION AND ORGANIZATION OF THE PROCEDURE

Preterm infants are always referred by neonatologist for percutaneous closure, usually after failure of medical therapy or when medical pharmacotherapy is contraindicated and/or failure to wean from the ventilator. Pre-procedure transthoracic echocardiography confirms the hemodynamic significance (left cavities dilation, functional mitral/aortic regurgitation, and ductal morphology) and transcatheter closure is usually performed in catheterization laboratory. In most centers the procedure is performed in the cardiac catheter lab, although in some centers with portable fluoroscopy equipment the procedure can be performed at the bedside, especially in very unstable patients unsafe to move or when there is no access to cardiac catheterization lab. Transcatheter closure at the bedside under echocardiography guidance-only has also been reported (44). Unfortunately, bedside procedure under echocardiography guidance has to be performed via trans-arterial route (femoral route) without fluoroscopy which carries increased risk of potentially severe life-threatening complications such as limb ischemia and more worryingly it has limited management options for disc embolization if it occurs (56). Hence, despite technical feasibility it is almost never performed on bedside in ELBW infants and smallest reported infant having this procedure successfully done was around 1,400 g. In comparison, when percutaneous PDA closure performed in in the catheter lab it has been performed successfully in infants as small as 700 g (50–52).

AVAILABLE DEVICES

Over the last few years, different devices have been used to close PDAs in premature babies (**Figure 1**). PDA coil-occlusion was initially achieved in selected low-weight infants with symptomatic PDA (44, 51). More recently, the Amplatzer Vascular Plug II (AVP II) was successfully implanted with good results (43, 50, 54). Unfortunately, this device is often not suitable for short ducts in extremely low-weight infants. In such cases the central disk, which is the same diameter than the proximal and distal disk can stretch and make the whole device too long, increasing the risk of LPA and/or aortic stenosis. The Amplatzer Vascular Plug IV has also been used but its length is also a limiting factor in extremely small infants (55). Similarly, the retention disks of the Amplatzer duct occluder II are too large for infants weighing <1,500 g. The Medtronic Micro Vascular Plug® (MVP), initially designed for occlusion of abnormal blood vessels, has shown excellent results for PDA closure in premature babies (47, 50). It is made of a nitinol framework covered partially by a polytetrafluoroethylene (PTFE) membrane at the proximal portion. It is delivered through a microcatheter with two sizes of 5.3 and 6.5 mm. The APO is currently the only dedicated device for this procedure. It is a self-expanding occlusion device with a central waist and retention disc on both ends, delivered through a 4-French delivery catheter. The largest size of the distal disks is 6.5 mm whereas the central waist is available in 3, 4, and 5 mm diameter and the length of the central waist varies between 2, 4, and 6 mm. Catheter and sheath diameters are measured in French (Fr) units and 1Fr = 1/3 mm or 0.013 inch. Wire diameter is measured in inches; 0.014, 0.018, and 0.021 wires are 0.014, 0.018, and 0.021 inch in diameter, respectively (49, 52).

DESCRIPTION OF THE PROCEDURE

Ultrasound-guided access of the femoral vein increases the likelihood of successful access and reduces the risk of local complications, especially inadvertent puncture of the femoral artery. Femoral artery access is not recommended and even contraindicated in extremely premature babies due to a high risk for vessel occlusion and potential ischemia of the lower limb (57). Aortic angiogram after device deployment is unnecessary when appropriate echocardiographic guidance can be performed. A 4Fr sheath is usually inserted in the femoral vein.

Heparin administration remains controversial (58). Whereas, some operators give no heparin, others would give 50–100 units/kg of unfractionated heparin bolus once access has been achieved. Prophylactic antibiotics are administered.

Under fluoroscopic guidance, a 3Fr multipurpose BALT catheter (Montmorency, France) is usually advanced over a 0.014 coronary wire through the inferior vena cava toward the right atrium. The coronary wire is advanced *via* right ventricle outflow tract and through the patent ductus arteriosus toward descending aorta. The 3Fcatheter is positioned in the descending aorta. Sathanandam et al. have reported a similar technique using a 4Fr angled glide catheter (Terumo, Japan) and a 0.035 Wholey wire (Medtronic, Minneapolis, MN, USA) to cross the PDA antegradely into the descending aorta (59). Other teams have used 4Fr Swan Ganz catheter instead of catheters described above (43).

If a 3Fr catheter is used to cross the PDA, then a 0.021 Fixed-Core Guide Wire (Cook Medical®, USA) is advanced in the descending aorta and the 3Fr catheter is directly exchanged with the 4Fr TorqVue® delivery sheath. This latest is often advanced over a microcatheter to minimize mismatch with the 0.021 wire. The tip of the TorqVue® sheath is placed in the descending

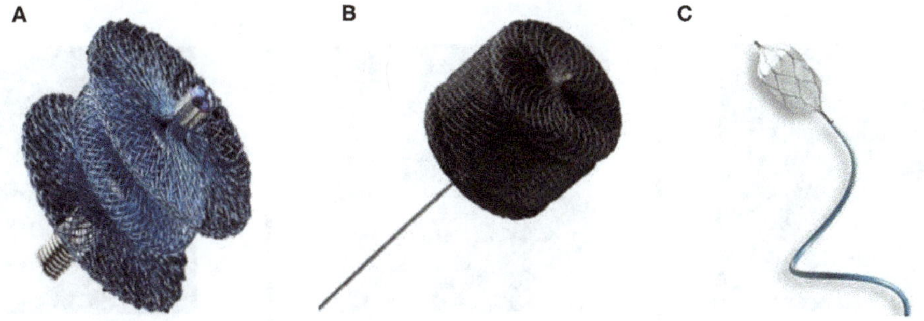

FIGURE 1 | Devices generally used for percutaneous PDA closure in premature babies. **(A)** Amplatzer Ductus Occluder II Additional Sizes / Piccolo Occluder (Abbott). **(B)** Amplatzer vascular plug II (Abbott). **(C)** MVP Microvascular Plug (Medtronic).

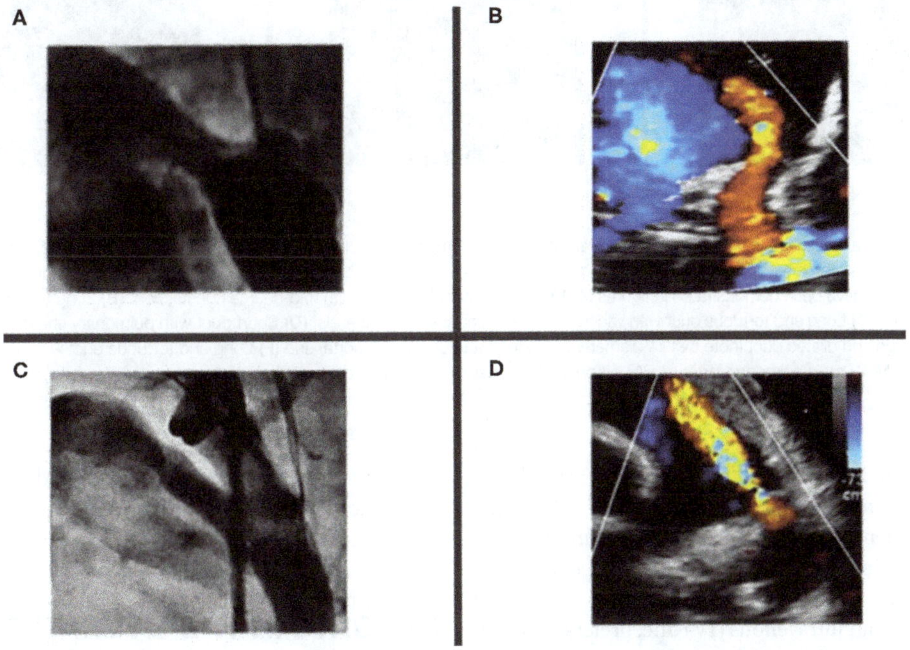

FIGURE 2 | Most common ductal morphology in premature babies undergoing percutaneous closure. **(A,B)** Showing type "C" tubular ductus without any constrictions at the aortic end or the pulmonary artery end. **(C,D)** Showing a "fetal type" ductus, which is typical long, wide and tortuous.

aorta, slightly lower than the PDA. A hand angiogram of 1.5–2 ml is performed in RAO and lateral projection or only in lateral projection in single plane laboratories. In some centers fluoroscopic guidance only is used (51, 53), although most centers routinely perform this procedure under angiography guidance to minimize the risk of complications. Most of the patients needing PDA closure had type C (tubular) and F (fetal) types of PDA morphology (54) (**Figure 2**).

The appropriate device is selected based on echocardiographic and angiographic measurements (**Figure 3**). As a rule, the shortest APO device is used to avoid protrusion of the device in aorta/pulmonary artery branches. In almost all cases only 2 mm or 4 mm-length devices are used.

The device is positioned under fluoroscopy guidance with the goal to implant the entire length of the device into the PDA. Successful positioning is defined by complete occlusion of the duct and the absence of aortic or LPA obstruction by echocardiography.

Following release of the device, echocardiographic evaluation is repeated, paying also particular attention to the tricuspid valve function. Follow-up echocardiography is performed within 24 h after procedure.

ANESTHESIA MANAGEMENT

Anesthesia in this high-risk population presents a number of challenges for the anesthesia team. The cardiac catheter laboratory (CCL) can be a hostile environment for these fragile patients. Ambient temperature cannot be easily controlled. The

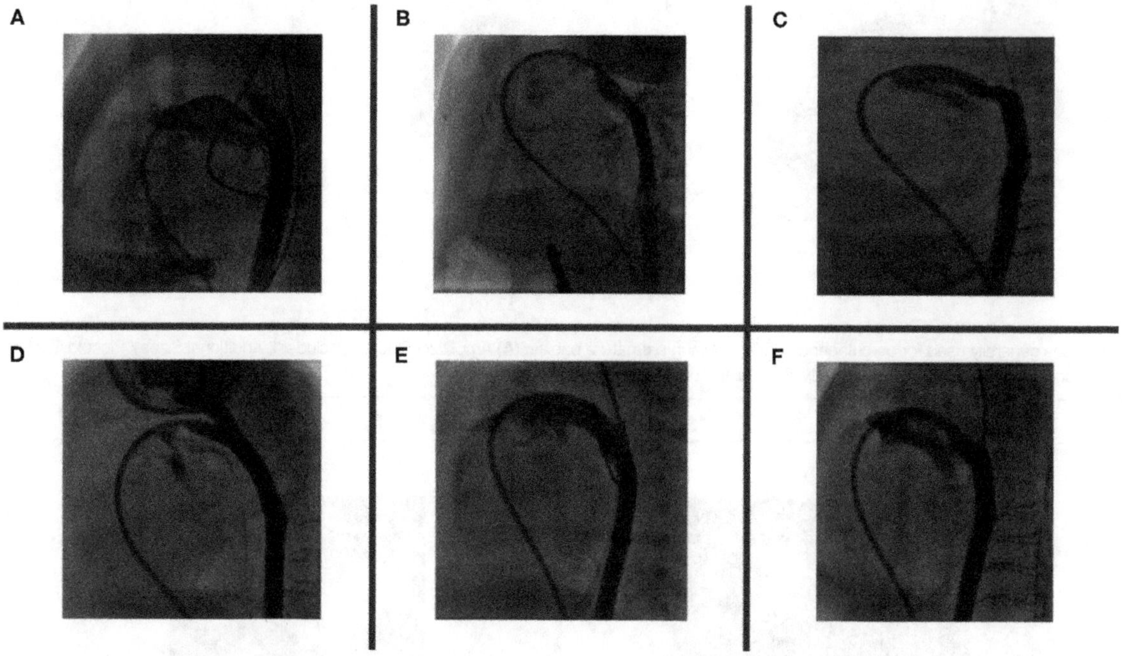

FIGURE 3 | PDA morphology and size are extremely variable in premature babies. Angiogram helps to delineate duct features, accurately measures both PDA's aortic and pulmonary ends and choose the most appropriate device. Angiogram performed through a catheter via RV—MPA—PDA—Descending aorta. Six types of described PDA morphologies have been demonstrated in figures **(A–F)**. **(A)** Relatively long duct with mid-course constriction. **(B)** Long and tortuous duct with pulmonary end constriction. **(C)** Long and tortuous duct with widely open pulmonary and aortic ends. **(D)** Short duct with pulmonary end constriction and LPA origin stenosis. **(E)** Extremely large and dilated duct (note that its diameter is bigger than descending aorta) and **(F)** Long and tortuous duct with variable diameter along its course (RV, right ventricle; MPA, main pulmonary artery; LPA, left pulmonary artery; PDA, patent ductus arteriosus).

warming blanket should be turned on prior to patient arrival and central patient temperature monitoring is mandatory. Imaging equipment makes patient access during the procedure difficult so patient positioning (arms up) should be optimized prior to allowing equipment in.

Ensure easy access to an intravenous (IV) line, preferably in an upper limb. Two IV lines are essential; one to continue dextrose containing maintenance fluid and the other for fluids and/or drugs required during the procedure. IV access should be secured in the NICU to minimize time in the cardiac catheter laboratory.

Accurate monitoring of end-tidal carbon dioxide ($ETCO_2$) can be difficult. It is advisable to have an endotracheal tube (ETT) with minimal leak and minimize circuit dead-space.

There are two periods of potential instability during the procedure however both are generally short-lived and respond quickly to the measures described. Firstly, when the device is positioned in the duct, there is a sudden drop in pulmonary blood flow with a corresponding drop in $ETCO_2$ measurements and peripheral saturations. It is advisable to briefly increase the inspired oxygen concentration to maintain acceptable saturation levels until the circulation adjusts. It may also help to temporarily lower the positive end-expiratory pressure to promote forward flow from the right ventricle.

The second is during echocardiography to confirm device position. This can impact significantly on ventilation requiring an increase in ventilatory pressures and the echocardiographer to echo intermittently to ensure adequate ventilation during assessment.

REPORTS IN THE LITERATURE ON VENOUS-ONLY ACCESS TCPC IN PREMATURE INFANTS

Morville et al. reported successful transcatheter closure of PDA in 32 out of 34 infants under 2,500 g and in their series two patients had major complications: (1) death from hemopericardium and (2) LPA obstruction that required surgical device removal (60). Zahn et al. reported successful PDA closure via transcatheter route in 20 out of 23 premature infants (mean weight 1,250 g; range 755–2,380) and two patients were reported to have complications: (1) LPA stenosis that required stent placement at 3 months of age and (2) transient descending aortic obstruction that was relieved by device manipulation (43, 61). In a small case series 16 patients, Baspinar et al. reported successful closure of PDA in 13 premature infants with a mean weight of 1,000 ± 300 g and three patients were reported to have significant complications including: (1) death from cardiac perforation in one patient and (2) device embolization in two patients, which were retrieved successfully by transcatheter route. These patients needed subsequent surgical closure of the PDA (62). Rodriguez

TABLE 1 | Success rate and major complications from transcatheter closure of PDA in preterm infants (43, 49, 50, 52, 60–62).

Author (ref)	Mean weight (grams)	No of procedures	Success rate	Major complications (no of cases)
Baspinar et al. (62)	1,700 ± 300 g	16	13/16 (81%)	Device embolization (2); Death from cardiac perforation (1)
Zahn et al. (43, 61)	1,250 g (range: 755–2,380 g)	23	20/23 (87%)	Transient descending aortic obstruction (1); LPA stenosis needing stenting (1)
Morville et al. (60)	<2,500 g; 17 under 1,200 g	34	32/34 (94%)	Death from hemopericardium (1); LPA obstruction requiring surgical device removal (1)
Sathanandam et al. (50)	<2,000 g	82	80/82 (98%)	Death from inferior vena cava laceration (1); Severe LPA stenosis needing device retrieval (1); Pericardial effusion needing drainage (1)
Rodriguez Ogando et al. (49)	1,260 g (range: 1,000–1,980 g)	27	27 (100%)	No major complications reported
Regan et al. (52)	1,200 g (range: 1,025–1,700 g)	64	63/64 (98%)	Severe LPA stenosis needing device retrieval (2); Aortic arch obstruction needing re-intervention (1);

Ogando et al. reported 100% success rate with PDA device closure in 27 preterm infants with a median weight of 1,260 g (range 1,000–1,980) and no major complications were reported (49).

In one of the largest published study so far, Sathanandam et al. reported successful closure of 80 out of 82 preterm infants weighing <2,000 g and three patients were reported to have major complications: (1) death from inferior vena cava laceration, (2) severe LPA stenosis needing manipulation of device, and (3) pericardial effusion needing drainage percutaneously (50).

Recently from one of the largest multi-center study involving 147 infants, 64 undergoing transcutaneous PDA closure or 83 with surgical ligation, Regan et al. reported that transcatheter closure of PDA offers sustained improvement in morbidity as compared to surgical ligation through a reduction in post-procedural mechanical ventilation time that is significant throughout the total NICU stay. They reported successful closure of PDA in 63 out of 64 preterm infants with a mean weight 1,200 g (range 1,025–1,700) and three patients were reported to have complications: (1) severe LPA stenosis needing device retrieval and (2) aortic arch obstruction needing re-intervention (51). Six cases had mild LPA stenoses due to protrusion of the device, with a maximum velocity of 2.5 m/s on CW Doppler interrogation, which all resolved within 3–12 months during the follow-up (52).

The results from these reports are encouraging and provide evidence that transcatheter closure PDA in preterm infants is feasible with an acceptable complications rate (**Table 1**) and at least study comparing results with surgical ligation demonstrate that outcomes were better with device closure and complications were less compared to surgical ligation (52). However, none of these reports provide long-term outcomes (especially death or BPD) and the impact on neurodevelopment is unknown.

COMPLICATIONS

One of the most frequent complications is left pulmonary artery (LPA) obstruction due to protrusion of the device. In a 1,000 g infant, the LPA diameter is ~3 mm whereas the APO retention discs for the 4 and 5 mm-devices are 5.25 and 6.5 mm, respectively. Despite the goal to implant the whole device inside the duct itself, protrusion of the proximal disk may occur especially in patients with a large duct and restriction at the pulmonary end. In cases with significant LPA stenosis (max velocity >2 m/s on continuous wave (CW) Doppler interrogation) diagnosed before the device is released it is recommended to reposition it or to change it for a shorter and/or a smaller device. Significant LPA stenosis has been described with AVP II requiring LPA stenting (61). When the LPA stenosis is mild, the device can sometimes be released as this will resolve in most of the cases during follow-up (49).

Coarctation of the aorta related to the device is an uncommon complication. It is often diagnosed with transthoracic echocardiography (TTE) during implantation of the device and repositioning is required in such cases. Similar to LPA stenosis, mild coarctation may resolve with patient's growth. However, significant coarctation may develop, necessitating surgical repair (52) (**Figure 4**).

Device embolization has also been reported during, immediately after and up to 9 days post procedure (48, 49, 63), usually in patients over 1,200 g with a large PDA. The device can be retrieved percutaneously in most cases through a 4Fr or 5Fr sheath (52).

Tricuspid valve injury has been reported and it is often due to chordae rupture from the catheter when the tricuspid valve is crossed.

Rupture and/or dissection of inferior vena cava has been reported as a fatal complication (50). Position of the wire during the femoral vein access should be checked by fluoroscopy before advancing any sheath to minimize this potentially life-threatening complication.

Morville et al. reported fatal cardiac perforation in a 680 g patient. During the procedure the right ventricle was perforated by a 4Fr catheter over a 0.018 Terumo wire, creating a hemopericardium (64). Use of 0.014 soft coronary wire should be advocated in the smallest patients.

There is an existing gap in knowledge in comparing the immediate post-PDA closure complication rates among those undergoing surgical ligation vs. transcatheter occlusion and at this stage no studies have been published comparing such data.

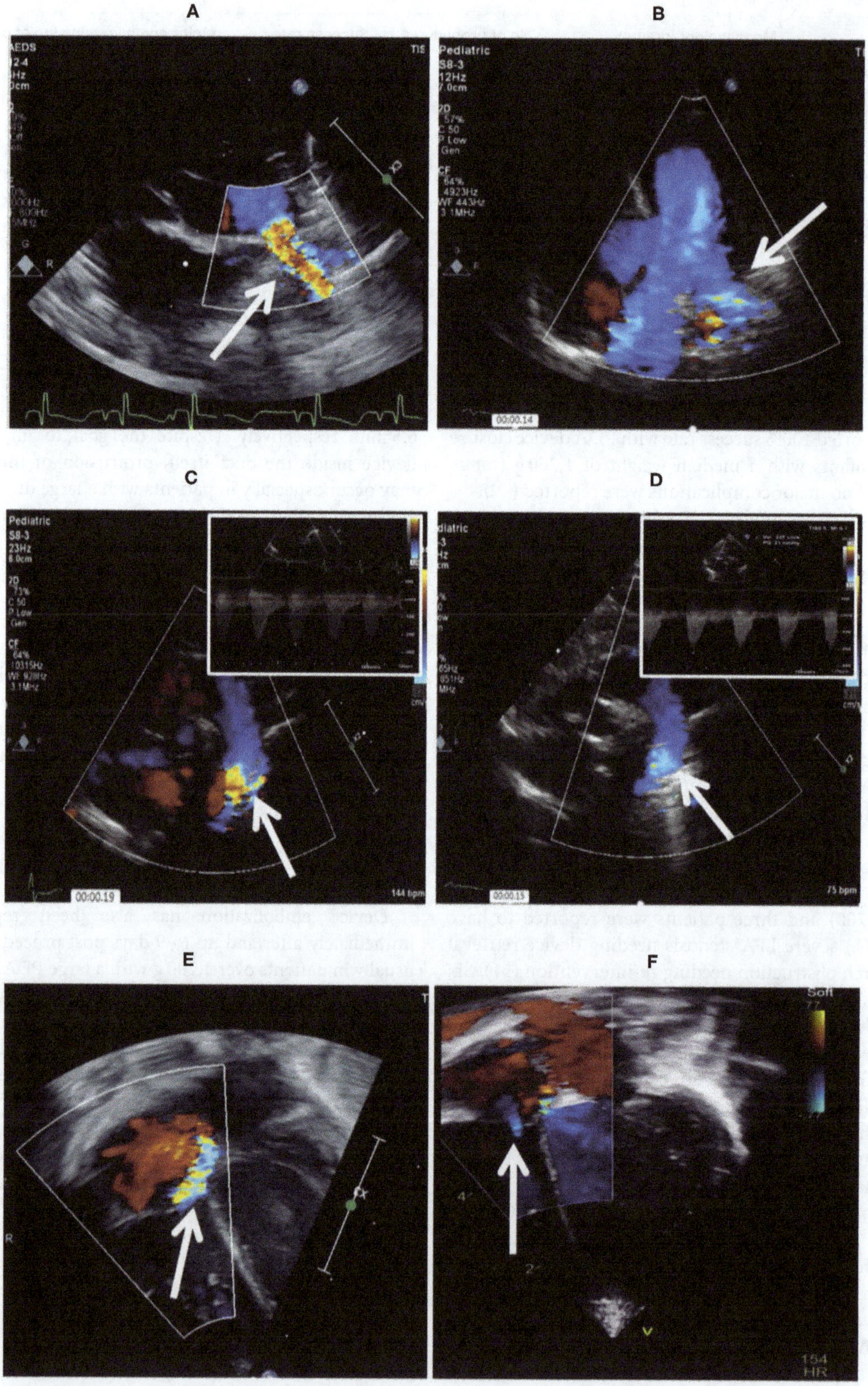

FIGURE 4 | Complications encountered after PDA device closure. **(A)** Shows LPA origin stenosis following percutaneous closure, which is fully resolved 5 months after follow-up **(B)**. **(C)** Mild aortic coarctation after device deployment, which is fully resolved after 11 months of follow-up **(D)**. **(E)** Tricuspid valve trauma noted after successful PDA device closure. **(F)** Tricuspid regurgitation is trivial 12 months after the procedure.

FUTURE DIRECTION

Transcatheter closure of PDA intuitively appear to be advantageous in ELBW infants. A refined an echocardiographic guided antegrade femoral venous approach, which can be performed at the bedside with little or no contrast and minimal radiation exposure has been developed. Early results from the US ADO II-AS multicenter clinical trial are encouraging. We are cautiously optimistic that ongoing modifications in device design and techniques may ultimately make this a routine bedside procedure performed in the neonatal intensive care unit. However, carefully designed prospective randomized trials studying short- and long-term outcomes will be necessary to determine whether this novel therapy should be the new standard of care. Whether early transcutaneous closure of PDA in ELBW infants will result in improved short- and long- term outcomes, less BPD, improved neurodevelopment, or better long term renal function remains to be seen.

CONCLUSION

Transcatheter PDA closure in preterm ELBW infants is technically feasible with high PDA occlusion success rates and acceptable complication rates. The current technique and available devices apply for most of the population, including extremely low birth weight infants. Although follow up studies report excellent short and medium term outcomes, they need to be further tested in the prospective, well-designed and probably randomized controlled trials comparing the results and outcomes of this technique vs. current treatment strategies including medical treatment. This innovative technique is being adopted in increasing number of centers across the globe, however further experience is needed. There is an urgent need for multicenter studies and registries to better clarify the results, optimal timing for this procedure, and to study the short-term and long-term outcomes before this can be considered as an alternative first line therapy, when PDA closure is required in ELBW infants.

AUTHOR CONTRIBUTIONS

YS and AF conceptualized the idea and prepared the draft manuscript. All authors contributed to the manuscript. All authors contributed to the article and approved the submitted version.

REFERENCES

1. Sellmer A, Bjerre JV, Schmidt MR, McNamara PJ, Hjortdal VE, Host B, et al. Morbidity and mortality in preterm neonates with patent ductus arteriosus on day 3. *Arch Dis Child Fetal Neonatal Ed.* (2013) 98:F505–10. doi: 10.1136/archdischild-2013-303816
2. Hamrick SEG, Hansmann G. Patent ductus arteriosus of the preterm infant. *Pediatrics.* (2010) 125:1020–30. doi: 10.1542/peds.2009-3506
3. Roze J-C, Cambonie G, Marchand-Martin L, Gournay V, Durrmeyer X, Durox M, et al. Association between early screening for patent ductus arteriosus and in-hospital mortality among extremely preterm infants. *JAMA.* (2015) 313:2441–8. doi: 10.1001/jama.2015.6734
4. Garland J, Buck R, Weinberg M. Pulmonary hemorrhage risk in infants with a clinically diagnosed patent ductus arteriosus: a retrospective cohort study. *Pediatrics.* (1994) 94:719–23.
5. Marshall DD, Kotelchuck M, Young TE, Bose CL, Kruyer L, O'Shea TM. Risk factors for chronic lung disease in the surfactant era: a North Carolina population-based study of very low birth weight infants. North Carolina Neonatologists Association. *Pediatrics.* (1999) 104:1345–50. doi: 10.1542/peds.104.6.1345
6. Dollberg S, Lusky A, Reichman B. Patent ductus arteriosus, indomethacin and necrotizing enterocolitis in very low birth weight infants: a population-based study. *J Pediatr Gastroenterol Nutr.* (2005) 40:184–8. doi: 10.1097/00005176-200502000-00019
7. Evans N, Kluckow M. Early ductal shunting and intraventricular haemorrhage in ventilated preterm infants. *Arch Dis Child Fetal Neonatal Ed.* (1996) 75:F183–6. doi: 10.1136/fn.75.3.F183
8. Noori S, McCoy M, Friedlich P, Bright B, Gottipati V, Seri I, et al. Failure of ductus arteriosus closure is associated with increased mortality in preterm infants. *Pediatrics.* (2009) 123:e138–44. doi: 10.1542/peds.2008-2418
9. Sankar MN, Bhombal S, Benitz WE. PDA: to treat or not to treat. *Congenit Heart Dis.* (2019) 14:46–51. doi: 10.1111/chd.12708
10. Weisz DE, McNamara PJ. Patent ductus arteriosus ligation and adverse outcomes: causality or bias? *J Clin Neonatol.* (2014) 3:67–75. doi: 10.4103/2249-4847.134670
11. Benitz WE. Treatment of persistent patent ductus arteriosus in preterm infants: time to accept the null hypothesis? *J Perinatol.* (2010) 30:241–52. doi: 10.1038/jp.2010.3
12. Fowlie PW, Davis PG, McGuire W. Prophylactic intravenous indomethacin for preventing mortality and morbidity in preterm infants. *Cochrane Database Syst Rev.* (2010) 2010:CD006181. doi: 10.1002/14651858.CD000174.pub2
13. Mosalli R, Alfaleh K. Prophylactic surgical ligation of patent ductus arteriosus for prevention of mortality and morbidity in extremely low birth weight infants. *Cochrane Database of Syst Rev.* (2008) 2008:CD006181. doi: 10.1002/14651858.CD006181.pub2
14. Kluckow M, Jeffery M, Gill A, Evans N. A randomised placebo-controlled trial of early treatment of the patent ductus arteriosus. *Arch Dis Child Fetal Neonatal Ed.* (2014) 99:F99–F104. doi: 10.1136/archdischild-2013-304695
15. Heuchan AM, Clyman RI. Managing the patent ductus arteriosus: current treatment options. *Arch Dis Child Fetal Neonatal Ed.* (2014) 99:F431–6. doi: 10.1136/archdischild-2014-306176
16. Bose CL, Laughon MM. Patent ductus arteriosus: lack of evidence for common treatments. *Arch Dis Child Fetal Neonatal Ed.* (2007) 92:F498–502. doi: 10.1136/adc.2005.092734
17. Trus T, Winthrop AL, Pipe S, Shah J, Langer JC, Lau GY. Optimal management of patent ductus arteriosus in the neonate weighing less than 800 g. *J Pediatr Surg.* (1993) 28:1137–9. doi: 10.1016/0022-3468(93)90148-E
18. Janz-Robinson EM, Badawi N, Walker K, Bajuk B, Abdel-Latif ME. Neurodevelopmental outcomes of premature infants treated for patent ductus arteriosus: a population-based cohort study. *J Pediatr.* (2015) 167:1025–32.e3. doi: 10.1016/j.jpeds.2015.06.054
19. Irmesi R, Marcialis MA, Anker JVD, Fanos V. Non-steroidal anti-inflammatory drugs (NSAIDs) in the management of patent ductus arteriosus (PDA) in preterm infants and variations in attitude in clinical practice: a flight around the world. *Curr Med Chem.* (2014) 21:3132–52. doi: 10.2174/0929867321666140304095434
20. Hammerman C, Bin-Nun A, Markovitch E, Schimmel MS, Kaplan M, Fink D. Ductal closure with paracetamol: a surprising new approach to patent ductus arteriosus treatment. *Pediatrics.* (2011) 128:e1618–21. doi: 10.1542/peds.2011-0359

21. Ohlsson A, Shah PS. Paracetamol (acetaminophen) for patent ductus arteriosus in preterm or low birth weight infants. *Cochrane Database Syst Rev.* (2020) 1:CD010061. doi: 10.1002/14651858.CD010061.pub4
22. Hutchings K, Vasquez A, Price D, Cameron BH, Awan S, Miller GG. Outcomes following neonatal patent ductus arteriosus ligation done by pediatric surgeons: a retrospective cohort analysis. *J Pediatr Surg.* (2013) 48:915–8. doi: 10.1016/j.jpedsurg.2013.02.003
23. Lee LCL, Tillett A, Tulloh R, Yates R, Kelsall W. Outcome following patent ductus arteriosus ligation in premature infants: a retrospective cohort analysis. *BMC Pediatr.* (2006) 6:15. doi: 10.1186/1471-2431-6-15
24. Koehne PS, Bein G, Alexi-Meskhishvili V, Weng Y, Buhrer C, Obladen M. Patent ductus arteriosus in very low birthweight infants: complications of pharmacological and surgical treatment. *J Perinat Med.* (2001) 29:327–34. doi: 10.1515/JPM.2001.047
25. Palder SB, Schwartz MZ, Tyson KR, Marr CC. Management of patent ductus arteriosus: a comparison of operative v pharmacologic treatment. *J Pediatr Surg.* (1987) 22:1171–4. doi: 10.1016/S0022-3468(87)80730-3
26. Raval M V, Laughon MM, Bose CL, Phillips JD. Patent ductus arteriosus ligation in premature infants: who really benefits, and at what cost? *J Pediatr Surg.* (2007) 42:69–75. doi: 10.1016/j.jpedsurg.2006.09.040
27. Weisz DE, Mirea L, Rosenberg E, Jang M, Ly L, Church PT, et al. Association of patent ductus arteriosus ligation with death or neurodevelopmental impairment among extremely preterm infants. *JAMA Pediatr.* (2017) 171:443–9. doi: 10.1001/jamapediatrics.2016.5143
28. Ting JY, Resende M, More K, Nicholls D, Weisz DE, El-Khuffash A, et al. Predictors of respiratory instability in neonates undergoing patient ductus arteriosus ligation after the introduction of targeted milrinone treatment. *J Thorac Cardiovasc Surg.* (2016) 152:498–504. doi: 10.1016/j.jtcvs.2016.03.085
29. McNamara PJ, Stewart L, Shivananda SP, Stephens D, Sehgal A. Patent ductus arteriosus ligation is associated with impaired left ventricular systolic performance in premature infants weighing less than 1000 g. *J Thorac Cardiovasc Surg.* (2010) 140:150–7. doi: 10.1016/j.jtcvs.2010.01.011
30. Jain A, Sahni M, El-Khuffash A, Khadawardi E, Sehgal A, McNamara PJ. Use of targeted neonatal echocardiography to prevent postoperative cardiorespiratory instability after patent ductus arteriosus ligation. *J Pediatr.* (2012) 160:584–9.e1. doi: 10.1016/j.jpeds.2011.09.027
31. Kabra NS, Schmidt B, Roberts RS, Doyle LW, Papile L, Fanaroff A. Neurosensory impairment after surgical closure of patent ductus arteriosus in extremely low birth weight infants: results from the trial of indomethacin prophylaxis in preterms. *J Pediatr.* (2007) 150:229–34. doi: 10.1016/j.jpeds.2006.11.039
32. Chorne N, Leonard C, Piecuch R, Clyman RI. Patent ductus arteriosus and its treatment as risk factors for neonatal and neurodevelopmental morbidity. *Pediatrics.* (2007) 119:1165–74. doi: 10.1542/peds.2006-3124
33. Weisz DE, More K, McNamara PJ, Shah PS. PDA ligation and health outcomes: a meta-analysis. *Pediatrics.* (2014) 133:e1024–46. doi: 10.1542/peds.2013-3431
34. Clyman RI, Couto J, Murphy GM. Patent ductus arteriosus: are current neonatal treatment options better or worse than no treatment at all? *Semin Perinatol.* (2012) 36:123–9. doi: 10.1053/j.semperi.2011.09.022
35. Vanhaesebrouck S, Zonnenberg I, Vandervoort P, Bruneel E, Van Hoestenberghe M-R, Theyskens C. Conservative treatment for patent ductus arteriosus in the preterm. *Arch Dis Child Fetal Neonatal Ed.* (2007) 92:F244–7. doi: 10.1136/adc.2006.104596
36. Kaempf JW, Wu YX, Kaempf AJ, Kaempf AM, Wang L, Grunkemeier G. What happens when the patent ductus arteriosus is treated less aggressively in very low birth weight infants? *J Perinatol.* (2012) 32:344–8. doi: 10.1038/jp.2011.102
37. Sung SI, Chang YS, Chun JY, Yoon SA, Yoo HS, Ahn SY, et al. Mandatory closure versus nonintervention for patent ductus arteriosus in very preterm infants. *J Pediatr.* (2016) 177:66–71.e1. doi: 10.1016/j.jpeds.2016.06.046
38. Wickremasinghe AC, Rogers EE, Piecuch RE, Johnson BC, Golden S, Moon-Grady AJ, et al. Neurodevelopmental outcomes following two different treatment approaches (early ligation and selective ligation) for patent ductus arteriosus. *J Pediatr.* (2012) 161:1065–72. doi: 10.1016/j.jpeds.2012.05.062
39. Semberova J, Sirc J, Miletin J, Kucera J, Berka I, Sebkova S, et al. Spontaneous closure of patent ductus arteriosus in infants </=1500 g. *Pediatrics.* (2017) 140:e20164258. doi: 10.1542/peds.2016-4258
40. Slaughter JL, Reagan PB, Newman TB, Klebanoff MA. comparative effectiveness of nonsteroidal anti-inflammatory drug treatment vs no treatment for patent ductus arteriosus in preterm infants. *JAMA Pediatr.* (2017) 171:e164354. doi: 10.1001/jamapediatrics.2016.4354
41. Benitz WE, Slaughter JL, Reagan PB, Newman TB, Klebanoff MA, Semberova J, et al. Patent ductus arteriosus in preterm infants. *Pediatrics.* (2016) 171:66–71.e1. doi: 10.1542/peds.2015-3730
42. Available online at: https://clinicaltrials.gov/ct2/results?term=pDA&Search=Apply&recrs=a&age
43. Zahn EM, Nevin P, Simmons C, Garg R. A novel technique for transcatheter patent ductus arteriosus closure in extremely preterm infants using commercially available technology. *Catheter Cardiovasc Interv.* (2015) 85:240–8. doi: 10.1002/ccd.25534
44. Bentham J, Meur S, Hudsmith L, Archer N, Wilson N. Echocardiographically guided catheter closure of arterial ducts in small preterm infants on the neonatal intensive care unit. *Catheter Cardiovasc Interv.* (2011) 77:409–15. doi: 10.1002/ccd.22637
45. Francis E, Singhi AK, Lakshmivenkateshaiah S, Kumar RK. Transcatheter occlusion of patent ductus arteriosus in pre-term infants. *JACC Cardiovasc Interv.* (2010) 3:550–5. doi: 10.1016/j.jcin.2010.01.016
46. Narin N, Pamukcu O, Baykan A, Sunkak S, Ulgey A, Uzum K. Percutaneous PDA closure in extremely low birth weight babies. *J Interv Cardiol.* (2016) 29:654–60. doi: 10.1111/joic.12352
47. Sathanandam S, Justino H, Waller BR 3rd, Radtke W, Qureshi AM. Initial clinical experience with the medtronic micro vascular plug in transcatheter occlusion of PDAs in extremely premature infants. *Catheter Cardiovasc Interv.* (2017) 89:1051–8. doi: 10.1002/ccd.26878
48. Wang-Giuffre EW, Breinholt JP. Novel use of the medtronic micro vascular plug for PDA closure in preterm infants. *Catheter Cardiovasc Interv.* (2017) 89:1059–65. doi: 10.1002/ccd.26855
49. Rodriguez Ogando A, Planelles Asensio I, de la Blanca ARS, Ballesteros Tejerizo F, Sanchez Luna M, Gil Jaurena JM, et al. Surgical ligation versus percutaneous closure of patent ductus arteriosus in very low-weight preterm infants: which are the real benefits of the percutaneous approach? *Pediatr Cardiol.* (2018) 39:398–410. doi: 10.1007/s00246-017-1768-5
50. Sathanandam S, Balduf K, Chilakala S, Washington K, Allen K, Knott-Craig C, et al. Role of transcatheter patent ductus arteriosus closure in extremely low birth weight infants. *Catheter Cardiovasc Interv.* (2019) 93:89–96. doi: 10.1002/ccd.27808
51. clinicaltrials.gov. *AMPLATZER Duct Occluder II Additional Sizes (ADO II AS).* NCT03055858 @clinicaltrials.gov. (2020). Available online at: https://www.clinicaltrials.gov/ct2/show/NCT03055858 (accessed August 5, 2020).
52. Regan W, Benbrik N, Sharma SR, Auriau J, Bouvaist H, Bautista C, et al. Improved ventilation in premature babies after transcatheter versus surgical closure of patent ducts arteriosus. *Int J Cardiol.* (2020) 311:22–7. doi: 10.1016/j.ijcard.2020.03.040
53. Kannan BRJ, Anil SR, Padhi SS, Kumar RK. Transcatheter management of patent ductus arteriosus in sick ventilated small infants. *Indian Heart J.* (2004) 56:232–4.
54. Philip R, Waller BR 3rd, Agrawal V, Wright D, Arevalo A, Zurakowski D, et al. Morphologic characterization of the patent ductus arteriosus in the premature infant and the choice of transcatheter occlusion device. *Catheter Cardiovasc Interv.* (2016) 87:310–7. doi: 10.1002/ccd.26287
55. Prsa M, Ewert P. Transcatheter closure of a patent ductus arteriosus in a preterm infant with an amplatzer vascular plug IV device. *Catheter Cardiovasc Interv.* (2011) 77:108–11. doi: 10.1002/ccd.22657
56. Almeida-Jones M, Tang NY, Reddy A, Zahn E. Overview of transcatheter patent ductus arteriosus closure in preterm infants. *Congenit Heart Dis.* (2019) 14:60–4. doi: 10.1111/chd.12712
57. Alexander J, Yohannan T, Abutineh I, Agrawal V, Lloyd H, Zurakowski D, et al. Ultrasound-guided femoral arterial access in pediatric cardiac catheterizations: A prospective evaluation of the prevalence, risk factors, and mechanism for acute loss of arterial pulse. *Catheter Cardiovasc Interv.* (2016) 88:1098–7. doi: 10.1002/ccd.26702
58. Monagle P, Chan AKC, Goldenberg NA, Ichord RN, Journeycake JM, Nowak-Gottl U, et al. Antithrombotic therapy in neonates and children: antithrombotic therapy and prevention of thrombosis, 9th ed: American

college of chest physicians evidence-based clinical practice guidelines. *Chest.* (2012) 141(Suppl.2):e737S–801S. doi: 10.1378/chest.11-2308

59. Sathanandam S, Agrawal H, Chilakala S, Johnson J, Allen K, Knott-Craig C, et al. Can transcatheter PDA closure be performed in neonates </=1000 grams? the memphis experience. *Congenit Heart Dis.* (2019) 14:79–84. doi: 10.1111/chd.12700
60. Morville P, Akhavi A. Transcatheter closure of hemodynamic significant patent ductus arteriosus in 32 premature infants by amplatzer ductal occluder additional size-ADOIIAS. *Catheter Cardiovasc Interv.* (2017) 90:612–7. doi: 10.1002/ccd.27091
61. Zahn EM, Peck D, Phillips A, Nevin P, Basaker K, Simmons C, et al. Transcatheter closure of patent ductus arteriosus in extremely premature newborns: early results and midterm follow-up. *JACC Cardiovasc Interv.* (2016) 9:2429–37. doi: 10.1016/j.jcin.2016.09.019
62. Baspinar O, Sahin DA, Sulu A, Irdem A, Gokaslan G, Sivasli E, et al. Transcatheter closure of patent ductus arteriosus in under 6 kg and premature infants. *J Interv Cardiol.* (2015) 28:180–9. doi: 10.1111/joic.12196
63. Backes CH, Cheatham SL, Deyo GM, Leopold S, Ball MK, Smith C V., et al. Percutaneous patent ductus arteriosus (PDA) closure in very preterm infants: feasibility and complications. *J Am Heart Assoc.* (2016) 5:1–10. doi: 10.1161/JAHA.115.002923
64. Morville P, Douchin S, Bouvaist H, Dauphin C. Transcatheter occlusion of the patent ductus arteriosus in premature infants weighing less than 1200 g. *Arch Dis Child Fetal Neonatal Ed.* (2018) 103:F198–201. doi: 10.1136/archdischild-2016-312582

19

Molecular and Mechanical Mechanisms Regulating Ductus Arteriosus Closure in Preterm Infants

Fahri Ovalı*

Division of Neonatology, Department of Pediatrics, Istanbul Medeniyet University, Istanbul, Turkey

***Correspondence:**
Fahri Ovalı
fovali@yahoo.com

Failure of ductus arteriosus closure after preterm birth is associated with significant morbidities. Ductal closure requires and is regulated by a complex interplay of molecular and mechanical mechanisms with underlying genetic factors. *In utero* patency of the ductus is maintained by low oxygen tension, high levels of prostaglandins, nitric oxide and carbon monoxide. After birth, ductal closure occurs first by functional closure, followed by anatomical remodeling. High oxygen tension and decreased prostaglandin levels mediated by numerous factors including potassium channels, endothelin-1, isoprostanes lead to the contraction of the ductus. Bradykinin and corticosteroids also induce ductal constriction by attenuating the sensitivity of the ductus to PGE2. Smooth muscle cells of the ductus can sense oxygen through a mitochondrial network by the role of Rho-kinase pathway which ends up with increased intracellular calcium levels and contraction of myosin light chains. Anatomical closure of the ductus is also complex with various mechanisms such as migration and proliferation of smooth muscle cells, extracellular matrix production, endothelial cell proliferation which mediate cushion formation with the interaction of blood cells. Regulation of vessel walls is affected by retinoic acid, TGF-β1, notch signaling, hyaluronan, fibronectin, chondroitin sulfate, elastin, and vascular endothelial cell growth factor (VEGF). Formation of the platelet plug facilitates luminal remodeling by the obstruction of the constricted ductal lumen. Vasa vasorum are more pronounced in the term ductus but are less active in the preterm ductus. More than 100 genes are effective in the prostaglandin pathway or in vascular smooth muscle development and structure may affect the patency of ductus. Hemodynamic changes after birth including fluid load and flow characteristics as well as shear forces within the ductus also stimulate closure. Current pharmacological treatment for the closure of a patent ductus is based on the blockage of the prostaglandin pathway mainly through COX or POX inhibition, albeit with some limitations and side effects. Further research for new agents aiming ductal closure should focus on a clear understanding of vascular biology of the ductus.

Keywords: ductus arteriosus, oxygen, vasa vasorum, hemodynamics, indomethacin, ibuprofen, acetaminophen, prostaglandins

Fetal circulation is a unique event, functionally different from pediatric and adult circulation. Ductus arteriosus (DA) is a small, simple vessel with just a few milimeters length and width, but has a profound impact on the survival of the fetus and newborn and plays an essential role in normal postnatal adaptation after birth. It functions as a bridge between two large vessels in fetal life, but sometimes it becomes the "bridge between life and death" in preterm infants. It has baffled scientists since ancient times, and beginning from Galen and Ibn-al Nafis, Vesalius, Leonardo Botallo and William Harvey have commented on its structure and function (1).

During fetal development, cardiovascular septation occurs during days 22–28 of gestation and looping of ventricles completes. At this stage, bilateral aortic arches and bilateral DA form but over the next week, the right aortic arch and ductus involutes. Ductus arteriosus arises from the left sixth embryonic arch; leaves the pulmonary artery very close to the bifurcation point and inserts at the transition zone between the aortic arch and descending aorta, distal to the origin of the left subclavian artery. Usually it has a tubular shape but may be funnel-shaped with a narrow end on the pulmonary side and a wide end on the aortic side (2). Although they all derive from the same embryonic tissue, histological structure of the DA is completely different from that of the aorta or pulmonary arteries. The walls of both great vessels are composed of mainly elastic layers, whereas DA wall is mainly muscular. The inner layer of its wall is composed of longitudinal arranged smooth muscle cells whereas the arrangement of outer layer is mainly circular. On the luminal side, a layer of intimal endothelial cells resides on an internal elastic lamina. This unique structure of the DA sets the stage for the constriction of the vessel after birth.

Ductus arteriosus needs to be remain open in fetal life, in order to sustain the "serial" circulation of the blood. Magnetic resonance studies show that 41% of combined ventricular output passes through the DA in fetal life (3). However, after birth, as the lungs begin to function, a "parallel" circulation is maintained, rendering DA non-functional. Initially it was thought that the ductus was a flabby structure that remained passively open. However, in fetal life, ductus in actively kept dilated by continuous intramural production of prostaglandins (4). The transition from intrauterine to extrauterine life is a critical period and dysregulation of this process may lead to cardiopulmonary instability. Cardiopulmonary adaptation is completed by the closure of DA, followed by closure of ductus venosus and lastly by foramen ovale. In 88% of normal term infants, the ductus is closed by the 8th week of life (5). Preterm infants are born before complete maturation of the cardiovascular system, and they manifest most of the characteristics of fetal life. In a retrospective study of 280 preterm infants who did not receive any therapy directed at closing the ductus, the median time to closure was 71 days in infants born <26 weeks; 13 days in infants born 26–27 weeks, 8 days in infants born 28–29 weeks and 6 days in infants born >30 weeks (6). This implies that extremely preterm infants will be subjected to a period of left-to-right shunting and complications relevant to this shunting.

Ductal closure occurs in two steps: The functional step (vasoconstriction) and the anatomical step (remodeling). Interestingly, the closure of DA resembles the process after vascular injury or atherosclerosis in the adult arteries (7). Understanding different mechanisms which are involved in maintaining ductal tone is essential to comprehend why preterm infants have a high incidence of ductal patency, why some of them do not respond to treatment and where to direct novel therapeutic approaches. On the other hand, it must be stated that most of the experiments and studies toward understanding the physiology of ductal closure are done in animals such as rats or lambs and extrapolated to humans. However, some mechanisms as well as their magnitudes may not be the same in humans.

DUCTAL PATENCY *IN UTERO*

Smooth muscle tone is regulated by phosphorylation/dephosphorylation of myosin light chain (MLC). MLC is phosphorylated by Calcium/calmodulin-dependent MLC-kinase (MLCK) and dephosphorylated by calcium independent MLC-phosphate (MLCP). Increased cytosolic calcium activates MLCK, which leads to MLC phosphorylation and vasoconstriction (8) (**Figure 1**). Patency of DA is regulated by counteractive forces causing vasodilation or vasoconstriction. In the fetus, DA needs to remain open, therefore vasodilating factors are more active than vasoconstrictive factors. Prostaglandins play a dominant role to oppose constriction. Since the pulmonary artery pressure is very high, the pressure within the DA is very high, preventing it from constriction.

Prostaglandins

Prostaglandins are synthesized from arachnidonic acid by cyclooxygenases COX1 and COX2 within the ductal muscle. Circulating prostaglandins, originated from the placenta contribute to the patency of DA (**Figure 2**). Prostaglandins are metabolized in the lung and low pulmonary blood flow in the fetus leads to reduced clearance of prostaglandins, increasing their concentration further.

Prostacylin (PGI_2) is the major arachnidonic acid product of the ductus but although it is more prevalent, it is less potent than prostaglandin E2 (PGE_2), which is the most important prostaglandin to regulate the patency of DA (9). PGE_2 interacts mainly with its receptor EP_4. EP_4 activates voltage-gated potassium channel (Kv) and outward K^+ current increases, thereby inducing membrane hyperpolarization, which inhibits Ca^{2+} influx via the voltage-gated L-type calcium channels (Ca_L) and decreases intracellular calcium (10). PGE_2also activates cyclic adenosine monophosphate (cAMP), which inturn activates protein kinase (PKA), which inhibits myosin light chain creatine kinase (MLCK). Inhibition of MLCK blocks phosphorylation of myosin light chains, which results in inhibition of vasoconstriction, hence vasodilation occurs (11–13) (**Figure 1**). *In utero* vasodilation of the ductus is maintained by dephosphorylation of MLC to MLCP. MLCP is enhanced due to the inhibitory effect of PKG on the Rho-kinase pathway. PKG also activates Kv channels, leading to hyperpolarization and inhibition of Ca^{2+} influx through Ca_L channels. Stimulation of sarcoplasmic reticulum calcium ATPase (SERCA), by PKG

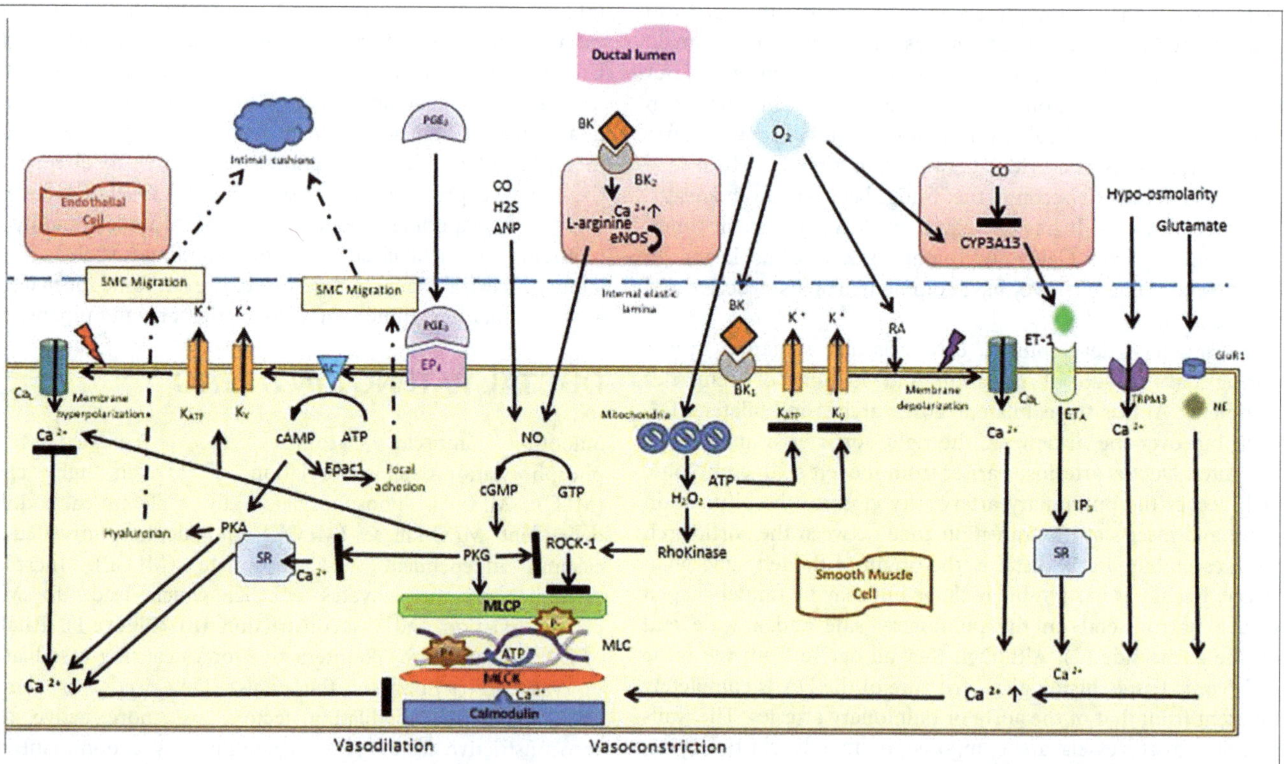

FIGURE 1 | Vasoconstrictive and vasodilatory effects in the ductal smooth muscle cell. Smooth muscle cells are lined with an internal elastic lamina, on which endothelial cells reşide. Vasodilation is maintained by the interaction of PGE2 with its receptor EP4, which triggers potassium outflow through voltage-sensitive potassium channels, which leads to membrane hyperpolarization. Thereby, calcium entry into the cells decreases and binding of calmodulin to MLCK is inhibited. cAMP and cGMP are also effective during this process. After birth, high oxygen tension, which is sensed through the mitochondria triggers the formation of H_2O_2 which blocks Rho-kinase pathway as well as potassium channels leading to membrane depolarization and calcium entry into cells. Calcium entry is also stimulated by endothelin-1, hypo-osmolarity and glutamate. Calcium activates MLCK, which leads to MLC phosphorylation and vasoconstriction. cAMP is also effective in smooth muscle migration and intimal cushion formation. AC, adenylyl cyclase; ANP, Atrial Natriuretic peptide; ATP, Adenosine Tri Phosphate; BK, Bradykinin; BK1, Bradykinin receptor; CaL, calcium channels; cAMP, cyclic adenosine monophosphate; cGMP, cyclic guanosin monophosphate; CO, Carbon monoxide; CYP3A13, cytochrome P450; eNOS, endogenous nitric oxide synthase; EP4, Prostaglandin receptor 4; ET-1, Endothelin-1; ETA, endothelin receptor A; epac, exchange protein activated cAMP; H2, Hydrogen sülfite; GluR1, glutamate receptor-1; KATP, KV, Voltage-dependent potassium channels; NE, Norepinephrine; MLC, Myosin Light Chain; MLCK, Myosin Light Chain Kinase; MLCP, Myosin Light Chain Phosphatase; NO, nitric oxide; PKA, cAMP-dependent protein kinase; PGE2, Prostaglandin E2; PKG, cGMP-dependent protein kinase; RA, Retinoic acid; ROCK-1, Rho-associated protein kinase-1; SR, Sarcoplasmic Reticulum; SMC, Smooth Muscle Cell; TRMP3, transient receptor potential melastatin 3 (Figure courtesy of Fahri Ovali).

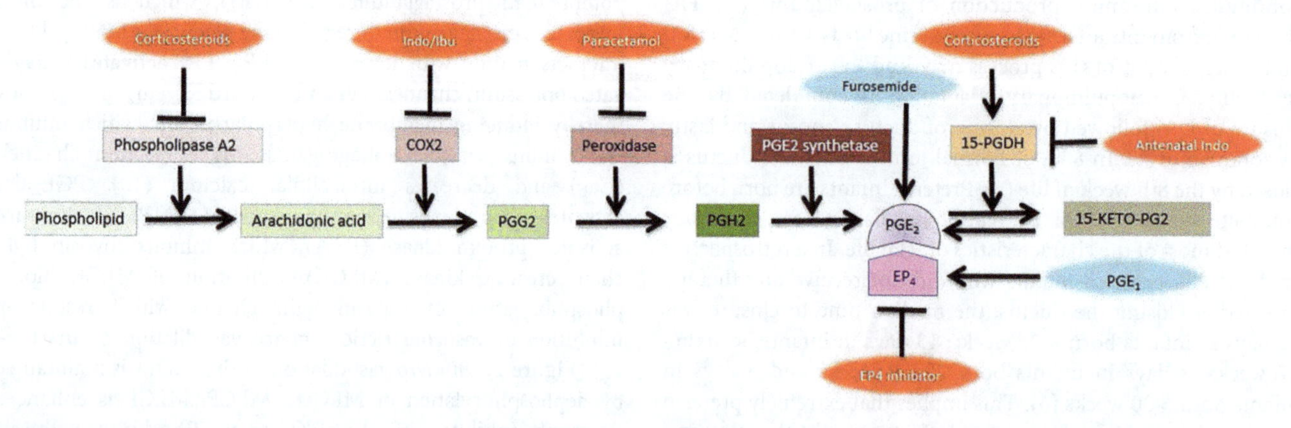

FIGURE 2 | Prostaglandin pathway and metabolism. Inhibitors of various steps are shown in red., COX-1, cyclooxygenase-1; EP4, Prostaglandin receptor 4; Indo, Indomethacin; Ibu, Ibuprofen; PG, prostaglandin; 15-PGDH, 15-hydroxyprostaglandin dehydrogenase; 15-KETO-PG2 (Figure courtesy of Fahri Ovali).

leads to uptake of Ca^{2+} in sarcoplasmic reticulum, lowering intracellular calcium (14, 15).

Nitric Oxide

Nitric oxide (NO) is produced by endothelial nitric oxide synthase in the luminal endothelium and endothelium of vasa vasorum and maintains the patency of DA by acting through cGMP. After its production, it diffuses into the SMC and binds with soluble guanylyl cyclase, producing cyclic guanosine monophosphate (cGMP). cGMP activates cGMP-dependent protein kinase (PKG), which induces vasodilation (16) (**Figure 1**). NO is also formed in small amounts in the SMC by inducible nitric oxide synthase (iNOS) and neuronal NOS, which contribute to ductal relaxation (17). Nitric oxide is used commonly in preterm infants for the management of pulmonary hypertension and may affect the patency of the ductus. PGE_2 and NO are coupled for reciprocal compensation such that inhibition of one of them increases the concentration of the other one (18). This might explain why some preterm infants fail to close their ductus in response to COX inhibitors.

Carbon Monoxide

Hem oxygenase 1 and hem oxygenase 2 which produce carbon monoxide (CO) are found in the endothelial and smooth muscle cells of the DA. CO dilates the ductus by inhibition of O_2 sensing cytochrome P450, thus interrupting endothelin-1 signaling (19, 20) (**Figure 1**). Carbon monoxide produced under physiological conditions seems to be negligible with regard to ductal patency but in cases of upregulation such as endotoxemia, it may have a relaxing effect on the ductus. Carbon monoxide is also formed in a molar ration during bilirubin production. Theoretically, high bilirubin levels may be associated with ductal patency. However, since high bilirubin levels are not allowed and treated accordingly in human neonates, this effect does not seem to be an important contributor to PDA. Similarly hydrogen sulfide inhibits DA tone (21).

Phosphodiesterase 3 (PDE_3) inhibitors such as milrinone and amrinone have positive inotrope and vasodilator effects. Inhibition of PDE_3 also induces dilation of the fetal and postnatal ductus arteriosus in humans. This effect is mediated by an increase in cAMP and cGMP in vascular smooth muscle (22) (**Figure 1**).

Transient receptor potential melastatin 3 (TRPM3) is expressed heavily in ductal SMC and acts as a calcium channel which increases intracellular Ca^{2+} independent of Ca_L channels. Progesterone is a natural inhibitor of TRPM3 and may prevent ductal closure *in utero* (23).

Factors that maintain ductal patency *in utero* are summarized in **Table 1** (24).

FUNCTIONAL CLOSURE

Functional closure of the ductus occurs by 8 h in 44% of normal term infants and almost 100% are closed by 72 h. (25). The rate and degree of this closure is determined by the balance of vasodilator and vasoconstrictive factors. Several changes in late gestation contribute to an increase in ductal tone.

Constriction of the ductus is maintained via3 factors:

a) Decreased concentration of prostaglandins by the loss of placental source and increased removal by the lungs, and decreased number of EP_4 receptors on the ductal wall.
b) Increased arterial oxygen pressure.
c) Decreased pulmonary vascular resistance resulting in decreased blood pressure within the lumen of the DA.

Decreased Prostaglandins

After the cord is clamped, PGE_2 concentrations drop rapidly due to removal of placental production and increased metabolism in the lungs (9). The metabolism of PGE_2in the lung is mediated by PG transporter, which controls the uptake of PGE_2into type II alveolar epithelial cells (26). In the alveolar epithelial cell, $PGE_2$is degraded reversibly to biologically inactive metabolite 15-keto-PGE_2 by 15-hydroxyprostaglandin dehydrogenase (15-PGDH) (27). The activity of 15-PGDH increases with increasing gestational age (28). 15-keto-$PGE_2$is metabolized irreversibly to 13, 14-dihydro- 15-keto-$PGE_2$by Δ-13-reductase. After birth, expression of EP_4 decreases and increased oxygen reduces the sensitivity of the ductus to PGE_2 (29). On the other hand, lungs also produce bradykinin (27). Bradykinin induces vasodilation *in utero*, but in higher concentrations, it induces vasoconstriction (30).

In the preterm infant, the sensitivity of DA to PGE_2 is higher than that in the term infant, which is attributed to increased binding to EP_2, EP_3, and EP_4 receptors (18). The catabolism of PGE_2 is slower due to low 15-PGDH activity in early gestation. The preterm ductus is also six times more sensitive to dilation to NO than the mature DA (31). Postnatal increase in oxygen might enhance NO production, which induces vasodilation (9).

Although PGE_2 is the most important agent in maintaining ductal patency in fetal life, there is some evidence that in late gestation, it may paradoxically prepare the ductus for postnatal closure. At that time, PGE_2 may promote the expression of some genes involved in vasoconstriction (32, 33). In late gestation, some phosphodiesterases that degrade cAMP are upregulated, which results in limited accumulation of cAMP and attenuates the vasodilator effects of PGE_2 (34).

Increased Oxygen

There are a number of oxygen sensing tissues in human body, such as fetoplacental arteries in the placenta, pulmonary artery, DA, adrenomedullary chromaffin cells, neuroepithelial body and carotid body. This oxygen-sensing and responding system is called the Homeostatic Oxygen Sensing System (HOSS) and should be considered one of the body's major systems such as cardiovascular, nervous or endocrine systems (35).

During fetal life, oxygen pressure in the ductal lumen is about 18–28 mmHg, which is suitable for maintaining the ductus open (36). After birth, arterial oxygen rises sharply to 80–100 mmHg, which leads to vasoconstriction of almost all vascular smooth muscle, with the exception of pulmonary artery (37). Oxygen-induced constriction begins within 4.6 ± 1.2 min after a rise in PaO_2 (38).

TABLE 1 | Factors that maintain ductal patency *in utero*.

Factors
Low oxygen tension
High levels of circulating prostaglandins
Increase in nitric oxide production
Increase in carbon monoxide production
High levels of circulating adenosine
Increase in intracellular cAMP and cGMP
Raised plasma concentrations of atrial natriuretic peptide
Activation of potassium channels Kv1.5, Kv1.2, Kv2.1, K_{ATP}, BKca

Oxygen-induced vasoconstriction is a multistep process. Oxygen sensing involves a change in redox state, determined by mitochondria and nicotinamide adenine dinucleonide phosphate (NADPH) oxidase. Proximal electron transport chain is the major oxygen sensor in the ductal SMC. This is reflected in the observation that electron transport chain inhibitors (i.e., rotenone and antimycin) mimic hypoxia and constrict the ductus, as well as activating the carotid body. When PO_2 rises, mitochondria respond by production of reactive O_2 species (ROS) especially H_2O_2, which changes the cellular redox potential and alters the function of redox-sensitive genes, second messenger systems and oxygen-sensitive potassium channels, which control SMC membrane potential. Production of adenosine triphosphate (ATP) through oxidative phosphorylation increases with rising oxygen levels and inhibits K_{ATP} channels (39). These channels compose of many subunits such as Kv1.2, Kv1.5, Kv2.1, Kv31b, Kv4.3, Kv9.3, and BKca (40).

Response to oxygen is mediated through potassium channels. Although the pulmonary artery and the ductus are continuous and have similar Kv channels, their response to oxygen is reversed. Hypoxia causes pulmonary artery vasoconstriction and ductal vasodilation. Reduced expression of Kv1.5 and Kv2.1 channels results in failure of ductal closure. It may be speculated that the failed response of premature infants' ductus to normoxia may be related to "deficient" Kv channels, reduced PGE_2induced gene expression of ion channels (41) and a gene transfer which restores K2.1 or Kv1.5 expression might be helpful for vasoconstriction (40).

Inhibition of potassium channels leads to membrane depolarization, influx of calcium into the cells through L type (Ca_L) and T type (Ca_T) calcium channels, and opening of inositol triposphate (IP3) sensitive sarcoplasmic reticulum calcium stores which release calcium (11, 42). This causes DA constriction without depolarization. Subsequent calcium entry through these channels promotes constriction of the DA.

L-type calcium channels are themselves oxygen-sensitive (43). T-type calcium channels also regulate calcium entry into the cells and they are upregulated with increased oxygenation (44). In response to oxygen, calcium may also enter the cell through reverse-mode function of the Na/Ca exchanger also. Maturation of the sensor, mediator and effectors goes in parallel (45).

Cytochrome P450 enzymes catalyze a number of reactions to modulate inflammation, angiogenesis and vascular tone. A member of this system also acts as a sensor for oxygen (46). Monooxygenase and lipooxygenase metabolites of arachidonic acid have the ability to respond to changes in oxygen tension (47). Stimulation of the endothelin A receptor and production of endothelin-1 (ET-1) mediates ductal constriction (48).

Isoprostanes are prostaglandin-like compounds which are produced in response to oxidative stress via non-enzymatically free radical mediated peroxidation of arachidonic acid, without the effect of COX enzymes. They increase as a response to increased arterial PO_2 and increased ROS and mediate inflammation as well as constriction of the DA (49).

Retinoic acid is also active in oxygen signaling and maternally administered vitamin A accelerates the development of oxygen sensing mechanism by increasing the expression of Cav1.2 and Cav3.1 in the rat DA (50).

Rho-kinase pathway is effective in sustaining the contractile state of the ductus. Increased ROS, mainly H_2O_2 in the mitochondria induces RhoB and Rho-associated protein kinase-1 (ROCK-1) expression, which promotes phosphorylation of myosin phosphatase inhibiting MLCP. Activation of the Rho-kinase pathway induces calcium sensitization, which sustains ductal constriction through positive feedback mechanism (51). Rho-kinase system balances MLCK and MLCP (**Figure 1**). Inhibitors of Rho-kinase such as fasudil lead to pulmonary vascular relaxation, thus pulmonary hypertension (52). In the preterm infant, mitochondrial ROS system is immature, and together with failure to upregulate Rho-kinase expression to oxygen, leads to ductal vasodilation. Exogenous H_2O_2 mimics the effects of increased oxygen.

Oxygen stimulates the release and synthesis of endothelin-1 (ET-1), acting on type A receptors (ET_A). Stimulation of these receptors induces IP_3 production by phospholipase c, which leads to an increase in intracellular Ca^{2+} (53). Endothelin receptor antagonists are found to inhibit ductal constriction (54).

In the preterm infant smooth muscle myosin isoforms are immature and the contractile capacity of the muscle cells are weak. L-type calcium channels are immature with impaired calcium entry into the cells. Reduced expression of Rho kinase expression and activity as well as oxygen sensing KV channels contribute to the ductus patency (45). Inhibition of these potassium channels by oxygen leads to SMC depolarization, opening of the voltage-gated L-type Ca channels, influx of calcium into the SMC and vasoconstriction. The preterm ductus has increased sensitivity to the vasodilating effects of prostaglandins and nitric oxide, which prevents constriction. This sensitivity is affected by increased cAMP signaling and decreased cAMP degradation by phosphodiesterases (55). High rates of response to PG inhibitors such as indomethacin and ibuprofen may be explained by this exaggerated sensitivity of the ductus to PGs. On the contrary, elevated levels of PGs during sepsis or necrotizing enterocolitis may mediate the re-opening of ductus in preterm infants (56).

Non-oxygen Pathways

In the preterm ductus energy metabolism begins to fall after birth, with decreased amounts of glucose, oxygen and adenosine triphosphate (ATP). This is not profound enough to cause cell death but interferes with the ability of the ductus to close (57).

Glutamate promotes ductal constriction by glutamate inotropic receptor subunit 1 (GluR1)-mediated noradrenalin production in animal models (58). It may be suggested that nutritional supply of glutamate may have a therapeutic role in the closure of PDA (59).

Caffeine is an adenosine receptor blocker, but it also affects several mechanisms involved in ductal closure. It increases cAMP, releases Ca^{+2} from endoplasmic reticulum, and inhibits the production and activity of prostaglandins. It is used frequently in extremely low birth weight infants for the prevention and treatment of apnea and bronchopulmonary dysplasia. However, it does not affect the contractile response of the ductus at therapeutic concentrations (60).

There is a transient decline in serum osmolarity after birth, which recovers to adult levels within a few days There is some evidence that hypo-osmolarity may mediate ductal closure. In preterm infants with hemodynamically significant PDA, osmolarity is 5 mOsm/L higher compared to non-hemodynamically significant PDA group (61). Hypo-osmotic receptor transient receptor potential melastatin 3 (TRPM3) is upregulated in the ductus and regulates calcium influx into the cells, promoting vasoconstriction. Rats with transient hypo-osmolarity after birth have increased rates of ductal closure (62).

B-type Natriuretic peptide (BNP) plays an important role in regulating the body fluid volume and blood pressure. It is secreted from the ventricles in response to increased cardiac stress and increases intracellular cGMP, inducing vasodilation. In PDA, the volume of left-to-right shunting is associated with the BNP level and higher levels predict a hemodynamically significant PDA and a poor response to indomethacinin preterm infants (63, 64). Bradykinin induces ductal constriction through BK-1 receptors (29).

Progesterone

Progesterone regulates prostaglandin synthesis and prostaglandin sensitivity of smooth muscle cells. Progesterone withdrawal in late pregnancy coincides with the increasing sensitivity of ductus arteriosus to constriction by indomethacin (65). This effect is similar to that of glucocorticoids (66). However, this effect seems to be pharmacological, rather than physiological (67).

In summary, the overall mechanism of functional closure of the ductus involves a drop in PGE_2 levels after birth, which impairs ductal vasodilation and a concomitant rise in oxygen which leads to vasoconstriction. Intracellular calcium increases, secondary to inhibition of Kv channels and K_{ATP} induced membrane depolarization. Increased calcium within the cell activates Ca^{2+}–Calmodulin dependent MLCK activation, which phosphorylates MLC (8). Calmodulin expression is upregulated after birth (68). Increased ET-1 synthesis releases intracellular calcium from the sarcoplasmic reticulum (69). Rho-kinase pathway inhibits MLCP, inducing calcium sensitization by reducing the requirement for calcium influx, maintaining vasoconstriction (9).

Factors that contribute to ductal constriction after birth are summarized in **Table 2** (23).

ANATOMIC CLOSURE AND REMODELING

The initial constriction of the ductus alone is insufficient for the permanent cessation of blood flow through it. Permanent anatomic closure is essential to prevent re-opening, which occurs through a process of remodeling. This process involves intimal cushion formation, disassembly of internal elastic lamina and loss of elastic fibers in the medial layer, migration and proliferation of the SMCs, extracellular matrix production and endothelial cell proliferation and finally blood cell interaction. Each step is related to each other and occurs in a sequential way. After complete anatomic closure, the ductus undergoes apoptosis and becomes the ligamentum arteriosum.

Vasa Vasorum

A substantial amount of nutrients of the ductal wall is provided by vasa vasorum, which supply the outer portion of the wall. Vasa vasorum enters the outer wall of the ductus and grow toward the lumen. They stop growing ~400–500 μm from the lumen. The distance between the lumen and the tip of vasa vasorum is called the avascular zone of the vessel. The thickness of the avascular zone defines the furthest distance that still maintain oxygen and nutrient homeostasis in the tissue. Vasa vasorums appear in the ductal wall only after wall thickness exceeds 400 μm which is not evident before 28 weeks of gestation (70, 71). The thickness of the ductal wall in the full term fetus is 1,000 μm. When the ductus constricts after birth, it increases up to 1,250 μm, in lieu of the lumen (9). In the preterm fetal ductus, the wall thickness is about 480 μm and it increases to 670 μm after birth, when constricted (9) (**Figure 3**). In the full-term ductus, the increased tissue pressure occurring during ductus constriction occludes the vasa vasorum and prevents flow of nutrients to the outer wall of the vessel. This results in the effective avascular zone expanding from 500 μm to the entire thickness of the vessel wall. When this occurs, the center of the ductus wall becomes profoundly ischemic (73). However, in the 24-week-old preterm infant, the ductus is only 200 μm thick. The vasa vasorum do not penetrate the muscle media. This thin walled ductus does not need the vasa vasorum for nutrient flow. As a result, there is no vulnerable region of the wall during closure of the ductus. The preterm ductus arteriosus is less likely to develop the severe degree of hypoxia that is necessary for ductal remodeling (74).

In the term infant, increased intramural pressure occludes vasa vasorum leading to the inhibition of provision of nutrients and oxygen to the muscular layer. Thereafter, the blood and hence the oxygen supply to the cellular layer subsides, leading to hypoxia and cell death (73). The profound hypoxia that follows induces local production of hypoxia inducible factors 1α and VEGF, inhibits the production of PGE_2 and results in apoptosis of SMCs. The proliferation of endothelial cells is mediated by VEGF. Adhesion of mononuclear cells is mediated by VEGF whereas the formation of the platelet plug is mediated by platelet-derived growth factor. This induces an inflammatory response and monocytes and macrophages begin to recruit

TABLE 2 | Factors that contribute to ductal constriction after birth.

High levels of oxygen
Low levels of circulating prostaglandins
Increase in endothelin-1
Activation of cytochrome P450
Rise in intracellular calcium
Decrease in intracellular cAMP and cGMP
Inhibition of potassium channels
Production of isoprostanes
Response to acethycholine
Response to norepinephrine
Activation of transient receptor potential channels
Activation of Rho-kinase family members
Release of angiotensin II

to the ductal wall, producing platelet-derived growth factor which is essential for migration and proliferation. During the initial functional vasoconstriction, loss of luminal blood flow causes hypoxia in the ductal muscle, inducing VEGF secretion (74).

Since the ductal vessel wall is very thin in the preterm infant, it does not contain vasa vasorum and the cells receive oxygen by diffusion from the lumen. This means that as long as luminal patency continues, the cells will receive oxygen and will fail to undergo anatomic remodeling. The preterm ductus requires a greater degree of constriction than that of the term infant in order to achieve a similar degree of hypoxia to trigger the cascade of events necessary for anatomic closure. At the same time, they will be responsive to prosglandins, and be susceptible to re-opening in case of prostaglandin surge as it happens in sepsis or necrotizing enterocolitis. In contrast, preterm ductus produces NO after birth, due to the growth of new vasa vasorum that synthesize NO (63). Therefore, the ductus becomes more dependent on vasodilators other than prostaglandins after the first few weeks. This is reflected in the decreased response to indomethacin with increasing postnatal age. In animal data, combined use of NO-synthase inhibitors with indomethacin produces a greater ductus constriction than indomethacin alone (75).

Elastic Fibers

The structure of the ductal wall is strikingly different from the aortic wall with regard to its elastic content. In great arteries, complex extracellular matrix and elastic fibers are essential to overcome the mechanical and hemodynamic stress of the pulsatile flow. Well-developed elastic fibers in the aorta prevents it from collapsing. However, in the ductal wall, there are very few and thin elastic fibers which do not prevent, but in fact facilitate ductal collapse. Ductal wall is composed of just a media layer which consists SMCs and a superficial thin internal elastic lamina (**Figure 3**). This lamina is also very prone to fragmentation. The intima layer contains the endothelial cells facing the lumen of the ductus. The structural features of the ductus prepares it for immediate closure after birth. Abnormalities of the elastic fibers and elastic lamina may be responsible for some of the PDA cases by preventing intimal cushion formation and collapse of the ductal wall (73).

In the ductal wall, there is less elastin binding protein leading to less elastin deposition. Moreover, increased chondroitin sulfate in the ductus leads to dissociation of tropoelastin from the cell surface, interfering with elastin fiber assembly further (76). Tropoelastin is a chemoattractant for SMCs. Lysl oxidase (LOX) catalyzes elastin cross-linking and it is degraded in the ductal cell when EP_4 receptor is stimulated by the prostaglandins (77). EP_4 is a Gs protein coupled receptor which increases intracellular cAMP by adenylyl cyclases. Signaling coupled with PGE_2 and EP_4 stimulates vascular dilation and intimal thickening.

Intimal Cushion Formation

After the functional phase, progressive intimal thickening and fragmentation of the internal elastic lamina occurs, ultimately forming protrusions which occlude the ductal lumen. During the remodeling process; endothelial cells and internal elastic lamina separate, leaving a subendothelial space in-between for the migration of SMCs and endothelial cells. Integrins, which are transmembrane receptors on the cell surface participate in the interaction of these cells, promoting Intimal cushion formation. In patients whose ductus is not closed, integrin expression is downregulated (78). Intimal thickening is due to the migration of smooth muscle cells from the media layer to the intima and to the proliferation of luminal endothelial cells. During this process, the first step is the migration of SMC from the media to the subendothelial layer, leading to neointimal cushion formation (79). SMC migration is mediated by PGE_2, Transforming Growth Factor Beta (TGFβ-1), notch signaling, Vascular Endothelial Growth Factor (VEGF) and fibronectin coupled with hyaluronan. The proliferation of SMCs is mediated by retinoic acid and notch signaling. Mounds are formed by expansion of the neointima by hyaluronan, which creates a suitable space for migrating SMC from the muscle into the intima and proliferating endothelial cells. The process begins with the accumulation of hyaluronan beneath the endothelial cells, accompanied by loss of laminin and type IV collagen and their separation from the internal elastic lamina. Influx of water into the hyaluronan widens the subendothelial space. Hyaluronan potentiates the migration of SMCs to the subendothelial space through hyaluronan binding protein, synthesized by SMCs (80). This wide space is suitable for SMC migration. Smooth muscle migration is facilitated by impaired elastin assembly and elastin fragmentation. Accumulation of hyaluronan is associated with increased production of TGFβ and prostaglandins via activation of adenylylcyclase 6 (81). Ductal SMCs also secrete fibronectin and chondroitin sulfate which facilitate the migration of these cells (82). SMC also secrete laminin, which is a promigratory protein (83).

In addition to its effects on vasodilation, PGE_2 stimulates SMC migration through exchange protein activated cAMP (epac) pathway in the ductal wall (84) (**Figure 1**). Cyclic AMP has 2 targets: protein kinase A (PKA) and epac. Epac is a guanine nucleotide exchange protein independent of PKA, which regulates the activity of small G proteins.

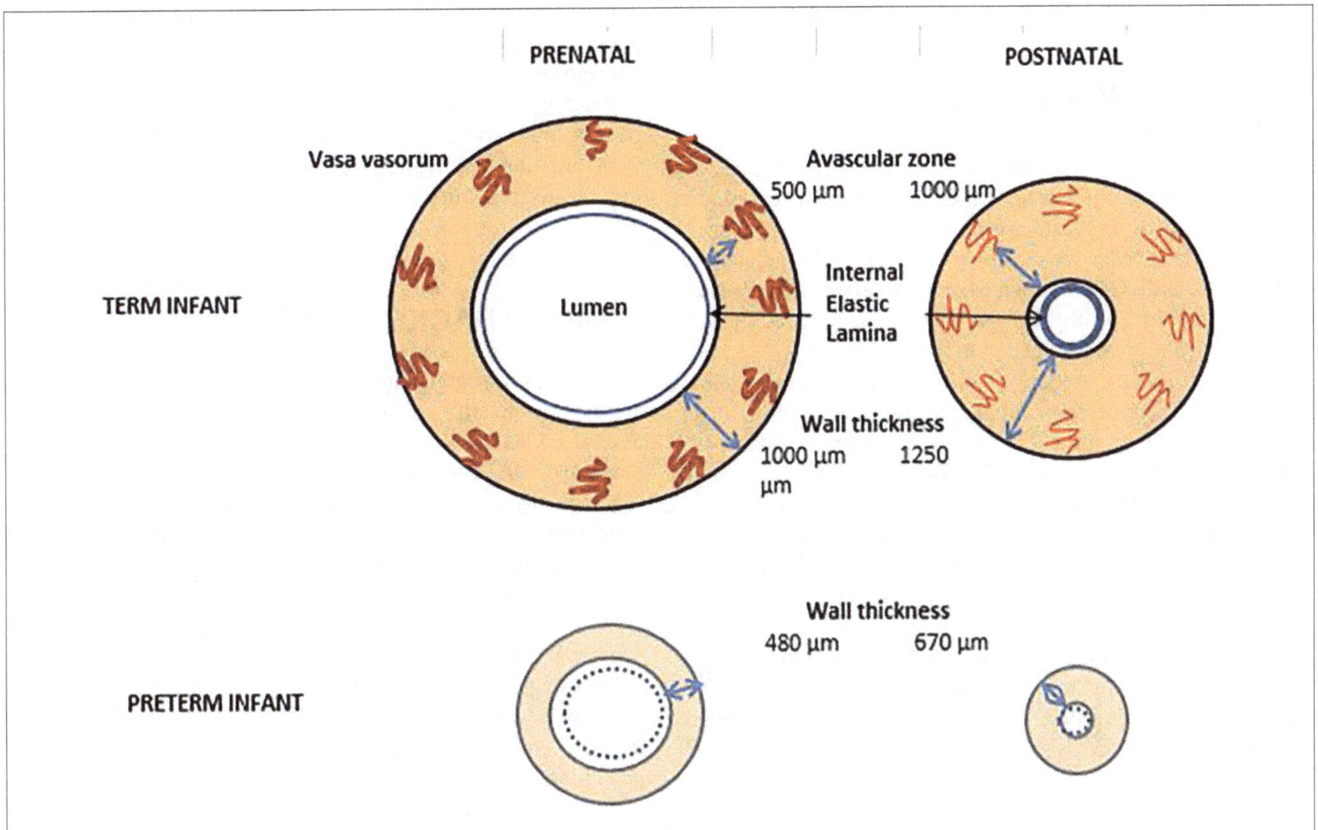

FIGURE 3 | Vaso vasorum in term and preterm infants before and after birth. By the obliteration of vaso vasorum, the thickness of the vaso vasorum increases after birth and the lumen shrinks. In the preterm infant, vaso vasorum are absent or very scarce and the elastic lamina is thin [Figure adapted from (72)].

It is upregulated during the perinatal period and promotes SMC migration without hyaluronan production (85). cAMP is degraded by phosphodiesterases (PDE) to 5'AMP. Activation of PDE can suppress cAMP mediated EP_4 signaling and PDE inhibitors can enhance it (12). Neointimal mounds are less well-developed in the preterm infant, rendering the occlusion of the lumen difficult.

Retinoic Acid

Retinoic acid stimulates the growth of SMCs and decreases apoptosis (86). Prenatal administration of vitamin A increases the production of fibronectin and hyaluronic acid, leading to intimal tickening, as well as the intracellular calcium response and the contractile response of the ductus to oxygen (50). This response is activated by the upregulation of α1G subunit of voltage-dependent calcium channel, which is activated by oxygen-induced inhibition of potassium channel (32). In other words, retinoic acid stimulates both functional and anatomic closure of the ductus. Early trials in human neonates concluded that administration of vitamin A after birth does not result in constriction of DA, but retinoic acid receptor activation may be have a therapeutic potential for treating PDA (87, 88). However, in a recent trial on preterm infants administering 10,000 units of Vitamin A on alternate days for 28 days, rate of PDA was significantly reduced (89).

TGF-β1

TGF-β1 binds the SMC through integrins to the extracellular matrix, slowing down the migration. This is necessary during the remodeling process for maintaining the tension to sustain DA contraction (90).

Interleukin-15

(IL-15) has many pro-inflammatory effects, but also inhibits SMC proliferation and hyaluronan accumulation during the remodeling process of the ductus. The up-regulation of IL-15 in the ductus is mediated through the prostaglandin pathway. IL-15 upregulates the expression of EP_4 mRNA, as well as stimulating angiogenesis through binding to endothelial cells (91). In late gestation, several factors try to promote the structural closure of the ductus in preparation for the postnatal life and IL-15 may balance this tendency by a counteractive mechanism (92).

Notch Signaling

Notch receptors are critical for cell differentiation and there are 4 Notch receptors in humans. Notch 2 and Notch3 receptors are abundant in smooth muscle and they regulate proliferation, migration and angiogenesis in the vasculature. A decrease in the number of Notch receptors in SMCs is associated with downregulation of gene expressions related to contractile elements (84). Notch signaling is required for contractile SMC differentiation in mice (91).

Extracellular Matrix Production and Proliferation

Extracellular matrix consists of hyaluronan, fibronectin, chondroitin sulfate and elastin, which are mediated by retinoic acid, TGFβ, PGE_2, IL-15, and oxygen (51).

Hyaluronan is effective in SMC migration and regulated by PGE_2, IL-15, and TGFβ. PGE_2-mediated EP_4 activation increases the cAMP production through protein kinase A (PKA), which stimulates hyaluronan production in the SMCs (93).

Fibronectin is secreted by the SMCs and promotes SMC migration in the process of intimal cushion formation. Ductal SMC produce twice more fibronectin than aortic SMCs (94). It is possible that preventing fibronectin dependent intimal thickening may be utilized for the patency of DA in congenital heart diseases (82). Other mediators which play an important role in the proliferation and migration of SMCs include versican, a hyaluronan-binding proteoglycan and tanacin, a hexameric glycoprotein (95, 96).

Chondroitin sulfate causes the release of elastin binding protein from the SMCs, impairing the elastin assembly and stabilizing the hyaluronan. Therefore, it indirectly promotes the migration of SMCs and upregulates the synthesis of fibronectin (97).

Elastin contributes to the patency of the ductus by maintaining the elasticity of the ductal wall. Its production is regulated by oxygen and PGE_2. Inhibition of elastogenesis by PGE_2 causes vascular collapse and ductal closure. Oxygen reduces elastin secretion in the SMCs. Stated otherwise, PGE_2 and oxygen stimulates elastogenesis, leading to vasodilation and patency of the ductus (72, 98).

Blood Cell Interactions

Vascular wall ischemia induces a local inflammatory response, which activates mononuclear cells in the blood. Leukocyte interactions with P-selectin and Intercellular Adhesion Molecule-1 (ICAM-1) is necessary for recruitment when physiologic shear forces are present and this interaction is only possible when the flow is very slow. Therefore, leukocytes can adhere to the ductal wall only after vasoconstriction and loss of ductal flow has occurred (99, 100) Monocytes and phagocytes adhere to the wall of the ductus via vascular cell adhesion molecule-1 (VCAM-1), whose expression increase after birth (7, 91). VEGF is a direct chemoattractant for monocytes (101). The magnitude of this adhesion is correlated by the extent of intimal cushion formation (102). Monocytes also stimulate PDGF-B, which is a mediator of smooth muscle migration (103).

During the initial process of vasoconstriction, detachment of endothelial cells triggers the adhesion of platelets to the "injured" site, forming a platelet plug, which further blocks the lumen. Mice with disrupted platelet function or administered antibody against platelets have impaired ductus remodeling (104). The effect of platelets on ductal closure is minimal in term infants but it is more pronounced in preterm infants. Since the intimal cushion formation is mainly triggered by hypoxia and the preterm ductus is less likely to become hypoxic when it constricts after birth, platelets play a more significant role in ductal plug formation and closure in this setting (105). It is reported that platelet-derived growth factor is lower in infants with PDA (106). Low platelet count is also correlated with hemodynamically significant PDA and delayed closure of the ductus (104, 107), whereas high platelet counts promote the initial constriction of the ductus (108).

GENETIC BACKGROUND

Although they originate from the same neural crest lineage, there are major transcriptional differences between the DA and aorta. Several studies highlight the effect of genetic predisposition to the patency of DA. These include either the prostaglandin pathway (i.e., smooth muscle contraction), or vascular smooth muscle development or structure. Most of these information is obtained through mouse models. Overall, there are more than 100 genes are effective in the development of DA (33, 109).

Arachidonic acid is metabolized by PGH_2 synthase to prostaglandin H_2, which in turn is metabolized by PGE synthase to prostaglandin E_2 (PGE_2). Prostaglandin endoperoxide synthase 1 (*Ptgs1* or *COX1*) and (*Ptgs2* or *COX2*) is the rate limiting enzyme in the production of prostaglandins from arachidonic acid. Mice deficient in *Ptgs1* have normal survival after birth whereas 35% of mice deficient in *Ptgs2* die shortly after birth because of PDA (110). If both are lacking, 100% of mice die in the first day (111). Prostaglandin E_2 binds to the cell through its receptor EP_4 (*Ptger4*) and mediates vascular smooth muscle relaxation and intimal thickening. Mice lacking these receptors die due to PDA (11). Furthermore, *Hpgd* gene encodes hydroxyprostaglandin dehydrogenase 15-(NAD) which is responsible for PGE_2 metabolism. The deletion of this gene leads to elevated levels of PGE, leaving the DA open and resulting in death (112). Mice deficient in prostaglandin transporter gene Slco2a1 also die within 2 days after birth (113).

The effects of prostaglandins are mediated through cyclic guanosine monophosphate (cGMP) and cyclic adenosine monophosphate (cAMP). Phosphodiesterases degrade these compounds and several genes have been proposed for phosphodiesterases. *Pde5a* mediates vasoconstriction in SMC of DA and its expression decreases in 6 h after birth (114).

The genes upregulated during ductal closure are phosphodiesterase 4B (PDE4B), desmin pyruvate dehydrogenase kinase isozyme 4 (PDK4), and insulin-like growth factor binding protein 3 (IGFBP3). Downregulated genes include cyclin-dependent kinase inhibitor 1C (CDKN1C) and alpha-2-glycoprotein1 (AZGP1). PDE4B limits the accumulation of cAMP, minimizing the vasodilator effect of endogenous prostaglandins. Therefore, increasing PDE4B would facilitate ductal constriction. Desmin is a component of the cytoskeleton and its increase indicates the maturation of SMCs. PDK4 and IGFBP3 regulate cell proliferation and apoptosis, which are operative in ductal closure. Increased transforming growth factor β-receptor II regulates PDK4 also (90, 115, 116). Wingless integrin pathway (Wnt), which is a part of IGFBP3 system plays a major role in ductal closure through upregulation of cyclooxygenase 2 and apoptotic processes mediated by macrophages (117).

Smooth muscle of the DA contracts in response to oxygen. Mice deficient in myosin heavy chain gene (*Myh11*) have delayed closure of DA (118). Myocardin regulates expression of genes for contractile proteins in smooth muscle cells (SMC) and selective deletion or ablation of *Mycocd* results in death (119). *Tcfap2b* is the gene which encodes the transcription factor in neural crest cells, from which the DA originates. Mice deficient in *Tcfap2b* die within the first day of life with PDA and pulmonary overload (120). The DA of these mice lack markers of differentiated SMCs such as calponin and hypoxia-inducible factor 2α (HIF2α) which are also involved in oxygen sensing, suggesting that *Tcfap2b* plays an important role in the development of SMCs (121). Some genes act together resulting in PDA. Whereas, the deletion of *Notch2* gene results in PDA in only 40% of cases, when combined with the deletion of *Notch3*, PDA is observed in 100% of cases (122). Deletion of the *Notch* ligand, *jag1* also results in lethal PDA on day 1 because of significant defects in SMC differentiation (123). On the other hand, deletion of the Brahma-related gene (Brg1-a) which is responsible for chromatin remodeling results in cardiovascular anomalies, including PDA (124). Genes involved in platelet production or adhesion such as *Nfe2* or *Itga2b* affect the complete occlusion and remodeling of the DA (104).

Changes in the expression of structural genes also affect the patency of DA. Vascular SMC contraction is mediated by myosin II. Myosin II has two components, namely heavy chains and light chains. The genes encoding these proteins such as *Myh11, Myl2, Myl5, Myl7,* and *Myl9* may be effective in the regulation of ductal patency, but more studies are needed to reach a definite conclusion (68, 125). Contraction of the myosin light chains requires phosphorylation and this step is regulated by the Rho-Rho kinase system. The gene encoding the RhoBGTPase (*Rhob*) and its effector *Rock2* is upregulated in the newborn DA and inhibition of this system may result in the patency of DA (38).

L-type calcium channels are essential for ductal closure and the genes encoding the Na/K ATPase (*Akq1b1*) and a subunit of L-type calcium channels (*Cacna2d1*) are highly expressed in the DA (126). Potassium channels control the resting membrane potential of SMCs and the genes encoding these channels (*Kcnk3* and *Abcc9*) are also upregulated in the DA (127). Large conductance calcium-activated potassium channels (*BKca*) are abundant in vascular smooth muscle and they are expressed significantly higher in DA (109). These ion channels may be promising targets for novel PDA therapies.

Vasoconstrictive effect of oxygen in the DA is mediated by endothelin-1 (ET-1). There are 2 membrane receptors for ET-1, ET_A receptor is encoded by the *Ednra* gene and ET_B receptor is encoded by the *Ednrb* gene. ET_B receptor functions as a scavenger for ET-1 and inhibits endothelin dependent vasoconstriction. Downregulation of this receptor would result in increased levels of ET-1, leading to vasoconstriction of the ductus, which takes place in late preterm infants (68, 126).

In humans, there are a number of syndromes associated with PDA, as well as non-syndromic PDA which are associated with single nucleotide polymorphisms (128). In twin studies, a familial component has been suggested for PDA in preterm infants (129). Consanguineous marriages provide insights to specific chromosome regions associated with increased susceptibility to PDA (130). A polymorphism in the estrogen receptor alpha gene ESR1 *rs2234693,* prostaglandin I2 synthase gene *(rs493694)* and another polymorphism in the interferon gamma gene *rs2430561* is associated with a decreased risk of PDA and bronchopulmonary dysplasia (131, 132). On the other hand, polymorphisms in the TNF receptor associated factor 1 TRAF1 (*rs1056567*) gene, angiotensin II type 1 receptor AGTR1 gene and TFAP2β (*rs987237*) gene, are associated with increased risk of PDA (133, 134). TFAP2β is also associated with altered levels of calcium and potassium channels in SMCs, which are essential for proper contraction (135). Angiotensin II is vasoconstrictive for the ductus and its receptor (*Agtr2*) is upregulated in late preterm infants also (128).

Although their significance remain to be elucidated, there are other genes involved in the development of matrix molecules of the DA, such as *Tcfab2b*, lysyl oxidase (*Lox*), and fibronectin (*Fn1*) genes which may draw attention in the future (128). Lysyl oxidase is a cross-linking enzyme for elastic fibers and stabilizes the extracellular matrix. Reduction of LOX activity is demonstrated in the pathogenesis of many vascular diseases (136). Activation of PGE_2-EP_4 pathway promotes the degradation of this enzyme, leading to poor elastogenesis, suggesting that control of elastogenesis is clinically important (72). Paradoxically, there are some data that indomethacin treatment of preterm infants may have an adverse effect on the inhibition of elastic fiber formation (72). Regulation of the LOX protein through PGE_2-EP_4 pathway may be a basis for further therapeutic strategies that target vascular elastogenesis (72).

MECHANICAL AND HEMODYNAMICAL FACTORS

Hemodynamic Changes After Birth

In fetal life, high pulmonary arterial pressure, coupled with low systemic resistance in the placenta results in right to left shunting of blood through the ductus so that a large proportion of blood coming from the umbilical circulation is directed to the systemic circulation without passing through the pulmonary vascular bed. During fetal life, 10–20% of total biventricular cardiac output enters the lungs but in late gestation, this increases to 30% (137). After birth, umbilical cord clamping increases the systemic resistance whereas ventilation of the lungs decreases the pulmonary vascular resistance and increases the pulmonary blood flow; the shunt through the ductus reverses to left to right. This sudden reversal of shunting across the DA rises the pulmonary blood flow even further. In term infant, dominant left to right shunting is achieved by 10 min after birth and it is entirely left to right by 24 h of age (138). In critical cyanotic congenital heart disease, patency of ductus is life-saving. In persistent pulmonary hypertension, high resistance in pulmonary arteries results in persistance of right to left shunting through the ductus. In the preterm neonate, if the ductus remains open, left to right shunting will occur both during systole and diastole and large amounts of blood would flood the lungs. This will expose the endothelium to increased shearing forces, which will induce the production of vasodilatory mediators such as nitric oxide, bradykinin, prostacyclin, and inactivate the production of vasoconstrictor mediators such as thromboxane, endothelin and leukotriens. Arachnidonic acid may be released from pulmonary tissue damaged by shear stress, secondary to mechanical ventilation. Prolonged mechanical ventilation can also induce the release of prostacyclin, often associated with increased ductal shunting (139). This would lead to alveolar edema, and increased need for respiratory support. Positive pressure ventilation during resuscitation, oxygen, and exogenous surfactant treatment induce a rapid fall in PVR. Especially in preterm infants <32 weeks, surfactant administration is associated with an increase in the right ventricular output and absolute ductal diameter (140, 141). Acute rise in pulmonary blood low causes a significant increase in left heart preload and rise in left atrial pressure which results in increased pressure in the left atrium and contraction of foramen ovale (142). The myocardium of the preterm infant is less contractile due to fewer contractile units, increased water content and immature sarcoplasmic reticulum (143). Thus, hemodynamic stability of the preterm infant is highly dependent on myocardial function, and a sudden increase in the workload of myocardium after birth may result in failure of the myocardium resulting in pulmonary overload and hypertension. In preterm infants, delayed cord clamping does not seem to affect the incidence of PDA (144). Early adrenal insufficiency may also have a role in prolonged ductal patency (145).

Fluid dynamics state that the shunt volume across a tubular structure is directly proportional to the 4th power of the radius of the tube (i.e., ductus) and the pressure gradient between both ends (i.e., aorta and pulmonary artery), and inversely proportional to the blood viscosity and length of the tube (i.e., ductus). Moreover, increased venous return from the lungs to the left ventricle will cause an increase in the left ventricular end-diastolic pressure, which will increase atrial natriuretic peptide (ANP), with evolution of pulmonary venous hypertension and pulmonary hemorrhage. On the other hand, left to right shunting at the ductus will decrease the systemic perfusion (i.e., ductal steal) leading to systemic hypoxia and organ dysfunction. Shorter diastolic time and increased myocardial oxygen demand may result in endocardial ischemia (142).

There is scarce information on the effects of dilation mediated by the mechanical force of the flow, or through shear forces and shear stress. Although there is no clear evidence, it may be speculated that there are some mechanosensors in the ductal wall, which can sense the biomechanical changes in the lumen and regulate ductal closure. The effect of laminar flow vs. turbulent flow across the ductus is also understudied. In case of laminar flow, endothelial cells are less likely to proliferate and nitric oxide synthase and prostacyclin are upregulated (146, 147). However, if turbulent flow develops, endothelial cells begin to upregulate vasoconstrictors such as endothelin-1 and adhesion molecules such as VCAM-1 and ICAM-1 (148, 149). Matrix modeling is an essential component of intimal cushion formation. Stretch of the ductal wall induces the release of angiotensin II from the endothelial cell, leading to smooth muscle proliferation and production of matrix metalloproteinases which trigger extracellular matrix remodeling and vasoconstriction (149, 150). Circumferential stretch also triggers phenotypic switching of SMCs from contractile to synthetic cells, which means more proliferation and migration of SMCs (150).

Fluid Load

A sharp decrease in pulmonary artery pressure, as it happens after surfactant replacement therapy may increase the left-to-right shunt through the ductus, leading to pulmonary overflow and hemorrhage. In preterm infants, increased pulmonary fluid and protein load is eliminated by an increased lung lymph flow, named as "edema safety factor." Therefore, ductal closure within the first 24 h of birth do not have any significant effect on the course of respiratory distress syndrome. However, if ductus remains open for several days, this compensation cannot be maintained and alteration in the pulmonary mechanics and pulmonary edema ensue. The impact of patent ductus arteriosus on patient outcomes seems to be a function of magnitude of shunt, rather than its mere presence. Closure of the ductus improves lung mechanics in these infants (151). Early ductal closure is associated with less pulmonary hemorrhages in preterm infants (152). Ibuprofen leads to increased expression of sodium channels and increased removal of fluid from the alveolar compartment (153). In some studies, fluid restriction is recommended as an alternative to treatment; such an approach may reduce pulmonary circulation but also compromises end organ flow in patients already suffering from ductal steal phenomenon (154). However, high (liberal) fluid intake is associated with an increased risk of PDA and BPD (155). Therefore, close monitoring of fluid intake and individualized treatment of infants are of utmost importance in preterm infants, especially in the first days of life.

Early Adrenal Function

Cortisol is central to the ability of the infant to attenuate its response to inflammation and is potent inhibitor of inflammatory edema. Animal and human studies have shown that adrenal insufficiency can lead to increased inflammatory response to injury and that glucocorticoids can affect patency of the ductus (156, 157). Glucocorticoids induce production of lipocortin which inhibits phospholipase A_2. Phospholipase A_2 stimulates the release of arachnidonic acid precursors needed for prostaglandin synthesis; thus in response to steroids, prostaglandin production is inhibited (158). Animal studies have shown that glucocorticoid administration decreases the sensitivity of ductal tissue to the dilating influence of PGE_2 (156). Sick infants do not have elevated serum corticol levels compared to well infants. These infants are also prone to developing bronchopulmonary dysplasia (159). Therefore, it is not surprising that patent ductus arteriosus is one of the most prominent risk factors in the development of bronchopulmonary dysplasia (160).

Effects of Surgical Ligation

Surgical ligation of the ductal immediately after birth increases the expression of genes involved in lung inflammation and decreases the expression of genes involved in epithelial sodium channels (161). Therefore, the pulmonary mechanics do not improve as much as expected. Furthermore, early ligation may slow down lung growth (162). On the other hand, in the presence of atelectasis, the persistence of left to right shunt through the PDA maintains an elevated arterial oxygen pressure in the lungs and after PDA ligation, a decrease in the systemic arterial pressure may be observed (163).

EFFECTS OF PHARMACOLOGICAL AGENTS

Oxygen is the most powerful agent for closure of the ductus. In numerous studies investigating the effect of different levels of oxygen on preterm morbidities, ductal closure was associated with high levels of oxygen but oxygen-related co-morbidities in these infants raised significant concerns (164). These trials including Surfactant, Positive Pressure, Pulse Oxymetry Randomized Trial (SUPPORT), Canadian Oxygen Trial (COT), and Benefits of Oxygen Saturation Targeting (BOOST) II trials have reported neurodevelopmental outcomes after various oxygen targeting, as well as other complications; however the discussion of these trials are out of the context of this article (165–167).

All available pharmacological treatments aiming for changing the ductal tone use the prostaglandin pathway by either the cyclooxygenase pathway (indomethacin and ibuprofen) or the peroxidase pathway (acetaminophen). The infant's gestational age, as well as the infant's race, ethnicity, growth, and exposure to antenatal corticosteroids modify the effects of prostaglandins and determine the rate of drug-induced closure (168, 169).

In the term infant PGE_2 receptors are down-regulated after birth. However, in the preterm infant, the production of receptors increases, rendering the ductus susceptible to vasodilation and resistant to indomethacin or ibuprofen. COX1 and COX2 expression increases with advancing maturity in the fetus (170, 171). COX inhibitors decrease vaso vasorum flow, leading to hypoperfusion and ischemic injury in the vessel wall (85). Preterm ductus also synthesizes other vasodilators such as NO, TNF-α, and IL-6 in response to wall hypoxia. Decreased ATP concentrations also prevent the ductus from contracting (172). Therefore, the preterm ductus becomes more resistant to treatment with constrictor agents (173).

Cyclooxygenase (COX) Inhibitors

Indomethacin and Ibuprofen non-selectively inhibit cyclooxygenase enzymes; thus preventing arachidonic acid conversion to prostaglandins (**Figure 2**). Both drugs are associated with increased amiloride-sensitive alveolar epithelial sodium channels, suggesting improved lung water clearance and lung compliance (174). Ductal sensitivity to indomethacin increases with gestational age. Response rate to indomethacin is about 5–10% in infants <27 weeks of gestation, whereas it is almost 100% above 34 weeks (175). Half-life of indomethacin is 4–5 h longer (i.e., 17 h) in preterm infants <32 weeks of gestation. It can be given by intravenous, oral, rectal or intraarterial route. Closure rates vary from 48 to 98.5%, depending upon the dose, method and duration of administration (176, 177). Early use of indomethacin within the first few days of life decreases the risk of pulmonary hemorrhage, intraventricular hemorrhage and the need for surgical ligation, although does not affect the development of BPD (178). If needed, a second course may be given, with a success rate of 40–50% (179). Since more courses are associated with periventricular leukomalacia, repeat doses are not recommended (180). Efficacy of indomethacin declines with decreasing gestational age and becomes doubtful at 22–23 weeks of gestation (176). Indomethacin have several side effects including renal failure, oliguria, proteinuria, hyperkalemia, cerebral white matter damage, necrotizing enterocolitis, intestinal perforation and platelet dysfunction (181).

Ibuprofen is a non-selective COX inhibitor with less side effects than those of indomethacin. It can be given orally or intravenously. Elimination is slower after oral administration and the rate of closure is also higher (182). Its efficacy for ductal closure is the same as indomethacin. Major side effects include gastrointestinal hemorrhage, oliguria, high bilirubin levels, and pulmonary hypertension (183, 184). These effects may vary depending on the relevant genetic polymorphisms (185).

Peroxidase (POX) Inhibitors

Paracetamol (Acetaminophen) inhibits POX enzyme which catalyzes the conversion of PG_2 to PGH_2, without any peripheral vasoconstriction (**Figure 2**). Although it is commonly discussed under the family of non-steroidal anti-inflammatory drugs, it does not have any anti-inflammatory effect (186). Its gastrointestinal tolerance is better than other NSAIDs and it lacks antiplatelet activity. Paracetamol induced POX inhibition is competitive and independent of COX activity (187). Paracetamol induced reduction in PGH_2 production can be counteracted by lipid peroxides and PGG_2 itself (188). The maturational difference in lipid hydroperoxide production in preterm newborns may contribute to paracetamol-induced ductal closure (188). Since the mechanism of action is different than that of indomethacin or ibuprofen, the efficacy of paracetamol in extremely low birth weight infants may be less than other NSAIDs, although solid evidence is lacking. On the other hand, its pharmacokinetics has not been well-studied in ductal closure. Inhibition of the POX dilators may lead to an increase in the pulmonary vascular resistance via peroxynitrite production (189). Furthermore, there are some data that paracetamol may synergistically enhance the inhibitory effects of other anti-inflammatory drugs on platelets (190). In preterm infants, very few cases of toxicity have been reported, which may be attributed to the low activity of cytochrome P450 in the immediate postnatal period, minimizing the formation of toxic metabolites (191). Meta-analysis comparing oral paracetamol vs. oral ibuprofen concluded that paracetamol confers comparable efficacy with fewer adverse effects (192). Paracetamol may be used as a rescue treatment for infants with persistent PDA (193). Due to the small number of studies, it is difficult do decide whether paracetamol is superior or inferior to other NSAIDs. Although there are no randomized controlled trials, there are some observational studies which suggest that paracetamol use in pregnancy or in early infancy might be associated with attention deficit/hyperactivity disorder, autism spectrum disorder or hyperactivity symptoms. Although the exact mechanism is unknown and a cause-effect relation is difficult to establish, a small but significant odds ratio is observed in many studies (194–196). However, another study suggests that there is not an increased risk of autism in these infants at 2-year follow-up (197). There is no data on the possible long-term neurodevelopmental effects of paracetamol use in preterm infants. Therefore, paracetamol should be used cautiously until further safety data exists.

Some authors have suggested to use a combination therapy of ibuprofen and paracetamol as a first line therapy for ductal closure. However, preliminary reports suggest that the effectiveness of combination therapy does not differ compared to monotherapy of either drug (198). In another study, in infants who failed two previous cycles of monotherapy, combination therapy with oral ibuprofen and oral paracetamol was effective in 9 infants out of 12 (199). Results of an ongoing randomized controlled trial are pending (https://clinicaltrials.gov/ct2/show/NCT03103022).

Other non-steroidal anti-inflammatory drugs such as aspirin, metamizol, nimesulid, and diclophenac have constrictor effects on the ductus (200–203).

Glucocorticoids have also vasoconstrictive effects on the ductus, as well as synergistic effects with non-steroidal anti-infective drugs (NSAIDs), as a result of decreasing the sensitivity of the ductal SMCs to prostaglandins (204) (**Figure 2**). In the preterm fetus, elevated levels of corticosteroids is associated with decreased sensitivity of the ductus to the vasodilating effects of prostaglandins and prenatal administration of corticosteroids, mainly for the prevention of respiratory distress syndrome have also decreased the incidence of PDA in these infants (205). Similarly, postnatal corticosteroid administration may constrict the ductus (206). Angiotensin II does not have a role in ductal closure after birth (207).

There are many substances and foods with anti-inflammatory and anti-oxidant properties, such as those rich in polyphenols or flavonoids. For example, 30–40% of solid extract of green tea composes of polyphenols, mainly catechins. They exert their anti-inflammatory effects through the inhibition of endogenous prostaglandins. Similar effects have been reported with black tea, resveratrol, mate tea, orange juice and dark chocolate (207). Excessive consumption of such foods by the pregnant woman may influence the dynamics of the DA, by inhibiting COX and PG synthesis pathway. The amount of flavonoids necessary to trigger clinically significant ductal closure remains to be determined (208).

Genetic therapies may include endothelin-signaling genes or blockage of potassium channels. Channel isoforms have distinct pharmacological and physiological characteristics, making them ideal targets for ductal-selective therapies (209). Glibenclamide is a non-specific K_{ATP} channel inhibitor, used for treating diabetes. It is shown that DA constricts in response to glibenclamide, and constriction is inhibited by diazoxide, a K_{ATP} channel activator (210). Children with Cantu syndrome, which is caused by mutations in the subgroup of K_{ATP} channel genes, have PDA, often resistant to medical treatment, requiring surgical closure most of the time (16). Agonist or antagonist molecules targeting K_{ATP} channels may modulate DA tone.

Novel treatment strategies for PDA include combined use of ibuprofen and paracetamol (211), EP_4 inhibition (212), NOS inhibition (213), enhancing ion channel expression (50), glutamate supplementation (59) especially in situations where COX inhibitors have proven to be ineffective.

Prostaglandin E1

PGE_1 is the main drug used for vasodilatatory effects of the ductus. PGE_1 binds to the EP_4receptor which increases intracellular cAMP. Milrinon is a phosphodiesterase 3 inhibitor, which can also increase cAMP levels and dilate the ductus (12).

Non-selective endothelin receptor antagonist TAK-044 and inhibition of Notch pathway may have vasodilating effects on the ductus (51, 91). Natriuretic peptide (NP) is an activator of PKG-cGMP and can prevent ductal closure also (51).

Antenatal corticosteroids are used for the maturation of preterm lung, but their effects on the development of patent ductus arteriosus, intracranial hemorrhage, and necrotizing enterocolitis are also well-studied (214). However, some reports conclude that the incidence of PDA is not effected significantly by antenatal corticosteroids (215). Antenatal steroids increase 15-PGDH activity, thereby promoting PGE_2 breakdown (216).

Antenatal $MgSO_4$ which is a calcium channel blocker may result in delayed ductal closure in infants (217). However, recent evidence in extremely low birth weight infants suggests that antenatal $MgSO_4$ exposure is not associated with an increased risk of hemodynamically significant PDA; in fact, it may be associated with a decreased likelihood of hemodynamically significant PDA (218). Diazoxide, which is a K_{ATP} channel activator may induce ductal opening (173). Furosemide increases renal PGE_2 production, thus dilating the ductus in animals but its effect is limited in humans (219).

CONCLUSION

Ductus arteriosus is an intriguing and complex vessel with many distinct features. Understanding the precise mechanisms of regulation of the ductus is essential in order to improve individual pharmacological treatments. The debate about PDA should not be "treat all" or "treat none," but rather, "who to treat." This approach necessitates individualized treatment. Treatments targeting endogenous ductus regulation pathways other than prostaglandins, such as cell cycle regulators, transcription factors, and epigenomic regulators should be developed. Since vascular constriction and ductal wall remodeling are required for complete closure, treatments that favor vasoconstriction and remodeling would also be ideal for infants with persistent PDA. Novel therapies for ductal closure in preterm infants should also focus on a clear understanding of genes which are operative on ductal patency, as new genome-wide studies uncover genes associated with PDA. Evolving pediatric clinical pharmacology heralds next generation solutions for unresolved issues of today, such as drugs with selective DA effects, without any side effects.

AUTHOR CONTRIBUTIONS

FO is responsible for the design, research, writing, and editing of the manuscript.

REFERENCES

1. Raju TN. From Galen to Gross and beyond: a brief history of the enigmatic ductus arteriosus. *J Perinatol.* (2019) 39:1442–8. doi: 10.1038/s41372-019-0517-4
2. Reese J. Towards a greater understanding of the ductus arteriosus. *Sem Perinatol.* (2018) 42:199–202. doi: 10.1053/j.semperi.2018.05.001
3. Prsa M, Sun L, Van Amerom J, Yoo SJ, Wortmann LG, Jaeggi E, et al. Reference ranges of blood flow in the majör vessels on the normal human fetal circulation at term by phase-contrast magnetic resonance imaging. *Circ Cardiovasc Imaging.* (2014) 7:663–70. doi: 10.1161/CIRCIMAGING.113.001859
4. Hammenman C. Patent ductus arteriosus. Clinical relevance of prostaglandins and prostaglandin inhibitors in PDA pathophysiology and treatment. *Clin Perinatol.* (1995) 22:457–79. doi: 10.1016/S0095-5108(18)30293-8
5. Matsui H, McCarthy KP, Ho SY. Morphology of the patent arterial duct: features relevant to treatment. *Images Paediatr Cardiol.* (2008) 10:27–38.
6. Semberova J, Sirc J, Miletin J, Kucera J, Berka I, Sebkova S, et al. Spontaneous closure of patent ductus arteriosus in infants ≤1500 g. *Pediatrics.* (2017) 140:e20164258. doi: 10.1542/peds.2016-4258
7. Newby AC, Zaltsman AB. Molecular mechanisms in intimal hyperplasia. *J Pathol.* (2000) 190:300–9. doi: 10.1002/(SICI)1096-9896(200002)190:3<300::AID-PATH596>3.0.CO;2-I
8. Somlyo AP, Somlyo AV. Ca2+ sensitivity of smooth muscle and nonmuscle myosin II modulated by G proteins, kinases and myosin phosphatase. *Physiol Rev.* (2003) 83:135–8. doi: 10.1152/physrev.00023.2003
9. Hundscheid T, vanden Boek M, van der Lee R, de Boode W. Understanding the pathobiology in patent ductus arteriosus in prematurity-beyond prostaglandins and oxygen. *Pediatr Res.* (2019) 86:28–38. doi: 10.1038/s41390-019-0387-7
10. Fan F, Ma A, Guan Y, Huo J, Hu Z, Tian H, et al. Effect of PGE_2 on DA tone by EP_4 modulating Kv channels with different oxygen tension between preterm and term. *Int J Cardiol.* (2011) 147:58–65. doi: 10.1016/j.ijcard.2009.07.045
11. Nguyen M, Camenisch T, Snouwaert JN, Hicks E, Coffman TM, Anderson PA, et al. The prostaglandin receptor EP_4 triggers remodelling of the cardiovascular system at birth. *Nature.* (1997) 390:78–81. doi: 10.1038/36342
12. Yokoyama U, Iwatsubo K, Umemura M, Fujita T, Ishikawa Y. The prostanoid EP_4 receptor and its signaling pathway. *Pharm Rev.* (2013) 65:1010–52. doi: 10.1124/pr.112.007195
13. Crichton CA, Smith GC, Smith GL. alpha-Toxin-permeabilised rabbit fetal ductus arteriosus is more sensitive to Ca^{2+} than aorta or main pulmonary artery. *Cardiovasc Res.* (1997) 33:223–9. doi: 10.1016/S0008-6363(96)00171-X
14. Lewis RS. Store-operated calcium channels: new perspectives on mechanism and function. *Cold Spring Harb Perspect Biol.* (2011) 3:a003970. doi: 10.1101/cshperspect.a003970
15. Clyman RI, Waleh N, Kajino H, Roman C, Mauray F. Calcium-dependent and calcium-sensitizing pathways in the mature and immature ductus arteriosus. *Am J Physiol Regul Integr Comp Physiol.* (2007) 293:R1650–6. doi: 10.1152/ajpregu.00300.2007
16. Francis SH, Busch JL, Corbin JD, Sibley D. cGMP-dependent protein kinases and cGMP phosphodiesterases in nitric oxide and cGMP action. *Pharm Rev.* (2010) 62:525–63. doi: 10.1124/pr.110.002907
17. Baragatti B, Brizzi F, Barogi S, Laubach VE, Sodini D, Shesely EG, et al. Interactions between NO, CO and an endothelium-derived hyperpolarizing factor (EDHF) in maintaining patency of the ductus arteriosus in the mouse. *Br J Pharm.* (2007) 151:54–62. doi: 10.1038/sj.bjp.0707211
18. Sodini D, Baragatti B, Barogi S, Laubach VE, Coceani F. Indomethacin promotes nitric oxide function in the DA in the mouse. *Br J Pharmacol.* (2008) 153:1631–40. doi: 10.1038/bjp.2008.36
19. van der Sterren S, Kleikers P, Zimmermann LJ, Villamor E. Vasoactivity of the gasotransmitters hydrogen sulfide and carbon monoxide in the chicken ductus arteriosus. *Am J Physiol Regul Integr Comp Physiol.* (2011) 301:R1186–98. doi: 10.1152/ajpregu.00729.2010
20. Coceani F, Kelsey L, Seidliz E, Mars GS, McLaughlin BE, Vreman HJ, et al. Carbon monoxide formation in the ductus arteriosus in the lamb: implications for regulation of muscle tone. *Br J Pharmacol.* (1997) 120:599–608. doi: 10.1038/sj.bjp.0700947
21. Majeed Y, Tumova S, Green BL, Seymour VAL, Woods DM, Agarwal AK, et al. Pregnenolone sulphate-independent inhibition of TRPM3 channels by progesterone. *Cell Calcium.* (2012) 51:1–11. doi: 10.1016/j.ceca.2011.09.005
22. Yasuda K, Koyama N, Nomura T, Makino Y, Murata M, Takenaka M, et al. Effects of phosphodiesterase 3 inhibitors to premature PDA (abstract). *J Japan Soc Premature Newborn Med.* (2004) 16:395.
23. Crockett SL, Berger CD, Shelton EL, Reese J. Molecular and mechanical factors contributing to ductus arteriosus patency and closure. *Congenital Heart Dis.* (2019) 14:15–20. doi: 10.1111/chd.12714
24. Park SM, Ahn CM, Hong SJ, Kim YH, Park JH, Shim WJ, et al. Acute changes of left ventricular hemodynamics and function during percutaneous coronary intervention in patients with unprotected left main coronary artery disease. *Heart Vessels.* (2015) 30:432–40. doi: 10.1007/s00380-014-0495-6
25. Nomura T, Lu R, Pucci ML, Schuster VL. The two-step model of prostaglandin signal termination: *in vitro* reconstitution with the prostaglandin transporter and prostaglandin 15 dehydrogenase. *Mol Pharm.* (2004) 65:973–8. doi: 10.1124/mol.65.4.973
26. Printz MP, Skidgel RA, Friedman WF. Studies of pulmonary prostaglandin biosynthetic and catabolic enzymes as fctors in ductus arteriosus patency and closure. Evidence for a shift in products with gestational age. *Pediatr Res.* (1984) 18:19–24.
27. Tsai MY, Einzig S. Prostaglandin catabolism in fetal and maternal tissues a study of 15-hydroxyprostaglandin dehydrogenase and delta 13 reductase with specific assay methods. *Prostaglandins Leukot Ess Fat Acids.* (1989) 38:25–30. doi: 10.1016/0952-3278(89)90143-9
28. Smith GC, McGrath JC. Prostaglandin E2 and fetal oxygen tension synergistically inhibit response of isolated fetal rabbit ductus arteriosus to norepinephrine. *J Cardiovasc Pharm.* (1991) 17:861–6. doi: 10.1097/00005344-199106000-00001
29. Bateson EA, Schulz R, Olley PM. Response of fetal rabbit ductus arteriosus to bradykinin: a role of nitric oxide, prostaglandins, and bradykinin receptors. *Pediatr Res.* (1999) 45:568–74. doi: 10.1203/00006450-199904010-00017
30. Clyman RI, Mauray F, Roman C, Heymann MA, Payne B. Effect of gestational age on ductus arteriosus response to circulating prostaglandin E2. *J Pediatr.* (1983) 102:907–11. doi: 10.1016/S0022-3476(83)80023-7
31. Clyman RI, Waleh N, Black SM, Riemer RK, Mauray F, Chen YQ. Regulation of ductus arteriosus patency by nitric oxide in fetal lambs: the role of gestation, oxygen tension and vasa vasorum. *Pediatr Res.* (1998) 43:633–44. doi: 10.1203/00006450-199805000-00012
32. Yokoyama U, Minamisawa S, Adachi-Akahane S, Akaike T, Naguro I, Funokoshi K, et al. Multiple transcripts of Ca2+channel alpha1-subunits and a novel spliced variant of the alpha1C-subunit in rat ductus arteriosus. *Am J Physiol Heart Circ Physiol.* (2006) 290:H1660–70. doi: 10.1152/ajpheart.00100.2004
33. Goyal R, Goyal D, Longo LD, Clyman RI. Microarray gene expression analysis in ovine ductus arteriosus during fetal development and birth transition. *Pediatr Res.* (2016) 80:610–8. doi: 10.1038/pr.2016.123

34. IchikawaY, Yokoyama U, Iwamoto M, Oshikawa J, Okumura S, Sato M, et al. Inhibition of phosphodiesterase type 3 dilates the rat ductus arteriosus without inducing intimal thickening. *Circ J.* (2012) 76:2456–64. doi: 10.1253/circj.CJ-12-0215
35. Weir EK, Lopez-Barneo J, Buckler KJ, Archer SL. Acute oxygen-sensing mechanisms. *N Engl J Med.* (2005) 353:2042–55. doi: 10.1056/NEJMra050002
36. Heymann MA, Rudolph AM. Control of the ductus arteriosus. *Physiology.* (1975) 55:62–78. doi: 10.1152/physrev.1975.55.1.62
37. Smith GC, McGrath JC. Indomethacin but not oxygen tension affects the sensitivity of isolated neonatal rabit ductus arteriosus, but not aorta to noradrenaline. *Cardiovas Res.* (1988) 22:910–5. doi: 10.1093/cvr/22.12.910
38. Kajimoto H, Hashimoto K, Bonnet SN, Heromy A, Harry G, Moudgil R, et al. Oxygen activates the Rho/Rho-kinase pathway and induces RhoB and ROCK-1 expression in human and rabbit ductus arteriosus by increasing mitochondria-derived reactive oxygen species. *Circulation.* (2008) 115:1777–88. doi: 10.1161/CIRCULATIONAHA.106.649566
39. Nakanishi T, Gu H, Hagiwara N, Momma K. Mechanisms of oxygen-induced contraction of ductus arteriosus isolated from the fetal rabbit. *Circ Res.* (1993) 72:1218–28. doi: 10.1161/01.RES.72.6.1218
40. Michelakis ED, Rebeyka I, Wu X, Nsair A, Tehabud B, Hashimoto K, et al. O2 sensing in the human ductus arteriosus regulation of voltage gated K+ channels in smooth muscle cells by a mitochondrial redox sensor. *Circ Res.* (2002) 91:478–86. doi: 10.1161/01.RES.0000035057.63303.D1
41. Thebaud B, Michelakis ED, Wu XC, Moudgil R, Kuzyk M, Dyck JR, et al. Oxygen-sensitive Kv channel gene transfer confers oxygen responsiveness to preterm rabbit and remodeled human ductus arteriosus: implications for infants with patent ductus arteriosus. *Circulation.* (2004) 110:1372–9. doi: 10.1161/01.CIR.0000141292.28616.65
42. Michealakis E, Rebeyka I, Bateson J, Olley P, Puttagunta L, Archer S. Voltage gated potassium channels in human ductus arteriosus. *Lancet.* (2000) 356:134–7. doi: 10.1016/S0140-6736(00)02452-1
43. Thebaud B, Wu XC, Kajimoto H, Bonnet S, Hashimoto K, Michelakis ED, et al. Developmental absence of the O2 sensitivity of L type calcium channels in preterm ductus arteriosus smooth muscle cells impairs O2 constriction contributing to patent ductus arteriosus. *Pediatr Res.* (2008) 63:176–81. doi: 10.1203/PDR.0b013e31815ed059
44. Akaike T, Jin MH, Yokoyama U, Izumi-Nakaseko H, Jiao Q, Iwasaki S, et al. T-type Ca2+ channels promote oxygenation induced closure of the rat ductus arteriosus not only by vasoconstriction but also by neointima formation. *J Biol Chem.* (2009) 284:24025–34. doi: 10.1074/jbc.M109.017061
45. Cogolludo AL, Moral-Sanz J, van der Sterren S, Frazziano G, van Cleef AN, Menéndez C, et al. Maturation of O2 sensing and signaling in the chicken ductus arterious. *Am J Physiol Lung Cell Mol Physiol.* (2009) 297:L619–30. doi: 10.1152/ajplung.00092.2009
46. Fleming I. Vascular cytochrome p450 enzymes: physiology and pathophysiology. *Trends Cardiovasc Med.* (2008) 18:20–5. doi: 10.1016/j.tcm.2007.11.002
47. Baragatti B, Coceani F. Arachidonic acid epoxygenase and 12(S) lipoxygenase: evidence of their concerted involvement in ductus arteriosus constriction to oxygen. *Can J Physiol Pharmacol.* (2011) 89:329–34. doi: 10.1139/y11-025
48. Coceani F, Kelsey L, Seidliz E. Evidence for an effector role of endothelin in closure of the ductus arteriosus at birth. *Can J Physiol Pharmacol.* (1992) 70:1061–4. doi: 10.1139/y92-146
49. Chen JX, O'Mara PW, Poole SD, Brown N, Ehinger NJ, Slaughter JC, et al. Isoprostanes as physiological mediators of transition to newborn life: novel mechanism regulating patency of the term and preterm ductus arteriosus. *Pediatr Res.* (2012) 72:122. doi: 10.1038/pr.2012.58
50. Wu GR, Jing S, Momma K, Nakanishi T. The effect of vitamin A on contraction of the ductus arteriosus in fetal rat. *Pediatr Res.* (2001) 49:747–54. doi: 10.1203/00006450-200106000-00006
51. Hung YC, Yeh JL, Hsu JH. Molecular mechanism for regulation postnatal ductus arteriosus closure. *Int J Mol Sci.* (2018) 19:1861. doi: 10.3390/ijms19071861
52. Hong Z, Hong F, Olschewski A, Cabrera JA, Varghese A, Nelson DP, et al. Role of store-operated calcium channels and calcium sensitization in normoxic contraction of the ductus arterisosus. *Circulation.* (2006) 114:1372–9. doi: 10.1161/CIRCULATIONAHA.106.641126
53. Akaike T, Minamisawa S. Role of ion channels in ductus arteriosus closure. *Hum Genet Embryo.* (2013) 3:116. doi: 10.4172/2161-0436.1000116
54. Takizawa T, Horikoshi E, Shen MH, Masaoka T, Takagi H, Yamamoto M, et al. Effects of TAK-044, a nonselective endothelin receptor antagonist, on the spontaneous and indomethacin- or methylene blue-induced constriction of the ductus arteriosus in rats. *J Vet Med Sci.* (2000) 62:505–9. doi: 10.1292/jvms.62.505
55. Waleh N, Kajino H, Marrache AM, Ginzinger D, Roman C, Seidner SR, et al. Prostaglandin E2–mediated relaxation of the ductus arteriosus: effects of gestational age on g protein-coupled receptor expression, signaling, and vasomotor control. *Circulation.* (2004) 110:2326–32. doi: 10.1161/01.CIR.0000145159.16637.5D
56. altered ductus Gonzalez A, Sosenko IR, Chandar J, Hummler H, Claure N, Bancalari E. Influence of infection on patent ductus arteriosus and chronic lung disease in premature infants weighing 1000 grams or less. *J Pediatr.* (1996) 128:470–8. doi: 10.1016/S0022-3476(96)70356-6
57. Levin M, McCurnin D, Seidner SR, Yoder B, Waleh N, Goldberg S, et al. Postnatal constriction, ATP depletion, and cell death in the mature and immature ductus arteriosus. *Am J Physiol Regul Integr Comp Physiol.* (2006) 290:R359–64. doi: 10.1152/ajpregu.00629.2005
58. Clyman RI, Teitel D, Padbury J, Roman C, Mauray F. The role of beta-adrenoreceptor stimulation and contractile state in the preterm lamb's response to arteriosus patency. *Pediatr Res.* (1988) 23:316–22. doi: 10.1203/00006450-198803000-00017
59. Fujita S, Yokoyama U, Ishiwata R, Aoki R, Nagao K, Masukawa D, et al. Glutamate promotes contraction of the rat ductus arteriosus. *Circ J.* (2016) 80:2388–96. doi: 10.1253/circj.CJ-16-0649
60. Clyman RI, Roman C. The effects of caffeine on the preterm sheep ductus arteriosus. *Pediatr Res.* (2007) 62:167–9. doi: 10.1203/PDR.0b013e3180a725b1
61. Çakir U, Tayman C. A mystery of patent ductus arteriosus and serum osmolality in preterm infants. *Am J Perinatol.* (2018) 36:641–6. doi: 10.1055/s-0038-1673397
62. Aoki R, Yokoyama U, Ichikawa Y, Taguri M, Kumagaya S, Ishiwata R, et al. Decreased serum osmolality promotes ductus arteriosus constriction. *Cardiovasc Res.* (2014) 104:326–36. doi: 10.1093/cvr/cvu199
63. Hu Y, Jin H, Jiang Y, Du J. Prediction of therapeutic response to cyclooxygenase inhibitors in preterm infants with patent ductus arteriosus. *Pediatr Cardiol.* (2018) 39:647–52. doi: 10.1007/s00246-018-1831-x
64. Mine K, Ohashi A, Tsuji S, Nakashima JI, Hirabayashi M, Kaneko K. B-type antriuretic peptide for assessment of haemodynamically significant patent ductus arteriosus in premature infants. *Acta Pediatr.* (2013) 102:e347–52. doi: 10.1111/apa.12273
65. Sharpe GL, Larsson KS, Thalme MB. Studies on closure of the ductus arteriosus. XII. *In vitro* effect of indomethacin and sodium salicylate in rats and rabbits. *Prostaglandins.* (1975) 9:585–95. doi: 10.1016/0090-6980(75)90064-7
66. Clyman RI, Mayray F, Roman C, Rudolph AM, Heyman M. Glucorticoids alter the sensitivity of the lamb ductus arteriosus to prostaglandin E2. *J Pediatr.* (1981) 98:126–8. doi: 10.1016/S0022-3476(81)80558-6
67. Pulkkinen MO, Momma K, Pulkkinen J. Constriction of fetal ductus arteriosus by progesterone. *Biol Neonate.* (1986) 50:270–3. doi: 10.1159/000242608
68. Costa M, Barogi S, Socci ND, Angeloni D, Maffei M, Baragatti B, et al. Gene expression in ductus arteriosus and aorta: comparison of birth and oxygen effects. *Physiol Genom.* (2006) 25:250–62. doi: 10.1152/physiolgenomics.00231.2005
69. Coceani F, Liu YA, Seidlitz E, Kelsey L, Kuwaki T, Ackerley C, et al. Deletion of the endothelin-A-receptor suppresses oxygen induced constriction but not postnatal closure of the ductus arteriosus. *J Cardiovasc Pharm.* (2000) 36:S75–7. doi: 10.1097/00005344-200036001-00025
70. Clyman RI, Seidner SR, Kajino H, Roman C, Koch CJ, Ferrara N, et al. VEGF regulates remodeling during permanent anatomic closure of the ductus arteriosus. *Am J Physiol.* (2002) 282:R199–206. doi: 10.1152/ajpregu.00298.2001

71. Kajino H, Goldberg S, Roman C, Liu BM, Mauray F, Qi Y, et al. Vasa vasorum hypoperfusion is responsible for medial hypoxia and anatomic remodeling in the newborn lamb ductus arteriosus. *Pediatr Res.* (2002) 51:228-35. doi: 10.1203/00006450-200202000-00017
72. Yokoyama U, Minamismawa S, Shioda A, Ishiwata R, Jin MH, Masuda M, et al. Prostaglandin E 2 inhibits elastogenesis in the ductus arteriosus via EP_4 signaling. *Circulation.* (2014) 129:487–96. doi: 10.1161/CIRCULATIONAHA.113.004726
73. Gitterberger-de Groot AC. Persistent ductus arteriosus: most probably a primary congenital malformation. *Br Heart J.* (1977) 39:610–8. doi: 10.1136/hrt.39.6.610
74. Clyman RI, Chan CY, Mauray F, Chen YQ, Cox W, Seidner SR, et al. Permanent anatomic closure of the ductus arteriosus in newborn baboons: the roles of postnatal constriction, hypoxia and gestation. *Pediatr Res.* (1999) 45:19–29. doi: 10.1203/00006450-199901000-00005
75. Seidner SR, Chen YQ, Oprysko PR, Mauray F, Tse MM, Lin E, et al. Combined prostaglandin and nitric oxide inhibition produces anatomic remadoling and closure of the ductus arteriosus in the premature newborn baboon. *Pediatr Res.* (2001) 50:365–73. doi: 10.1203/00006450-200109000-00012
76. Hinek A, Mecham RP, Keeley F, Rabinovitch M. Impaired elastin fiber assembly related to reduced 67-kD elastin-binding protein in fetal lamb DA and in cultured aortic smooth muscle cells treated with chondroitin sulfate. *J Clin Invest.* (1991) 88:2083–94. doi: 10.1172/JCI115538
77. Hsieh YT, Liu NM, Ohmori E, Yokota T, Kajimura I, Akaike T, et al. Transcription profiles of the DA in Brown-Norway rats with irregular elastic fiber formation. *Circ J.* (2014) 78:1224–33. doi: 10.1253/circj.CJ-13-1029
78. Clyman RI, Goetzman BW, Chen YQ, Mauray F, Kramer RH, Pytela R, et al. Changes in endotehial cell and smooth muscle cell integrin expression during closure of the ductus arteriosus: an immunohistochemical comparison of the fetal, preterm newborn and full term newborn rhesus monkey ductus. *Pediatr Res.* (1996) 40:198–208. doi: 10.1203/00006450-199608000-00004
79. Francalanci P, Camassei FD, Orzalesi M, Danhaive O, Callea F. CD44-v6 expression in smooth muscle cells in the postnatal remodeling process of ductus arteriosus. *Am J Cardiol.* (2006) 97:1056–9. doi: 10.1016/j.amjcard.2005.10.046
80. Boudreau N, Turley E, Rabinovitch M. Fibronectin, hyaluronan, and a hyaluronan binding protein contribute to increased DA smooth muscle cell migration. *Dev Biol.* (1991) 143:235–47. doi: 10.1016/0012-1606(91)90074-D
81. Yokoyama U, Minamisawa S, Katayama A, Tang T, Suzuki S, Iwatsubo K, et al. Differential regulation of vascular tone and remodeling via stimulation of type 2 and type 6 adenylyl cyclases in the ductus arteriosus. *Circ Res.* (2010) 106:1882–92. doi: 10.1161/CIRCRESAHA.109.214924
82. Mason CA, Bigras JL, O'Blenes SB, Zhou B, McIntyre B, Nakamura N, et al. Gene transfer *in utero* biologically engineers a patent DA in lambs by arresting fibronectin-dependent neointimal formation. *Nat Med.* (1999) 5:176–82. doi: 10.1038/5538
83. Clyman RI. Mechanisms regulating closure of the ductus arteriosus. In: Polin R, Abman SH, Rowitch DH, Benitz WE, Fox WW, editors. *Fetal and Neonatal Physiology.* New York, NY: Elsevier (2019). p. 57:592–9.
84. Lezoulach F, Fazal L, Laudette M, Conte C. Cyclic AMP sensor EPAC proteins and their role in cardiovascular function and disease. *Circ Res.* (2016) 118:881–97. doi: 10.1161/CIRCRESAHA.115.306529
85. Bos JL. Epac: a new cAMP target and new avenues in cAMP research. *Nat Rev Mol Cell Biol.* (2003) 4:733–8. doi: 10.1038/nrm1197
86. Wu LH, Xu SJ, Teng JY, Wu W, Ye DY, Wu XZ. Differential response of human fetal smooth muscle cells from arterial dut to retinoid acid. *Acta Pharmacol Sin.* (2008) 29:413–20. doi: 10.1111/j.1745-7254.2008.00766.x
87. Ravishankar C, Nafday S, Green RS, Kamenir S, Lorber R, Stacewicz-Sapuntzakis M, et al. A trial of vitamin A therapy to facilitate ductal closure in premature infants. *J Pediatr.* (2003) 143:644–48. doi: 10.1067/S0022-3476(03)00501-8
88. Momma K, Toyono M, Miyagawa-Tomita S. Accelerated maturation of fetal ductus arteriosus by maternally administered vitamin A in rats. *Pediatr Res.* (1998) 43:629–32. doi: 10.1203/00006450-199805000-00011
89. Basu S, Khanna P, Srivastava R, Kumar A. Oral vitamin A supplemantation in very low birth weight neonates: a randomized controlled trial. *Eur J Pediatr.* (2019) 178:1255–65. doi: 10.1007/s00431-019-03412-w
90. Tannenbaum JE, Waleh NS, Mauray F, Breuss J, Pytela R, Karemer RH, Clyman RI. Transforming growth factor beta 1 inhibits fetal lab ductus arteriosus smooth muscle cell migration. *Pediatr Res.* (1995) 37:561–70. doi: 10.1203/00006450-199505000-00001
91. Wu JR, Yeh JL, Liou SF, Dai ZK,Wu BN, Hsu JH. Gamma-secretase inhibitor prevents proliferation and migration of ductus arteriosus smooth muscle cells through the Notch3-HES1/2/5 pathway. *Int J Biol Sci.* (2016) 12:1063–73. doi: 10.7150/ijbs.16430
92. Giri JG, Ahdieh M, Einsenman J, Schanebeck K, Grabstein K, Kumaki S, et al. Utilization of the beta and gamma chains of the IL-2 receptor by the novel cytokine IL-15. *EMBO J.* (1994) 13:2822–30. doi: 10.1002/j.1460-2075.1994.tb06576.x
93. Yokoyama U, Minamisawa S, Quan H, Ghatak S, Akaike T, Segi-Nishida E, et al. Chronic activation of the prostaglandin receptor EP_4 promotes hyaluronan-mediated neointimal formation in the ductus arteriosus. *J Clin Invest.* (2006) 116:3026–34. doi: 10.1172/JCI 28639
94. Rabinovich M. Cell-extracellular matrix interactions in the ductus arteriosus and perinatal pulmonary circulation. *Semin Perinatol.* (1996) 20:531–41. doi: 10.1016/S0146-0005(96)80067-X
95. Evanko SP, Angello JC, Wight TN. Formation of hyaluronan and versican rich pericellular matrix is required for proliferation and migration of vascular smooth muscle cells. *ArterioscIerThromb Vasc Biol.* (1999) 19:1004–13. doi: 10.1161/01.ATV.19.4.1004
96. Cowan KN, Jones PL, Rabinovitch M. Elastase and matrix metalloproteinase inhibitors induce regression, and tenascin C antisense prevents progression of vascular disease. *J Clin Invest.* (2000) 105:21–34. doi: 10.1172/JCI6539
97. Hinek A, Boyle J, Rabinovitch M. Vascular smooth muscle cell detachment from elastin and migration through elastic laminae is promoted by chondroitin sulfate indnuced shedding of the 67 kDa cell surface elastin binding protein. *Exp Cell Res.* (1992) 203:344–53. doi: 10.1016/0014-4827(92)90008-V
98. Kawakami S, Minamisawa S. Oxygenation decreases elastin secretion from rat ductus arteriosus smooth muscle cells. *Pediatr Int.* (2015) 57:541–5. doi: 10.1111/ped.12684
99. Waleh N, Seidner S, McCurnin D, Yoder B, Liu BM, Roman C, et al. The role of monocyte-derived cells and inflammation in baboon ductus arteriosus remodeling. *Pediatr Res.* (2005) 57:254–26. doi: 10.1203/01.PDR.0000148278.64777.EF
100. Johnston B, Issekutz TB, Kubes P. The alpha 4-integrin supports leukocyterolling and adhesion in chronically inflamed postcapillary venules *in vivo*. *J Exp Med.* (1996) 183:1995. doi: 10.1084/jem.183.5.1995
101. Barleon B, Sozzani S, Zhou D, Weich HA, Mantovani A, Marme D. Migration of human monocytes in response to vascular endothelial growth factor (VEGF) is mediated via the VEGF receptor flt-1. *Blood.* (1996) 87:3336–43. doi: 10.1182/blood.V87.8.3336.bloodjournal8783336
102. Waleh N, Seidner S, McCurnin D, Giavedoni L, Hodara V, Goelz S, et al. Anatomic closure of the premature patent ductus arteriosus: the role of CD14/CD163+ mononuclear cells and ascular endothelial growth factor (VEGF) in neointimal mound formation. *Pediatr Res.* (2020) 70:332–8. doi: 10.1203/PDR.0b013e3182294471
103. Jackson CL, Raines EW, Ross R, Reidy MA. Role of endogenous platelet-derived growth factor in arterial smooth muscle cell migration after balloon catheterinjury. *Arterioscler Thromb.* (1993) 13:1218–122. doi: 10.1161/01.ATV.13.8.1218
104. Echtler K, Stark K, Lorenz M, Kerstan S, Walch A, Jennen L, et al. Platelets contribute to postnatal occlusion of the ductus arteriosus *Nat Med.* (2019) 16:75–82. doi: 10.1038/nm.2060
105. Clyman R, Cherntob S. Vessel remodeling in the newborn: platelets fill the gap. *Nat Med.* (2010) 16:33–4. doi: 10.1038/nm0110-33
106. Engür D, Kaynak-Türkmen M, Deveci M, Yenisey C. Platelets and platelet derived growth factor in closure of ductus arteriosus. *Turk J Pediatr.* (2015) 57:242–7.
107. Dani C, Poggi C, Fontanell G. Relationship between platelet count and volume and spontaneous and pharmacological closure o of ductur arteriosus in preterm infants. *Am J Perinatol.* (2013) 30:359–64. doi: 10.1055/s-0032-1324702

108. Shah NA, Hills NK, Waleh N, McCurnin D, Seidner S, Chemto S, et al. Relationship between circulating platelet counts and ductus arteriosus patency after indomethacin treatment. *J Pediatr.* (2011) 158:919–23. doi: 10.1016/j.jpeds.2010.11.018
109. Shelton EL, Ector G, Galind CL, Hooper CW, Brown N, Wilkerson I, et al. Transcriptional profiling reveals ductus arteriosus specific genes that regulate vascular tone. *Physiol Genomics.* (2014) 46:457–66. doi: 10.1152/physiolgenomics.00171.2013
110. Loftin CD, Trivedi DB, Tiano HF, Clark JA, Lee CA, Epstein JA, et al. Failure of ductus arteriosus closure and remodeling in neonatal mice deficient in cyclooxygenase-1 and cyclooxygenase-2. *Proc Natl Acad Sci USA.* (2001) 98:1059–64. doi: 10.1073/pnas.98.3.1059
111. Reese J, Paria BC, Brown N, Zhao X, Morrow JD, Dey SK. Coordinated regulation of fetal and maternal prostaglandins directs successful birth and postnatal adaptation in the mouse. *Proc Natl Acad Sci USA.* (2000) 97:9759e64. doi: 10.1073/pnas.97.17.9759
112. Ment LR, Vohr B, Allan W, Westerveld M, Sparrow SS, Schneider KC, et al. Outcome of children in the indomethacin intraventricular hemorrhage prevention trial. *Pediatrics.* (2000) 105:485–91. doi: 10.1542/peds.105.3.485
113. Coggins KG, Latour A, Nguyen MS, Audoly L, Coffman TM, et al. Metabolism of PGE_2 by prostaglandin dehydrogenase is essential for remodeling the ductus arteriosus. *Nat Med.* (2002) 8:91–2. doi: 10.1038/nm0202-91
114. Nagar S, Walther S, Blanchard RL. Sulfotransferase (SULT) 1A1 polymorphic variants *1, *2, and *3 are associated with altered enzymatic activity, cellular phenotype, and protein degradation. *Mol Pharmacol.* (2006) 69:2084–92. doi: 10.1124/mol.105.019240
115. Grassian AR, Metallo CM, Coloff JL, Stephanopoulos G, Brugge JS. Erk regulation of pyruvate dehydrogenase flux through PDK4 modulates cell proliferation. *Genes Dev.* (2011) 25:1716–33. doi: 10.1101/gad.16771811
116. Sun Y, Daemen A, Hatzivassiliou G, Arnott D, Wilson C, Zhuang G, et al. Metabolic and transcriptional profiling reveals pyruvate dehydrogenase kinase 4 as a mediator of epithelial-mesenchymal transition and drug resistance in tumor cells. *Cancer Metab.* (2014) 2:20. doi: 10.1186/2049-3002-2-20
117. Kurihara T, Kubota Y, Ozawa Y, Takubo K, Noda K, Simon MC, et al. von Hippel-Lindau protein regulates transition from the fetal to the adult circulatory system in retina. *Development.* (2010) 137:1563–71. doi: 10.1242/dev.049015
118. Morano I, Chai GX, Baltas LG, Lamounier-Zepter V, Lutsch G, Kott M, et al. Smooth-muscle contraction without smooth-muscle myosin. *Nat Cell Biol.* (2000) 2:371–5. doi: 10.1038/35014065
119. Huang J, Cheng L, Li J, Chen M, Zhou D, Lu MM, et al. Myocardin regulates expression of contractile genes in smooth muscle cells and is required for closure of the ductus arteriosus in mice. *J Clin Invest.* (2008) 118:515–25. doi: 10.1172/JCI33304
120. Zhao F, Bosserhoff AK, Buettner R, Moser M. A heart-hand syndrome gene: Tfap2b plays a critical role in the development and remodeling of mouse ductus arteriosus and limb patterning. *PLoS ONE.* (2011) 6:e22908. doi: 10.1371/journal.pone.0022908
121. Ivey KN, Sutcliffe D, Richardson J, Clyman RI, Garcia JA, Srivastava D. Transcriptional regulation during development of the ductus arteriosus. *Circ Res.* (2008) 103:388–95. doi: 10.1161/CIRCRESAHA.108.180661
122. Baeten JT, Jackson AR, McHugh KM, Lilly B. Loss of Notch2 and Notch3 in vascular smooth muscle causes patent ductus arteriosus. *Genesis.* (2015) 53:738e48. doi: 10.1002/dvg.22904
123. Feng X, Krebs LT, Gridley T. Patent ductus arteriosus in mice with smooth muscle-specific Jagl deletion. *Development.* (2010) 137:4191e9. doi: 10.1242/dev.052043
124. Zhang M, Chen M, Kim JR, Zhou J, Jones RE, Tune JD, et al. SWI/SNF complexes containing Brahma or Brahma-related gene 1 play distinct roles in smooth muscle development. *Mol Cell Biol.* (2011) 31:2618–31. doi: 10.1128/MCB.01338-10
125. Coceani F, Scebba F, Angeloni D. Gene profiling in ductus arteriosus and aorta: a question of consistency. *J Physiol Sci.* (2011) 61:443–4. doi: 10.1007/s12576-011-0161-z
126. Bokenkamp R, DeRuiter MC, van Munsteren C, Gittenfactor-de Groot AC. Insights into the pathogenesis and genetic background of patency of the ductus arteriosus. *Neonatology.* (2010) 98:6–17. doi: 10.1159/000262481
127. Tang B, Li Y, Nagaraj C, Morty RE, Gabor S, Stacher E, et al. Endothelin-1 inhibits background two-pore domain channel TASK-1 in primary human pulmonary artery smooth muscle cells. *Am J Respir Cell Mol Biol.* (2009) 41:476–83. doi: 10.1165/rcmb.2008-0412OC
128. Lewis TR, Shelton EL, Van Driest SL, Kannankeril PJ, Reese J. Genetics of the patent ductus arteriosus (PDA) and pharmacogenetics of PDA treatment. *Semin Fetal Neonatal Med.* (2018) 23:232–8. doi: 10.1016/j.siny.2018.02.006
129. Lavoie PM, Pham C, Jang KL. Heritability of bronchopulmonary dysplasia, defined according to the consensus statement of the national institutes of health. *Pediatrics.* (2008) 122:479–85. doi: 10.1542/peds.2007-2313
130. Mani A, Meraji SM, Houshyar R, Radhakrishnan J, Mani A, Ahangar M, et al. Finding genetic contributions to sporadic disease: a recessive locus at 12q24 commonly contributes to patent ductus arteriosus. *Proc Natl Acad Sci USA.* (2002) 99:15054e9. doi: 10.1073/pnas.192582999
131. Derzbach L, Treszl A, Balogh A, Vasarhelyi B, Tulassay T, Rigó JJ. Gender dependent association between perinatal morbidity and estrogen receptor-alpha Pvull polymorphism. *J Perinat Med.* (2005) 33:461–2. doi: 10.1515/JPM.2005.082
132. Bokodi G, Derzbach L, Banyasz I, Tulassay T, Vasarhelyi B. Association of interferon gamma $T^{+}874A$ and interleukin 12 p40 promoter CTCTAA/GC polymorphism with the need for respiratory support and perinatal complications in low birthweight neonates. *Arch Dis Child Fetal Neonatal Ed.* (2007) 92:F25–9. doi: 10.1136/adc.2005.086421
133. Dagle JM, Lepp NT, Cooper ME, Schaa KL, Kelsey KJP, et al. Determination of genetic predisposition to patent ductus arteriosus in preterm infants. *Pediatrics.* (2009) 123:1116–23. doi: 10.1542/peds.2008-0313
134. Treszi A, Szabo M, Dunai G, Nobilis A, Kocsis I, Machay T, et al. Angiotensin II type 1 receptor A1166C polymorphism and prophylactic indomethacin treatment induced ductus arteriosus closure in very low birth weight neonates. *Pediatr Res.* (2003) 54:753–5. doi: 10.1203/01.PDR.0000088016.67117.39
135. Waleh N, Hodnick R, Jhaveri N, McConaghy S, Dagle J, Seidner S, et al. Patterns of gene expression in the ductus arteriosus are related to environmental and genetic risk factors for persistent ductus patency. *Pediatr Res.* (2010) 68:292–7. doi: 10.1203/PDR.0b013e3181ed8609
136. Smit-Mungo LI, Kagan HM. Lysyl oxidase: properties, regulation and multiple functions in biology. *Matrix Biol.* (1998) 16:387–98. doi: 10.1016/S0945-053X(98)90012-9
137. *Neonatal Ed.* (2014) 99:F408–12. Rasanen J, Wood DC, Debbs RH, Cohen J, Weiner S, Huhta JC. Reactivity of the human fetal pulmonary circulation to maternal hyperoxygenation increases during the second half ou pregnancy: a randomized study. *Circulation.* (1998) 97:257–62. doi: 10.1161/01.CIR.97.3.257
138. van Vonderen JJ, te Pas AB, Kolster-Bijdevaate C, van Lith JM, Blom NA, Hooper SB, et al. Non-invasive measurements of ductus arteriosus flow directly after birth. *Arch Dis Child Fetal Nenatal Ed.* (2014) 99:F408–12. doi: 10.1136/archdischild-2014-306033
139. Hammerman C, Aramburo MJ. Effects of hyperventilation on prostacyclin formation and on pulmonary vasodilation after GBS induced pulmonary hypertension. *Pediatr Res.* (1991) 29:282–7. doi: 10.1203/00006450-199103000-00012
140. Haworth SG. Pulmonary endothelium in the perinatal period. *Pharmacol Rep.* (2006) 58:153–64.
141. Sehgal A, Mak W, Dunn M, Kelly E, Whyte H, McCrindle B, et al. Haemodynamic changes after delivery room surfactant administration to verye low birth weight infants. *Arch Dis Cild Fetal Neonatal Ed.* (2010) 95:F345–51. doi: 10.1136/adc.2009.173724
142. Deshpande P, Baczynski M, McNamara P, Jain M. Patent ductus arteriosus: the physiology of transition. *Semin Fetal Neonatal Med.* (2018) 23:225–31. doi: 10.1016/j.siny.2018.05.001
143. Rychik J. Fetal cardiovascular physiology. *Pediatr Cardiol.* (2004) 25:201–9. doi: 10.1007/s00246-003-0586-0
144. Kresch MJ. Management of the third stage of labor: How delayed umbilical cord clamping can affect neonatal outcome. *Am J Perinatol.* (2017) 34:1375–81. doi: 10.1055/s-0037-1603733

145. Chung HR. Adrenal and thyroid function in the fetus and preterm infant. *Korean J Pediatr.* (2014) 57:425–33. doi: 10.3345/kjp.2014.57.10.425
146. Okahara K, Sun B, Kambayashi J. Upregulation of prostacyclin synthesis-related gene expression by shear stress in vascular endothelial cells. *Arterioscler Thromb Vasc Biol.* (1998) 18:1922–26. doi: 10.1161/01.ATV.18.12.1922
147. Uematsu M, Ohara Y, Navas JP, Nishida K, Murphy TJ, Alexander RW, et al. Regulation of endothelial cell nitric oxide synthase mRNA expression by shear stress. *Am J Physiol.* (1995) 269(Pt. 1):C1371–8. doi: 10.1152/ajpcell.1995.269.6.C1371
148. Chappell DC, Varner SE, Nerem RM, Medford RM, Alexander RW. Oscillatory shear stress stimulates adhesion molecule expression in cultured human endothelium. *Circ Res.* (1998) 82:532–9. doi: 10.1161/01.RES.82.5.532
149. Conway DE, Williams MR, Eskin SG, McIntire LV. Endothelial cell responses to atheroprone flow are driven by two separate flow components: low time-average shear stress and fluid flow reversal. *Am J Physiol Heart Circ Physiol.* (2010) 298:H367–74. doi: 10.1152/ajpheart.00565.2009
150. Mantella LE, Quan A, Verma S. Variability in vascular smooth muscle cell stretch-induced responses in 2D culture. *Vasc Cell.* (2015) 7:7. doi: 10.1186/s13221-015-0032-0
151. Gerhardt T, Bancalari E. Lung compliance in newborns with patent ductus arteriosus before and after surgical ligation. *Biol Neonate.* (1980) 38:96–105. doi: 10.1159/000241348
152. Clyman RI. Commentary: recommendations for the postnatal use of indomethacin. An analysis of four separate treatment strategies. *J Pediatr.* (1996) 128:601–7. doi: 10.1016/S0022-3476(96)80123-5
153. Clyman RI. Mechanisms regulating the ductus arteriosus. *Biol Neonate.* (2006) 89:330–5. doi: 10.1159/000092870
154. De Buyst J, Rakza T, Pennaforte T, Johansson AB, Storme L. Hemodynamic effects of fluid irestriction in preterm infants with significant patent ductus arteriosus. *J Pediatr.* (2012) 161:404–8. doi: 10.1016/j.jpeds.2012.03.012
155. Stephens BE, Gargus RA, Walden RV, Mance M, Nye J, McKinley L, et al. Fluid regimens in the first week of life may increase risk of patent ductus arteriosus in extremely low birth weight infants. *J Perinatol.* (2008) 28:123–8. doi: 10.1038/sj.jp.7211895
156. Clyman RI, Mauray F, Roman C, Heymann MA, Ballard PL, Rudolph AM, et al. Effects of antenatal glucocorticoid administration on ductus arteriosus of preter lambs. *Am J Physiol.* (1981) 100:H415–20. doi: 10.1152/ajpheart.1981.241.3.H415
157. Padbury JF, Ervin MG, Polk DH. Extrapulmonary effects of antenatally administered steroids. *J Pediatr.* (1996) 128:167–72. doi: 10.1016/S0022-3476(96)70384-0
158. Lundgren J, Hirata F, Marom Z, Logun C, Steel L, Kaliner, et al. Dexamethasone inhibits respirotary glyconjugate secretion from feline airways *in vitro* by the induction of lipocortin (lipomodilin) synthesis. *Am Rev Respir Dis.* (1988) 106:801–5.
159. Watterberg KL, Scott SM, Backstrom C, Gifford KL, Cook KL. Link between early adrenal function and respiratory outcome in preterm infants: Airway infllammation and patent ductus arteriosus. *Pediatrics.* (2000) 105:320–4. doi: 10.1542/peds.105.2.320
160. Gürsoy T, Hayran M, Derin H, Ovali FA. Clinical scoring system to predict the development of bronchopulmonary dysplasia. *Am J Perinatol.* (2015). 32:659–66. doi: 10.1055/s-0034-1393935
161. Waleh N, McCurnin DC, Yoder BA, Shaul PW, Clyman RI. Patent DA ligation alters pulmonary gene expression in preterm baboons. Pediatr Res. *Pediatr Res.* (2011) 69:212–216. doi: 10.1203/PDR.0b013e3182084f8d
162. Chang LY, McCurnin D, Yoder B Shaul PW, Clyman RI. Ductus arteriosus ligation alveolar growth in preterm baboons with a patent DA. *Pediatr Res.* (2008) 63:299–302. doi: 10.1203/PDR.0b013e318163a8e4
163. Dawes GS, Mott JC, Widdicombe JG. The patency of the ductus arteriosus in newborn lambs and its physiological consequences. *J Physiol.* (1955) 128:361–83. doi: 10.1113/jphysiol.1955.sp005313
164. Noori S, Patel D, Friedlich P, Siassi B, Seri I, Ramanathan R. Effects of low oxygen saturation limits on the ductus arteriosus in extremely low birth weight infants. *J Perinatol.* (2009) 29:553–7. doi: 10.1038/jp.2009.60
165. SUPPORT study group of the Eunice Kennedy Shriver NICHD Neonatal Research Network. Finer NN, Carlo WA, Walsh MC, Rich W, Gantz MG, et al. Target ranges of oxygen saturation in extremely preterm infants. *N Eng J Med.* (2010) 362:1959–69. doi: 10.1056/NEJMoa0911781
166. BOOSTII United Kingdom Collaborative Group, BOOSTII Australia Collaborative Group. BOOSTII New Zealand Collaborative Group. Stenson BJ, Tarnow Mordi WO, Darlow BA, et al. Oxygen saturation and outcomes in preterm infants. *N Engl J Med.* (2013) 368:2094–104. doi: 10.1056/NEJMoa1302298
167. Schmidt B, Whyte RK, Asztalos EV, Moddemann D, Poets C, Rabi Y, et al. Effects of targeting higher vs lower arterial oxygen saturations on death or disability in extremely preterm infants: a randomized clinical trial. *JAMA.* (2013) 309:2111–20. doi: 10.1001/jama.2013.5555
168. Shelton EL, Waleh N, Plosa EJ, Benjamin JT, Milne GL, Hooper CW, et al. Effects of antenatal betamethasone on preterm human and mouse ductus arteriosus: comparison with baboon data. *Pediatr Res.* (2018) 84:458–65. doi: 10.1038/s41390-018-0006-z
169. Waleh N, Barrette AM, Dagle JM, Momany A, Jin C, Hills NK, et al. Effects of advancing gestation and non-Caucasian race on ductus arteriosus gene expression. *J Pediatr.* (2015) 167:1033–41. doi: 10.1016/j.jpeds.2015.07.011
170. Trivedi DB, Sugimoto Y, Loftin CD. Attenuated cyclooxygenase 2 expression contributes to patent ductus arteriosus in preterm mice. *Pediatr Res.* (2006) 60:669–74. doi: 10.1203/01.pdr.0000246480.13170.c0
171. Rheinlander C, Weber SC, Sarioglu N, Strauss E, Obladen M. Changing expression of cyclooxygenases and prostaglandin receptor EP_4 during development of the human ductus arteriosus. *Peditar Res.* (2006) 60:270–5. doi: 10.1203/01.pdr.0000233066.28496.7c
172. Levin M, Goldberg S, Lindqvist A, Swärd A, Roman C, Liu BM, et al. ATP depletion and cell death in the neonatal lamb ductus arteriosus. *Pediatr Res.* (2005) 57:801–5. doi: 10.1203/01.PDR.0000157791.95954.56
173. van der Lugt NM, Lopriore E, Bokenkamp R, Smits-Wintjens VE, Steggerda SJ, Walther FJ. Repeated courses of ibuprofen are effective in closure of a patent DA. *Eur J Pediatr* (2012) 171:1673–7. doi: 10.1007/s00431-012-1805-6
174. Jensen EA, Dysart KC, Gantz MG, Carper B, Higgins RD, Keszler M, et al. Association between use of prophylactic indomethacin and the risk for bronchopulmonarydysplasia in extremely preterm infants. *J Pediatr.* (2017) 186:34–40. doi: 10.1016/j.jpeds.2017.02.003
175. Vermillon ST, Scardo JA, Lashus AG, Wiles HB. The effecs of indomethacin tocolysis on fetal ductus arteriosus constriction with advancing gestational ageb. *Am J Obstet Gynecol.* (1997) 177:256–9. doi: 10.1016/S0002-9378(97)70184-4
176. Pacifici GM. Clinical pharmacology of indomethacin in preterm infants: implications in patent ductus arteriosus closure. *Paediatr Drugs.* (2013) 15:363–76. doi: 10.1007/s40272-013-0031-7
177. Gersony WM, Peckham GJ, Ellison RC, Miettinen OS, Nadas AS. Effects of indomethacin in premature infants with patent ductus arteriosus: results of a national collaborative study. *J Pediatr.* (1983) 102:895–906. doi: 10.1016/S0022-3476(83)80022-5
178. Clyman RI. The role of patent ductus arteriosus and its treatments in the development of bronchopulmonary dysplasia. *Semin Perinatal.* (2013) 37:102–7. doi: 10.1053/j.semperi.2013.01.006
179. Godambe S, Newby B, Shah V, Shah PS. Effect of indomethacin on closure of ductus arteriosus in very-low-birthweight neonates. *Acta Paediatr.* (2006) 95:1389–93. doi: 10.1080/08035250600615150
180. Sangem M, Asthana S, Amin S. Multiple courses of indomethacin and neonatal outcomes in premature infants. *Pediatr Cardiol.* (2008) 29:878–84. doi: 10.1007/s00246-007-9166-z
181. Mitra S, Florez D, Tamayo ME, Aune D, Mbuagbaw L, Veroniki A, et al. Effectiveness and safety of treatments used for the management of patent ductus arteriosus (PDA) in preterminfants: A protocol for a systematic review and network meta-analysis. *BMJ Open.* (2016) 6:e011271. doi: 10.1136/bmjopen-2016-011271
182. Ohlsson A, Walia R, Shah SS. Ibuprofen for the treatment of patent ductus arteriosus in preterm or low birth weight (or both) infants. *Cochrane Database Syst Rev.* (2015) 2:CD003481. doi: 10.1002/14651858.CD003481.pub6
183. Hirt D, Van OB, Treluyer JM, Langhendries JP, Marguglio A, Eisinger MJ, et al. An optimized ibuprofen dosing scheme for preterm neonates with patent ductus arteriosus, based on a population pharmacokinetic and pharmacodynamic study. *Br J Clin Pharmacol.* (2008) 65:629–36. doi: 10.1111/j.1365-2125.2008.03118.x
184. Gournay V, Roze JC, Kuster A, Daoud P, Cambonie G, Hascoet JM, et al. Prophylactic ibuprofen versus placebo in very premature

infants: a randomised, double-blind, placebo-controlled trial. *Lancet.* (2004) 364:1939–44. doi: 10.1016/S0140-6736(04)17476-X

185. Bardanzellu F, Neroni P, Dessi A, Fanos V. Patacatemol in patentductus arteriosus treatment: efficacious and safe? *Biomed Res Intern.* (2017) 2017:1438038. doi: 10.1155/2017/1438038
186. Jozwiak-Bebenista M, Nowak JZ. Paracetamol: mechanism of action, applications and safety concern. *Acta Poloniae Pharma Drug Res.* (2014) 71:11–23.
187. Smith WL, DeWitt DL, Garavito RM. Cyclooxygenases: structural, cellular and molecular biology. *Annu Rev Biochem.* (2000) 69:145–82. doi: 10.1146/annurev.biochem.69.1.145
188. Allegaert K, Anderson B, Simons S, van Overmeire B. Paracetamol to induce ductus arteriosus closure: is it valid? *Arch Dis Child.* (2013) 98:462–6. doi: 10.1136/archdischild-2013-303688
189. Hostovsky LT, Pan J, McNamara PJ, Belik J. Acetaminophen increases pulmonary and systemic vasomotor tone in the newborn rat. *Pediatr Res.* (2019) 87:1171–6. doi: 10.1038/s41390-019-0725-9
190. Munsterhjelm E, Munsterhjelm NM, Niemi TT, Ylikorkala O, Neuvonen PJ, Rosenberg PH. Dose dependent inhibition of platelet function by acetaminophen in healthy volunteers. *Anesthesiology.* (2005) 103:712–17. doi: 10.1097/00000542-200510000-00009
191. Beringer RM, Thompson JP, Parry S, Stoddart PA. Intravenous paracetamol overdose: two case reports and a change to national treatment guidelines. *Arch Dis Child.* (2011) 96:307–8. doi: 10.1136/adc.2010.192005
192. Huang X, Wang F, Wang K. paracetamol versus ibuprofen for the treatment of patent ductus arteriosus in preterm neonates: a meta-analysis of randomized controlled trials. *J Matern Fetal Neonatal Med.* (2018) 31:2216–22. doi: 10.1080/14767058.2017.1338263
193. Jasani B, Weisz DE, McNamara PJ. Evidence-based use of acetaminophen for hemodynamically significant ductus arteriosus in preterm infants. *Semin Perinatol.* (2018) 42:243–52. doi: 10.1053/j.semperi.2018.05.007
194. Masarwa R, Levine H, Görelik E, Reif S, Perlman A, Matok I. Prenatal exposure to acetaminophen and risk for attention deficit hyperactivity disorder and autistic spectrum disorder: a systematic review, meta-analysis and meta-regression analysis of cohort studies. *Am J Epidemiol.* (2018) 87:1817–27. doi: 10.1093/aje/kwy086
195. Chen MH, Pan TL, Wang PW, Hsu JW, Huang KL, Su TP, et al. Prenatal exposure to acetaminophen and the risk of attention deficit hyperactivity disorder: A nationwide study in Taiwan. *J Clin Psychiatry.* (2019) 80:18m12612. doi: 10.4088/JCP.18m12612
196. Bittker SS, Bell KR. Acetaminophen, antibiotics, ear infection, breastfeeding, vitamin D drops and autism: an epidemiological study. *Neuropsychiatr Dis Treat.* (2018) 14:1399–414. doi: 10.2147/NDT.S158811
197. Juujarvi S, Kallankari H, Patsi P, Leskinen M, Saarela T, Hallman M, et al. Follow-up study of the early, randomized paracetamol trial to preterm infant, found no adverse reactions at the two-years corrected age. *Acta Paediatr.* (2019) 108:452–8. doi: 10.1111/apa.14614
198. Kimani S, Surak A, Miller M, Bhattacharya S. Use of combination therapy with acetaminophen and ibuprofen for closure of patent ductus arteriosus in preterm neonates. *Pediatr Child Health.* (2020). doi: 10.1093/pch/pxaa057. [Epub ahead of print].
199. Yurttutan S, Bozkaya A, Hudayioglu F, Oncel MY. The effect of combined therapy for treatment of monotherapy-resistant PDA in preterm infants. *J Matern Neonatal Med.* (2018) 32:1–4. doi: 10.1080/14767058.2018.1481043
200. Paladini D, Marasini M, Volpe P. Severe ductal constriction in the third trimester fetus fflowing maternal self-medication with nimesulide. *Ultrasound Obstet Gynecol.* (2005) 25:357–61. doi: 10.1002/uog.1873
201. Fridman E, Mangel L, Mandel D, Beer G, Kapusta L, Marom R. Effects of maternal aspirin treatment on hemodynamically significant patent ductus arteriosus in preterm infants-pilot study. *J Matern Fetal Neonatal Med.* (2020). doi: 10.1080/14767058.2020.1736028. [Epub ahead of print].
202. Schiessl B, Schneider KT, Zimmermann A, Kainer F, Friese K, Oberhoffer R. Peranatal constriction of the fetal ductus arteriosus-related to maternal pain medication? *Z Geburtshilfe Neonatol.* (2005) 209:65–8. doi: 10.1055/s-2005-864116
203. Rein AJ, Nadjari M, Elchalal U, Nir A. Contraction of fetal ductus arteriosus induced by diclofenac. Case report. *Fetal Diagn Ther.* (1999) 14:24–5. doi: 10.1159/000020882
204. Levey R, Matitiau A, Ben Arie A, Milman D, Or Y, Hagay Z. Indomethacin and corticosteroids: an additive constrictive effect on the fetal ductus arteriosus. *Am J Perinatol.* (1999) 16:379–83. doi: 10.1055/s-1999-6814
205. Momma K, Mishihara S, Ota Y. Constriction of the fetal DA by glucocorticoid hormones. *Pediatr Res.* (1981) 15:19–21. doi: 10.1203/00006450-198101000-00005
206. Vermont Oxford Network Steroid Study Group. Early postnatal dexamethasone therapy for the prevention of chronic lung disease. *Pediatrics.* (2001) 108:741–8. doi: 10.1542/peds.108.3.741
207. Pagni E, Baragatti B, Scebba F, Coceani F. Functional closure of the DA at birth: evidence against an intermediary role of angiotensin II. *Pharmacology.* (2014) 93:120–5. doi: 10.1159/000358013
208. Zielinsky P, Piccoli AL, Langer Manica JJ, Nicoloso LHS. New insights on fetal ductal constriction: role of maternal ingestion of polyhenol-rich foods. *Expert Rev Cardiovas Ther.* (2010) 8:291–8. doi: 10.1586/erc.09.174
209. Kharade SV, Nichols C, Denton JS. The shifting landscape of K_{ATP} channelopathies and the need for sharper therapeutics. *Future Med Chem.* (2016) 8:789–802. doi: 10.4155/fmc-2016-0005
210. Toyoshima K, Momma K, Ishii T, Nakanishi T. Dilatation of the ductus arteriosus by diazoxide in fetal and neonatal rats. *Pediatr Int.* (2017) 59:1246–51. doi: 10.1111/ped.13424
211. Dzialowski EM. Comparative physiology of the ductus arteriosus among vertebrates. *Semin Perinatol.* (2018) 42:203–11. doi: 10.1053/j.semperi.2018.05.002
212. Sakuma T, Akaike T, Minamisawa S. Prostaglandin E2 receptor EP_4 inhibition contracts rat ductus arteriosus. *Circ J.* (2018) 83:209–16. doi: 10.1253/circj.CJ-18-0761
213. Takizawa T, Kihara T, Kamata A. Increased constriction of the ductus arteriosus with combined administration of indomethacin and L-NAME in fetal rats. *Biol Neonate.* (2001) 80:64–7. doi: 10.1159/000047122
214. Bevilacqua E, Brunelli R, Anceschi MM. Review and meta-analysis: benefits and risks of multiple courses of antenatal corticosteroids. *J Matern Fetal Neonatal Med.* (2010) 23:244–60. doi: 10.3109/14767050903165222
215. Travers CP, Carlo WA, McDonald S, Das A, Bell EF, Ambalavanan N, et al. Mortality and pulmonary outcomes of extremely preterm infants exposed to antenatal corticosteroids. *Am J Obstet Gynecol.* (2018) 218:130e1–13. doi: 10.1016/j.ajog.2017.11.554
216. Tsai MY, Brown DM. Effect of dexamethasone on fetal lung 15-hydroxyprostaglandin dehydrogenase: possible mechanism for the prevention of patent ductus arteriosus by maternal dexamethasone therapy. *Prostaglandins Leukot Med.* (1987) 27:237–45. doi: 10.1016/0262-1746(87)90074-6
217. del Moral T, Gonzalez-Quintero VH, Claure N, Vanbuskirk S, Bancalari E. Antenatal exposure to magnesium sulfate and the incidence of patent ductus arteriosus in extremely low birth weight infants. *J Perinatol.* (2007) 27:154–7. doi: 10.1038/sj.jp.7211663
218. Qasim A, Jain SK, Aly AM. Antenatal magnesium sulfate exposure and hemodynamically significant patent ductus arteriosus in premature infants. *AJP Rep.* (2019) 9:e353–6. doi: 10.1055/s-0039-3400316
219. Toyoshima K, Momma K, Nakanishi T. *In vivo* dilatation of the ductus arteriosus induced by furosemide in the rat. *Pediatr Res.* (2010) 67:173–6. doi: 10.1203/PDR.0b013e3181c2df30

20

Current Controversy on Platelets and Patent Ductus Arteriosus Closure in Preterm Infants

Hannes Sallmon [1,2], Natalie Timme [1], Begüm Atasay [3], Ömer Erdeve [3], Georg Hansmann [4], Yogen Singh [5,6], Sven C. Weber [1†] and Elaine L. Shelton [7,8†]*

[1] Department of Pediatric Cardiology, Charité University Medical Center, Berlin, Germany, [2] Department of Congenital Heart Disease/Pediatric Cardiology, Deutsches Herzzentrum Berlin (DHZB), Berlin, Germany, [3] Division of Neonatology, Department of Pediatrics, Ankara University School of Medicine, Ankara, Turkey, [4] Department of Pediatric Cardiology and Intensive Care Medicine, Medizinische Hochschule Hannover, Hanover, Germany, [5] Department of Neonatology and Pediatric Cardiology, Cambridge University Hospitals, Cambridge, United Kingdom, [6] University of Cambridge School of Clinical Medicine, Cambridge, United Kingdom, [7] Department of Pediatrics, Vanderbilt University Medical Center, Nashville, TN, United States, [8] Department of Pharmacology, Vanderbilt University Medical Center, Nashville, TN, United States

***Correspondence:**
Hannes Sallmon
hannes.sallmon@charite.de

†These authors have contributed equally to this work and share senior authorship

Platelets are critically involved in murine patent ductus arteriosus (PDA) closure. To date, the clinical significance of these findings in human preterm infants with PDA is still controversial. We discuss the available study data on the role of platelets for PDA closure in preterm infants: Several mostly retrospective studies have yielded conflicting results on whether thrombocytopenia contributes to failed spontaneous ductal closure. The same applies to investigations on the role of thrombocytopenia as a risk factor for unsuccessful ductus arteriosus closure by pharmacological treatment with cyclooxygenase inhibitors. Nonetheless, recent meta-analyses have concluded that thrombocytopenia constitutes an independent risk factor for both failed spontaneous and pharmacological PDA closure in preterm infants. However, the available investigations differ in regard to patient characteristics, diagnostic strategies, and treatment protocols. Several studies suggest that impaired platelet function rather than platelet number is critically involved in failure of ductus arteriosus closure in the preterm infant. A recent randomized-controlled trial on platelet transfusions in preterm infants with PDA failed to show any benefit for liberal vs. restrictive transfusion thresholds on PDA closure rates. Importantly, liberal transfusions were associated with an increased rate of intraventricular hemorrhage, and thus should be avoided. In conclusion, the available evidence suggests that thrombocytopenia and platelet dysfunction contribute to failure of spontaneous and pharmacological PDA closure in preterm infants. However, these platelet effects on PDA seem to be of only moderate clinical significance. Furthermore, platelet transfusions in thrombocytopenic preterm infants in order to facilitate PDA closure appear to cause more harm than good.

Keywords: platelets, thrombocytopenia, very low birth weight, patent ductus arteriosus, hemodynamics

INTRODUCTION

After birth, a persistently patent ductus arteriosus (PDA) is usually associated with left-to-right shunt; and subsequently, variable degrees of pulmonary overcirculation, systemic hypotension, and malperfusion (1). In preterm infants, the consequences of a hemodynamically significant PDA (hsPDA) are frequently associated with several severe cardiopulmonary complications such as left ventricular volume overload, pulmonary edema, impairment of lung compliance, and abdominal-renal malperfusion due to the ductal steal (1–3). Thus, understanding the mechanisms that contribute to ductus arteriosus (DA) closure is of pivotal importance in order to provide tailored care to at-risk neonates (4, 5).

In 2010, Echtler et al. (6) reported that platelets contribute to ductal closure and subsequent vascular remodeling in mice. By means of intravital microscopy, they showed that platelets are recruited to the luminal aspect of the ductal endothelium within minutes after birth and that formation of a platelet-plug within the DA contributes to ductal remodeling. In addition, by using two murine models of genetic disruption of platelet biogenesis and function ($Nfe^{-/-}$ and $Itga2b^{-/-}$ mice), the authors demonstrated that platelet dysfunction was associated with hsPDA (as assessed by a quantification of pulmonary blood flow using radiolabeled microspheres). Similar results were observed when an antibody directed against platelet collagen receptor GPVI was administered, thus indicating that both GPVI and GPIIb/IIIa contribute to platelet-triggered DA closure. In addition, the authors showed that administration of cyclooxygenase inhibitors (ibuprofen or indomethacin) was not sufficient to compensate for impaired platelet function in their murine model (6). Of note, mouse ductuses are remarkably similar to human ductuses, but they lack prominent intimal cushions, which protrude into the vessel lumen and contribute to vessel closure and permanent remodeling. Therefore, platelets may play a larger role in mouse vs. human duct occlusion due to the lack of intimal cushions.

Taken together, the experimental results above suggest that platelets play a pivotal role in ductus arteriosus closure. However, the clinical significance of these findings in human preterm infants is still controversial and has not been confirmed *in vivo* (7). Here, we discuss the available data on the current controversy on platelets and PDA and their clinical implications in preterm infants.

THE EFFECTS OF THROMBOCYTOPENIA AND PLATELET TRANSFUSIONS ON SPONTANEOUS AND PHARMACOLOGICAL DUCTUS ARTERIOSUS CLOSURE

Low platelet counts are frequently observed among preterm infants (8, 9) and the role of platelets in spontaneous or pharmacological PDA closure has been explored by several groups yielding conflicting results. In addition to their animal results, Echtler et al. (6) also reported on a small cohort of 123 preterm infants, in which low platelet counts within the first 24 h after birth were associated with a higher incidence of PDA. However, another small study ($n = 211$) failed to confirm these results in a Japanese cohort of preterm infants (10). Similarly, Shah et al. could not find any association between low platelet counts during the 1st week of life and incidence of PDA, but they observed a decreased incidence of PDA when platelet counts were consistently > 230/nL. Of note, all infants in this study received prophylactic indomethacin within the first 15 h of life (11). Consistently, two other studies did not confirm any significant associations between thrombocytopenia and a higher incidence of PDA/hsPDA or later PDA treatment failure (12, 13). In contrast, data from several other investigators suggest that thrombocytopenia within the 1st week of life did contribute to prolonged ductal patency (14–17) and a meta-analysis from 2015, which included 11 cohort studies involving 3,479 infants, concluded that low platelet counts within the 1st day(s) of life were marginally but significantly associated with PDA/hsPDA (18).

In terms of platelets and pharmacological DA closure, several authors reported that low platelet counts within the 1st day(s) of life were not predictive of later pharmacological treatment failure in infants with hsPDA (14, 15, 19, 20). However, recent studies have yielded conflicting results on whether a positive association between higher platelet counts just before or during cyclooxygenase inhibitor therapy and PDA closure rates exists. For example, while platelet counts before pharmacological therapy were not predictive of PDA treatment success rates, low platelet counts during pharmacological treatment were associated with an increased rate of treatment failure in a cohort of 471 preterm infants. In this study, only infants with hsPDA on day of life 3–5 received cyclooxygenase inhibitor treatment (hemodynamically significant if (i) a respiratory setback with a supplemental oxygen requirement >30% and/or mechanical ventilation, (ii) a LA/Ao ratio ≥1.4 in the echocardiogram and/or (iii) ductal diameter ≥2.5 mm, and/or (iv) a decreased end-diastolic flow in the anterior cerebral artery with a resistance index ≥0.85) (21). In addition, two reports on indomethacin found that higher platelet counts just before treatment initiation were associated with higher success rates (22, 23), while others were unable to demonstrate such an association (24, 25). Nonetheless, similar to the results obtained for spontaneous ductal closure (18), a recent meta-analysis (eight studies including 1,087 infants) revealed a moderate but significant association between pretreatment thrombocytopenia and failure of pharmacological PDA closure (26). Of note, cyclooxygenase inhibitors are known to adversely affect platelet plug formation in adults. The few available data from preterm infants suggest that inhibition of platelet plug formation in neonates may occur, but seem to be of limited clinical significance under cyclooxygenase inhibitor treatment (27). However, one might speculate that even moderate alterations in platelet function may become relevant in severely thrombocytopenic infants.

Taken together, the combined evidence suggests the existence of a moderate but detectable impact of platelets on both spontaneous and pharmacological PDA closure in preterm infants. However, it should be noted, that most studies were retrospective in nature, and thus, even the positive studies cannot conclude on any causality as relevant confounding factors might have been missed by the analyses. In addition, the remarkable heterogeneity in study design (selection criteria, genetic background, and timing of platelet counts), diagnostic protocols (timing of echocardiography and criteria used to define hemodynamic significance), and differences in treatment approaches (timing, dosage, and application route) may have influenced the comparability of the available studies (18, 26, 28).

A recent randomized-controlled trial on platelet transfusions addressed the clinical implications of the aforementioned associations between low platelet counts and failure of hsPDA closure in preterm infants (<35 weeks of gestational age) (29). The authors compared liberal platelet-transfusion criteria (platelet counts were maintained >100,000 /μL) vs. restrictive criteria (platelet count < 20,000/μL, clinical bleed, platelet count < 50,000/μL and requiring a major non-neurosurgical procedure, or platelet count < 100,000/μL and requiring a neurosurgical procedure), and the impact of either approach on hsPDA closure ($n = 22$ in each group). All subjects received standard co-treatment with nonsteroidal anti-inflammatory drugs. There was no significant difference in the time required to achieve PDA closure (median of 72 h in both groups, $p = 0.697$). However, 41% of all infants in the liberal transfusion group were found to develop intraventricular hemorrhage (IVH, any grade), while IVH was only seen in 4.5% of the infants allocated to the restrictive transfusion group ($p = 0.009$) (29). Potential mechanisms that might contribute to the increased rate of IVH in liberally transfused infants include hemodynamic alterations due to volume challenge by transfusions and a possible modification of periventricular capillary function by transfused platelets.

PLATELET INDICES AND PDA

Considering the contradictory results on platelet counts and their possible associations with PDA incidence and treatment success, several experts have speculated that platelet indices such as mean platelet volume (MPV), platelet distribution width (PDW), or platelet mass (calculated by multiplying platelet count by MPV) may be more useful in predicting PDA and/or treatment response. Alyamac Dizdar et al. (14) reported that high PDW values within the first 3 days of life were associated with PDA. Similar to Dani et al. (15) they did not find any association between MPV and PDA incidence or treatment response. Another group reported consistently higher PDW values in infants with hsPDA within the first 24 h after birth, but did not find any association between MPV, platelet mass, or platelet counts and hsPDA, respectively (20). However, such an association between higher platelet mass and MPV and hsPDA closure has been reported by others (30). Another group from Turkey did not find any relationship between platelet counts, MPV, or platelet mass and successful hsPDA closure by ibuprofen (19). In addition to MPV, PDW, and platelet mass, other hematologic indices, such as red cell distribution width-to-platelet ratio (RPR) and platelet-to-lymphocyte-ratio (PLR) have been proposed as markers for hsPDA and treatment response (31–33).

In summary, the aforementioned studies (and recent meta-analyses) on platelet indices and PDA have revealed inconsistent or even conflicting results, which were probably, at least in part, due to differences in study designs, treatment protocols, and the definition of hsPDA (28, 34). Furthermore, hematologic indices might be affected by several conditions, such as inflammation, hypoxia and/or volume status, and thus likely represent surrogate markers of neonatal well-being rather than being specific indicators of PDA/hsPDA, e.g., higher PDW values are thought to reflect altered platelet function/activation (35).

PLATELET FUNCTION AND PDA CLOSURE IN PRETERM INFANTS

Previous studies investigating the role of thrombocytopenia in spontaneous or pharmacological ductus arteriosus closure have provided controversial results. However, several investigations have consistently identified sepsis/inflammation, lower gestational age, and feto-maternal conditions such as preeclampsia as risk factors for failure of DA closure in preterm infants. Since all these factors are associated with altered platelet function, it has been speculated that platelet function, rather than platelet number, is the key determinant of PDA closure in neonates (36, 37). A significant association between lower platelet count, higher CRP level and incidence of PDA has been demonstrated, with CRP being the only independent predictive factor for PDA in a regression model (38). These findings support the theory of a combined effect of one common cause (e.g., sepsis) on both platelet number and function and failure of DA closure. A proteomics-based study on human neonatal plasma identified six differentially expressed proteins (platelet factor 4, fibrinogen, von Willebrand factor, collagen, mannose binding lectin-associated serine protease-2, fibronectin), which were associated with PDA. Interestingly, those proteins are closely related to platelet activation and plasmatic coagulation cascades (39).

Recent observational studies have also confirmed a relationship between altered platelet function and failure of DA closure in human preterm infants. Collagen-ADP closure times > 130 s (PFA-100) are more frequently observed in infants with PDA as compared to those without PDA, and longer collagen-ADP closure times represent an independent risk factor for ductal patency (40). In addition, lower median levels of platelet-derived growth factor (PDGF) were found in those infants who later required pharmacological PDA therapy vs. those who did not require such treatment (41). The same group of authors also proposed the usage of platelet-rich plasma in preterm infants with PDA as an experimental approach for PDA treatment (42–44). Recently, other investigators found lower PDGF levels in very immature infants (22–27 weeks) with failure of spontaneous DA closure (45). In addition, Ghirardello et al. (46) assessed thromboelastography at birth in VLBW infants with PDA ($n = 151$). In their study, thromboelastography at birth did not predict persistence of PDA. However, infants who failed

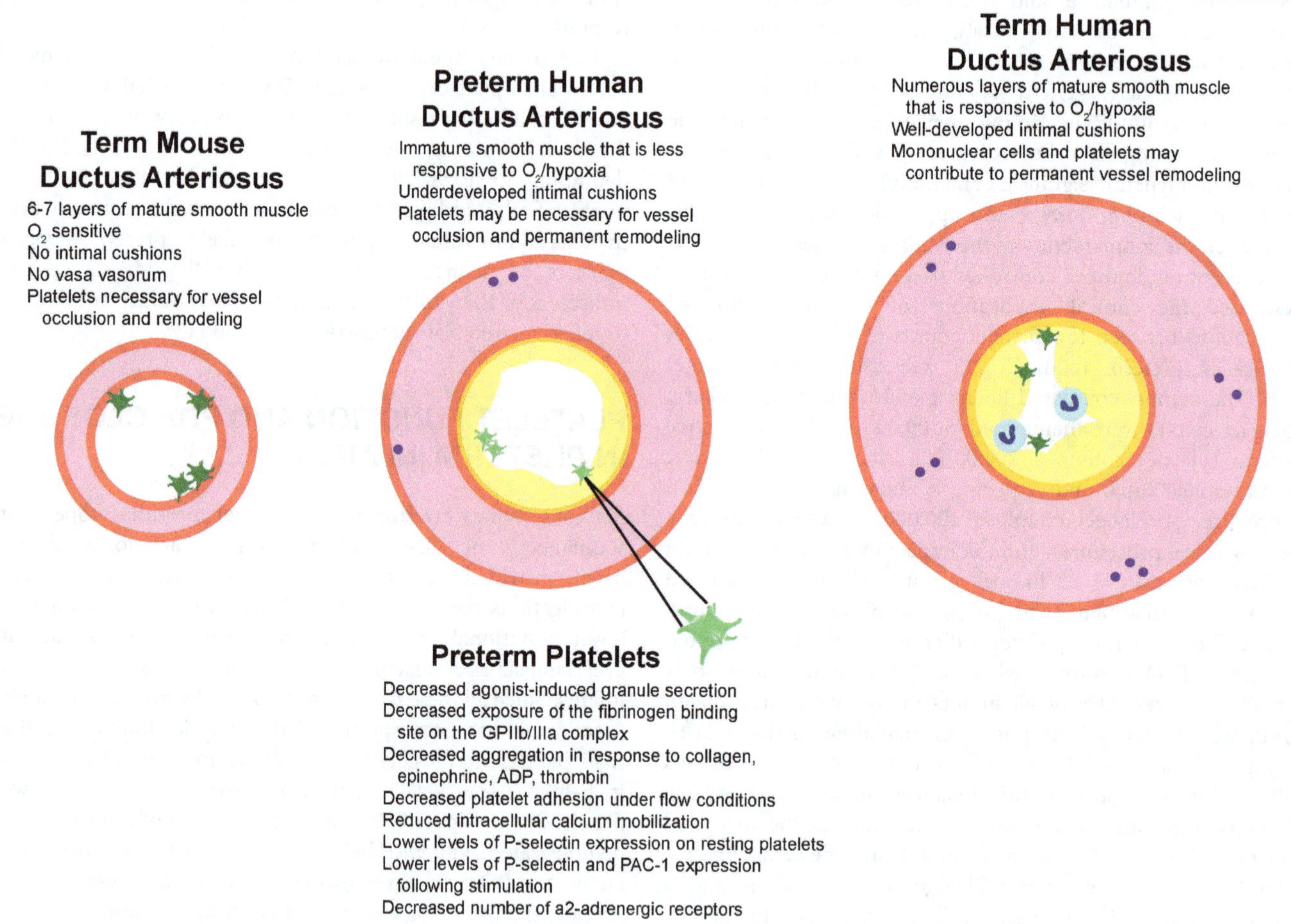

FIGURE 1 | Structural factors that play a role in ductus arteriosus closure. Illustrated are the structural features known to regulate ductus closure in mice, preterm infants, and term-gestation infants. Mice have mature smooth muscle cells (pink) that constrict robustly in response to oxygen but lack intimal cushions (yellow), which may explain why platelets (green) are required for vessel occlusion and remodeling. Term-gestation infants have a thick medial layer composed of mature smooth muscle cells that are very sensitive to oxygen-induced constriction. They also have prominent vasa vasorum (purple circles) which results in local ischemic areas and hypoxic signaling during closure. A platelet plug and mononuclear cells (blue circles) adhere to the lumen during closure and promote formation of a permanent seal and remodeling. In contrast, several structural factors contribute to failed ductal closure in preterm infants. The preterm ductus has an underdeveloped media containing immature smooth muscle cells and less vasa vasorum, making it less sensitive to oxygen/hypoxia signaling. Preterm vessels also lack prominent intimal cushions and have preterm platelets. Characteristics of preterm human platelets that are associated with an enhanced vulnerability to dysfunction, which in turn might contribute to higher rates of ductal patency in immature preterm infants are also listed. ADP, adenosine di-phosphate; GPIIb/IIIa, glycoprotein IIb/IIIa; PAC-1, procaspase activating compound 1 which detects activated GPIIb/IIIa.

medical treatment exhibited signs of an enhanced fibrinolysis (46). While the exact mechanisms and the clinical consequences of these findings are yet to be examined, they further indicate a role of the neonatal coagulation system in ductal closure.

It should be noted that the hemostatic system and especially platelet function in infants differ from that of adults—a fact that needs to be taken into account when designing future studies on the impact of platelet function on neonatal diseases such as PDA (47, 48). Despite developmental "defects" in platelet function, healthy full-term infants show a more effective primary hemostasis than healthy adults in whole blood tests of primary hemostasis such as bleeding time and PFA-100 (49). This has been attributed to several factors, including high levels of large von Willebrand factor (vWF) multimers, high hematocrit, and high mean corpuscular volume (MCV) values, which compensate for the impaired platelet function in newborns (47, 49).

Platelet function may play an even larger role in closure of the preterm ductus, given that preterm vessels are often structurally underdeveloped (lack fully-formed intimal cushions) and less responsive to oxygen-induced vasoconstriction. However, in preterm infants below 30 weeks of gestational age platelet function is further impaired when compared to full-term infants (**Figure 1**). For example, preterm platelets show a decreased number of α2-adrenergic receptors, decreased calcium mobilization, and impaired signal transduction causing a decreased agonist-induced granule secretion and exposure of the fibrinogen binding site on the GPIIb/IIIa complex (49). More immature preterm infants also exhibit lower levels of P-selectin expression on resting platelets (50) and lower levels of P-selectin and PAC-1 following stimulation with platelet agonists (49). They also show decreased platelet adhesion and aggregation in response to platelet agonists such as collagen, epinephrine, ADP, and thrombin and longer bleeding and closure times by PFA-100 (49, 51, 52). Similar results on the developmental maturation of platelet function have recently been reported in murine fetuses. Interestingly, these investigators reported rapid platelet aggregate formation when adult platelets where transfused into the fetal circulation. However, in line with the later prospective trial by Kumar et al. (29), a retrospective analysis on the effect of platelet transfusions on PDA closure rates in preterm infants failed to demonstrate any influence of transfusions on ductal closure (53).

In addition to developmental differences in platelet function between preterm infants, term infants and adults, it is known that newly released platelets (immature platelets) differ in their functional properties as compared to older, more mature platelets (54). It has recently been shown that a lower number of mature platelets during the latter half of the 1st week of life was associated with PDA in preterm infants, while immature platelets were not independently associated with PDA (55). Importantly, a mathematical model of platelet turnover in preterm infants demonstrated significantly shorter population survival values for immature platelets and shorter platelet life spans in thrombocytopenic vs. non-thrombocytopenic neonates, indicating a preferential depletion of older, more mature platelets in thrombocytopenic infants (56).

Of note, the interaction of platelets with other circulating and tissue resident blood cells has been studied in common cardiovascular diseases such as atherosclerosis, but not in human PDA. For example, platelet–neutrophil complexes (PNCs) are increased in patients with acute myocardial infarction, in association with increased levels of neuronal guidance protein semaphorin 7A (57). Mononuclear cells contribute to ductal closure (58, 59), but their direct or paracrine interaction with platelets and other circulating blood cells in human PDA is still unclear. Likewise, red blood cells affect bleeding and thrombosis, and interact with cellular and molecular components of the hemostatic system; however, platelet-erythrocyte interactions have not been investigated in preterm infants with PDA (60).

CONCLUSIONS

The identification of platelets as contributors to ductal closure in neonates represents a conceptual breakthrough in developmental vascular medicine. Developmentally regulated platelet-endothelial interactions contribute to normal cardiovascular transition from fetal to postnatal life (6, 7, 36). In addition, thrombocytopenia and impaired platelet function seem to impact spontaneous and pharmacological PDA closure in preterm infants, linking platelets to a specific neonatal cardiovascular disease. While the clinical implications of these findings are still controversial, during the last decade, they have stipulated further research efforts on the specific developmental differences between neonatal and adult megakaryopoiesis, platelet formation and function, and their respective roles in neonatal health and disease (61). For example, the role of platelets in retinopathy of prematurity has been recently elucidated by several investigators (62–64).

In light of the recently observed practice changes toward a less frequent and less proactive treatment approach to managing preterm PDA, clinicians still face the difficult questions on how to decide which infants will benefit from PDA closure; and on when and how PDA closure should be attempted or facilitated [(1, 2, 4)—please also refer to other articles in this special issue]. Despite the experimental and epidemiologic evidence for an association between platelets and ductal closure, current clinical evidence strongly suggests, that platelet transfusions for facilitating PDA closure in preterm thrombocytopenic infants cause more harm than good (29, 65).

Thus, further research is required to elucidate the complex interplay between PDA, shunt, circulating blood cells, including platelets, and adverse outcomes of PDA in order to define accurate biomarkers and the optimal therapeutic strategies for this still elusive condition in the most vulnerable population of preterm infants (1, 66).

AUTHOR CONTRIBUTIONS

HS, NT, SW, and ES drafted the manuscript and prepared display items. All other authors reviewed and critically revised the manuscript. All authors contributed to the article and approved the final version as submitted.

REFERENCES

1. Hamrick SEG, Sallmon H, Rose AT, Porras D, Shelton EL, Reese J, et al. Patent ductus arteriosus of the preterm infant. *Pediatrics.* (2020) 146:e20201209. doi: 10.1542/peds.2020-1209
2. Sallmon H, Koehne P, Hansmann G. Recent advances in the treatment of preterm newborn infants with patent ductus arteriosus. *Clin Perinatol.* (2016) 43:113–29. doi: 10.1016/j.clp.2015.11.008
3. Smith A, El-Khuffash AF. Defining "haemodynamic significance" of the patent ductus arteriosus: do we have all the answers? *Neonatology.* (2020) 117:225–32. doi: 10.1159/000506988
4. Crockett SL, Berger CD, Shelton EL, Reese J. Molecular and mechanical factors contributing to ductus arteriosus patency and closure. *Congenit Heart Dis.* (2019) 14:15–20. doi: 10.1111/chd.12714
5. Mitra S, McNamara PJ. Patent ductus arteriosus-time for a definitive trial. *Clin Perinatol.* (2020) 47:617–39. doi: 10.1016/j.clp.2020.05.007
6. Echtler K, Stark K, Lorenz M, Kerstan S, Walch A, Jennen L, et al. Platelets contribute to postnatal occlusion of the ductus arteriosus. *Nat Med.* (2010) 16:75–82. doi: 10.1038/nm.2060
7. Clyman R, Chemtob S. Vessel remodeling in the newborn: platelets fill the gap. *Nat Med.* (2010) 16:33–5. doi: 10.1038/nm0110-33
8. Sallmon H, Sola-Visner M. Clinical and research issues in neonatal anemia and thrombocytopenia. *Curr Opin Pediatr.* (2012) 24:16–22. doi: 10.1097/MOP.0b013e32834ee5cc

9. Cremer M, Sallmon H, Kling PJ, Buhrer C, Dame C. Thrombocytopenia and platelet transfusion in the neonate. *Semin Fetal Neonatal Med.* (2016) 21:10–8. doi: 10.1016/j.siny.2015.11.001
10. Fujioka K, Morioka I, Miwa A, Morikawa S, Shibata A, Yokoyama N, et al. Does thrombocytopenia contribute to patent ductus arteriosus? *Nat Med.* (2011) 17:29–30; author reply −1. doi: 10.1038/nm0111-29
11. Shah NA, Hills NK, Waleh N, McCurnin D, Seidner S, Chemtob S, et al. Relationship between circulating platelet counts and ductus arteriosus patency after indomethacin treatment. *J Pediatr.* (2011) 158:919–23.e1–2. doi: 10.1016/j.jpeds.2010.11.018
12. Sallmon H, Weber SC, Huning B, Stein A, Horn PA, Metze BC, et al. Thrombocytopenia in the first 24 hours after birth and incidence of patent ductus arteriosus. *Pediatrics.* (2012) 130:e623–30. doi: 10.1542/peds.2012-0499
13. Bas-Suarez MP, Gonzalez-Luis GE, Saavedra P, Villamor E. Platelet counts in the first seven days of life and patent ductus arteriosus in preterm very low-birth-weight infants. *Neonatology.* (2014) 106:188–94. doi: 10.1159/000362432
14. Alyamac Dizdar E, Ozdemir R, Sari FN, Yurttutan S, Gokmen T, Erdeve O, et al. Low platelet count is associated with ductus arteriosus patency in preterm newborns. *Early Hum Dev.* (2012) 88:813–6. doi: 10.1016/j.earlhumdev.2012.05.007
15. Dani C, Poggi C, Fontanelli G. Relationship between platelet count and volume and spontaneous and pharmacological closure of ductus arteriosus in preterm infants. *Am J Perinatol.* (2013) 30:359–64. doi: 10.1055/s-0032-1324702
16. Kulkarni VV, Dutta S, Sundaram V, Saini SS. Preterm thrombocytopenia and delay of ductus arteriosus closure. *Pediatrics.* (2016) 138:e20161627. doi: 10.1542/peds.2016-1627
17. Brunner B, Hoeck M, Schermer E, Streif W, Kiechl-Kohlendorfer U. Patent ductus arteriosus, low platelets, cyclooxygenase inhibitors, and intraventricular hemorrhage in very low birth weight preterm infants. *Pediatr.* (2013) 163:23–8. doi: 10.1016/j.jpeds.2012.12.035
18. Simon SR, van Zogchel L, Bas-Suarez MP, Cavallaro G, Clyman RI, Villamor E. Platelet counts and patent ductus arteriosus in preterm infants: a systematic review and meta-analysis. *Neonatology.* (2015) 108:143–51. doi: 10.1159/000431281
19. Akar S, Karadag N, Gokmen Yildirim T, Toptan HH, Dincer E, Tuten A, et al. Does platelet mass influence the effectiveness of ibuprofen treatment for patent ductus arteriosus in preterm infants? *J Matern Fetal Neonatal Med.* (2016) 29:3786–9. doi: 10.3109/14767058.2016.1145207
20. Demirel G, Yilmaz A, Vatansever B, Tastekin A. Is high platelet distribution width in the first hours of life can predict hemodynamically significant patent ductus arteriosus in preterm newborns? *J Matern Fetal Neonatal Med.* (2020) 33:2049–53. doi: 10.1080/14767058.2018.1536743
21. Sallmon H, Weber SC, Dirks J, Schiffer T, Klippstein T, Stein A, et al. Association between platelet counts before and during pharmacological therapy for patent ductus arteriosus and treatment failure in preterm infants. *Front Pediatr.* (2018) 6:41. doi: 10.3389/fped.2018.00041
22. Boo NY, Mohd-Amin I, Bilkis AA, Yong-Junina F. Predictors of failed closure of patent ductus arteriosus with indomethacin. *Singapore Med J.* (2006) 47:763–8.
23. Ahamed MF, Verma P, Lee S, Vega M, Wang D, Kim M, et al. Predictors of successful closure of patent ductus arteriosus with indomethacin. *J Perinatol.* (2015) 35:729–34. doi: 10.1038/jp.2015.33
24. Mitra S, Wahab MG. Indomethacin dose-interruption and maternal chorioamnionitis are risk factors for indomethacin treatment failure in preterm infants with patent ductus arteriosus. *J Clin Neonatol.* (2015) 4:250–5.
25. Murphy DP, Lee HC, Payton KS, Powers RJ. Platelet count and associated morbidities in VLBW infants with pharmacologically treated patent ductus arteriosus. *J Matern Fetal Neonatal Med.* (2016) 29:2045–8. doi: 10.3109/14767058.2015.1076785
26. Mitra S, Chan AK, Paes BA, Thrombosis, Hemostasis in Newborns G. The association of platelets with failed patent ductus arteriosus closure after a primary course of indomethacin or ibuprofen: a systematic review and meta-analysis. *J Matern Fetal Neonatal Med.* (2017) 30:127–33. doi: 10.3109/14767058.2016.1163684
27. Schmutz N, Lambert DK, Henry E, Christensen RD. Ibuprofen lysine administration to neonates with a patent ductus arteriosus: effect on platelet plug formation assessed by *in vivo* and *in vitro* measurements. *J Perinatol.* (2009) 29:39–43. doi: 10.1038/jp.2008.122
28. González-Luis G, Ghirardello S, Bas-Suárez P, Cavallaro G, Mosca F, Clyman RI, et al. Platelet counts and patent ductus arteriosus in preterm infants: an updated systematic review and meta-analysis. *Front Pediatr.* (2021) 8:613766. doi: 10.3389/fped.2020.613766
29. Kumar J, Dutta S, Sundaram V, Saini SS, Sharma RR, Varma N. Platelet transfusion for PDA closure in preterm infants: a randomized controlled trial. *Pediatrics.* (2019) 143:e20182565. doi: 10.1542/peds.2018-2565
30. Demir N, Peker E, Ece I, Agengin K, Bulan KA, Tuncer O. Is platelet mass a more significant indicator than platelet count of closure of patent ductus arteriosus? *J Matern Fetal Neonatal Med.* (2016) 29:1915–8. doi: 10.3109/14767058.2015.1067296
31. Karabulut B, Arcagok BC, Simsek A. Utility of the platelet-to-lymphocyte ratio in diagnosing and predicting treatment success in preterm neonates with patent ductus arteriosus. *Fetal Pediatr Pathol.* (2019). doi: 10.1080/15513815.2019.1686786. [Epub ahead of print].
32. Ozer Bekmez B, Tayman C, Buyuktiryaki M, Cetinkaya AK, Cakir U, Derme T. A promising, novel index in the diagnosis and follow-up of patent ductus arteriosus: red cell distribution width-to-platelet ratio. *J Clin Lab Anal.* (2018) 32:e22616. doi: 10.1002/jcla.22616
33. Guler Kazanci E, Buyuktiryaki M, Unsal H, Tayman C. Useful platelet indices for the diagnosis and follow-up of patent ductus arteriosus. *Am J Perinatol.* (2019) 36:1521–7. doi: 10.1055/s-0039-1688821
34. Ding R, Zhang Q, Duan Y, Wang D, Sun Q, Shan R. The relationship between platelet indices and patent ductus arteriosus in preterm infants: a systematic review and meta-analysis. *Eur J Pediatr.* (2020). doi: 10.1007/s00431-020-03802-5. [Epub ahead of print].
35. Budzianowski J, Pieszko K, Burchardt P, Rzezniczak J, Hiczkiewicz J. The role of hematological indices in patients with acute coronary syndrome. *Dis Markers.* (2017) 2017:3041565. doi: 10.1155/2017/3041565
36. Sallmon H, Weber SC, von Gise A, Koehne P, Hansmann G. Ductal closure in neonates: a developmental perspective on platelet-endothelial interactions. *Blood Coagul Fibrinolysis.* (2011) 22:242–4. doi: 10.1097/MBC.0b013e328344c5ed
37. Engur D. Regarding platelets and ductus: is it platelet function rather than number that matters for ductal closure? *Pediatr Neonatol.* (2018) 59:640–1. doi: 10.1016/j.pedneo.2018.08.006
38. Meinarde L, Hillman M, Rizzotti A, Basquiera AL, Tabares A, Cuestas E. C-reactive protein, platelets, and patent ductus arteriosus. *Platelets.* (2016) 27:821–3. doi: 10.1080/09537104.2016.1203398
39. Hou HT, Xi Z, Wang J, Liu LX, Zhang JF, Yang Q, et al. Altered plasma proteins released from platelets and endothelial cells are associated with human patent ductus arteriosus. *J Cell Physiol.* (2019) 234:6842–53. doi: 10.1002/jcp.27433
40. Kahvecioglu D, Erdeve O, Akduman H, Ucar T, Alan S, Cakir U, et al. Influence of platelet count, platelet mass index, and platelet function on the spontaneous closure of ductus arteriosus in the prematurity. *Pediatr Neonatol.* (2018) 59:53–7. doi: 10.1016/j.pedneo.2017.01.006
41. Engur D, Kaynak-Turkmen M, Deveci M, Yenisey C. Platelets and platelet-derived growth factor in closure of the ductus arteriosus. *Turk J Pediatr.* (2015) 57:242–7.
42. Ali Engur M, Engur D. Platelet-rich plasma for patent ductus arteriosus: an orthopaedic surgeon's perspective. *Cardiol Young.* (2014) 24:385–7. doi: 10.1017/S1047951114000146
43. Sallmon H, Barikbin P, Koehne P, von Gise A, Hansmann G. Platelet-rich plasma for the treatment of patent ductus arteriosus: not quite ready for prime time. *Cardiol Young.* (2015) 25:139–40. doi: 10.1017/S1047951114001516
44. Engür D, Engür MA. Response to commentary: platelet-rich plasma for patent ductus arteriosus in the era of organ-targeted therapy, author reply. *Cardiol Young.* (2015) 25:141–2. doi: 10.1017/S1047951114001784
45. Olsson KW, Larsson A, Jonzon A, Sindelar R. Exploration of potential biochemical markers for persistence of patent ductus arteriosus in preterm infants at 22-27 weeks' gestation. *Pediatr Res.* (2019) 86:333–8. doi: 10.1038/s41390-018-0182-x
46. Ghirardello S, Raffaeli G, Crippa BL, Gulden S, Amodeo I, Consonni D, et al. The thromboelastographic profile at birth in very preterm

newborns with patent ductus arteriosus. *Neonatology.* (2020) 117:316–23. doi: 10.1159/000507553
47. Sitaru AG, Holzhauer S, Speer CP, Singer D, Obergfell A, Walter U, et al. Neonatal platelets from cord blood and peripheral blood. *Platelets.* (2005) 16:203–10. doi: 10.1080/09537100400016862
48. Haley KM, Recht M, McCarty OJ. Neonatal platelets: mediators of primary hemostasis in the developing hemostatic system. *Pediatr Res.* (2014) 76:230–7. doi: 10.1038/pr.2014.87
49. Israels SJ, Rand ML, Michelson AD. Neonatal platelet function. *Semin Thromb Hemost.* (2003) 29:363–72. doi: 10.1055/s-2003-42587
50. Wasiluk A, Mantur M, Szczepanski M, Kemona H, Baran E, Kemona-Chetnik I. The effect of gestational age on platelet surface expression of CD62P in preterm newborns. *Platelets.* (2008) 19:236–8. doi: 10.1080/09537100701882046
51. Linder N, Shenkman B, Levin E, Sirota L, Vishne TH, Tamarin I, et al. Deposition of whole blood platelets on extracellular matrix under flow conditions in preterm infants. *Arch Dis Child Fetal Neonatal Ed.* (2002) 86:F127–30. doi: 10.1136/fn.86.2.F127
52. Saxonhouse MA, Garner R, Mammel L, Li Q, Muller KE, Greywoode J, et al. Closure times measured by the platelet function analyzer PFA-100 are longer in neonatal blood compared to cord blood samples. *Neonatology.* (2010) 97:242–9. doi: 10.1159/000253755
53. Margraf A, Nussbaum C, Rohwedder I, Klapproth S, Kurz ARM, Florian A, et al. Maturation of platelet function during murine fetal development *in vivo*. *Arterioscler Thromb Vasc Biol.* (2017) 37:1076–86. doi: 10.1161/ATVBAHA.116.308464
54. Lador A, Leshem-Lev D, Spectre G, Abelow A, Kornowski R, Lev EI. Characterization of surface antigens of reticulated immature platelets. *J Thromb Thrombolysis.* (2017) 44:291–7. doi: 10.1007/s11239-017-1533-x
55. Sallmon H, Metze B, Koehne P, Opgen-Rhein B, Weiss K, Will JC, et al. Mature and immature platelets during the first week after birth and incidence of patent ductus arteriosus. *Cardiol Young.* (2020) 30:769–73. doi: 10.1017/S1047951120000943
56. Kulshrestha M, Sola-Visner M, Widness JA, Veng-Pedersen P, Mager DE. Mathematical model of platelet turnover in thrombocytopenic and nonthrombocytopenic preterm neonates. *Am J Physiol Heart Circ Physiol.* (2015) 308:H68–73. doi: 10.1152/ajpheart.00528.2013
57. Köhler D, Granja T, Volz J, Koeppen M, Langer HF, Hansmann G, et al. Red blood cell-derived semaphorin 7A promotes thrombo-inflammation in myocardial ischemia-reperfusion injury through platelet GPIb. *Nat Commun.* (2020) 11:1315. doi: 10.1038/s41467-020-14958-x
58. Waleh N, Seidner S, McCurnin D, Yoder B, Liu BM, Roman C, et al. The role of monocyte-derived cells and inflammation in baboon ductus arteriosus remodeling. *Pediatr Res.* (2005) 57:254–62. doi: 10.1203/01.PDR.0000148278.64777.EF
59. Waleh N, Seidner S, McCurnin D, Giavedoni L, Hodara V, Goelz S, et al. Anatomic closure of the premature patent ductus arteriosus: the role of CD14+/CD163+ mononuclear cells and VEGF in neointimal mound formation. *Pediatr Res.* (2011) 70:332–8. doi: 10.1203/PDR.0b013e3182294471
60. Weisel JW, Litvinov RI. Red blood cells: the forgotten player in hemostasis and thrombosis. *J Thromb Haemost.* (2019) 17:271–82. doi: 10.1111/jth.14360
61. Davenport P, Liu ZJ, Sola-Visner M. Changes in megakaryopoiesis over ontogeny and their implications in health and disease. *Platelets.* (2020) 31:692–9. doi: 10.1080/09537104.2020.1742879
62. Cakir B, Liegl R, Hellgren G, Lundgren P, Sun Y, Klevebro S, et al. Thrombocytopenia is associated with severe retinopathy of prematurity. *JCI Insight.* (2018) 3:e99448. doi: 10.1172/jci.insight.99448
63. Lundgren P, Lundberg L, Hellgren G, Holmstrom G, Hard AL, Smith LE, et al. Aggressive posterior retinopathy of prematurity is associated with multiple infectious episodes and thrombocytopenia. *Neonatology.* (2017) 111:79–85. doi: 10.1159/000448161
64. Jensen AK, Ying GS, Huang J, Quinn GE, Binenbaum G. Longitudinal study of the association between thrombocytopenia and retinopathy of prematurity. *J AAPOS.* (2018) 22:119–23. doi: 10.1016/j.jaapos.2017.11.009
65. Sola-Visner MC. Platelet transfusions in neonates - less is more. *N Engl J Med.* (2019) 380:287–8. doi: 10.1056/NEJMe1813419
66. Gillam-Krakauer M, Hagadorn JI, Reese J. Pharmacological closure of the patent ductus arteriosus: when treatment still makes sense. *J Perinatol.* (2019) 39:1439–41. doi: 10.1038/s41372-019-0518-3

21

Voice and Exercise Related Respiratory Symptoms in Extremely Preterm Born Children After Neonatal Patent Ductus Arteriosus

Merete S. Engeseth [1,2*], *Mette Engan* [2,3], *Hege Clemm* [2,3], *Maria Vollsæter* [2,3], *Roy M. Nilsen* [1], *Trond Markestad* [2], *Thomas Halvorsen* [2,3] and *Ola D. Røksund* [1,3]

[1] *Department of Health and Functioning, Western Norway University of Applied Sciences, Bergen, Norway,* [2] *Department of Clinical Science, University of Bergen, Bergen, Norway,* [3] *Department of Pediatrics and Adolescent Medicine, Haukeland University Hospital, Bergen, Norway*

***Correspondence:**
Merete S. Engeseth
msen@hvl.no

Objective: To investigate voice characteristics and exercise related respiratory symptoms in extremely preterm born 11-year-old children, focusing particularly on associations with management of a patent ductus arteriosus (PDA).

Study design: Prospective follow-up of all children born in Norway during 1999–2000 at gestational age <28 weeks or with birthweight <1,000 g. Neonatal data were obtained prospectively on custom-made registration forms completed by neonatologists. Voice characteristics and exercise related respiratory symptoms were obtained at 11 years by parental questionnaires.

Result: Questionnaires were returned for 228/372 (61%) eligible children, of whom 137 had no history of PDA. PDA had been noted in 91 participants, of whom 36 had been treated conservatively, 21 with indomethacin, and 34 with surgery. Compared to the children treated with indomethacin or conservatively, the odds ratio (95% confidence interval) for the surgically treated children were 3.4 (1.3; 9.2) for having breathing problems during exercise, 16.9 (2.0; 143.0) for having a hoarse voice, 4.7 (1.3; 16.7) for a voice that breaks when shouting, 4.6 (1.1; 19.1) for a voice that disturbs singing, and 3.7 (1.1; 12.3) for problems shouting or speaking loudly. The significance of surgery *per se* was uncertain since the duration of mechanical ventilation was associated with the same outcomes.

Conclusion: Extremely preterm born children with a neonatal history of PDA surgery had more problems with voice and breathing during exercise in mid-childhood than those whose PDA had been handled otherwise. The study underlines the causal heterogeneity of exercise related respiratory symptoms in preterm born children.

Keywords: patent ductus arteriosus, extremely premature infant, extremely low birth weight infant, voice quality, respiratory symptoms, cohort study

INTRODUCTION

Extremely preterm (EP) birth may lead to long-term complications, including respiratory problems of various etiologies (1). Survival at this early stage requires respiratory interventions, such as oxygen treatment and positive pressure ventilation, often with endotracheal intubation and mechanical ventilation (2, 3). Most of these lifesaving measures also cause various types of airway injuries with long-term consequences, challenging the diagnostic skills of health care providers (4–6).

Asthma, by far the most prevalent airway disorder, tends to be a first diagnostic option in young people with airway symptoms, often solely based on parental reports (7, 8). This practice inevitably leads to diagnostic errors, and is particularly unfortunate in EP-born individuals, given their wide causal repertoire (9–11). For example, bronchial obstruction and hyperresponsiveness are well described features after EP-birth as well as in asthma (12–16). Although linked to different immunological profiles (14, 16–19), large proportions of EP-born children are exposed to asthma medication (20). Recent literature has highlighted that also upper airway pathology creates respiratory symptoms that are misunderstood as asthma in EP-born children (21–23). We should keep in mind that the larynx is the narrowest part of the airway tree, representing a large proportion of total airway resistance (24). Thus, even minor injuries might hamper airflow when ventilatory requirements are high, such as during exercise. The larynx might be traumatized from repeated intubations or from prolonged use of mechanical ventilation (21, 25, 26). Moreover, surgical treatment of a patent ductus arteriosus (PDA) has been linked to left vocal cord paralysis (LVCP) in several studies, explained by the close proximity between the PDA and the left recurrent laryngeal nerve (11, 27, 28). Few studies have investigated symptoms of upper airway abnormalities in EP-born children (21, 26). We need more knowledge on these issues in order to develop evidence based guidelines for work-up of respiratory complaints in this group. Previous studies have suggested a role for laryngoscopy (11, 29–31); however, this notion needs support from more studies.

In this study, we used parental reports of voice abnormalities and exercise related respiratory symptoms to explore potential presence of upper airway pathology in a nationwide cohort of 11-year-old children born extremely preterm. Further, we investigated associations between these symptoms and neonatal PDA and its management.

MATERIALS AND METHODS

Study Population

This investigation was part of a Norwegian nationwide prospective cohort study of all children born with gestational age (GA) 23^0–27^6 weeks or birth weight (BW) below 1,000 g born during 1999–2000 (2). Of 638 children, 174 were stillborn or died in the delivery room, 86 died in the neonatal intensive care unit (NICU), and two declined participation (2). Three children died after discharge from NICU and one died later during the follow-up period, leaving 372 children eligible for inclusion. A "clinically significant PDA" had been diagnosed in 143 survivors, of whom 47 had undergone PDA surgery (**Figure 1**).

Sources and Collection of Data

Information on the neonatal characteristic and clinical course in the NICU was obtained from compulsory notifications to the Medical Birth Registry of Norway and custom-made study registration forms (2). GA was based on ultrasound at 17–18 weeks of gestation. Small for gestational age (SGA) was defined as a BW less than the 5th· percentile for GA and gender according to Norwegian growth curves (32). Bronchopulmonary dysplasia (BPD) was defined as still dependency on oxygen supplementation at 36 weeks' GA. The respiratory medical history of this cohort has been published (20, 33). PDA was diagnosed at the discretion of the participating NICUs, with algorithms based on echocardiographic assessment of the left atrium to the aortic root ratio (above 1.3–1.5 depending on clinical situation) and clinical signs as listed by Evans in 1993 (bounding hyper dynamic pulses and signs of cardiac or respiratory insufficiency) (34). Infants with a diagnosed PDA were treated either conservatively with fluid retention, diuretics, or unspecified symptomatic support, or the PDA was actively treated with either indomethacin or surgical closure performed by suture or clip.

At 11 years of age, data on previous and current symptoms were obtained from parental questionnaires. The questions: "*Does the child have breathing problems beyond what is normal during physical exertion?*" and "*Does the child make 'scraping sounds' or other abnormal sounds from the throat during physical exertion?*" were custom made for the project. The questions regarding exercise related wheeze, asthma (ever) and use of asthma medications were obtained from the International Study of Asthma and Allergies in Childhood questionnaire (ISAAC) (35). Current asthma was defined as [1] a physician's diagnosis of asthma combined with either respiratory symptoms or use of asthma medication in the previous 12 months, *or* [2] asthma medication and symptoms in the past 12 months even if no recall of prior physician's diagnosis. Asthma medication included inhaled corticosteroids, short or long acting β2-agonists and oral leukotriene modifiers. The six questions about voice characteristics were based on the Voice Handicap Index version 5 questionnaire (36). All questions were translated to Norwegian language, and the questions analyzed in this study are described in **Supplementary Table I.**

Statistical Methods

Outcome variables were voice characteristics and exercise related respiratory symptoms obtained from questionnaires at age 11 years. We investigated these binary outcomes in relation to a neonatal history of PDA vs. no PDA, and in relation to the mode of treatment in the children with a neonatal history of PDA. Those who underwent surgical closure (labeled "surgery") were compared with those who did not undergo surgery ("no-surgery"). The "no-surgery" group included children who had been treated conservatively or with indomethacin, as initial analyses comparing the conservative and the indomethacin group showed that they did not differ in terms of neonatal

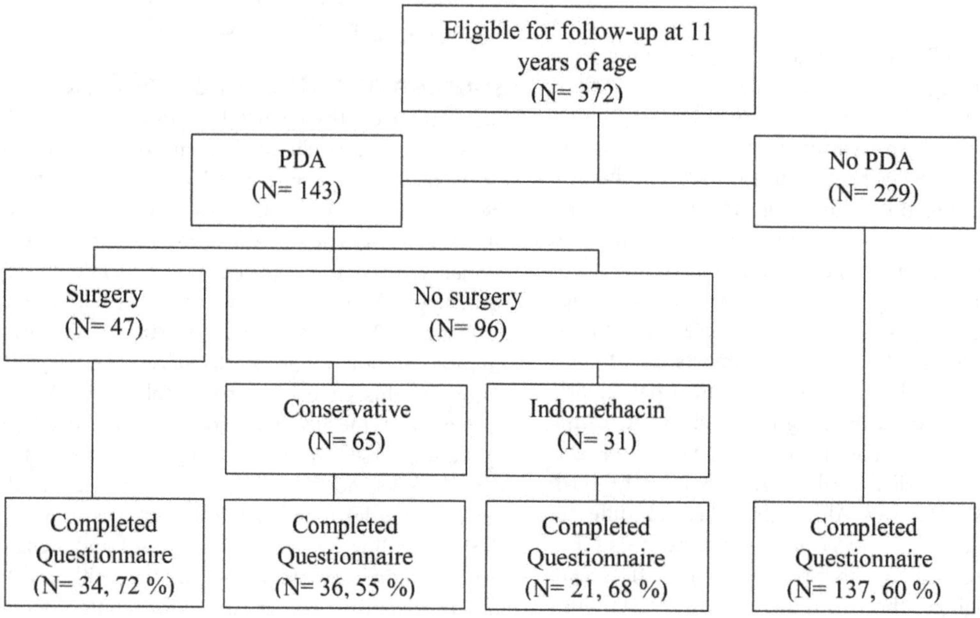

Abbreviations: Conservative: children who had PDA and was treated conservatively with fluid retention, diuretics or unspecified symptomatic support, Indomethacin: children who had PDA and received indomethacin treatment, N: number of subjects, No surgery: children who had PDA and was treated conservatively or treated with indomethacin, PDA: patent ductus arteriosus; Surgery: children receiving surgical PDA treatment.

FIGURE 1 | Follow-up of a national cohort of all 372 children born extremely preterm in Norway during 1999 and 2000 at a gestational age <28 weeks and/or with a birth weight <1,000 g, according to management of patent ductus arteriosus in the neonatal period.

variables and outcomes. Questions with graded response alternatives were transposed to dichotomous variables (no/yes) (**Supplementary Table I**).

Group differences were tested using independent samples *t*-test and chi-square test or Fischer's exact test, as appropriate. We further investigated associations by odds ratios (OR) with 95% confidence intervals (CI) using binary logistic regression. The ORs were estimated with crude and adjusted models, adjusted for days on mechanical ventilation and GA. We did not present analyses with adjustment for postnatal steroids because there is no causal link between use of postnatal steroids and PDA surgery. Potential confounders were adjusted for one by one in order to avoid that the total number of variables entered into the final regression equations exceeded 1/10 of the number of events. All analyses were performed using IBM SPSS statistics version 24 for Windows.

Ethics

The regional ethical committee of Western Norway approved the study (REC number 2009/2271). Informed written consents were obtained from the participant's parents.

RESULTS

Subjects

Questionnaires were returned for 228 of the 372 (61%) eligible children; including 91 of 143 children with a neonatal history of PDA and 137 of 228 children without PDA. Among the 91 children with PDA, 34 (37%) were treated with surgery, 36 (40%) received conservative treatment, and 21 (23%) received indomethacin (**Figure 1**). Six children in the surgery group had received indomethacin. Among the surgically treated children, those lost to follow-up had lower GA and BW, and spent more days on invasive mechanical ventilation. Further details on neonatal characteristics of children who were assessed and lost to follow-up at 11 years of age are presented in **Supplementary Table II**.

Perinatal Characteristics

The children with a neonatal history of a PDA had lower GA, were more often intubated at birth, received more postnatal steroids and surfactant, had spent more days on continuous positive airway pressure (CPAP) and had more often developed BPD compared to children without PDA (**Table 1**). Those with PDA who were treated with surgical closure were born at lower GA, had spent more days on mechanical ventilation, and more often received postnatal steroids compared to the children with PDA who were not treated with surgery.

Questionnaire Based Data of Respiratory and Voice Related Symptoms at 11 Years of Age

Our data showed that exercise related respiratory symptoms or voice problems were more common in children with- than

TABLE 1 | Neonatal characteristics of 228 extremely premature born children (<28 weeks GA/ <1,000 g BW) participating at the follow-up at 11 years of age.

	No PDA (N = 137)	PDA (N = 91)	PDA, no surgery (N = 57)	PDA, surgery (N = 34)	Mean difference (95% CI) No PDA vs. PDA	p	Mean difference (95% CI) no surgery vs. surgery	p
Characteristics, mean (SD)								
GA (weeks)	27.07 (1.7)	26.07 (1.4)	26.32 (1.3)	25.6 (1.4)	1.03 (0.6–1.4)	**<0.01**	0.73 (0.15–1.31)	**0.01**
Birth weight (gram)	865 (166.1)	866 (162.8)	886 (154.5)	832 (172.9)	−0.95 (-44.6–43.0)	0.97	53.5 (-16.1–123.0)	0.13
Start of PDA treatment, days after birth §								
Indomethacin			10.7 (7.4)	9.5 (5.2)				
PDA Surgery				13.4 (9.6)				
Days on invasive mechanical ventilation								
Mean (SD)	7.1 (15.7)	11.1 (14.0)	8.1 (9.3)	16.2 (18.6)	−3.96 (−7.8–0.04)	0.05	8.1 (1.2–15.0)	**0.02**
Median (range)	2 (0–113)	6 (0–83)	5 (0–44)	10.0 (0–83)				
Days on CPAP	22.8 (18.8)	28.4 (19.4)	29.7 (19.7)	26.1 (18.8)	−5.5 (−10.5; −0.6)	**0.03**	3.69 (−4.7–12.0)	0.38
Characteristics N (%)								
SGA	36 (26)	8 (9)	7 (12)	1 (3)		**0.001**		0.25
Sex (female)	63 (46)	41 (45)	28 (49)	13 (38)		0.185		0.31
BPD (O_2-suppl. at 36 weeks GA)	49 (36)	62 (68)	35 (61)	27 (79)		**<0.001**		0.08
Tracheal intubation at birth*	83 (64)	75 (82)	45 (79)	30 (88)		**0.001**		0.42
Surfactant	103 (75)	85 (93)	54 (95)	31 (91)		**<0.001**		0.67
Prenatal steroids	103 (75)	57 (63)	36 (63)	21 (62)		**0.04**		0.89
Postnatal steroids	37 (27)	45 (50)	23 (40)	22 (65)		**0.001**		**0.03**
Cerebral Palsy at 5 years of age	6 (4)	6 (7)	4 (7)	2 (6)		0.55		0.99

Independent t-test, chi-square test or Fischer's exact test was used as appropriate.
BPD, bronchopulmonary dysplasia; CI, confidence interval; CPAP, continuous positive airway pressure. GA, gestational age; IMV, invasive mechanical ventilation; PDA, patent ductus arteriosus; SD, standard deviation; SGA, small for gestational age.
**Missing data: Tracheal intubation at birth: Eight cases missing from the "no PDA" group and two cases missing from the "PDA"/"PDA, no surgery" groups. §Start of PDA treatment: Data are missing for nine children regarding age at day of PDA surgery. 21 children in the "PDA, no surgery" group received indomethacin treatment and six children in the "PDA, surgery" group received indomethacin treatment before surgery. Values in bold indicates a p-value of less than 0.05.*

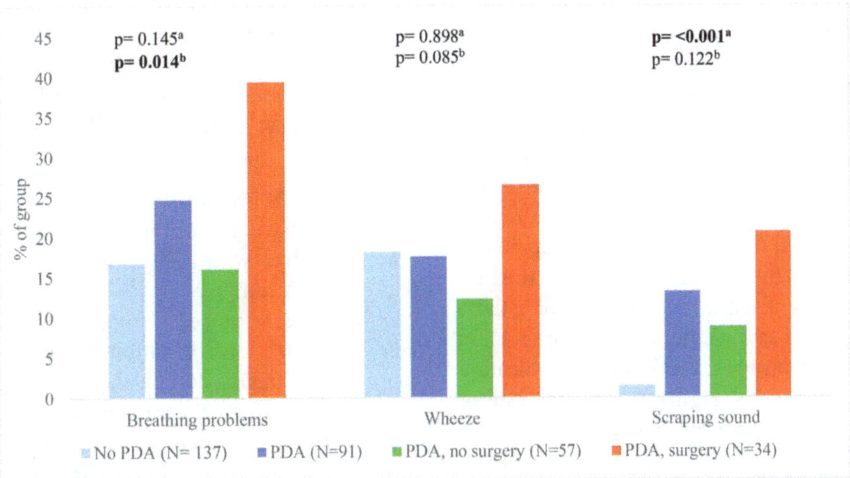

P-values for group differences between PDA vs. no PDA[a] and surgery vs. no surgery[b]. Breathing problems: proportion who answered "a little more than normal" or "a lot more than normal" to question 1: "Does the child have breathing problems beyond what is normal during physical exertion? Wheeze: Proportion who answered "yes" to question 2: "During the last 12 months, has the child had heavy breathing or wheezing from the chest during or after physical exercise or play?" Scraping sound: proportion who answered "a little" or "a lot" to question 3: "Does the child make «scraping sounds» or other abnormal sounds from the throat during physical exertion?" Abbreviations: PDA: patent ductus arteriosus.

FIGURE 2 | Reported respiratory symptoms during or after physical activity among a national cohort of extremely preterm born children at 11 years of age according to diagnosis and treatment of patent ductus arteriosus in the neonatal period.

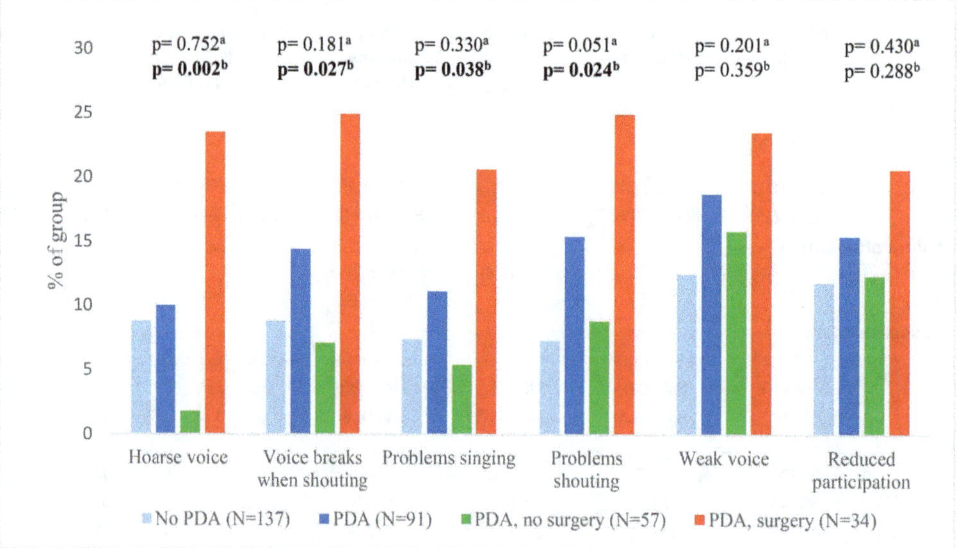

P-values for group differences between no PDA vs. PDA[a] and no surgery vs. surgery[b]. The bar graphs represents the proportion who answered affirmative ("A little", "Moderately", "A lot more" or "Extremely") to the following questions: Hoarse voice: "Is the child`s voice more hoarse compared to other children at the same age?", Voice cracks when shouting: "Does the voice «crack» when the child shouts?", Problems singing: "Does the voice influence the child`s participation in singing?", Problems shouting: " Does the child have problems with shouting or talking with a loud voice?", Weak voice: "Is the child`s voice so weak or unclear that it limits the possibility of being heard in a noisy environment?", Reduced participation: "Is the child`s voice influencing participation in school or regular social activities?" Abbreviations: PDA: patent ductus arteriosus.

FIGURE 3 | Reported voice characteristics among a national cohort of extremely preterm born children at the age of 11 years according to diagnosis and management of patent ductus arteriosus in the neonatal period.

without a neonatal history of PDA. However, differences were only statistically significant for scraping sound during physical exertion (**Figures 2, 3**). There were no important differences in reports of asthma or use of asthma medications (**Figure 4**).

In children who had a neonatal history of PDA, surgical closure was associated with more frequent reports of breathing problems during physical exertion (**Figure 2**) and voice related symptoms (**Figure 3**) compared to the no-surgery group. There were no differences between the surgery group and the no-surgery group regarding current asthma, current use of asthma medication or ever having had asthma, but a higher proportion of the surgery group had previously received asthma medication compared to the no-surgery group (**Figure 4**). In total, one or more symptoms related to respiration during exertion or voice were reported for 20 (61%) of the participants in the surgery group and 17 (31%) in the no-surgery group ($p = 0.006$).

Logistic Regression Analyses

Exercise Related Respiratory Symptoms

The odds ratio (OR) for having scraping sounds during physical exertion was increased among children with a PDA diagnosis (OR: 10.25; 95% CI: 2.24–47.0; $p = 0.03$) compared to the group without PDA, but not for other symptoms (not shown in tables). Among children with PDA, the crude odds of having breathing problems during physical exertion were higher in the surgery group relative to the no-surgery group (**Table 2**). After adjustment for number of days on mechanical ventilation, the OR of having breathing problems during physical exertion was still increased, but confidence intervals were wide. Adjusting for GA did not have impact on the OR.

Voice Characteristics

The OR for having symptoms related to voice was not increased among children with a PDA diagnosis, compared to the group without PDA. Among children with PDA, the crude odds of having a hoarse voice, a voice that breaks when shouting, a voice that affects participation in singing or a voice that leads to problems talking loudly/shout, were higher in the surgery group compared to the no-surgery group (**Table 3**). Adjusted for number of days on mechanical ventilation, the ORs were no longer increased for any of the voice characteristics. Adjusted for GA, the ORs were still increased for having a hoarse voice or a voice that cracks when shouting.

DISCUSSION

We found that voice and exercise related respiratory symptoms were more common in 11-year-old children born extremely preterm with a neonatal history of PDA surgery, compared to children whose PDA had been managed otherwise. However, the significance of surgery *per se* remains uncertain since adjusting

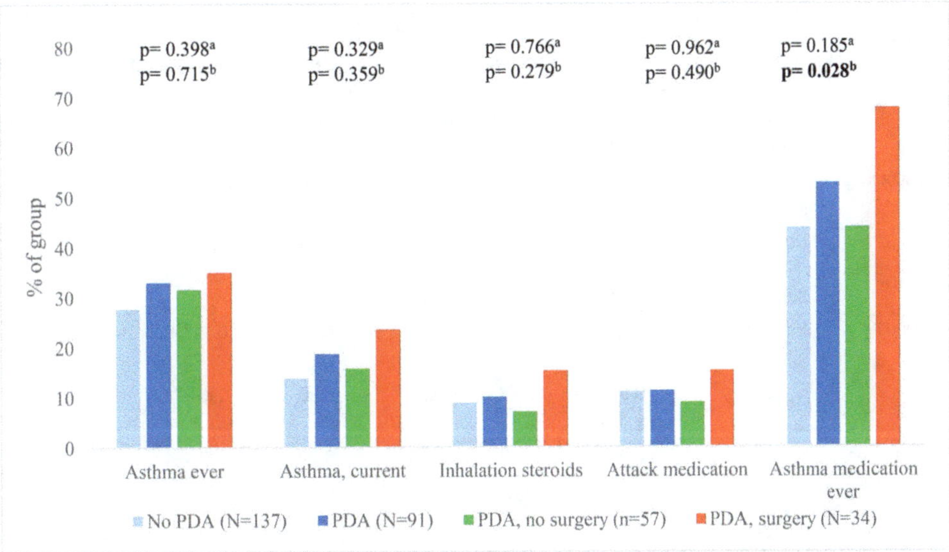

P-values for group differences between no PDA vs. PDA[a] and no surgery vs. surgery [b]. Asthma ever: parent reporting that the child has had asthma. Asthma, current: a doctor's diagnosis of asthma combined with either respiratory symptoms or use of asthma medication in the previous 12 months, or asthma medication and symptoms in the past 12 months even if no recall of prior doctor's diagnosis. Inhalation steroids: current use of inhaled corticosteroids. Attack medication: current use of short- or long acting β2-agonists. Asthma medication ever: use of inhaled corticosteroids, short or long acting β2-agonists and oral leukotriene modifiers after discharge from neonatal intensive care unit, but not current use. Abbreviations: PDA: patent ductus arteriosus.

FIGURE 4 | Reports of asthma and use of asthma medications among a national cohort of extremely preterm born children at 11 years of age according to diagnosis and treatment of patent ductus arteriosus in the neonatal period.

TABLE 2 | The odds ratio of having respiratory symptoms during or after physical activity at 11 years of age in a national cohort of extremely preterm born children according to treatment for patent ductus arteriosus (no surgery vs. surgery) in the neonatal period.

	PDA treatment	*N* (%)	Crude OR (95% CI)	*p*	aOR1 (95% CI)	*p*	aOR2 (95% CI)	*p*
Breathing problems	No surgery	9/56 (16)	3.4 (1.3–9.2)	**0.02**	2.6 (0.9–7.4)	0.08	3.2 (1.1–9.0)	**0.03**
	Surgery	13/33 (39)						
Wheeze	No surgery	7/57 (12)	2.6 (0.9–7.7)	0.09	2.5 (0.8–7.9)	0.11	2.8 (0.9–8.8)	0.08
	Surgery	9/34 (27)						
Scraping sound	No surgery	5/57 (9)	2.7 (0.8–9.3)	0.12	1.8 (0.5–6.8)	0.41	2.4 (0.7–8.7)	0.17
	Surgery	7/34 (21)						

Breathing problems: proportion who answered "a little more than normal" or "a lot more than normal" to question 1: "Does the child have breathing problems beyond what is normal during physical exertion?" Wheeze: Proportion who answered "yes" to question 2: "During the last 12 months, has the child had heavy breathing or wheezing from the chest during or after physical exercise or play?" Scraping sound: proportion who answered "a little" or "a lot" to question 3: "Does the child make ≪scraping sounds≫ or other abnormal sounds from the throat during physical exertion?" aOR1, adjusted for total number of days on invasive mechanical ventilation. aOR2, adjusted for gestational age; CI, confidence interval; OR, odds ratio; PDA, patent ductus arteriosus. Values in bold indicates a p-value of less than 0.05.

for days of mechanical ventilation significantly weakened the associations.

Previous studies have described that EP-born children with left vocal fold paralysis (LVCP) following PDA surgery had prolonged dependency of mechanical ventilation compared to surgically treated children without LVCP (11, 28, 37, 38). Unfortunately, the respective duration of mechanical ventilation before vs. after surgery could not be estimated in our study. Thus, prolonged mechanical ventilation in the surgery group could be *caused* by a possible LVCP or other complications following surgery (39). However, it could also reflect *confounding by indication*; i.e., those treated surgically were also those with the most severe disease, therefore spending most days ventilated (40). Both mechanisms might have been operative, but we do not have data to disentangle this scenario. Days on mechanical ventilation was associated with symptoms in all subgroups, also in those with no history of PDA, although at a lower odds ratio. The observed association (co-linearity) between days on mechanical ventilation and surgical PDA treatment complicates interpretations of the regression models. We therefore report both adjusted and unadjusted data in **Tables 2, 3**. However, taken together the data indicate that neonatal PDA surgery leads to more voice and

TABLE 3 | The odds ratio of having voice symptoms at 11 years of age in a national cohort of extremely preterm born children according to treatment (no surgery vs. surgery) for patent ductus arteriosus in the neonatal period.

	PDA treatment	*N* (%)	Crude OR (95% CI)	*p*	aOR1 (95% CI)	*p*	aOR2 (95% CI)	*p*
Hoarse voice	No surgery	1/56 (2)	16.9 (2.0–143)	**0.009**	9.6 (1.0–93.8)	0.05	14.1 (1.6–122)	**0.02**
	Surgery	8/34 (24)						
Voice cracks when the child shouts	No surgery	4/56 (7)	4.7 (1.3–16.7)	**0.017**	3.2 (1.2–20.7)	0.10	3.9 (1.1–14.4)	**0.04**
	Surgery	9/34 (27)						
Voice influences participation in singing	No surgery	3/56 (5)	4.6 (1.1–19.1)	**0.04**	2.8 (0.6–13.1)	0.19	3.7 (0.9–16.2)	0.08
	Surgery	7/34 (21)						
Problems shouting or talking loudly	No surgery	5/57 (9)	3.7 (1.1–12.3)	**0.03**	2.6 (0.7–9.3)	0.14	3.2 (0.9–10.9)	0.07
	Surgery	9/34 (27)						
Weak or unclear voice	No surgery	9/57 (16)	1.6 (0.6–4.8)	0.36	1.0 (0.3–3.4)	0.96	1.5 (0.5–4.6)	0.46
	Surgery	8/34 (24)						
Voice influences participation in school or social activities	No surgery	7/57 (12)	1.9 (0.6–5.8)	0.29	1.3 (0.4–4.4)	0.73	1.8 (0.5–5.8)	0.35
	Surgery	7/34 (21)						

N (%) represents proportion who answered affirmative ("A little," "Moderately," "A lot more" or "Extremely") to the following questions: Hoarse voice: "Is the child's voice more hoarse compared to other children at the same age? Voice cracks when the child shouts: Does the voice ≪crack≫ when the child shouts?," Voice influences participation in singing: "Does the voice influence the child's participation in singing?," Problems shouting or talking loudly: "Does the child have problems with shouting or talking with a loud voice?," Weak or unclear voice: "Is the child's voice so weak or unclear that it limits the possibility of being heard in a noisy environment?," Voice influences participation in school or social activities: "Is the child's voice influencing participation in school or regular social activities?." aOR1, adjusted for total number of days on invasive mechanical ventilation; aOR2, adjusted for gestational age; CI, confidence interval; OR, odds ratio; PDA, patent ductus arteriosus. Values in bold indicates a p-value of less than 0.05.

exercise related respiratory symptoms in mid-childhood, possibly influenced also by prolonged mechanical ventilation.

Management of PDA in EP-born neonates is debated. Options include a conservative approach, pharmacologic intervention, or surgical ligation, the latter usually used as a last resort (41, 42). Knowledge on long-term outcomes must count in these discussions. There are few studies reporting on voice characteristics and exercise related respiratory symptoms in children and adults exposed to neonatal PDA surgery (30). Although LVCP is a well-described complication, an unknown fraction may pass unnoticed or are misinterpreted during the neonatal period as symptoms may be vague, transient and uncharacteristic (27, 29, 37, 38, 43). Importantly, we know that pediatric LVCP does not usually recover (11, 44–46). Therefore, symptoms may continue to be overlooked or erroneously related to other disorders or even to malingering, later in life. We do not have research based data to substantiate this notion. However, early life events are rarely considered by respiratory specialists (5), and LVCP is probably not on top of the physicians' list when trying to interpret airway symptoms. In a regional study of 11 EP born adults who had undergone PDA surgery in the 1980s, seven had LVCP of whom six reported trouble with their voice. None of them were comfortable with singing or speaking loudly, and all disclosed prolonged inspirium, wheeze or stridor when tested on a treadmill (11). Importantly, three of them had a long history of "difficult-to-treat asthma," but they could substantially reduce medication after receiving the LVCP diagnosis. In our study, we found no association between PDA surgery and current asthma medication; however, a higher proportion of the surgically treated children had used asthma medication. Thus, breathing problems could initially have been perceived as asthma, and medication subsequently stopped due to lack of effect.

In the present study, we also identified children with respiratory and voice related symptoms among children with no history of PDA, or who had not undergone PDA surgery, implying that these symptoms are of multi-factorial origin. Prolonged mechanical ventilation is associated with subglottic stenosis and injury to the vocal cords (47), which may lead to stridor and affect voice (48). Walz et al. (25) found that prolonged intubation (more than 4 weeks) was associated with long-term reduced voice quality. In univariate analysis, both the presence of a PDA and surgical closure of a PDA were associated with lower score on voice related quality of life. In multivariate analysis, PDA did not contribute to the model, but PDA surgery was not included. French et al. (26) reported that 58% of school aged children born before 25 weeks' gestation had moderate to severe hoarseness, and that the number of intubations (more than five) was associated with voice disorders. The authors suggested that the voice abnormalities could be related to laryngeal injury from endotracheal intubation. As only three of the 67 tested children had undergone PDA surgery, they argued that surgery could not have contributed to the voice problems in their cohort (26). Simpson et al. (21) found that 25/35 very preterm born children presented with dysphonia at 11 years of age, and increased dysphonia severity was predicted by lower GA, increased number of intubations and days of mechanical ventilation. Only three subjects had undergone PDA surgery, but they represented 3/14 subjects with moderate to severe dysphonia. Presence of dysphonia was associated with reports of previous wheeze, asthma diagnosis and former use of asthma medications. However, there was no difference in lung function between groups with- or without dysphonia, and the authors suggested upper airway pathology and dysfunctional breathing contributing to increased reports of respiratory symptoms (21).

The major limitations of this study were the relatively small sample size and the fact that we relied on parental observation of respiratory and voice related symptoms. We know from asthma research that there are differences between parents' and children's perceptions (49). However, in this age group parental information is usually what we have to go by in clinical work. As in all follow-up studies, attrition influences interpretation; in our case underlined by differences between responders and non-responders listed in the appendix. Importantly, laryngoscopies had not been performed, precluding knowledge as to whether LVCP, or other laryngeal abnormalities contributed to the increased odds of respiratory and voice related symptoms in the PDA surgery group. Inability to ascertain why infants exposed to PDA surgery needed more days on mechanical ventilation challenged attempts to interpret the role of this variable in the regression models and thus in the causal chain leading to symptoms.

CONCLUSION

Extremely preterm born school-children who had undergone neonatal PDA surgery had more voice and exercise related respiratory symptoms than children exposed to other modes of PDA treatment. Although these symptoms are likely to have a compound etiology, when present in children exposed to neonatal PDA surgery, they must prompt a search for upper airway abnormalities, and not lead to empirical prescription of asthma medication. We must not forget early life events when dealing with respiratory symptoms.

ETHICS STATEMENT

The studies involving human participants were reviewed and approved by The Regional Commitee for Medical and Health Research Ethics west (REC number 2009/2271). Written informed consent to participate in this study was provided by the participants' legal guardian/next of kin.

AUTHOR'S NOTE

Preliminary data from this study was presented as an abstract at The European Respiratory Congress in 2018, where copyright is retained by the author or employer [as part of the conditions of the author(s)'s employment].

AUTHOR CONTRIBUTIONS

TH, TM, OR, MV, and HC designed the data collection instruments, collected the data, contributed to interpretation of the data, and reviewed and revised the manuscript for important intellectual content. ME contributed to the analyses and interpretation of the data, and reviewed and revised the manuscript for important intellectual content. RN contributed to the statistical analyses and interpretation of the data, and reviewed and revised the manuscript for important intellectual content. MSE carried out the statistical analyses and the interpretation of the data, drafted the article, and reviewed and revised the manuscript. All authors approved the final manuscript as submitted and agree to be accountable for all aspects of the work.

REFERENCES

1. Priante E, Moschino L, Mardegan V, Manzoni P, Salvadori S, Baraldi E. Respiratory outcome after preterm birth: a long and difficult journey. *Am J Perinatol.* (2016) 33:1040–2. doi: 10.1055/s-0036-1586172
2. Markestad T, Kaaresen PI, Rønnestad A, Reigstad H, Lossius K, Medbø S, et al. Early death, morbidity, and need of treatment among extremely premature infants. *Pediatrics.* (2005) 115:1289–98. doi: 10.1542/peds.2004-1482
3. Stoll BJ, Hansen NI, Bell EF, Walsh MC, Carlo WA, Shankaran S, et al. Trends in care practices, morbidity, and mortality of extremely preterm neonates, 1993–2012. *JAMA.* (2015) 314:1039–51. doi: 10.1001/jama.2015.10244
4. Baraldi E, Filippone M. Chronic lung disease after premature birth. *N Engl J Med.* (2007) 357:1946–55. doi: 10.1056/NEJMra067279
5. Bolton CE, Bush A, Hurst JR, Kotecha S, McGarvey L, Stocks J, et al. Are early life factors considered when managing respiratory disease? A British thoracic society survey of current practice. *Thorax.* (2012) 67:1110. doi: 10.1136/thoraxjnl-2012-202637
6. Bolton CE, Bush A. Coming now to a chest clinic near you. *Thorax.* (2013) 68:707–8. doi: 10.1136/thoraxjnl-2013-203836
7. Looijmans-van den Akker I, van Luijn K, Verheij T. Overdiagnosis of asthma in children in primary care: a retrospective analysis. *Br J Gen Practice.* (2016) 66:e152–7. doi: 10.3399/bjgp16X683965
8. Reddel HK, Pedersen S. *Global Strategy for Asthma Management and Prevention.* (2018). Available online at: https://ginasthma.org/2018-gina-report-global-strategy-for-asthma-management-and-prevention/
9. Bush A, Fleming L. Is asthma overdiagnosed? *Arch Dis Childhood.* (2016) 101:688–9. doi: 10.1136/archdischild-2015-309053
10. Hull JH. Not all wheeze is asthma: time for patients to exercise their rights. *Thorax.* (2015) 70:7–8. doi: 10.1136/thoraxjnl-2014-206096
11. Roksund OD, Clemm H, Heimdal JH, Aukland SM, Sandvik L, Markestad T, et al. Left vocal cord paralysis after extreme preterm birth, a new clinical scenario in adults. *Pediatrics.* (2010) 126:e1569–77. doi: 10.1542/peds.2010-1129
12. Doyle LW, Andersson S, Bush A, Cheong JLY, Clemm H, Evensen KAI, et al. Expiratory airflow in late adolescence and early adulthood in individuals born very preterm or with very low birthweight compared with controls born at term or with normal birthweight: a meta-analysis of individual participant data. *Lancet Resp Med.* (2019) 7:677–86. doi: 10.1016/S2213-2600(18) 30530-7
13. Kotecha S, Clemm H, Halvorsen T, Kotecha SJ. Bronchial hyper-responsiveness in preterm-born subjects: a systematic review and meta-analysis. *Pediatr Aller Immunol.* (2018) 29:715–25. doi: 10.1111/pai.12957
14. Halvorsen T, Skadberg BT, Eide GE, Roksund O, Aksnes L, Oymar K. Characteristics of asthma and airway hyper-responsiveness after premature birth. *PediatrAller Immunol.* (2005) 16:487–94. doi: 10.1111/j.1399-3038.2005.00314.x
15. Vollsaeter M, Skromme K, Satrell E, Clemm H, Roksund O, Øymar K, et al. Children born preterm at the turn of the millennium had better lung function than children born similarly preterm in the early 1990s. *PLoS ONE.* (2015) 10:1–17. doi: 10.1371/journal.pone.0144243
16. Filippone M, Carraro S, Baraldi E. The term "asthma" should be avoided in describing the chronic pulmonary disease of prematurity. *EurRespirJ.* (2013) 42:1430–1. doi: 10.1183/09031936.00055913

17. Filippone M, Bonetto G, Corradi M, Frigo AC, Baraldi E. Evidence of unexpected oxidative stress in airways of adolescents born very pre-term. *Eur Respir J.* (2012) 40:1253–9. doi: 10.1183/09031936.00185511
18. Course CW, Kotecha S, Kotecha SJ. Fractional exhaled nitric oxide in preterm-born subjects: a systematic review and meta-analysis. *Pediatr Pulmonol.* (2019) 54:595–601. doi: 10.1002/ppul.24270
19. Baraldi E, Bonetto G, Zacchello F, Filippone M. Low exhaled nitric oxide in school-age children with bronchopulmonary dysplasia and airflow limitation. *Am J Respir Crit Care Med.* (2005) 171:68–72. doi: 10.1164/rccm.200403-298OC
20. Skromme K, Vollsaeter M, Oymar K, Markestad T, Halvorsen T. Respiratory morbidity through the first decade of life in a national cohort of children born extremely preterm. *BMC Pediatrics.* (2018) 18:102. doi: 10.1186/s12887-018-1045-7
21. Simpson SJ, Champion Z, Hall GL, French N, Reynolds V. Upper airway pathology contributes to respiratory symptoms in children born very preterm. *J Pediatr.* (2019) 213:46–51. doi: 10.1016/j.jpeds.2019.06.048
22. Reynolds V, Meldrum S, Simmer K, Vijayasekaran S, French N. Voice problems in school-aged children following very preterm birth. *Arch Dis Childhood.* (2016) 101:556–60. doi: 10.1136/archdischild-2015-309441
23. Reynolds V, Meldrum S, Simmer K, Vijayasekaran S, French N. Laryngeal pathology at school age following very preterm birth. *Int J Pediatr Otorhinolaryngol.* (2015) 79:398–404. doi: 10.1016/j.ijporl.2014.12.037
24. Savard P, Cole P, Miljeteig H, Haight JS. Laryngeal resistance to respiratory airflow in humans. *Laryngoscope.* (1993) 103:785–92. doi: 10.1288/00005537-199307000-00012
25. Walz P, Hubbell M, Elmaraghy C. Voice related quality of life in pediatric patients with a history of prematurity. *Int J Pediatr Otorhinolaryngol.* (2014) 78:1010–4. doi: 10.1016/j.ijporl.2014.03.023
26. French N, Kelly R, Vijayasekaran S, Reynolds V, Lipscombe J, Buckland A, et al. Voice abnormalities at school age in children born extremely preterm. *Pediatrics.* (2012) 131:e733–e9. doi: 10.1542/peds.2012-0817
27. Nichols BG, Jabbour J, Hehir DA, Ghanayem NS, Beste D, Martin T, et al. Recovery of vocal fold immobility following isolated patent ductus arteriosus ligation. *Int J Pediatr Otorhinolaryngol.* (2014) 78:1316–9. doi: 10.1016/j.ijporl.2014.05.019
28. Benjamin JR, Smith PB, Cotten CM, Jaggers J, Goldstein RF, Malcolm WF. Long-term morbidities associated with vocal cord paralysis after surgical closure of a patent ductus arteriosus in extremely low birth weight infants. *J Perinatol.* (2010) 30:408–13. doi: 10.1038/jp.2009.124
29. Smith ME, King JD, Elsherif A, Muntz HR, Park AH, Kouretas PC. Should all newborns who undergo patent ductus arteriosus ligation be examined for vocal fold mobility? *Laryngoscope.* (2009) 119:1606–9. doi: 10.1002/lary.20148
30. Engeseth MS, Olsen NR, Maeland S, Halvorsen T, Goode A, Roksund OD. Left vocal cord paralysis after patent ductus arteriosus ligation: a systematic review. *Paediatr Respir Rev.* (2018) 27:74–85. doi: 10.1016/j.prrv.2017.11.001
31. Strychowsky JE, Rukholm G, Gupta MK, Reid D. Unilateral vocal fold paralysis after congenital cardiothoracic surgery: a meta-analysis. *Pediatrics.* (2014) 133:e1708–23. doi: 10.1542/peds.2013-3939
32. Skjærven R, Gjessing HK, Bakketeig LS. Birthweight by gestational age in Norway. *Acta Obstet Gynecol Scand.* (2000) 79:440–9. doi: 10.1080/j.1600-0412.2000.079006440.x
33. Skromme K, Leversen K, Eide G, Markestad T, Halvorsen T. Respiratory illness contributed significantly to morbidity in children born extremely premature or with extremely low birthweights in 1999–2000. *Acta Paediatr.* (2015) 104:1189–98. doi: 10.1111/apa.13165
34. Evans N. Diagnosis of patent ductus arteriosus in the preterm newborn. *Arch Dis Childhood.* (1993) 68:58–61. doi: 10.1136/adc.68.1_Spec_No.58
35. Beasley R. Worldwide variation in prevalence of symptoms of asthma, allergic rhinoconjunctivitis, and atopic eczema: ISAAC. *Lancet.* (1998) 351:1225–32. doi: 10.1016/S0140-6736(97)07302-9
36. Jacobson B, Johnson A, Grywalski C. The Voice Handicap Index (VHI): development and validation. *Am J Speech Lang Pathol.* (1997) 6:66–70. doi: 10.1044/1058-0360.0603.66
37. Clement WA, El-Hakim H, Phillipos EZ, Cote JJ. Unilateral vocal cord paralysis following patent ductus arteriosus ligation in extremely low-birth-weight infants. *Arch Otolaryngol Head Neck Surg.* (2008) 134:28–33. doi: 10.1001/archoto.2007.2
38. Pereira KD, Webb BD, Blakely ML, Cox CS Jr, Lally KP. Sequelae of recurrent laryngeal nerve injury after patent ductus arteriosus ligation. *Int J Pediatr Otorhinolaryngol.* (2006) 70:1609–12. doi: 10.1016/j.ijporl.2006.05.001
39. El-Khuffash AF, Jain A, McNamara PJ. Ligation of the patent ductus arteriosus in preterm infants: understanding the physiology. *J Pediatr.* (2013) 162:1100–6. doi: 10.1016/j.jpeds.2012.12.094
40. Weisz D, Mirea L, Resende M, Ly L, Church P, Kelly E, et al. Outcomes of surgical ligation after unsuccessful pharmacotherapy for patent ductus arteriosus in neonates born extremely preterm. *J Pediatrics.* (2018) 195:292–6. doi: 10.1016/j.jpeds.2017.11.029
41. Jain A, Shah PS. Diagnosis, evaluation, and management of patent ductus arteriosus in preterm neonates. *JAMA Pediatr.* (2015) 169:863–72. doi: 10.1001/jamapediatrics.2015.0987
42. Ngo S, Profit J, Gould JB, Lee HC. Trends in patent ductus arteriosus diagnosis and management for very low birth weight infants. *Pediatrics.* (2017) 139:e20162390. doi: 10.1542/peds.2016-2390
43. Davis J, Baciewicz F, Suriyapa S, Vauthy P, Polamreddy R, Bruce Barnett B. Vocal cord paralysis in premature infants undergoing ductal closure. *Ann Thorac Surg.* (1988) 46:214–5. doi: 10.1016/S0003-4975(10)65901-2
44. Truong MT, Messner AH, Kerschner JE, Scholes M, Wong-Dominguez J, Milczuk HA, et al. Pediatric vocal fold paralysis after cardiac surgery: rate of recovery and sequelae. *Otolaryngol Head Neck Surg.* (2007) 137:780–4. doi: 10.1016/j.otohns.2007.07.028
45. Henry BM, Hsieh WC, Sanna B, Vikse J, Taterra D, Tomaszewski KA. Incidence, risk factors, and comorbidities of vocal cord paralysis after surgical closure of a patent ductus arteriosus: a meta-analysis. *Pediatr Cardiol.* (2019) 40:116–25. doi: 10.1007/s00246-018-1967-8
46. Jabbour J, Robey T. Resolution of vocal fold immobility in preterm infants. *Int J Pediatr Otorhinolaryngol.* (2017) 103:83–6. doi: 10.1016/j.ijporl.2017.10.007
47. Vijayasekaran S, Lioy J, Maschhoff K. Airway disorders of the fetus and neonate: An overview. *Sem Fetal Neonatal Med.* (2016) 21:220–9. doi: 10.1016/j.siny.2016.03.004
48. Chisholm AG, Johnson RF. Stridor in the primary care setting. *Curr Treat Options Peds.* (2018) 4:456–66. doi: 10.1007/s40746-018-0144-x
49. Asmussen L, Weiss KB, Elfring D, Olson LM. Parent and child reports of asthma symptoms, activity limitations and emotional distress: early results from the child health information reporting project (CHIRP). *J Allergy Clin Immunol.* (2004) 113(2 Suppl.):S182. doi: 10.1016/j.jaci.2004.01.092

22

Size of Patent Ductus Arteriosus and Echocardiographic Markers of Shunt Volume in Preterm Infants Based on Postnatal Age

*Eui Kyung Choi, Kyu Hee Park and Byung Min Choi**

Department of Pediatrics, Korea University College of Medicine, Seoul, South Korea

Correspondence:
Byung Min Choi
cbmin@korea.ac.kr

Objective: This study was conducted in order to compare the strength of correlation between echocardiographic markers of shunt volume and patent ductus arteriosus (PDA) diameter based on postnatal age.

Methods: This retrospective study focused on preterm infants (aged <32 weeks of gestation) admitted to the Neonatal Intensive Care Unit of Korea University Ansan Hospital, between April 2014 and December 2017, who studied serial targeted neonatal echocardiography (TNE) for PDA during hospitalization. The association between echocardiographic characteristics and duct size was divided into the following days: within 3 days (very early, VE), 4–7 days after birth (early, E), and after 8 days of birth (late, L).

Results: We found 113 assessments conducted on 57 infants in the VE period, 92 assessments on 40 infants in the E period, and 342 assessments on 37 infants in the L period. Median gestational age and birth weight were 28^{+2} weeks of gestation and 1,115 g, respectively. In the univariate regression analysis, we found a statistically significant correlation between PDA diameter and all TNE markers in the E and L days, but not in the VE period. Only ductal velocity [coefficient of determination (R^2) = 0.224], antegrade left pulmonary artery diastolic flow velocity (R^2 = 0.165), left ventricular output (LVO)/superior vena cava (SVC) flow ratio (R^2 = 0.048), and E/A wave ratio (R^2 = 0.092) showed weak correlations with PDA diameter in the VE period. The slopes of the regressions showed significant changes based on postnatal age in the maximum ductal velocity, left atrium/aorta ratio, LVO/SVC flow ratio, and LVO.

Conclusions: It is difficult to predict the echocardiographic markers of shunt volume based on the PDA diameter in preterm infants younger than 4 days. A better understanding of the changes in the hemodynamic consequences of PDA based on postnatal age is needed when considering treatment.

Keywords: preterm infant, hemodynamically significant patent ductus arteriosus, patent ductus arteriosis, early targeted treatment, echocardiography

INTRODUCTION

Echocardiography is currently the preferred tool to screen neonates with hemodynamically significant patent ductus arteriosus (hsPDA) in the early postnatal period, owing to its potential benefits in the prevention of pulmonary hemorrhage or intra ventricular hemorrhage (1). The investigation is indicated for clinically suspected PDA, especially in very low birth weight neonates during the initial 24 to 72 h immediately following birth (2–4).

This transitional period is more complicated in preterm infants who have immature organ systems, thereby necessitating surfactant administration, ventilatory support, and vasoactive medications. The preterm left ventricular myocardium is exposed to an abrupt increase in afterload while being relatively immature; therefore, it may be less tolerant to the concurrent changes in preload conditions caused by the presence of pathologic atrial and ductal shunts. Therefore, defining hsPDA and deciding on the treatment may be complicated in the early postnatal period (5–7).

Since hsPDA is determined by both ductal size and shunt volume markers of pulmonary over circulation and systemic hypoperfusion in targeted neonatal echocardiography (TNE), the most common definition of hsPDA is based on the transductal diameter (2, 8, 9). Recently, Fernando de Freitas Martins et al. evaluated the correlation between ductal diameter and individual echocardiographic markers of shunt volume in preterm infants older than 7 days (10). However, there is lack of information regarding differences in the association between PDA diameter and shunt volume markers in the early postnatal period.

The aim of the present study was to compare the strength of association between echocardiographic markers of shunt volume and PDA diameter based on postnatal age and categorized as very early (VE, within 3 days after birth), early (E, 4–7 days after birth), and late (L, >8 days after birth) days.

MATERIALS AND METHODS

We retrospectively reviewed the medical records of 128 preterm infants who were born at <32 weeks of gestation and were admitted to the neonatal intensive care unit of Korea University Ansan Hospital between April 2014 and December 2017. Infants with major congenital anomalies (except PDA and patent foramen ovale), chromosomal abnormalities, and incomplete medical records were excluded. An additional exclusion criterion was the absence of data on TNE assessment of hemodynamic significance of the PDA during hospitalization.

The study was approved by the Institutional Review Board of the Korea University Ansan Hospital (2019AS0223).

Echocardiography Assessment

All infants delivered before 32 weeks of gestation underwent echocardiographic screening to identify congenital heart anomalies. After screening, we decided to study serial TNE assessments when the infants had PDA-related clinical signs or an established shunt, defined as evidence of left-to-right dominant transductal flow to ensure sufficient shunt flow. We performed standardized TNE assessment of hemodynamic significance of the PDA with pulmonary over circulation, myocardial performance, and/or systemic hypoperfusion to decide on the course of treatment. Given the direct vaso constricting effect of ibuprofen, TNE assessments were always performed before each dose of the medication. All study measurements were recorded by a single operator using the Vivid q system (GE Healthcare, Haifa, Israel) and a 10-Hz probe. Analysis of the recorded echocardiographic markers was performed by a blinded investigator. The mean variability between measurements was within 20% for all parameters, and 90% of the measures were approximately within 15% of each other.

Two-dimensional, M-mode, pulse, and color flow Doppler imaging were performed. PDA diameter was measured at its narrowest point, usually at the pulmonary end. We measured additional parameters, including ductal velocity (Vmax, peak velocity of transductal flow was assessed by pulse- and continuous-wave Doppler), end diastolic velocity of the left pulmonary artery (LPA), ratio of the left atrial diameter to aortic root diameter (LA/Ao, measured from the long axis parasternal view at the level of the aortic valve, using M-mode), ratio of mitral inflow E wave peak velocity to A wave peak velocity (E/A wave ratio, trans-mitral valve flow was assessed by pulse-wave Doppler at the tips of the mitral valve leaflets from an apical four-chamber view), left ventricular output (LVO, calculated based on heart rate, aortic diameter, and velocity time integral), and the percentage of retrograde diastolic flow in the descending aorta distal to PDA.

Clinical Data

The medical records of all eligible infants were reviewed to obtain neonatal demographic and clinical data. Birth and clinical characteristics were collected, including gestational age (GA) and birth weight at delivery, sex, mode of delivery, 5-min Apgar score, the use of antenatal steroids, and premature membrane rupture. The following clinical outcomes were also recorded: surfactant use in respiratory distress syndrome, PDA treatment with intravenous ibuprofen or surgical ligation, necrotizing enter colitis with radiologic evidence of pneumatosis intestinalis, intra ventricular hemorrhage classified according to the Papile classification, bronchopulmonary dysplasia (defined as the requirement for supplemental oxygen with a fraction of inspired oxygen of more than 0.21 for 28 days of life), treated retinopathy of prematurity, and death before discharge.

The policies of management to PDA in our NICU were "symptomatic treatment" and/or "early targeted treatment." The cyclooxygenase inhibitor was administered intravenously after confirming the diagnosis of hsPDA. Early targeted treatment based on echocardiographic parameters may allow for the selection of high-risk preterm infants prior to the duct becoming clinically significant. The clinical signs of PDA were based on the following features: (1) the presence of a systolic or continuous murmur; (2) a bounding pulse or a hyperactive precordial pulse; (3) difficulty in maintaining the blood pressure, i.e., hypotension (the lower limit of normal mean arterial pressure was regarded to corrected gestational age) without response to loading fluid and infusion of dopamine; (4) a worsening ventilator status; and (5) chest radiographic evidence, i.e., pulmonary congestion or cardiomegaly (a cardiothoracic ratio >60%) with increased pulmonary flow. Symptomatic PDA was defined as the presence of two of these five signs with the confirmation of a large left to right ductal flow by color flow Doppler echocardiography (11).

Statistical Analysis

Statistical analyses were performed using IBM SPSS 20 and R statistical software. Continuous variables were analyzed using either the *t* test or the Mann–Whitney *U* test/Kruskal–Wallis test for normal or skewed distributions. Proportions were tested using the chi-squared test and Fisher's exact test. *p* values of <0.05 were considered statistically significant. Data are presented as mean ± standard deviation (SD), median with interquartile range (IQR), or rate.

The association between PDA size and each of the echocardiographic markers was assessed using the Pearson correlation coefficient, followed by a linear regression analysis. The association was divided into VE, E, and L days as explained previously. The coefficient of determination (R^2) was used to determine the strength of the association for each marker. We used the *F* test and *t* test to compare the coefficients and slopes across different regressions.

RESULTS

A total of 128 preterm infants born at <32 weeks of gestation were identified, and 64 were excluded due to the presence of congenital defects, chromosomal abnormality, and absence of TNE data. A total of 547 TNE assessments in 64 infants with PDA were analyzed. We found 113 assessments conducted on 57 infants in the VE period, 92 assessments on 40 infants in the E period, and 342 assessments on 37 infants in the L period (**Figure 1**). Median GA and birth weight were 28^{+2} weeks (IQR, 26^{+4}-29^{+6} weeks) and 1,115 g (IQR, 950–1,397 g) (**Table 1**). The median number of TNE assessments per infant was 6 (IQR, 3–13). These were performed at a median of 2 days (range, 0–3) after birth in the VE period, 5 days (range, 4–7) after birth in the E period, and 18 days (range, 8–63) after birth in the L period. No difference was observed in the GA and birth weight of infants among the three periods. There were significant differences in the TNE assessments between the groups according to postnatal age, except E/A wave ratio, and in the use of mechanical ventilator depending on the different postnatal days (77.1 vs. 47.8 vs. 35.9%, $p < 0.05$). There were no significant differences in receiving treatment among the three periods (**Table 2**).

In the univariate regression analysis, we found a statistically significant correlation between PDA diameter and all TNE markers in the E and L days, but not in the VE period. Only ductal velocity ($R^2 = 0.224$, $p < 0.05$), antegrade LPA diastolic flow ($R^2 = 0.165$, $p < 0.05$), LVO/superior vena cava (SVC) flow ratio ($R^2 = 0.048$, $p < 0.05$), and E/A wave ratio ($R^2 = 0.092$, $p < 0.05$) showed weak correlations with PDA diameter in the VE period. The LA/Ao ratio ($R^2 = 0.010$, $p = 0.291$) and LVO ($R^2 = 0.028$, $p = 0.078$) did not correlate with PDA diameter in the VE period; however, there were strong correlations in the E ($R^2 = 0.230$, $p < 0.05$ and $R^2 = 0.344$, $p < 0.05$, respectively) and L days ($R^2 = 0.311$, $p < 0.05$ and $R^2 = 0.272$, $p < 0.05$, respectively) (**Table 3**). The regression lines in the scatter plots of PDA diameter and each of the TNE markers

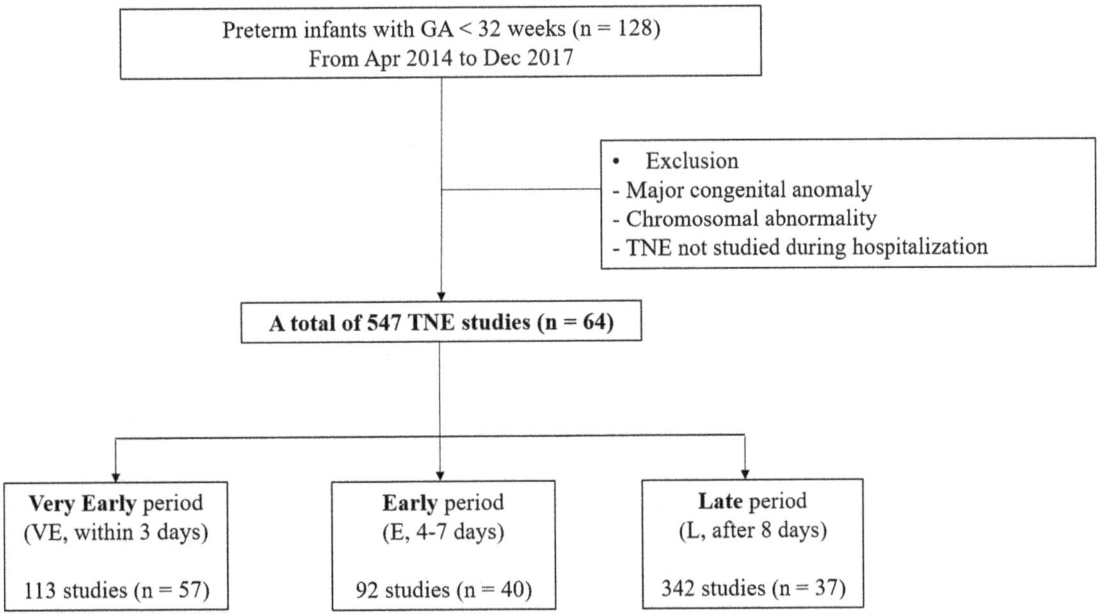

FIGURE 1 | Flowchart of the study population.

are outlined in **Figure 2**. *P*-values were analyzed to test the difference in the regression lines and slopes among groups. The regression lines of all echocardiographic markers except IVRT were significantly different between the VE and L days (**Table 4**). The slopes of the regressions showed significant changes depending on the time of birth for the maximum ductal velocity, LA/Ao ratio, LVO/SVC flow ratio, and LVO (**Table 5**). The slopes of the regressions for all markers except the maximum ductal velocity were statistically equivalent between the E and L days.

TABLE 1 | Demographics and outcomes.

Characteristics and outcomes	Values
Gestational age, weeks, median (IQR)	28^{+2} (26^{+4}-29^{+6})
Birth weight, g, median (IQR)	1,115 (950–1,397)
Number of echocardiograms, median (IQR)	6 (3–13)
Male sex, *n* (%)	44 (68.8)
PPROM, *n* (%)	17 (26.6)
Antenatal steroids (complete), *n* (%)	36 (56.3)
Surfactant administration, *n* (%)	57 (89.1)
Bronchopulmonary dysplasia, *n* (%)	37 (57.8)
Necrotizing enterocolitis, *n* (%)	5 (7.8)
Intraventricular hemorrhage grades 3–4, *n* (%)	7 (10.9)
Retinopathy of prematurity (laser/bevacizumab), *n* (%)	1 (1.6)
Death, *n* (%)	5 (7.8)
PDA, *n* (%)	
No treatment	19 (29.7)
Pharmacological treatment	30 (46.9)
Pharmacological treatment and ligation	6 (9.3)
Ligation	2 (3.1)

DISCUSSION

This study focused on the diameter of the PDA and its association with echocardiographic consequences of the shunt volume at the very early stages of life. It is difficult to estimate the echocardiographic markers of the ductal shunt and systemic hypoperfusion based on the PDA diameter in preterm infants younger than 4 days.

McNamara and Sehgal suggested a PDA staging system using clinical signs and echocardiographic parameters to understand the impact of the ductal shunt and PDA treatment (12, 13). However, their echocardiographic parameters have not been widely adopted in standard practice because of their extensive number of parameters and difficulties (14). Conventional echocardiographic markers such as PDA diameter do not predict neonatal outcomes, and it remains the routinely used parameter in clinical settings (15, 16). Based on the observations of our study, the PDA staging system was not correlated with the PDA diameter in the early period. We speculate that the impact of the PDA in echocardiography is less significant in the first 3 days of life due to the immediate transitional phase. The magnitude of the transductal shunt not only relates to the transductal diameter but also is affected by pulmonary and systemic vascular resistance and the compensatory ability of the immature myocardium depending on the time of birth (13). This result closely aligned with an earlier study reporting that clinical signs are not reliable in the first few days of life (17).

El-Khuffash et al. (18) proposed the use of another PDA severity score on day 2 after birth to predict the later occurrence of CLD/death. They suggested a predictive score within the first 48 h of life that could correlate with PDA-related morbidity, including GA, PDA diameter, LVO, maximum shunt velocity across PDA, and LV A wave. This suggestion is in accordance with the findings of our study, wherein the aforementioned factors showed a reliable correlation with the PDA diameter,

TABLE 2 | Clinical characteristics and echocardiographic markers of shunt volume based on postnatal age.

	Very early (*n* = 113)	Early (*n* = 92)	Late (*n* = 342)	*p*
Numbers of infants during the period, *n*	57	40	37	
Gestational age, weeks, median (IQR)	28^{+2} (26^{+4}-29^{+6})	27^{+6} (26^{+4}-29^{+6})	27^{+1} (26^{+0}-30^{+0})	0.536
Birth weight, g, median (IQR)	1,115 (950–1,415)	1,095 (940–1,367)	1,040 (880–1,315)	0.491
Mechanical ventilation during assessments, *n* (%)	87/113 (77.1)	44/92 (47.8)	123/342 (35.9)	<0.001
Pharmacological treatment for PDA, *n* (%)	30/58 (53.6)	23/40 (59.0)	22/37 (61.1)	0.492
PDA diameter (cm)	1.20 (1.03–1.50)	1.06 (0.90–1.31)	1.28 (1.00–1.68)	0.000
Ductal velocity max (m/s)	1.55 (1.18–2.19)	2.06 (1.48–2.50)	2.28 (1.68–2.92)	0.000
Antegrade LPA diastolic flow (cm/s)	23.88 (18.54–31.05)	24.55 (20.28–29.63)	27.23 (23.50–33.43)	0.000
Left atrial:aortic ratio	1.24 (1.18–1.33)	1.30 (1.20–1.38)	1.40 (1.27–1.50)	0.000
LVO/SVC flow ratio	1.57 (1.29–2.03)	1.63 (1.33–1.98)	1.93 (1.55–2.32)	0.000
E wave/A wave ratio	0.81 (0.77–0.86)	0.80 (0.76–0.87)	0.80 (0.75–0.85)	0.227
IVRT (ms)	59.15 (51.76–66.54)	51.81 (48.06–59.15)	48.06 (44.36–53.60)	0.000
Retrograde diastolic flow (%)	0 (0–23.56)	0 (0–18.23)	0 (0–17.92)	0.000
Left ventricular output (ml/kg/min)	202.0 (169.5–240.0)	240.5 (192.8–293.0)	296.0 (236.8–376.3)	0.000

Data are presented as median with interquartile range (IQR) for non-normally distributed variables. p values were obtained by Kruskal-Wallis test. PDA, patent ductus arteriosus; LPA, left pulmonary artery; LVO, left ventricular output; SVC, superior vena cava; IVRT, isovolumic relaxation time.

TABLE 3 | Univariate regression analysis of PDA diameter and echocardiographic markers of shunt volume based on postnatal age.

Markers	Very early			Early			Late		
	R^2	β coefficient correlation	p	R^2	β coefficient	p	R^2	β coefficient	p
Ductal velocity Vmax (m/s)	0.224	−0.777	0.000	0.091	−0.529	0.003	0.000	0.024	0.823
Antegrade LPA diastolic flow (cm/s)	0.166	10.632	0.000	0.144	8.502	0.000	0.175	9.192	0.000
LA/Ao ratio	0.010	0.036	0.291	0.230	0.145	0.000	0.311	0.210	0.000
LVO/SVC flow ratio	0.048	0.293	0.020	0.083	0.360	0.006	0.183	0.584	0.000
E wave/A wave ratio	0.059	0.083	0.010	0.160	0.135	0.000	0.033	0.062	0.001
IVRT (ms)	0.009	−2.990	0.325	0.099	−8.976	0.002	0.155	−7.043	0.000
Retrograde diastolic flow (%)	0.021	5.272	0.122	0.167	10.800	0.000	0.087	7.073	0.000
LVO (ml/kg/min)	0.028	24.206	0.078	0.344	92.591	0.000	0.272	128.940	0.000

LA/Ao, ratio of the left atrial diameter to aortic root diameter.

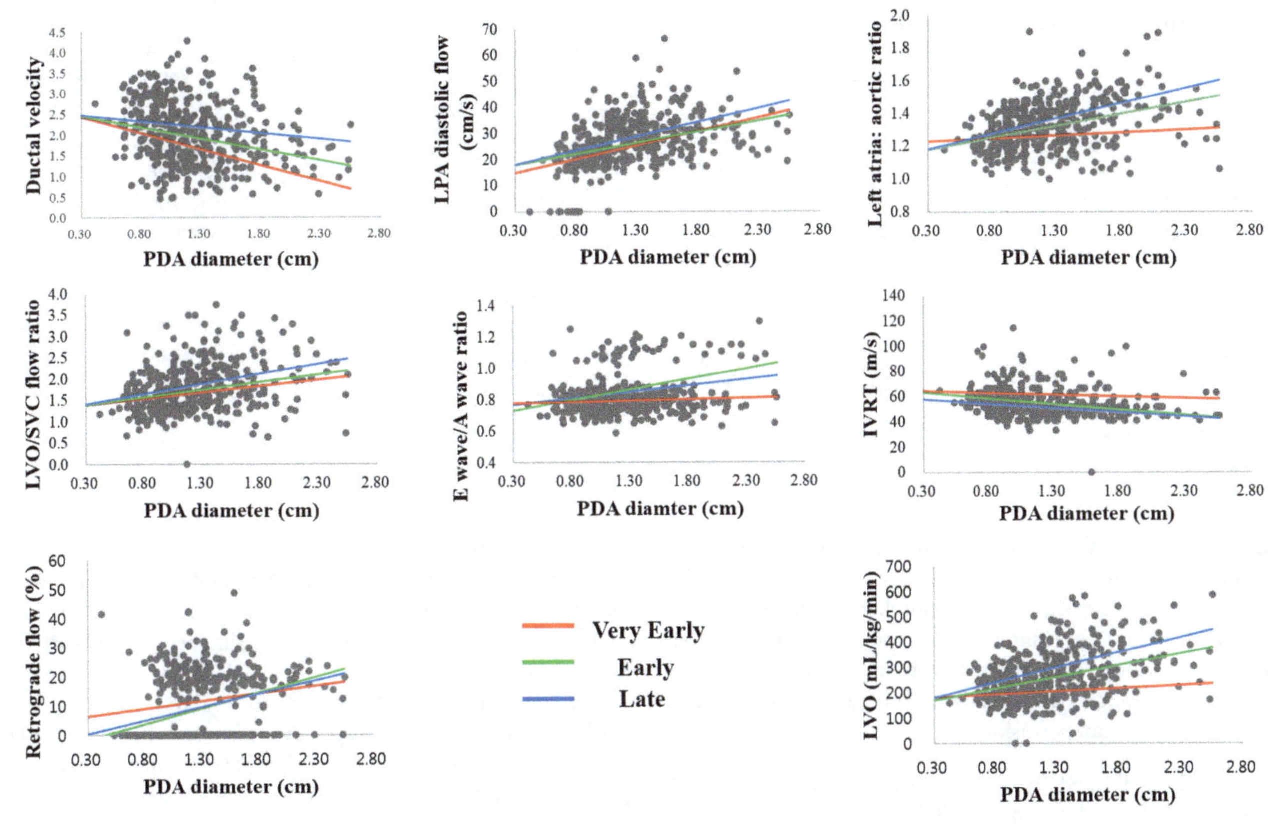

FIGURE 2 | Scatterplots showing the association between the echocardiographic markers with PDA diameter in the three periods.

despite being in the VE period. These factors could be predictive of the hemodynamic significance that can guide treatment decisions in the early period.

The treatment intervention for PDA in preterm infants varies from the conservative approach ("wait and watchful") to the active, early treatment approach. Recent evidence suggests that mortality may depend on the management of PDA, and a moderate approach is associated with optimal outcomes (19). While in some infants a careful "wait and watchful" strategy may be the best option, other infants may need treatment to minimize the comorbidities in the early postnatal period (20). Also, for extremely preterm infants in the transitional period, echocardiographic assessment for hsPDA is very important for the conservative management of hemodynamically unstable infants. Our report is the first to directly investigate the strength of association between echocardiographic markers of shunt volume and PDA diameter based on postnatal age in preterm infants. Our results might help to select newborns in the early postnatal period that should be treated in order to improve their clinical outcomes without a significant increase of markers of

TABLE 4 | Comparing the linear regression lines by analysis of the covariance.

	Very early vs. early		Early vs. late		Very early vs. late	
	t	*p*	*t*	*p*	*t*	*p*
Ductal velocity Vmax (m/s)	4.61,728	0.011	8.832,969	0.000	39.4,595	0.000
Antegrade LPA diastolic flow (cm/s)	0.847,749	0.430	3.744,606	0.024	15.20,804	0.000
LA/Ao ratio	0.686,919	0.504	1.676,959	0.188	5.061,182	0.007
LVO/SVC flow ratio	6.722,909	0.002	8.450,433	0.000	48.53,806	0.000
E wave/A wave ratio	0.317094	0.729	5.835,583	0.003	13.93,361	0.000
IVRT (ms)	0.845,727	0.431	2.88,524	0.057	0.919,061	0.397
Retrograde diastolic flow (%)	8.801,438	0.000	9.717,368	0.000	72.00,497	0.000
LVO (ml/kg/min)	2.446,328	0.089	1.066,506	0.345	5.463,855	0.005

p value <0.05 means the lines are significantly different.

TABLE 5 | Comparing the slopes of linear regression lines by analysis of the covariance.

	Very early vs. early		Early vs. late		Very early vs. late	
	t	*p*	*t*	*p*	*T*	*p*
Ductal velocity Vmax (m/s)	−1.12842	0.260	−2.3712	0.018	−3.780218	0.000
Antegrade LPA diastolic flow (cm/s)	0.6711137	0.503	−0.2831184	0.777	0.6102204	0.542
LA/Ao ratio	−2.390946	0.018	−1.766935	0.078	−4.738054	0.000
LVO/SVC flow ratio	−0.3765719	0.707	−1.503919	0.133	−2.057582	0.040
E wave/A wave ratio	−1.131472	0.260	1.799364	0.073	0.5451293	0.586
IVRT (ms)	1.419482	0.157	−0.8386917	0.402	1.715798	0.0869
Retrograde diastolic flow (%)	−1.266117	0.207	1.324976	0.186	−0.6051878	0.545
LVO (ml/kg/min)	−3.544158	0.000	−1.51831	0.130	−4.679049	0.000

p value <0.05 means the slopes are significantly different.

pulmonary over circulation and/or systemic hypoperfusion. PDA symptoms and echocardiography results are insignificant in the first few days of life; therefore, comprehensive interpretation is essential before any intervention including conservative management, along with assessment of other factors such as GA at birth, clinical risk, ventilation requirements, cardiac biomarkers, and organ perfusion.

Our study is limited by its retrospective design and small sample size. The indication for TNE evaluation was at the discretion of the attending neonatologist, which may have introduced a selection bias toward sicker patients. Although we did not report the clinical effectiveness of PDA treatment at any of the included periods, the clinical effectiveness of treatments of PDA cannot be concluded because of the retrospective design. Of note, there were no significant differences in receiving treatment among the three periods. Since the rates of hsPDA vary widely by center, our results may not be generalizable to other centers where the rates of hsPDA differ from ours. There is an urgent need of prospective randomized controlled trials to assess the effectiveness of targeted treatment of hsPDA in matched conditions, including the timing, medications used, GA, and PDA severity in order to assess the association between PDA treatment and outcomes in preterm infants.

In conclusion, we found a significantly weaker association between PDA diameter and echocardiographic parameters of shunt volume in the VE days after birth than in the other periods. It is difficult to predict the echocardiographic markers of ductal shunt by the PDA diameter in infants younger than 4 days. A prospective study identifying the proper criteria for beneficial PDA treatment, especially in the early period after birth, is of paramount importance.

ETHICS STATEMENT

The studies involving human participants were reviewed and approved by Institutional Review Board of the Korea University Ansan Hospital. Written informed consent from the participants' legal guardian/next of kin was not required to participate in this study in accordance with the national legislation and the institutional requirements.

AUTHOR CONTRIBUTIONS

EC: primary author and responsible for data collection, data analysis, and manuscript writing. KP: data collection. BC:

writing of the manuscript draft, editing, critical revision of the manuscript, and responsible for the overall content. All authors provided contributions and have read and approved the final version.

ACKNOWLEDGMENTS

The authors wish to thank Prof. Jae Hyung Cha for the invaluable help in the statistical analysis.

REFERENCES

1. Kluckow M, Seri I, Evans N. Functional echocardiography: an emerging clinical tool for the neonatologist. *J Pediatr.* (2007) 150:125–30. doi: 10.1016/j.jpeds.2006.10.056
2. van Laere D, van Overmeire B, Gupta S, El-Khuffash A, Savoia M, McNamara PJ, et al. Application of NPE in the assessment of a patent ductus arteriosus. *Pediatr Res.* (2018) 84:46–56. doi: 10.1038/s41390-018-0077-x
3. Kwinta P, Rudzinski A, Kruczek P, Kordon Z, Pietrzyk JJ. Can early echocardiographic findings predict patent ductus arteriosus? *Neonatology.* (2009) 95:141–8. doi: 10.1159/000153098
4. Roze JC, Cambonie G, Marchand-Martin L, Gournay V, Durrmeyer X, Durox M, et al. Association between early screening for patent ductus arteriosus and in-hospital mortality among extremely preterm infants. *JAMA.* (2015) 313:2441–8. doi: 10.1001/jama.2015.6734
5. Mertens L, Seri I, Marek J, Arlettaz R, Barker P, McNamara P, et al. Targeted neonatal echocardiography in the neonatal intensive care unit: practice guidelines and recommendations for training. *Eur J Echocardiogr.* (2011) 12:715–36. doi: 10.1016/j.echo.2011.07.014
6. Noori S, McCoy M, Anderson MP, Ramji F, Seri I. Changes in cardiac function and cerebral blood flow in relation to peri/intraventricular hemorrhage in extremely preterm infants. *J Pediatr.* (2014) 164:264–70 e1–3. doi: 10.1016/j.jpeds.2013.09.045
7. Osborn DA, Evans N, Kluckow M. Left ventricular contractility in extremely premature infants in the first day and response to inotropes. *Pediatr Res.* (2007) 61:335–40. doi: 10.1203/pdr.0b013e318030d1e1
8. Sehgal A, Menahem S. Interparametric correlation between echocardiographic markers in preterm infants with patent ductus arteriosus. *Pediatr Cardiol.* (2013) 34:1212–7. doi: 10.1007/s00246-013-0640-5
9. Hsu KH, Nguyen J, Dekom S, Ramanathan R, Noori S. Effects of patent ductus arteriosus on organ blood flow in infants born very preterm: a prospective study with serial echocardiography. *J Pediatr.* (2020) 216:95–100 e2. doi: 10.1016/j.jpeds.2019.08.057
10. de Freitas Martins F, Ibarra Rios D, MH FR, Javed H, Weisz D, Jain A, et al. Relationship of patent ductus arteriosus size to echocardiographic markers of shunt volume. *J Pediatr.* (2018) 202:50–5 e3. doi: 10.1016/j.jpeds.2018.06.045
11. Shin J, Lee EH, Lee JH, Choi BM, Hong YS. Individualized ibuprofen treatment using serial B-type natriuretic peptide measurement for symptomatic patent ductus arteriosus in very preterm infants. *Korean J Pediatr.* (2017) 60:175–80. doi: 10.3345/kjp.2017.60.6.175
12. Sehgal A, Paul E, Menahem S. Functional echocardiography in staging for ductal disease severity: role in predicting outcomes. *Eur J Pediatr.* (2013) 172:179–84. doi: 10.1007/s00431-012-1851-0
13. McNamara PJ, Sehgal A. Towards rational management of the patent ductus arteriosus: the need for disease staging. *Arch Dis Child Fetal Neonatal Ed.* (2007) 92:F424–7. doi: 10.1136/adc.2007.118117
14. Singh Y, Fraisse A, Erdeve O, Atasay B. Echocardiographic diagnosis and hemodynamic evaluation of patent ductus arteriosus in extremely low gestational age newborn (ELGAN) infants. *Front Pediatr.* (2020) 8:573627. doi: 10.3389/fped.2020.573627
15. Evans N. Current controversies in the diagnosis and treatment of patent ductus arteriosus in preterm infants. *Adv Neonatal Care.* (2003) 3:168–77. doi: 10.1016/S1536-0903(03)00143-7
16. Knight DB. The treatment of patent ductus arteriosus in preterm infants. A review and overview of randomized trials. *Semin Neonatol.* (2001) 6:63–73. doi: 10.1053/siny.2000.0036
17. Alagarsamy S, Chhabra M, Gudavalli M, Nadroo AM, Sutija VG, Yugrakh D. Comparison of clinical criteria with echocardiographic findings in diagnosing PDA in preterm infants. *J Perinat Med.* (2005) 33:161–4. doi: 10.1515/JPM.2005.030
18. El-Khuffash A, James AT, Corcoran JD, Dicker P, Franklin O, Elsayed YN, et al. A patent ductus arteriosus severity score predicts chronic lung disease or death before discharge. *J Pediatr.* (2015) 167:1354–61 e2. doi: 10.1016/j.jpeds.2015.09.028
19. Isayama T, Kusuda S, Reichman B, Lee SK, Lehtonen L, Norman M, et al. Neonatal intensive care unit-level patent ductus arteriosus treatment rates and outcomes in infants born extremely preterm. *J Pediatr.* (2020) 220:34–9 e5. doi: 10.1016/j.jpeds.2020.01.069
20. Terrin G, Di Chiara M, Boscarino G, Versacci P, Di Donato V, Giancotti A, et al. Echocardiography-Guided management of preterms with patent ductus arteriosus influences the outcome: a cohort study. *Front Pediatr.* (2020) 8:582735. doi: 10.3389/fped.2020.582735

23

Spontaneous Closure of the Ductus Arteriosus in Preterm Infants

Johan C. A. de Klerk[1], *Aline G. J. Engbers*[1,2], *Floor van Beek*[1], *Robert B. Flint*[1,3], *Irwin K. M. Reiss*[1], *Swantje Völler*[2,4] *and Sinno H. P. Simons*[1*]

[1] Division of Neonatology, Department of Pediatrics, Erasmus UMC—Sophia Children's Hospital, Rotterdam, Netherlands, [2] Division of Systems Biomedicine and Pharmacology, Leiden Amsterdam Center for Drug Research (LACDR), Leiden University, Leiden, Netherlands, [3] Department of Hospital Pharmacy, Erasmus UMC, Rotterdam, Netherlands, [4] Division of BioTherapeutics, Leiden Amsterdam Center for Drug Research (LACDR), Leiden University, Leiden, Netherlands

***Correspondence:**
Sinno H. P. Simons
s.simons@erasmusmc.nl

The optimal management strategy for patent ductus arteriosus in preterm infants remains a topic of debate. Available evidence for a treatment strategy might be biased by the delayed spontaneous closure of the ductus arteriosus in preterm infants, which appears to depend on patient characteristics. We performed a systematic review of all literature on PDA studies to collect patient characteristics and reported numbers of patients with a ductus arteriosus and spontaneous closure. Spontaneous closure rates showed a high variability but were lowest in studies that only included preterm infants with gestational ages below 28 weeks or birth weights below 1,000 g (34% on day 4; 41% on day 7) compared to studies that also included infants with higher gestational ages or higher birth weights (up to 55% on day 3 and 78% on day 7). The probability of spontaneous closure of the ductus arteriosus keeps increasing until at least 1 week after birth which favors delayed treatment of only those infants that do not show spontaneous closure. Better prediction of the spontaneous closure of the ductus arteriosus in the individual newborn is a key factor to find the optimal management strategy for PDA in preterm infants.

Keywords: patent ductus arteriosus, spontaneous closure, preterm infants, systematic review, VLBW, ELBW

INTRODUCTION

After preterm birth, the ductus arteriosus often remains open. Patent ductus arteriosus (PDA) in preterm infants has been associated with prolonged ventilation, bronchopulmonary dysplasia (BPD), and necrotizing enterocolitis potentially caused by pulmonary overcirculation and systemic hypoperfusion (1). It is unclear if these associations reflect a causal relationship or if PDA is a marker of poor condition and outcome, because outcomes of well-designed and controlled trials are still awaited (2). Treatment options include fluid restriction, pharmacological intervention with non-steroidal anti-inflammatory drugs (NSAIDs) or paracetamol, or closing the duct by surgical ligation or heart catheterization. All of these therapeutic options have their side-effects or specific risks in preterm infants. As a consequence, there is an ongoing worldwide discussion about the optimal management of PDA in preterm infants (3). This discussion is complicated by the lack of extensive knowledge on the (patho)physiology of the ductus arteriosus in preterm infants.

Intrauterine, the ductus arteriosus is needed and remains open due to the hypoxic fetal environment and by prostaglandins E2 (PGE2) produced by the placenta (4). Vasodilatation is further enhanced by nitric oxide (NO) produced by the wall of the ductus arteriosus (5). Upon term birth, the ductus arteriosus normally closes within hours. This is the result of different complex physiologic mechanisms that include changes in pulmonary and systemic vascular resistance, increase in arterial oxygen pressure, decreasing levels of prostaglandins and changes in different mediators and growth factors (6). After preterm birth, however, the ductus arteriosus frequently remains patent. Even after functional closure of the ductus arteriosus, either spontaneous or by pharmacological treatment, it might re-open in preterm infants afterwards caused by infection or increased inflammation (7).

Although the high levels of prostaglandins produced by the placenta also drop after preterm birth, the ductus arteriosus seems to remain much more sensitive to both PGE2 and NO in preterm infants compared to term born infants, due to increased expression of—and binding to—prostaglandin receptors in the ductal wall (5, 8). In addition to that, oxygenation and vascular resistance after preterm birth are hampered by an immature cardiovascular system and insufficient breathing whereas oxygen targets are decreased to prevent retinopathy of prematurity (9).

A substantial part of the preterm infants with PDA still seems to show delayed ductus closure without any intervention (10). The advantage of a wait-and-see PDA treatment strategy above intervention in the 1st days after birth (<72 h) may be that only those newborns without spontaneous ductus arteriosus closure are exposed to treatment and its potential side effects. On the other hand, early treatment strategy may be favored because the pharmacological closure rate seems to be highest on the 1st days of life (11, 12). Despite the limited studies on delayed treatment with NSAIDs and paracetamol, this late treatment seems less effective (13, 14). NSAIDs and paracetamol may enhance the spontaneous closure process. Therefore, the discussion on management of PDA in preterm infants cannot neglect the spontaneous closure, although a clear overview of the spontaneous closure rates is yet lacking. In this study, we aimed to provide such an overview of all available data from PDA studies to investigate and analyze the rates of spontaneous closure of the PDA.

METHODS

To retrieve all relevant evidence on the physiological spontaneous ductus arteriosus closure in preterm infants, we performed a thorough literature search. All studies published after 1990 that met both of the following criteria were considered eligible: (1) trials of any form including randomized controlled trials (RCTs), controlled clinical trials, quasi experimental studies [(un)controlled before and after studies], prospective and retrospective cohort studies and case-control studies and (2) trials with a clearly described timing of echocardiography to identify the presence or absence of a ductus arteriosus. Case series and case reports were excluded, as well as studies that reported on spontaneous closure after discharge. To examine spontaneous closure of the PDA, data on spontaneous closure before any intervention were collected and analyzed.

Search Strategy

A literature search was performed in collaboration with an experienced librarian. The search was done in MEDLINE, EMBASE, Cochrane central, Web of science, and Google Scholar until 2018 and included only English written articles. The following search terms were used "patent ductus arteriosus," "PDA," "preterm," "VLBW," and/or "prematurity." A more detailed search strategy for each library is available in **Supplementary File 1**.

The retrieved titles, abstracts, and full text were screened by two independent reviewers (JdK and FvB) to assess their eligibility according to pre-established criteria. Duplicate publications were excluded. The data extraction was done by the same two independent reviewers (JdK and FvB). Discrepancies were either resolved by discussion or by consulting a third reviewer (SS).

Data Synthesis

We developed a data extraction sheet, pilot-tested it on 10 randomly-selected included studies, and refined it accordingly. One review author (JdK) extracted the following data from included studies and the second author (FvB) checked the extracted data. Disagreements were resolved by discussion between the two review authors; if no agreement could be reached, it was planned a third author (SS) would decide. The data that was used included the following: total number of included neonates, their gestational age and birth weight, timing of the echocardiographic evaluation, and the number of neonates with closed ductus arteriosus at those times. Because only baseline reports of the occurrence of PDA were included, before any intervention for PDA was initiated, no bias of individual studies was expected.

Articles were categorized based on the inclusion criteria that were used in the studies for gestational age (GA) and birth weight (BW). Based on frequently used inclusion cut-off values of GA and BW, four different groups were defined prior to data collection: group 1: GA < 28 weeks and/or BW < 1,000 g, group 2: GA < 30 weeks and/or BW < 1,250 g, group 3: GA < 32 weeks and/or BW < 1,500 g, and group 4: GA < 37 weeks and/or BW < 2,500 g. If only GA or BW was given as inclusion criterion, this determined the category of the article, if both GA and BW were given as inclusion criteria, GA was leading for categorization. Studies were only included in one group: those included in group 1 were not included in groups 2–4, studies in group 2 were not included in group 3 and 4, and studies in group 3 were not included in group 4.

Data Analysis

The primary outcome of this systematic review was the rate of spontaneous closure of the ductus arteriosus in preterm infants as evaluated by echocardiography. A closed ductus arteriosus is defined as a ductus arteriosus that shows complete closure or no doppler flow on echocardiography as reported in the original reports. The closure rate was calculated as the part of patients with a closed ductus within a certain cohort (number of patients with a closed ductus divided by the total number of patients) at a time-point. To further explore how the observed trends were correlated to the maturational status of the patient, different subgroup analyses were performed for the different GA and BW groups.

R Software (V 3.5.1) was used in R Studio (V 1.1.643) to group, summarize, and visualize the data. The percentage of patients with PDA was plotted against postnatal age. To differentiate spontaneous closure between the different GA and BW groups, a linear smoothed line weighted by the total number of patients of each study was drawn. Mean percentages of patients with PDA of studies that performed an echocardiography on postnatal day 3 (between 72 and 95.9 h) and day 7 (between 168 and 191.9 h) were calculated, and were weighted by the number of patients in each study. These time-points were included because the ductus is mostly evaluated during the 1st days of life (<72 h) and administered courses of pharmacotherapy normally take 3 or 6 days.

RESULTS

Our literature search resulted in a retrieval of 8,173 records. After removing the duplicates 3,607 remained. Reading of the titles and abstracts resulted in 332 eligible articles. The arguments for exclusion of 233 articles after full text screening are listed in **Supplementary File 2**. The clinical characteristics of the included studies are summarized in **Supplementary File 3**. All studies were published between 1990 and 2018. Ninety-nine articles with a total of 29,532 patients were included in the analysis. In **Figure 1**, a flow diagram is presented of the studies retrieved for this review. **Figure 2** presents the reported percentages of patients with a PDA for each individual study with increasing postnatal ages. On PNA day 3 (all reported outcomes observed between 72 and 96 h of life), the mean reported percentage of patients that experienced spontaneous closure of the ductus arteriosus weighted by the number of patients was 47% (range 9–96%). On PNA day 7 (168–192 h) this percentage increased to 61% (11–100%).

Subgroup Analysis

In **Table 1**, the reported characteristics of all studies are presented per group, as well as the percentages of PDA closure at postnatal age days 3 and 7 and the studies and number of patients these are based on.

Eleven different articles were included in group 1 which contained preterm infants with a gestational age under 28 weeks and/or birth weight under 1,000 g (15–20, 54, 63–66). The median of reported mean or median GAs of the 17,156 patients in group 1 was 26.0 (range of mean/median 25.5–26.6) weeks. The median birth weight was 832 (range of medians 802–851) g. Exact numbers for gestational ages and birth weights were not available for three studies (19, 63, 66). Two of the 11 studies performed multiple cardiac ultrasounds to evaluate the PDA, ranging from 24 h until 61 days of postnatal age (15, 18). Seven of the 11 studies performed their first ultrasound at day 3 after birth.

Twenty articles were included in group 2 (GA < 30 weeks and/or BW < 1,250 g) (11, 21–29, 67–76). The median of the reported mean or median GA of the 2,980 patients in group 2 was 28.0 (range 26.2–28.8). The median of the reported mean or median birth weight was 1,028 (range 797–1,259) g. The exact gestational ages and birth weights were not available for four studies (28, 29, 69, 74). Seven of the 20 studies performed multiple cardiac ultrasounds to evaluate the PDA (21, 24, 25, 27, 67, 72, 73). The echocardiography was performed between 5 h and 28 days of postnatal age in all studies.

Forty-nine studies that included a total of 6,946 patients were eligible for group 3 (GA < 32 weeks and/or BW < 1,500 g) (30–45, 55–59, 77–103, 132). The median GA was 28.6 (range 26–31) weeks. The median birth weight was 1,120 (range 794–1,595) g. Exact gestational ages and birth weights were not available for nine studies (35, 38, 41, 42, 44, 85, 96, 100, 104). Multiple cardiac ultrasounds where performed in 14 of the 49 studies and were performed between 6 and 338 h of postnatal age.

Nineteen studies used GA < 37 weeks and/or birthweight < 2,500 g as inclusion criteria (group 4), in which a total of 2,450 patients were included (46–53, 60–62, 105–112). The median gestational age was 30.9 (range 28.1–31.2) weeks. The median birth weight was 1,479 (range 950–1,917) g. Gestational ages and/or birth weights were not available for six studies (47, 50, 53, 105, 107, 109). Six of the 19 studies performed multiple cardiac ultrasounds at varying post-natal ages between 24 and 168 h.

In **Figures 3** and **4** the reported percentage of preterm infants with PDA are presented for each subgroup with a postnatal age up to 3 and 7 days, respectively. To account for the large differences in number of patients (range 18–15,971), the size of the dots is scaled by the square root of the number of patients. At postnatal age day 3 (72–95.9 h), mean percentage of PDA closure was 34% for group 1, weighted by the number of patients in each study (range 9–71%). In group 2, this percentage was 47% (33–98%), and in group 3 this was 48% (22–65%). In group 4, the weighted mean was 55% at PNA 3 (15–97%).

At PNA 7, the weighted average of patients with a closed PDA was 41% for group 1 (11–97%). Of group 2, only one study was available with a reported percentage of closure at PNA 7, which was 77% (20 of 26 patients) (24). In group 3, the weighted average closure was 63% (38–100%) at PNA day 7, and for group 4 this was 78% (67–97%). Comparing **Figures 2–4** clearly show that with increasing postnatal ages the spontaneous closure continuous and PDA rates decrease. This is most obvious in the studies that also included the oldest groups of infants.

DISCUSSION

In this review, spontaneous closure rates of the ductus arteriosus in preterm neonates were systematically evaluated in 99 studies that represented 29,532 patients. As expected, we observed increasing rates of ductus closure with post-natal age and higher spontaneous closure rates in studies that also included

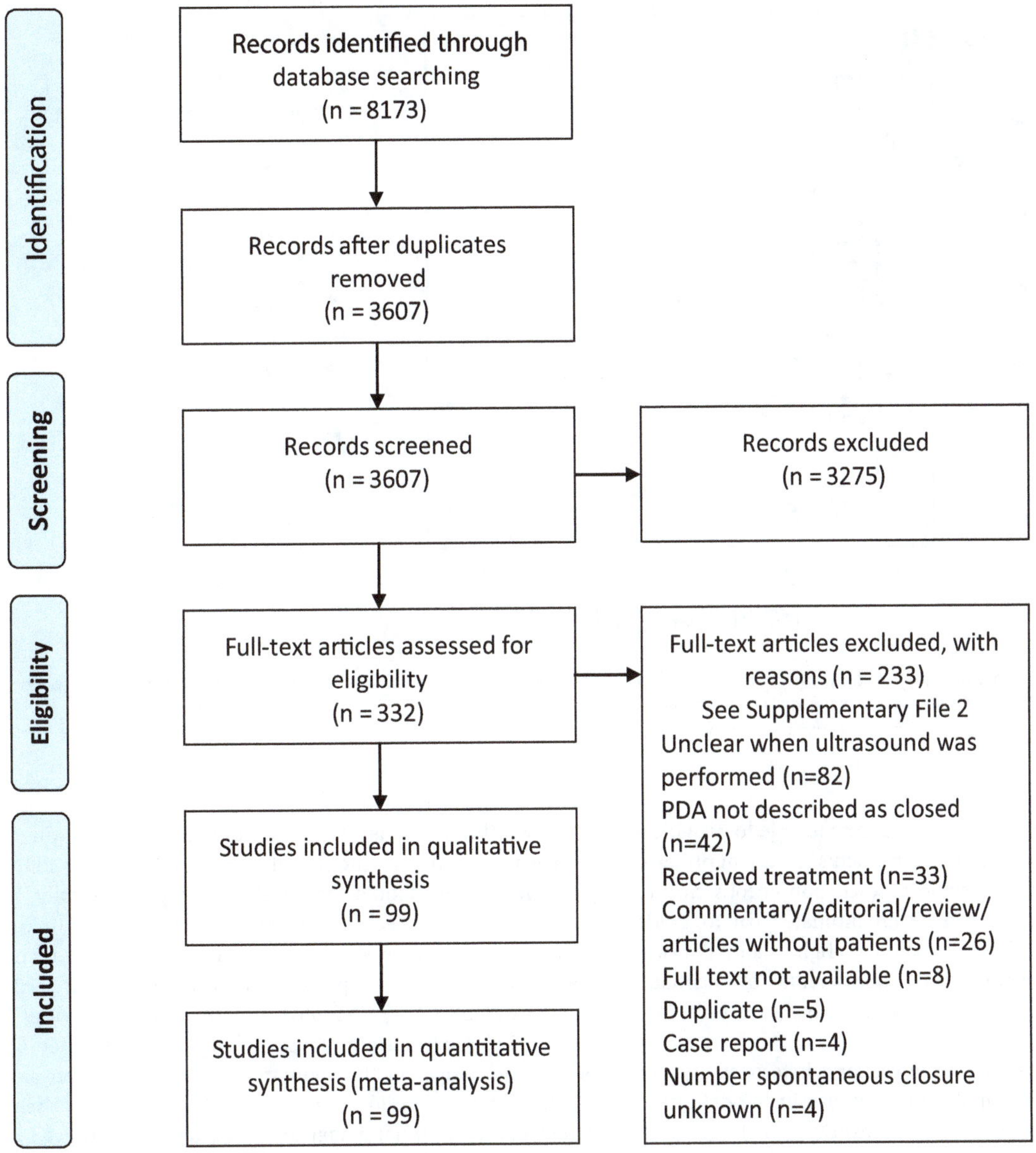

From: Moher D, Liberati A, Tetzlaff J, Altman DG, The PRISMA Group (2009). *P*referred *R*eporting *I*tems for *S*ystematic Reviews and *M*eta-*A*nalyses: The PRISMA Statement. PLoS Med 6(7): e1000097. doi:10.1371/journal.pmed1000097

For more information, visit www.prisma-statement.org.

FIGURE 1 | Flow diagram of the studies retrieved for this review.

patients with higher gestational ages. Spontaneous closure, however, occurs not only in the 1st day of life, but continues throughout the 1st week of life. Our systematic review revealed 34% spontaneous closure on the 3rd day of life (72–96 h) in the studies that only included the youngest group of infants (<28 weeks of GA and/or birthweight <1,000 g). If older infants were also included in studies, these closure rates increased up to 55%. At PNA day 7 (168–192 h) the ductus arteriosus was closed in 41% of the newborns in studies of the youngest infants and up to 78% in the studies that also included older gestational age groups. Because of a lack of detailed reports in the individual studies on subgroups of patients and the lack of longitudinal

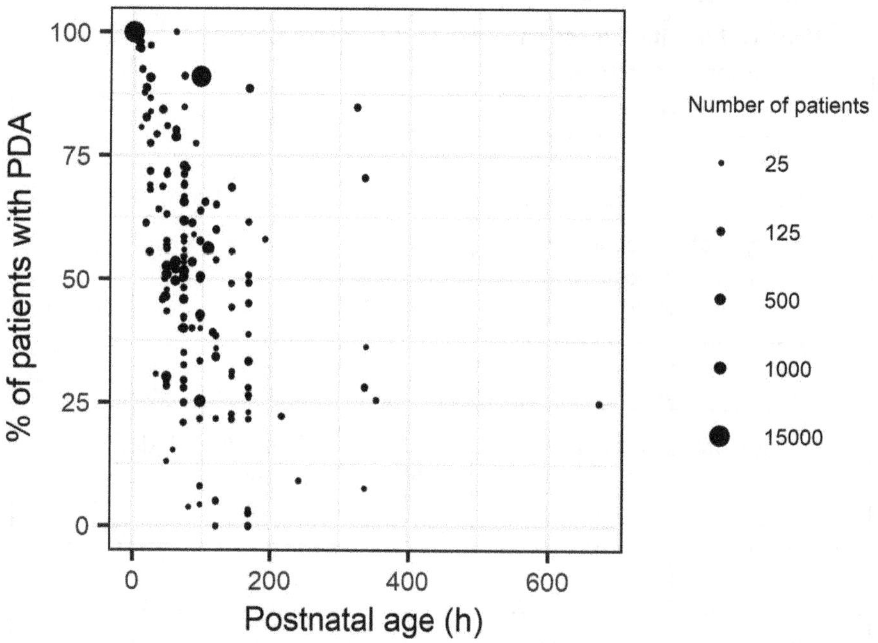

FIGURE 2 | Reported percentages of closure of patent ductus arteriosus of all included studies, up to a postnatal age of 28 days. Each dot represents a reported percentage, whose size represents the square root of the total number of patients of that observation.

assessment of the ductus arteriosus we were unable to provide a mathematical function of spontaneous ductus closure in preterm infants. Such a function that could predict spontaneous closure in an individual patient would be an ultimate goal to guide PDA management in individual patients. High quality datasets with repeated echocardiographic assessments of neonatal patients treated in current neonatal intensive care units are needed first.

Studies that reported on PDA showed large heterogeneity, not only in included patient populations, but also in the definition of a hemodynamically significant PDA (hsPDA) (113). It is quite clear that the significance of a PDA is not only determined by the diameter of the ductus, as was used in the current review, but also by the pulmonary vascular resistance. The lack of consensus on the definition of a hsPDA is partly based on the lack of validated echocardiographic markers and cutoff values. van Laere et al. (114) proposed to standardize essential echocardiographic measurements for the assessment of hemodynamic significance of a PDA. These consist of evaluation of the ductus arteriosus itself (including the diameter, flow direction, and velocity), indices of pulmonary overcirculation (La:Ao, left pulmonary artery diastolic flow) and indices of systemic shunt effect (flow pattern in aorta descendens, tructus coeliacus, or middle cerebral artery) (114). The LA:Ao ratio, ductal diameter and diastolic flow in the left pulmonary artery are easy to measure and seem the most accurate and easy to determine markers for a hsPDA (115). In our aim to select those infants that would not show spontaneous closure and might actually need PDA treatment these markers would be useful.

Currently, there is no international consensus on PDA management. It is unclear if, how and when PDA in preterm infants should be treated. More specifically, it is unclear if PDA needs treatment because it is unknown which preterm infants might benefit more from treatment than others. Therefore, prophylaxis, early treatment (<24 h), late treatment (72 h), symptomatic treatment and wait and see strategies are currently used alongside each other (116). Better knowledge on the spontaneous closure and physiology of the ductus arteriosus in preterm infants may help to determine the optimal management strategy. This is even more important as prophylactic as well as therapeutic treatment strategies are associated with risks for adverse effects, such as intraventricular hemorrhages and decreased renal function that might have severe consequences in these vulnerable patients. Treatment of the PDA, pharmacologically or surgically, should therefore be reserved for those patients who may benefit from it.

Next to the ongoing discussion on the type of drug being either ibuprofen, indomethacin, or acetaminophen (117–124), the timing of treatment initiation varies widely between studies, and might explain reported differences in efficacy. As spontaneous ductus closure increases with PNA, part of ductus closure reported in prophylactic and early treatment studies may be due to spontaneous closure rather than drug treatment. Efficacy of PDA pharmacotherapy seems to decrease, with post-natal age, even if dosages are increased with PNA to correct for increased clearance with age (10, 13). This suggests either a certain window of opportunity for PDA

TABLE 1 | Summary of reported mean or median gestational age and birthweight of the included studies, and reported percentages of PDA closure at postnatal age days 3 and 7.

	Group 1	Group 2	Group 3	Group 4	All studies
Inclusion criteria	GA < 28 weeks and/or birth weight <1,000 g	GA < 30 weeks and/or birth weight <1,250 g	GA < 32 weeks and/or birth weight <1,500 g	GA < 37 weeks and/or birth weight <2,500 g	
Number of studies	11	20	49	19	99
Total number of patients	17,156	2,980	6,946	2,450	29,532
Gestational Age					
Mean (weeks) [median (range)] (*n*)	26.0 [25.5–26.6] (8)	28.0 [26.2–28.8] (13)	28.4 [26.0–30.0] (22)	30.8 [30.2–31.1] (7)	28.1 [25.5–31.2] (50)
Median [median (range)]	–	28.0 [-] (2)	29 [27–31] (15)	31.0 [28.1–31.0] (5)	29.0 [27.0–31.0] (22)
Not reported (*n*)	3	5	12	7	27
Birth weight					
Mean [median (range)]	818 [802–851] (8)	1,028 [(797–1,259] (13)	112 [794–1,371] (22)	1,543 [1,355–1,917] (7)	1,082 [794–1,917] (50)
Median [median (range)]	–	1,060–1,062 (2)	1,160 [980–1,595] (15)	1,475 [950–1,640] (5)	1,160 [950–1,640] (22)
Not reported (*n*)	3	5	12	7	27
Postnatal age of cardiac ultrasound					
Median postnatal age in h (range)	72 (18–1,464)	72 (5–672)	79 (6–3,864)	72 (24–1,632	72 (5–3,864)
Percentage of PDA closure at postnatal age 3 (72–95.9 h)					
Weighted mean percentage of patients with PDA (range)	34% (9–71)	47% (33–98)	48% (22–65)	55% (15–79)	47% (9–96)
Number of studies with reported percentage	6	9	16	8	39
Total number of patients	646	978	1,709	621	3,954
Study references	(15–20)	(21–29)	(30–45)	(46–53)	(15–53)
Percentage of PDA closure at postnatal age 7 (168–191.9 h)					
Weighted mean percentage of patients with PDA (range)	41% (11–97)	77 % (-)	63% (38–100)	78% (67–97)	61% (11–100)
Number of studies with reported percentage	2	1	8	5	16
Total number of patients	228	26	550	181	985
Study references	(18, 54)	(24)	(30, 33, 43, 55–59)	(46, 50, 60–62)	(18, 24, 30, 33, 43, 46, 50, 54–62)

Separated by groups based on inclusion criteria.

treatment during the physiological process that is involved in the spontaneous closure of the ductus arteriosus or the need for higher drug exposures at older ages. Such a window can only be identified if the rate of spontaneous closure is well-characterized, and efficacy studies can correct for the chance of spontaneous closure.

With the current review, we have summarized the evidence that spontaneous closure is less likely to occur in preterm neonates with the lowest gestational ages. Nevertheless, in another significant number of preterm infants the ductus arteriosus although delayed, closes spontaneously within the first 150 h of life. The presented review was limited by the lack of detailed reports of PDA for different gestational age groups in the included studies. While the literature was systematically reviewed we were unfortunately unable to provide statistical analysis due to complexity of outcome data. This also resulted in overlap of patients in the different groups. All studies only had an upper limit of gestational age and/or bodyweight without a lower limit for gestational age/weight. As a consequence, the gestational age/weight range of inclusion criteria of the included studies increases from group 1 to 4. Therefore, the actual difference in the occurrence of spontaneous closure between different GA groups is bigger than observed in the present study. As other widely used measures for ductus closure, such as LA:Ao

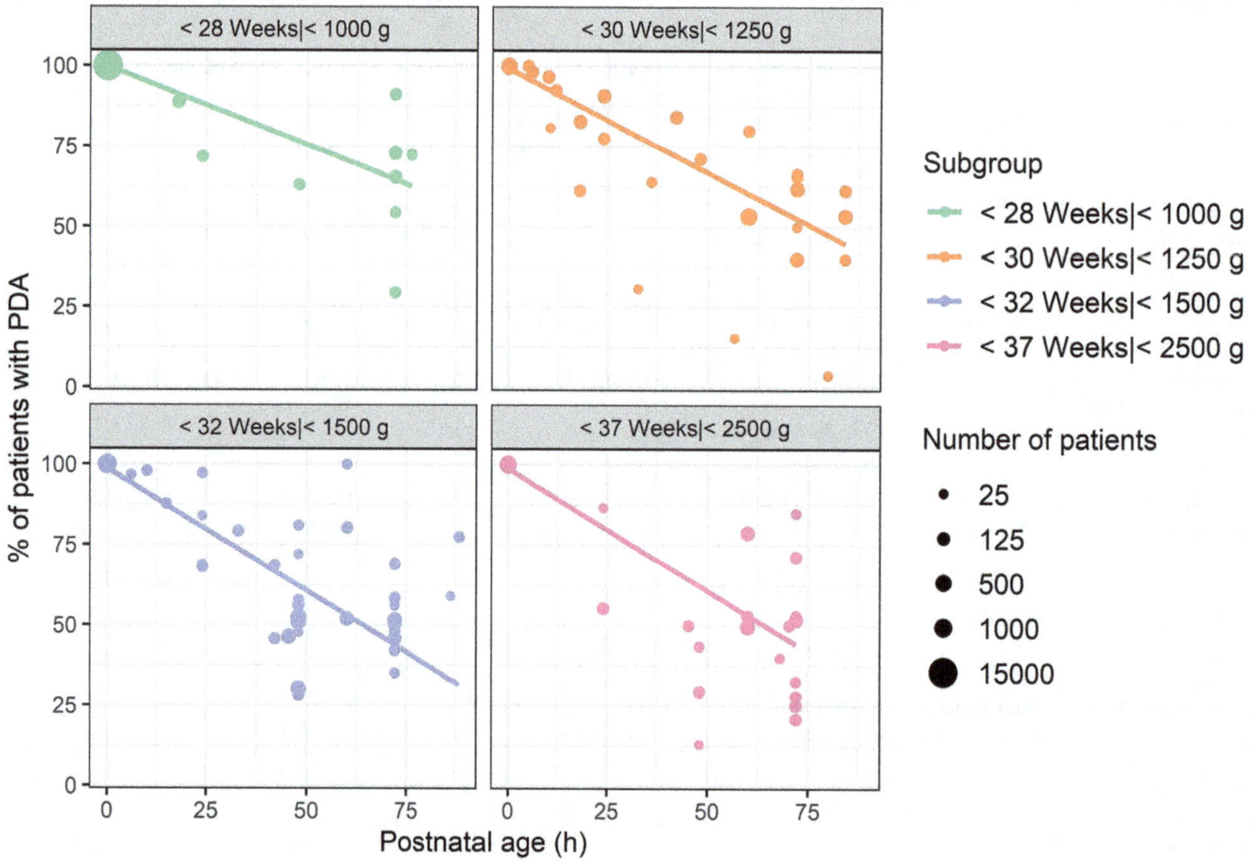

FIGURE 3 | Reported percentages of patients with patent ductus arteriosus up to a postnatal age of 4 days, grouped by mean or median gestational age or birthweight if gestational age was unreported. Each dot represents one observation at the reported postnatal age. The size of the dots represents square root of the number of patients of each observation. Lines represent a linear smooth weighted by the number of patients of each observation.

ratio were mostly missing, we defined a closed ductus as a ductus that was visually closed or when there was no doppler flow visible on echocardiography. As discussed previously, a better definition of a hsPDA might be desirable and might lead to a more precise estimation of incidence- and closure-rates. In this study, we presented the relationships between spontaneous closure rate and PNA as linear relationships. In reality, the spontaneous closure rate is probably highest on the 1st day and decreases with an asymptotic shape since in some patients the spontaneous closure will not occur, or the percentage of patients with PDA might even go up if the ductus arteriosus reopens. With the available data, it is not possible to determine whether the reported numbers of PDA at high postnatal ages (**Figure 2**) are due to non-closure or re-opening because seventy of the 99 articles performed only one echocardiography. Therefore, there were insufficient data to study potential reopening of the ductus arteriosus in this review. The patency of the ductus arteriosus is regulated by the balance of vasodilating (prostaglandin E2, nitric oxide) and vasoconstrictor (oxygen) factors (6). Preterm neonates are more sensitive to the vasodilating factors compared to the term neonates (5). There is some evidence suggesting that genetic variations may play a role in the occurrence of PDA in preterm infants. In a large cohort of 1,013 preterm neonates Dagle et al. (125) found that several single nucleotide polymorphisms that were associated with PDA. For future meta-analyses, it might thus be of interest to include genetic variations to determine their influence on spontaneous closure.

Our systematic review was based on the assumption that gestational age is a more important factor compared to birthweight for patent ductus arteriosus in preterm infants. Villamor-Martinez et al. (126) showed that small for gestational age (SGA) infants showed a significantly reduced risk of PDA, but their review was complicated by the heterogeneity of studies. As SGA infants also show a much higher clearance of ibuprofen compared to appropriate weight for age newborns these patients form a special population that need additional attention in future PDA studies (127).

A next step could be to find markers to repeatedly monitor closure and pathophysiology of the ductus arteriosus. These could include the continuously available perfusion index to identify a hemodynamic significant PDA (51, 128) or urinary prostaglandine levels (129). Neutrophil gelatinase-associated lipocalin and heart-type fatty acid-binding protein are two

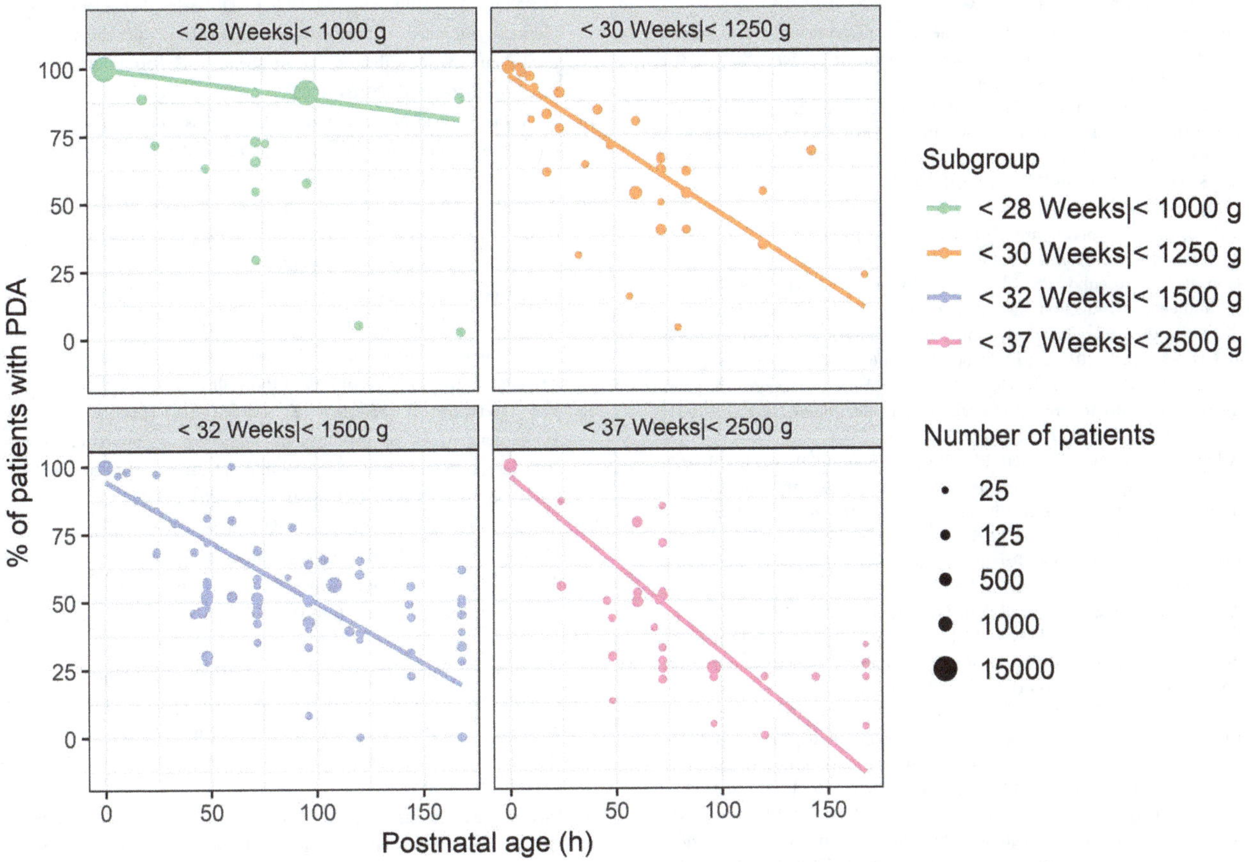

FIGURE 4 | Reported percentages of patients with patent ductus arteriosus up to a postnatal age of 8 days, grouped by mean or median gestational age or birthweight if gestational age was unreported. Each dot represents one observation at the reported postnatal age. The size of the dots represents square root of the number of patients of each observation. Lines represent a linear smooth weighted by the number of patients of each observation.

peptides that can be measured in urine and also appear to be promising future markers to quantify the effect of a PDA on systemic perfusion, which makes the ductus arteriosus more hemodynamic significant (130, 131). Relevant risk factors could help to predict those patients whose ductus arteriosus will remain open and for whom pharmacological treatment might be needed.

Spontaneous closure rates increase with both gestational age and postnatal age. This review showed that in 34% of the most premature infants (GA < 28 weeks and/or BW < 1,000 g), the ductus arteriosus had spontaneously closed on the 3rd day of life (72–96 h). This increased to 41% at PNA day 7. As patients with a GA < 28 weeks have the lowest chance of spontaneous closure of the ductus arteriosus in the 1st days of life, studies on PDA management should therefore focus on these most premature patients.

AUTHOR CONTRIBUTIONS

JK is responsible for the study design, data collection and extraction, and writing and editing the article. AE is responsible for the data analysis and writing the article. SV helped with the analysis and edited the manuscript. FB performed the data collection and extraction. RF supervised the design and edited the manuscript. IR supervised the design and edited the manuscript. SS supervised the study design, data collection, and contributed with the editing of the article. All authors contributed to the article and approved the submitted version.

ACKNOWLEDGMENTS

We would like to thank W. G. Kramer for his help in the literature search.

REFERENCES

1. Clyman RI. The role of patent ductus arteriosus and its treatments in the development of bronchopulmonary dysplasia. *Semin Perinatol.* (2013) 37:102–7. doi: 10.1053/j.semperi.2013.01.006
2. Hundscheid T, Onland W, Overmeire B Van, Dijk P, Kaam AHLC Van, Dijkman KP, et al. Early treatment versus expectative management of patent ductus arteriosus in preterm infants: a multicentre, randomised, non-inferiority trial in Europe (BeNeDuctus trial). *BMC Pediatr.* (2018) 18:262. doi: 10.1186/s12887-018-1215-7
3. Laughon M, Bose C, Clark R. Treatment strategies to prevent or close a patent ductus arteriosus in preterm infants and outcomes. *J Perinatol.* (2007)

27:164–70. doi: 10.1038/sj.jp.7211662
4. Hung YC, Yeh JL, Hsu JH. Molecular mechanisms for regulating postnatal ductus arteriosus closure. *Int J Mol Sci.* (2018) 19:1861. doi: 10.3390/ijms19071861
5. Hundscheid T, van den Broek M, van der Lee R, de Boode WP. Understanding the pathobiology in patent ductus arteriosus in prematurity-beyond prostaglandins and oxygen. *Pediatr Res.* (2019) 86:28–38. doi: 10.1038/s41390-019-0387-7
6. Chiruvolu A, Jaleel MA. Pathophysiology of patent ductus arteriosus in premature neonates. *Early Hum Dev.* (2009) 85:143–6. doi: 10.1016/j.earlhumdev.2008.12.006
7. Gonzalez A, Sosenko IRS, Chandar J, Hummler H, Claure N, Bancalari E. Influence of infection on patent ductus arteriosus and chronic lung disease in premature infants weighing 1000 grams or less. *J Pediatr.* (1996) 128:470–8. doi: 10.1016/S0022-3476(96)70356-6
8. Bardanzellu F, Neroni P, Dessì A, Fanos V. Paracetamol in patent ductus arteriosus treatment: efficacious and safe? *Biomed Res Int.* (2017) 2017:1438038. doi: 10.1155/2017/1438038
9. Askie LM, Darlow BA, Davis PG, Finer N, Stenson B, Vento M, et al. Effects of targeting lower versus higher arterial oxygen saturations on death or disability in preterm infants. *Cochrane Database Syst Rev.* (2017) 2017:CD011190. doi: 10.1002/14651858.CD011190.pub2
10. Benitz WE, Fetus CON. Patent ductus arteriosus in preterm infants. *Pediatrics.* (2016) 137:1–6. doi: 10.1542/peds.2015-3730
11. Aranda JV, Clyman R, Cox B, Van Overmeire B, Wozniak P, Sosenko I, et al. A randomized, double-blind, placebo- controlled trial on intravenous ibuprofen L-lysine for the early closure of nonsymptomatic patent ductus arteriosus within 72 hours of birth in extremely low-birth-weight infants. *Am J Perinatol.* (2009) 26:235–46. doi: 10.1055/s-0028-1103515
12. Kluckow M, Jeffery M, Gill A, Evans N. A randomised placebo-controlled trial of early treatment of the patent ductus arteriosus. *Arch Dis Child Fetal Neonatal Ed.* (2014) 99:F99–104. doi: 10.1136/archdischild-2013-304695
13. de Klerk JCA, van Paassen N, van Beynum IM, Flint RB, Reiss IKM, Simons SHP. Ibuprofen treatment after the first days of life in preterm neonates with patent ductus arteriosus. *J Matern Neonatal Med.* (2019) 1–7. doi: 10.1080/14767058.2019.1667323. [Epub ahead of print].
14. Roofthooft DWE, Van Beynum IM, Helbing WA, Reiss IKM, Simons SHP. Paracetamol for ductus arteriosus closure: not always a success story. *Neonatology.* (2013) 104:170. doi: 10.1159/000353451
15. Rolland A, Shankar-Aguilera S, Diomandé D, Zupan-Simunek V, Boileau P. Natural evolution of patent ductus arteriosus in the extremely preterm infant. *Arch Dis Child Fetal Neonatal Ed.* (2015) 100:F55–8. doi: 10.1136/archdischild-2014-306339
16. Narayanan M, Cooper B, Weiss H, Clyman RI. Prophylactic indomethacin: factors determining permanent ductus arteriosus closure. *J Pediatr.* (2000) 136:330–7. doi: 10.1067/mpd.2000.103414
17. Gournay V, Roze JC, Kuster A, Daoud P, Cambonie G, Hascoet JM, et al. Prophylactic ibuprofen versus placebo in very premature infants: a randomised, double-blind, placebo-controlled trial. *Lancet.* (2004) 364:1939–44. doi: 10.1016/S0140-6736(04)17476-X
18. Dani C, Bertini G, Pezzati M, Poggi C, Guerrini P, Martano C, et al. Prophylactic ibuprofen for the prevention of intraventricular hemorrhage among preterm infants: a multicenter, randomized study. *Pediatrics.* (2005) 115:1529–35. doi: 10.1542/peds.2004-1178
19. Erdeve O, Yurttutan S, Altug N, Ozdemir R, Gokmen T, Dilmen U, et al. Oral versus intravenous ibuprofen for patent ductus arteriosus closure: a randomised controlled trial in extremely low birthweight infants. *Arch Dis Child Fetal Neonatal Ed.* (2012) 97:F279–83. doi: 10.1136/archdischild-2011-300532
20. Polat TB, Celik IH, Erdeve O. Early predictive echocardiographic features of hemodynamically significant patent ductus arteriosus in preterm VLBW infants. *Pediatr Int.* (2016) 58:589–94. doi: 10.1111/ped.12915
21. Reller MD, Laird MR, Rice MJ, McDonald RW. Timing of ductal closure in very low birth weight premature infants without respiratory distress. *J Pediatr.* (1991) 119:976–7. doi: 10.1016/S0022-3476(05)83060-4
22. Parikh R, Negrine RJS, Chikermane A, Rasiah SV, Ewer AK. Assessment of myocardial function in preterm infants with patent ductus arteriosus using tissue Doppler imaging. *Cardiol Young.* (2014) 25:70–5. doi: 10.1017/S1047951113001595
23. Bin-Nun A, Mimouni FB, Fink D, Sela H, Hammerman C. Elevated nucleated red blood cells at birth predict hemodynamically significant patent ductus arteriosus. *J Pediatr.* (2016) 177:313–5. doi: 10.1016/j.jpeds.2016.07.005
24. De Waal K, Phad N, Lakkundi A, Tan P. Post-transitional adaptation of the left heart in uncomplicated, very preterm infants. *Cardiol Young.* (2017) 27:1167–73. doi: 10.1017/S1047951116002687
25. de Waal K, Phad N, Boyle A. Left atrium function and deformation in very preterm infants with and without volume load. *Echocardiography.* (2018) 35:1818–26. doi: 10.1111/echo.14140
26. Kahvecioglu D, Erdeve O, Akduman H, Ucar T, Alan S, Çakir U, et al. Influence of platelet count, platelet mass index, and platelet function on the spontaneous closure of ductus arteriosus in the prematurity. *Pediatr Neonatol.* (2018) 59:53–7. doi: 10.1016/j.pedneo.2017.01.006
27. Van Overmeire B, Allegaert K, Casaer A, Debauche C, Decaluwé W, Jespers A, et al. Prophylactic ibuprofen in premature infants: a multicentre, randomised, double-blind, placebo-controlled trial. *Lancet.* (2004) 364:1945–9. doi: 10.1016/S0140-6736(04)17477-1
28. Braulio R, Gelape CL, Araújo FD da R, Brandão KN, Abreu LDG, Costa PHN, et al. Indicadores para o tratamento cirúrgico na persistência do ducto arterial em neonatos prematuros na primeira semana de vida. *Braz J Cardiovasc Surg.* (2013) 28:504–8. doi: 10.5935/1678-9741.20130082
29. Oncel MY, Yurttutan S, Erdeve O, Uras N, Altug N, Oguz SS, et al. Oral paracetamol versus oral ibuprofen in the management of patent ductus arteriosus in preterm infants: A randomized controlled trial. *J Pediatr.* (2014) 164:510–4.e1. doi: 10.1016/j.jpeds.2013.11.008
30. Skelton R, Evans N, Smythe J. A blinded comparison of clinical and echocardiographic evaluation of the preterm infant for patent ductus arteriosus. *J Paediatr Child Health.* (1994) 30:406–11. doi: 10.1111/j.1440-1754.1994.tb00689.x
31. Su BH, Watanabe T, Shimizu M, Yanagisawa M. Echocardiographic assessment of patent ductus arteriosus shunt flow pattern in premature infants. *Arch Dis Child Fetal Neonatal Ed.* (1997) 77:36–40. doi: 10.1136/fn.77.1.F36
32. El-Khuffash A, Barry D, Walsh K, Davis PG, Molloy EJ. Biochemical markers may identify preterm infants with a patent ductus arteriosus at high risk of death or severe intraventricular haemorrhage. *Arch Dis Child Fetal Neonatal Ed.* (2008) 93:407–13. doi: 10.1136/adc.2007.133140
33. Nemerofsky SL, Parravicini E, Bateman D, Kleinman C, Polin RA, Lorenz JM. The ductus arteriosus rarely requires treatment in infants > 1000 grams. *Am J Perinatol.* (2008) 25:661–6. doi: 10.1055/s-0028-1090594
34. Sangtawesin C, Sangtawesin V, Lertsutthiwong W, Kanjanapattanakul W, Khorana M, Ayudhaya JKN. Prophylaxis of symptomatic patent ductus arteriosus with oral ibuprofen in very low birth weight infants. *J Med Assoc Thai.* (2008) 91(Suppl 3):28–34.
35. Gokmen T, Erdeve O, Altug N, Oguz SS, Uras N, Dilmen U. Efficacy and safety of oral versus intravenous ibuprofen in very low birth weight preterm infants with patent ductus arteriosus. *J Pediatr.* (2011) 158:549–54. doi: 10.1016/j.jpeds.2010.10.008
36. De Carolis MP, Romagnoli C, Polimeni V, Piersigilli F, Zecca E, Papacci P, et al. Prophylactic ibuprofen therapy of patent ductus arteriosus in preterm infants. *Eur J Pediatr.* (2000) 159:364–8. doi: 10.1007/s004310051288
37. Sellmer A, Bjerre JV, Schmidt MR, McNamara PJ, Hjortdal VE, Høst B, et al. Morbidity and mortality in preterm neonates with patent ductus arteriosus on day 3. *Arch Dis Child Fetal Neonatal Ed.* (2013) 98:F505–10. doi: 10.1136/archdischild-2013-303816

38. Akar S, Karadag N, Gokmen Yildirim T, Toptan HH, Dincer E, Tuten A, et al. Does platelet mass influence the effectiveness of ibuprofen treatment for patent ductus arteriosus in preterm infants? *J Matern Neonatal Med.* (2016) 29:3786–9. doi: 10.3109/14767058.2016.1145207
39. Härkin P, Härmä A, Aikio O, Valkama M, Leskinen M, Saarela T, et al. Paracetamol accelerates closure of the ductus arteriosus after premature birth: a randomized trial. *J Pediatr.* (2016) 177:72–7.e2. doi: 10.1016/j.jpeds.2016.04.066
40. Van Der Laan ME, Roofthooft MTR, Fries MWA, Berger RMF, Schat TE, Van Zoonen AGJF, et al. A hemodynamically significant patent ductus arteriosus does not affect cerebral or renal tissue oxygenation in preterm infants. *Neonatology.* (2016) 110:141–7. doi: 10.1159/000445101
41. Demir N, Peker E, Ece I, Balahoroglu R, Tuncer O. Efficacy and safety of rectal ibuprofen for patent ductus arteriosus closure in very low birth weight preterm infants. *J Matern Neonatal Med.* (2017) 30:2119–25. doi: 10.1080/14767058.2016.1238897
42. Sellmer A, Bech BH, Bjerre JV, Schmidt MR, Hjortdal VE, Esberg G, et al. Urinary neutrophil gelatinase-associated lipocalin in the evaluation of patent ductus arteriosus and AKI in very preterm neonates: a cohort study. *BMC Pediatr.* (2017) 17:7. doi: 10.1186/s12887-016-0761-0
43. Yum SK, Moon CJ, Youn YA, Lee JY, Sung IK. Echocardiographic assessment of patent ductus arteriosus in very low birthweight infants over time: prospective observational study. *J Matern Neonatal Med.* (2018) 31:164–72. doi: 10.1080/14767058.2016.1278207
44. Heyman E, Morag I, Batash D, Keidar R, Baram S, Berkovitch M. Closure of patent ductus arteriosus with oral ibuprofen suspension in premature newborns: a pilot study. *Pediatrics.* (2003) 112(5). doi: 10.1542/peds.112.5.e354
45. Schmitz L, Stiller B, Koch H, Koehne P, Lange P. Diastolic left ventricular function in preterm infants with a patent ductus arteriosus: a serial Doppler echocardiography study. *Early Hum Dev.* (2004) 76:91–100. doi: 10.1016/j.earlhumdev.2003.11.002
46. Shortland DB, Gibson NA, Levene MI, Archer LNJ, Evans DH, Shaw DE. Patent ductus arteriosus and cerebral circulation in preterm infants. *Dev Med Child Neurol.* (1990) 32:386–93. doi: 10.1111/j.1469-8749.1990.tb16957.x
47. Kulkarni VV, Dutta S, Sundaram V, Saini SS. Preterm thrombocytopenia and delay of ductus arteriosus closure. *Pediatrics.* (2016) 138:e20161627. doi: 10.1542/peds.2016-1627
48. Babaei H, Nemati R, Daryoshi H. Closure of patent ductus arteriosus with oral acetaminophen in preterm neonates: a randomized trial. *Biomed Res Ther.* (2018) 5:2034–44. doi: 10.15419/bmrat.v5i02.418
49. Bagheri MM, Bahman-Bijari B, Torabi-Nejad MH, Niknafs P, Mousavi H, Sabzevari F, et al. Is prophylactic parenteral paracetamol effective to diminish incidence of PDA in preterm neonates? A randomized trial. *Iran J Pediatr.* (2018) 28:10–3. doi: 10.5812/ijp.11735
50. Ding Y, Wang X, Wu Y, Li H, Xu J, Wang X. Effects of prophylactic oral ibuprofen on the closure rate of patent ductus arteriosus in premature infants. *Medicine.* (2018) 97:1–8. doi: 10.1097/MD.00000000000 12206
51. Khositseth A, Muangyod N, Nuntnarumit P. Perfusion index as a diagnostic tool for patent ductus arteriosus in preterm infants. (2013) 104:250–4. doi: 10.1159/000353862
52. Byung MC, Kee HL, Baik LE, Kee HY, Young SH, Chang SS, et al. Utility of rapid B-type natriuretic peptide assay for diagnosis of symptomatic patent ductus arteriosus in preterm infants. *Pediatrics.* (2005) 115:e255–61. doi: 10.1542/peds.2004-1837
53. van Overmeire B, Brus F, van Acker KJ, van der Auwera JC, Schasfoort M, Elzenga NJ, et al. Aspirin versus indomethacin treatment of patent ductus arteriosus in preterm infants with respiratory distress syndrome. *Pediatr Res.* (1995) 38:886–91. doi: 10.1203/00006450-199512000-00010
54. Liebowitz M, Clyman RI. Prophylactic indomethacin compared with delayed conservative management of the patent ductus arteriosus in extremely preterm infants: effects on neonatal outcomes. *J Pediatr.* (2017) 187:119–26.e1. doi: 10.1016/j.jpeds.2017.03.021
55. Vieux R, Desandes R, Boubred F, Semama D, Guillemin F, Buchweiller MC, et al. Ibuprofen in very preterm infants impairs renal function for the first month of life. *Pediatr Nephrol.* (2010) 25:267–74. doi: 10.1007/s00467-009-1349-9
56. Martinovici D, Vanden Eijnden S, Unger P, Najem B, Gulbis B, Maréchal Y. Early NT-proBNP is able to predict spontaneous closure of patent ductus arteriosus in preterm neonates, but not the need of its treatment. *Pediatr Cardiol.* (2011) 32:953–7. doi: 10.1007/s00246-011-0020-y
57. Letshwiti JB, Sirc J, O'Kelly R, Miletin J. Serial N-terminal pro-brain natriuretic peptide measurement as a predictor of significant patent ductus arteriosus in preterm infants beyond the first week of life. *Eur J Pediatr.* (2014) 173:1491–6. doi: 10.1007/s00431-014-2350-2
58. Chen HL, Yang RC, Lee W-T, Lee PL, Hsu JH, Wu JR, et al. Lung function in very preterm infants with patent ductus arteriosus under conservative management: an observational study. *BMC Pediatr.* (2015) 15:1–6. doi: 10.1186/s12887-015-0480-y
59. Suzumura H, Nitta A, Tanaka G, Arisaka O. Diastolic flow velocity of the left pulmonary artery of patent ductus arteriosus in preterm infants. *Pediatr Int.* (2001) 43:146–51. doi: 10.1046/j.1442-200x.2001.01365.x
60. Nuntnarumit P, Chongkongkiat P, Khositseth A. N-terminal-pro-brain natriuretic peptide: a guide for early targeted indomethacin therapy for patent ductus arteriosus in preterm infants. *Acta Paediatr Int J Paediatr.* (2011) 100:1217–21. doi: 10.1111/j.1651-2227.2011.02304.x
61. Ding YJ, Han B, Yang B, Zhu M. NT-proBNP plays an important role in the effect of ibuprofen on preterm infants with patent ductus arteriosus. *Eur Rev Med Pharmacol Sci.* (2014) 18:2596–8.
62. Puddy VF, Amirmansour C, Williams AF, Singer DRJ. Plasma brain natriuretic peptide as a predictor of haemodynamically significant patent ductus arteriosus in preterm infants. *Clin Sci.* (2002) 103:75–7. doi: 10.1042/cs1030075
63. Su BH, Lin HC, Chiu HY, Hsieh HY, Chen HH, Tsai YC. Comparison of ibuprofen and indometacin for early-targeted treatment of patent ductus arteriosus in extremely premature infants: a randomised controlled trial. *Arch Dis Child Fetal Neonatal Ed.* (2008) 93:F94–9. doi: 10.1136/adc.2007.120584
64. Candel-Pau J, Sillo Á, Salinas F, Redon E, Menduiña Q, Albert DC. Early versus conventional treatment for patent ductus arteriosus in preterm infants. *Am J Perinatol.* (2013) 30:289–96. doi: 10.1055/s-0032-1324696
65. Steiner M, Salzer-Muhar U, Swoboda V, Unterasinger L, Baumgartner S, Waldhoer T, et al. Preterm infants who later require duct ligation show different vital signs and pH in early postnatal life. *Acta Paediatr Int J Paediatr.* (2015) 104:e7–13. doi: 10.1111/apa.12814
66. Lee JH, Greenberg RG, Quek BH, Clark RH, Laughon MM, Smith PB, et al. Association between early echocardiography, therapy for patent ductus arteriosus, and outcomes in very low birth weight infants. *Cardiol Young.* (2017) 27:1732–9. doi: 10.1017/S1047951117001081
67. Breatnach CR, Franklin O, James AT, McCallion N, El-Khuffash A. The impact of a hyperdynamic left ventricle on right ventricular function measurements in preterm infants with a patent ductus arteriosus. *Arch Dis Child Fetal Neonatal Ed.* (2017) 102:F446–50. doi: 10.1136/archdischild-2016-311189
68. Elsayed Y, Seshia M, Baier RJ, Dakshinamurti S. Serial serum brain-type natriuretic peptide (BNP) identifies compromised blood flow in infants with hemodynamically significant patent ductus arteriosus. *J Pediatr Neonatal Individ Med.* (2017) 6:1–10.
69. Gomez-Pomar E, Makhoul M, Westgate PM, Ibonia KT, Patwardhan A, Giannone PJ, et al. Relationship between perfusion index and patent ductus arteriosus in preterm infants. *Pediatr Res.* (2017) 81:775–9. doi: 10.1038/pr.2017.10
70. Romagnoli V, Pedini A, Santoni M, Scutti G, Colaneri M, Pozzi M, et al. Patent ductus arteriosus in preterm infants born before 30 weeks' gestation: high rate of spontaneous closure after hospital discharge. *Cardiol Young.* (2018) 28:995–1000. doi: 10.1017/S1047951118000641
71. Küçük M, Bagci O, IGde M. The fate of patent ductus arteriosus is not affected by platelet count and mean platelet volume in premature infants < 32 gestational weeks. *Turkiye Klin Cardiovasc Sci.* (2018) 30:53–7. doi: 10.5336/cardiosci.2018-62380

72. Ment LR, Oh W, Ehrenkranz RA, Philip AGS, Vohr B, Allan W, et al. Low-dose indomethacin and prevention of intraventricular hemorrhage: a multicenter randomized trial. *Pediatrics.* (1994) 93:543–50.
73. Groves AM, Kuschel CA, Knight DB, Skinner JR. Does retrograde diastolic flow in the descending aorta signify impaired systemic perfusion in preterm infants? *Pediatr Res.* (2008) 63:89–94. doi: 10.1203/PDR.0b013e31815b4830
74. Kalra VK, DeBari VA, Zauk A, Kataria P, Myridakis D, Kiblawi F. Point-of-care testing for B-type natriuretic peptide in premature neonates with patent ductus arteriosus. *Ann Clin Lab Sci.* (2011) 41:131–7.
75. Alan S, Karadeniz C, Okulu E, Kilic A, Erdeve O, Ucar T, et al. Management of patent ductus arteriosus in preterm infants: clinical judgment might be a fair option. *J Matern Neonatal Med.* (2013) 26:1850–4. doi: 10.3109/14767058.2013.801956
76. Dani C, Poggi C, Fontanelli G. Relationship between platelet count and volume and spontaneous and pharmacological closure of ductus arteriosus in preterm infants. *Am J Perinatol.* (2013) 30:359–64. doi: 10.1055/s-0032-1324702
77. Koch J, Hensley G, Roy L, Brown S, Ramaciotti C, Rosenfeld CR. Prevalence of spontaneous closure of the ductus arteriosus in neonates at a birth weight of 1000 grams or less. *Pediatrics.* (2006) 117:1113–21. doi: 10.1542/peds.2005-1528
78. Rakza T, Magnenant E, Klosowski S, Tourneux P, Bachiri A, Storme L. Early hemodynamic consequences of patent ductus arteriosus in preterm infants with intrauterine growth restriction. *J Pediatr.* (2007) 151:624–8. doi: 10.1016/j.jpeds.2007.04.058
79. Strauss T, Pessach I, Jacoby E, Schushan-Eisen I, Mazkereth R, Kuint J. Carina angle measurements for diagnosis of patent ductus arteriosus in preterm infants. *Neonatology.* (2011) 99:224–30. doi: 10.1159/000315862
80. Dhuper S, Kim R, Weichbrod L, Mahdi E, Shah N, Kona S, et al. NT-proBNP levels improve the ability of predicting a hemodynamically significant patent ductus arteriosus in very low-birth-weight infants. *J Clin Neonatol.* (2012) 1:82. doi: 10.4103/2249-4847.96758
81. Desandes R, Jellimann JM, Rouabah M, Haddad F, Desandes E, Boubred F, et al. Echocardiography as a guide for patent ductus arteriosus ibuprofen treatment and efficacy prediction. *Pediatr Crit Care Med.* (2012) 13:324–7. doi: 10.1097/PCC.0b013e31822882b5
82. Alyamac Dizdar E, Ozdemir R, Nur Sari F, Yurttutan S, Gokmen T, Erdeve O, et al. Low platelet count is associated with ductus arteriosus patency in preterm newborns. *Early Hum Dev.* (2012) 88:813–6. doi: 10.1016/j.earlhumdev.2012.05.007
83. Sallmon H, Weber SC, Hüning B, Stein A, Horn PA, Metze BC, et al. Thrombocytopenia in the first 24 hours after birth and incidence of patent ductus arteriosus. *Pediatrics.* (2012) 130:e623–30. doi: 10.1542/peds.2012-0499
84. Brunner B, Hoeck M, Schermer E, Streif W, Kiechl-Kohlendorfer U. Patent ductus arteriosus, low platelets, cyclooxygenase inhibitors, and intraventricular hemorrhage in very low birth weight preterm infants. *J Pediatr.* (2013) 163:23–8. doi: 10.1016/j.jpeds.2012.12.035
85. Visconti LF, Morhy SS, Deutsch ADA, Tavares GMP, Wilberg TJM, Rossi F de S. Clinical and echocardiographic characteristics associated with the evolution of the ductus arteriosus in the neonate with birth weight lower than 1,500g. *Einstein (Sao Paulo).* (2013) 11:317–23. doi: 10.1590/S1679-45082013000300010
86. Grass B, Baumann P, Arlettaz R, Fouzas S, Meyer P, Spanaus K, et al. Cardiovascular biomarkers pro-atrial natriuretic peptide and pro-endothelin-1 to monitor ductus arteriosus evolution in very preterm infants. *Early Hum Dev.* (2014) 90:293–8. doi: 10.1016/j.earlhumdev.2014.03.002
87. Occhipinti F, De Carolis MP, De Rosa G, Bersani I, Lacerenza S, Cota F, et al. Correlation analysis between echocardiographic flow pattern and N-terminal-pro-brain natriuretic peptide for early targeted treatment of patent ductus arteriosus. *J Matern Neonatal Med.* (2014) 27:1800–4. doi: 10.3109/14767058.2014.880879
88. Trevisanuto D, Zaninotto M, Lachin M, Altinier S, Plebani M, Ferrarese P, et al. Effect of patent ductus arteriosus and indomethacin treatment on serum cardiac troponin T levels in preterm infants with respiratory distress syndrome. *Eur J Pediatr.* (2000) 159:273–6. doi: 10.1007/s004310050069
89. König K, Guy KJ, Drew SM, Barfield CP. B-type and N-terminal pro-B-type natriuretic peptides are equally useful in assessing patent ductus arteriosus in very preterm infants. *Acta Paediatr Int J Paediatr.* (2015) 104:e139–42. doi: 10.1111/apa.12892
90. Breatnach CR, Franklin O, McCallion N, EL-Khuffash A. The effect of a significant patent ductus arteriosus on doppler flow patterns of preductal vessels: an assessment of the brachiocephalic artery. *J Pediatr.* (2017) 180:279–81.e1. doi: 10.1016/j.jpeds.2016.09.029
91. Demir N, Peker E, Ece I, Agengin K, Bulan KA, Tuncer O. Is platelet mass a more significant indicator than platelet count of closure of patent ductus arteriosus? *J Matern Neonatal Med.* (2016) 29:1915–8. doi: 10.3109/14767058.2015.1067296
92. Dix L, Molenschot M, Breur J, de Vries W, Vijlbrief D, Groenendaal F, et al. Cerebral oxygenation and echocardiographic parameters in preterm neonates with a patent ductus arteriosus: an observational study. *Arch Dis Child Fetal Neonatal Ed.* (2016) 101:F520–6. doi: 10.1136/archdischild-2015-309192
93. Elsayed Y, Seshia M, Soni R, Buffo I, Baier RJ, McNamara PJ, et al. Pre-symptomatic prediction of morbitidies in preterm infants with patent ductus arteriosus by targeted neonatal echocardiography and brain-type natriuretic peptide. *J Pediatr Neonatal Individ Med.* (2016) 5:1–10.
94. Engür D, Deveci M, Türkmen MK. Early signs that predict later haemodynamically significant patent ductus arteriosus. *Cardiol Young.* (2016) 26:439–45. doi: 10.1017/S1047951115000372
95. Mochammading, Kaban RK, Yanuarso PB, Djer MM. Prostaglandin E2 and patent ductus arteriosus in premature infants. (2016) 56:8–14. doi: 10.14238/pi56.1.2016.02
96. Arlettaz R, Archer N, Wilkinson AR. Closure of the ductus arteriosus and development of pulmonary branch stenosis in babies of less than 32 weeks gestation. *Arch Dis Child Fetal Neonatal Ed.* (2001) 85. doi: 10.1136/fn.85.3.F197
97. Oliveira AGS, Soares P, Flor-de-Lima F, Neves AL, Guimarães H. PDA management in VLBW infants: experience of a level III NICU. *J Pediatr Neonatal Individ Med.* (2016) 5:1–9.
98. Tauber K, Granina E, Doyle R, Munshi U. Gestational and postnatal age influence B-type natriuretic peptide level used in diagnosis of a hemodynamically significant patent ductus arteriosus in preterm infants. *J Clin Neonatol.* (2016) 5:143. doi: 10.4103/2249-4847.191241
99. Valerio E, Valente MR, Salvadori S, Frigo AC, Baraldi E, Lago P. Intravenous paracetamol for PDA closure in the preterm: a single-center experience. *Eur J Pediatr.* (2016) 175:953–66. doi: 10.1007/s00431-016-2731-9
100. Ledo A, Aguar M, Núñez-Ramiro A, Saénz P, Vento M. Abdominal near-infrared spectroscopy detects low mesenteric perfusion early in preterm infants with hemodynamic significant ductus arteriosus. *Neonatology.* (2017) 112:238–45. doi: 10.1159/000475933
101. Demirel G, Yılmaz A, Vatansever B, Tastekin A. Is high platelet distribution width in the first hours of life can predict hemodynamically significant patent ductus arteriosus in preterm newborns? *J Matern Fetal Neonatal Med.* (2020) 33:2049–53. doi: 10.1080/14767058.2018.1536743
102. Van Overmeire B, Van De Broek H, Van Laer P, Weyler J, Vanhaesebrouck P. Early versus late indomethacin treatment for patent ductus arteriosus in premature infants with respiratory distress syndrome. *J Pediatr.* (2001) 138:205–11. doi: 10.1067/mpd.2001.110528
103. Sanjeev S, Pettersen M, Lua J, Thomas R, Shankaran S, L'Ecuyer T. Role of plasma B-type natriuretic peptide in screening for hemodynamically significant patent ductus arteriosus in preterm neonates. *J Perinatol.* (2005) 25:709–13. doi: 10.1038/sj.jp.7211383
104. Dix LML, Blok CA, Lemmers PMA, Van Der Aa N, Molenschot MC, Vreman HJ, et al. Early end-tidal carbon monoxide levels, patency of the ductus arteriosus and regional cerebral oxygenation in preterm infants. *Neonatology.* (2014) 105:161–5. doi: 10.1159/000356167
105. Olukman O, Ozdemir R, Karadeniz C, Calkavur S, Mese T, Vergin C. Is there a relationship between platelet parameters and patency of ductus arteriosus in preterm infants? *Blood Coagul Fibrinolysis.* (2017) 28:8–13. doi: 10.1097/MBC.0000000000000520
106. Khositseth A, Nuntnarumit P, Chongkongkiat P. Echocardiographic parameters of patent ductus arteriosus in preterm infants. *Indian Pediatr.* (2011) 48:773–8. doi: 10.1007/s13312-011-0127-5

107. Lago P, Bettiol T, Salvadori S, Pitassi I, Vianello A, Chiandetti L, et al. Safety and efficacy of ibuprofen versus indomethacin in preterm infants treated for patent ductus arteriosus: a randomised controlled trial. *Eur J Pediatr.* (2002) 161:202–7. doi: 10.1007/s00431-002-0915-y

108. Khosroshahi AJ, Kianfar A, Aharanjani BM, Zanjani KS. Usefulness of serum brain natriuretic peptide level for screening hemodynamically significant patent ductus arteriosus in preterm neonates. *Iran J Pediatr.* (2014) 24:766–9.

109. Van Overmeire B, Follens I, Hartmann S, Creten WL, Van Acker KJ. Treatment of patent ductus arteriosus with ibuprofen. *Arch Dis Child Fetal Neonatal Ed.* (1997) 76:1–6. doi: 10.1136/fn.76.3.F179

110. Nuntnarumit P, Khositseth A, Thanomsingh P. N-terminal probrain natriuretic peptide and patent ductus arteriosus in preterm infants. *J Perinatol.* (2009) 29:137–42. doi: 10.1038/jp.2008.185

111. Terek D, Yalaz M, Ulger Z, Koroglu OA, Kultursay N. Medical closure of patent ductus arteriosus does not reduce mortality and development of bronchopulmonary dysplasia in preterm infants. *J Res Med Sci.* (2014) 19:1074–9.

112. Mine K, Ohashi A, Tsuji S, Nakashima JI, Hirabayashi M, Kaneko K. B-type natriuretic peptide for assessment of haemodynamically significant patent ductus arteriosus in premature infants. *Acta Paediatr Int J Paediatr.* (2013) 102:347–52. doi: 10.1111/apa.12273

113. Zonnenberg I, De Waal K. The definition of a haemodynamic significant duct in randomized controlled trials: A systematic literature review. *Acta Paediatr Int J Paediatr.* (2012) 101:247–51. doi: 10.1111/j.1651-2227.2011.02468.x

114. van Laere D, van Overmeire B, Gupta S, El Khuffash A, Savoia M, McNamara PJ, et al. Application of NPE in the assessment of a patent ductus arteriosus. *Pediatr Res.* (2018) 84:46–56. doi: 10.1038/s41390-018-0077-x

115. El Hajjar M, Vaksmann G, Rakza T, Kongolo G, Storme L. Severity of the ductal shunt: a comparison of different markers. *Arch Dis Child Fetal Neonatal Ed.* (2005) 90:419–22. doi: 10.1136/adc.2003.027698

116. Ngo S, Profit J, Gould JB, Lee HC. Trends in patent ductus arteriosus diagnosis and management for very low birth weight infants. *Pediatrics.* (2017) 139:e20162390. doi: 10.1542/peds.2016-2390

117. Lamp KC, Reynolds MS. Indomethacin for prevention of neonatal intraventricular hemorrhage. *DICP.* (1991) 25:1344–8. doi: 10.1177/106002809102501213

118. Fowlie PW, Davis PG. Cochrane review: prophylactic intravenous indomethacin for preventing mortality and morbidity in preterm infants. *Evidence Based Child Health A Cochrane Rev J.* (2010) 5:416–71. doi: 10.1002/ebch.526

119. Jensen EA, Dysart KC, Gantz MG, Carper B, Higgins RD, Keszler M, et al. Association between use of prophylactic indomethacin and the risk for bronchopulmonary dysplasia in extremely preterm infants. *J Pediatr.* (2017) 186:34–40.e2. doi: 10.1016/j.jpeds.2017.02.003

120. Pacifici GM. Differential renal adverse effects of ibuprofen and indomethacin in preterm infants: a review. *Clin Pharmacol Adv Appl.* (2014) 6:111–6. doi: 10.2147/CPAA.S59376

121. Ferguson JM. Pharmacotherapy for patent ductus arteriosus closure. *Congenit Heart Dis.* (2018) 14:52–6. doi: 10.1111/chd.12715

122. Ohlsson A, Shah SS. Ibuprofen for the prevention of patent ductus arteriosus in preterm and/or low birth weight infants. *Cochrane Database Syst Rev.* (2020) 2020:1–60. doi: 10.1002/14651858.CD004213.pub5

123. Mitra S, Florez ID, Tamayo ME, Mbuagbaw L, Vanniyasingam T, Veroniki AA, et al. Association of placebo, indomethacin, ibuprofen, and acetaminophen with closure of hemodynamically significant patent ductus arteriosus in preterm infants a systematic review and meta-analysis. *JAMA J Am Med Assoc.* (2018) 319:1221–38. doi: 10.1001/jama.2018.1896

124. Aikio O, Härkin P, Saarela T, Hallman M. Early paracetamol treatment associated with lowered risk of persistent ductus arteriosus in very preterm infants. *J Matern Neonatal Med.* (2014) 27:1252–6. doi: 10.3109/14767058.2013.854327

125. Dagle JM, Ryckman KK, Spracklen CN, Momany M, Cotten CM, Levy J, et al. Genetic variants associated with patent ductus arteriosus in extremely preterm infants. (2019) 39:401–8. doi: 10.1038/s41372-018-0285-6

126. Villamor-Martinez E, Kilani MA, Degraeuwe PL, Clyman RI, Villamor E. Intrauterine growth restriction and patent ductus arteriosus in very and extremely preterm infants: a systematic review and meta-analysis. *Front Endocrinol.* (2019) 10:1–11. doi: 10.3389/fendo.2019.00058

127. Engbers AGJ, Klerk JCA De Flint RB, Völler S, Reiss IKM, Andriessen P, et al. Enantiomer specific pharmacokinetics of ibuprofen in preterm neonates with patent ductus arteriosus. (2020) 1–12. doi: 10.1111/bcp.14298. [Epub ahead of print].

128. Terek D, Altun Koroglu O, Ulger Z, Yalaz M, Kultursay N. The serial changes of perfusion index in preterm infants with patent ductus arteriosus: is perfusion index clinically significant? *Minerva Pediatr.* (2016) 68:250–5.

129. Antonucci R, Cuzzolin L, Arceri A, Dessì A, Fanos V. Changes in urinary PGE2 after ibuprofen treatment in preterm infants with patent ductus arteriosus. *Eur J Clin Pharmacol.* (2009) 65:223–30. doi: 10.1007/s00228-008-0586-3

130. Tosse V, Pillekamp F, Verde P, Hadzik B, Sabir H, Mayatepek E, et al. Urinary NT-proBNP, NGAL, and H-FABP may predict hemodynamic relevance of patent ductus arteriosus in very low birth weight infants. *Neonatology.* (2012) 101:260–6. doi: 10.1159/000334826

131. Lavery AP, Meinzen-Derr JK, Anderson E, Ma Q, Bennett MR, Devarajan P, et al. Urinary NGAL in premature infants. *Pediatr Res.* (2008) 64:423–8. doi: 10.1203/PDR.0b013e318181b3b2

132. El-Khuffash A, Higgins M, Walsh K, Molloy EJ. Quantitative assessment of the degree of ductal steal using celiac artery blood flow to left ventricular output ratio in preterm infants. *Neonatology.* (2008) 93:206–12. doi: 10.1159/000110869

Permissions

All chapters in this book were first published by Frontiers; hereby published with permission under the Creative Commons Attribution License or equivalent. Every chapter published in this book has been scrutinized by our experts. Their significance has been extensively debated. The topics covered herein carry significant findings which will fuel the growth of the discipline. They may even be implemented as practical applications or may be referred to as a beginning point for another development.

The contributors of this book come from diverse backgrounds, making this book a truly international effort. This book will bring forth new frontiers with its revolutionizing research information and detailed analysis of the nascent developments around the world.

We would like to thank all the contributing authors for lending their expertise to make the book truly unique. They have played a crucial role in the development of this book. Without their invaluable contributions this book wouldn't have been possible. They have made vital efforts to compile up to date information on the varied aspects of this subject to make this book a valuable addition to the collection of many professionals and students.

This book was conceptualized with the vision of imparting up-to-date information and advanced data in this field. To ensure the same, a matchless editorial board was set up. Every individual on the board went through rigorous rounds of assessment to prove their worth. After which they invested a large part of their time researching and compiling the most relevant data for our readers.

The editorial board has been involved in producing this book since its inception. They have spent rigorous hours researching and exploring the diverse topics which have resulted in the successful publishing of this book. They have passed on their knowledge of decades through this book. To expedite this challenging task, the publisher supported the team at every step. A small team of assistant editors was also appointed to further simplify the editing procedure and attain best results for the readers.

Apart from the editorial board, the designing team has also invested a significant amount of their time in understanding the subject and creating the most relevant covers. They scrutinized every image to scout for the most suitable representation of the subject and create an appropriate cover for the book.

The publishing team has been an ardent support to the editorial, designing and production team. Their endless efforts to recruit the best for this project, has resulted in the accomplishment of this book. They are a veteran in the field of academics and their pool of knowledge is as vast as their experience in printing. Their expertise and guidance has proved useful at every step. Their uncompromising quality standards have made this book an exceptional effort. Their encouragement from time to time has been an inspiration for everyone.

The publisher and the editorial board hope that this book will prove to be a valuable piece of knowledge for researchers, students, practitioners and scholars across the globe.

List of Contributors

Yogen Singh
Department of Pediatrics—Pediatric Cardiology and Neonatal Medicine, Cambridge University Hospitals NHS Foundation Trust, Cambridge, United Kingdom
University of Cambridge School of Clinical Medicine, Cambridge, United Kingdom

Alain Fraisse
Pediatric Cardiology Services, Royal Brompton Hospital, London, United Kingdom
Imperial College London, National Heart and Lung Institute, London, United Kingdom

Begüm Atasay and Ömer Erdeve
Division of Neonatology, Department of Pediatrics, Ankara University School of Medicine, Ankara, Turkey

Maurice J. Huizing and Eduardo Villamor
Department of Pediatrics, Maastricht University Medical Centre (MUMC+), School for Oncology and Developmental Biology (GROW), Maastricht, Netherlands

Moreyba Borges-Luján and Gema E. González-Luis
Department of Neonatology, Complejo Hospitalario Universitario Insular Materno-Infantil (CHUIMI) de Canarias, Las Palmas de Gran Canaria, Spain

Genny Raffaeli
Neonatal Intensive Care Unit, Fondazione IRCCS Cà Granda Ospedale Maggiore Policlinico, Milan, Italy
Department of Clinical Sciences and Community Health, Università degli Studi di Milano, Milan, Italy

Jaap A. Bakker
Department of Clinical Chemistry and Laboratory Medicine, Leiden University Medical Center, Leiden, Netherlands

Rob M. Moonen
Department of Pediatrics, Zuyderland Medical Center, Heerlen, Netherlands

Giacomo Cavallaro
Neonatal Intensive Care Unit, Department of Clinical Sciences and Community Health, Fondazione IRCCS Cà Granda Ospedale Maggiore Policlinico, Università degli Studi di Milano, Milan, Italy

Pilar Bas-Suárez
Department of Pediatrics, Hospital Vithas Santa Catalina, Las Palmas de Gran Canaria, Spain

Fuat Emre Canpolat, Gülsüm Kadıoğlu Şimşek, Mehmet Büyüktiryaki, Nazmiye Bengü Karaçağlar, Sarkhan Elbayiyev and H. Gözde Kanmaz Kutman
NICU, Department of Neonatology, Ankara City Hospital, University of Health Sciences, Ankara, Turkey

James Webbe
Neonatal Medicine, Imperial College London, London, United Kingdom

Thowfique Ibrahim, Abdul Alim Abdul Haium, Suresh Chandran, Mei Chien Chua and Victor Samuel Rajadurai
Department of Neonatology, KK Women's and Children's Hospital, Singapore, Singapore
Duke-NUS Medical School, Singapore, Singapore
Department of Neonatology, National University of Singapore, Singapore, Singapore
Lee Kong Chian School of Medicine, Singapore, Singapore

Sarah Jane Tapawan and Rowena Dela Puerta
Department of Neonatology, KK Women's and Children's Hospital, Singapore, Singapore

John C. Allen Jr.
Duke-NUS Medical School, Singapore, Singapore

Caterina Coviello, Iuri Corsini and Valentina Leonardi
Division of Neonatology, Careggi University Hospital of Florence, Florence, Italy

Maria Luisa Tataranno
Department of Neonatology, University Medical Center Utrecht, Utrecht, Netherlands

Mariangela Longini, Francesco Bazzini and Giuseppe Buonocore
Department of Pediatrics, Obstetrics and Reproductive Medicine, University of Siena, Siena, Italy

Carlo Dani
Division of Neonatology, Careggi University Hospital of Florence, Florence, Italy
Department of Neurosciences, Psychology, Drug Research and Child Health, Careggi University Hospital of Florence, Florence, Italy

Emel Okulu and Saadet Arsan
Division of Neonatology, Department of Pediatrics, Ankara University School of Medicine, Ankara, Turkey

Zehra Arslan
Department of Neonatology, Etlik Zubeyde Hanim Women's Health Teaching and Research Hospital, University of Health Sciences, Ankara, Turkey

Nihal Demirel
Division of Neonatology, Department of Pediatrics, Ankara Yildirim Beyazit University School of Medicine, Ankara, Turkey

Huseyin Kaya and Ismail Kursad Gokce
Division of Neonatology, Department of Pediatrics, Inonu University School of Medicine, Malatya, Turkey

Sabahattin Ertugrul
Division of Neonatology, Department of Pediatrics, Dicle University School of Medicine, Diyarbakir, Turkey

Ferda Ozlu and Huseyin Simsek
Division of Neonatology, Department of Pediatrics, Cukurova University School of Medicine, Adana, Turkey

Yalcin Celik
Division of Neonatology, Department of Pediatrics, Mersin University School of Medicine, Mersin, Turkey

Hilal Ozkan and Nilgun Köksal
Division of Neonatology, Department of Pediatrics, Uludag University School of Medicine, Bursa, Turkey

Baris Akcan and Munevver Turkmen
Division of Neonatology, Department of Pediatrics, Adnan Menderes University School of Medicine, Aydin, Turkey

Kiymet Celik
Neonatal Intensive Care Unit, Diyarbakir Gazi Yasargil Training and Research Hospital, Diyarbakir, Turkey

Didem Armangil
Neonatal Intensive Care Unit, Koru Hospital, Ankara, Turkey

Ali Bulbul
Department of Neonatology, University of Health Sciences, Sisli Etfal Hamidiye Training and Research Hospital, Istanbul, Turkey

Kadir Serafettin Tekgunduz
Division of Neonatology, Department of Pediatrics, Ataturk University School of Medicine, Erzurum, Turkey

Mehmet Yekta Oncel
Division of Neonatology, Department of Pediatrics, Izmir Katip Celebi University School of Medicine, Izmir, Turkey

Funda Tuzun
Division of Neonatology, Department of Pediatrics, Dokuz Eylul University School of Medicine, Izmir, Turkey

Ebru Ergenekon
Division of Neonatology, Department of Pediatrics, Gazi University School of Medicine, Ankara, Turkey

Hacer Ergin
Division of Neonatology, Department of Pediatrics, Pamukkale University School of Medicine, Denizli, Turkey

Merih Cetinkaya and Gokhan Buyukkale
Department of Neonatology, University of Health Sciences, Kanuni Sultan Suleyman Training and Research Hospital, Istanbul, Turkey

Ilker Gonen, Aslan Babayigit, Beril Yasa, Seyma Memur and Seda Yilmaz Semerci
Department of Neonatology, Kanuni Sultan Suleyman Training and Research Hospital, Health Sciences University, Istanbul, Turkey

Helen Bornaun
Department of Pediatric Cardiology, Kanuni Sultan Suleyman Training and Research Hospital, Health Sciences University, Istanbul, Turkey

Chang Liu, Xingwang Zhu and Dinggang Li
Department of Neonatology, Children's Hospital of Chongqing Medical University, Chongqing, China
National Clinical Research Center for Child Health and Disorders, Chongqing, China
Ministry of Education Key Laboratory of Child Development and Disorders, Chongqing, China

Yuan Shi
Department of Neonatology, Children's Hospital of Chongqing Medical University, Chongqing, China
National Clinical Research Center for Child Health and Disorders, Chongqing, China
Ministry of Education Key Laboratory of Child Development and Disorders, Chongqing, China
Chongqing Key Laboratory of Pediatrics, Chongqing, China

Flaminia Bardanzellu, Alessandra Atzei, Paola Neroni and Vassilios Fanos
Neonatal Intensive Care Unit, Department of Surgical Sciences, Azienda Ospedaliero-Universitaria and University of Cagliari, Cagliari, Italy

Cristina Piras
Department of Biomedical Sciences, University of Cagliari, Cagliari, Italy

Karl Wilhelm Olsson, Sawin Youssef, Mattias Kjellberg and Richard Sindelar
Department of Women's and Children's Health, Uppsala University, Uppsala, Sweden

Renske Raaijmakers
Division of Neonatology, Department of Pediatrics, Sahlgrenska University Hospital, Gothenburg, Sweden

Ming-Chun Yang and Yung-Ning Yang
Department of Pediatrics, E-Da Hospital, Kaohsiung City, Taiwan
School of Chinese Medicine for Post Baccalaureate, I-Shou University, Kaohsiung City, Taiwan
School of Medicine for International Students, I-Shou University, Kaohsiung City, Taiwan

Hsien-Kuan Liu
Department of Pediatrics, E-Da Hospital, Kaohsiung City, Taiwan
School of Medicine for International Students, I-Shou University, Kaohsiung City, Taiwan

Hsuan-Yin Wu
School of Medicine for International Students, I-Shou University, Kaohsiung City, Taiwan
Division of Cardiovascular Surgery, Department of Surgery, E-Da Hospital, Kaohsiung City, Taiwan

Shu-Leei Tey and Chien-Yi Wu
Department of Pediatrics, E-Da Hospital, Kaohsiung City, Taiwan
School of Chinese Medicine for Post Baccalaureate, I-Shou University, Kaohsiung City, Taiwan

Jiunn-Ren Wu
Department of Pediatrics, E-Da Hospital, Kaohsiung City, Taiwan

María Carmen Bravo, Rebeca Sánchez, Ana Isabel Blanco and Adelina Pellicer
Department of Neonatology, La Paz University Hospital, Madrid, Spain

Itsaso Losantos
Division of Statistics, La Paz University Hospital, Madrid, Spain

Gema González-Luis
Department of Neonatology, Complejo Hospitalario Universitario Insular Materno-Infantil (CHUIMI) de Canarias, Las Palmas de Gran Canaria, Spain

Stefano Ghiradello and Fabio Mosca
Neonatal Intensive Care Unit, Department of Clinical Sciences and Community Health, Fondazione IRCCS Cà Granda Ospedale Maggiore Policlinico, Università degli Studi di Milano, Milan, Italy

Ronald I Clyman
Cardiovascular Research Institute, Department of Pediatrics, University of California, San Francisco, San Francisco, CA, United States

Sarah Parkerson
Department of Pediatrics, University of Tennessee, Memphis, TN, United States

Ranjit Philip and Shyam Sathanandam
Division of Pediatric Cardiology, University of Tennessee, Memphis, TN, United States

Ajay Talati
Division of Neonatology, University of Tennessee, Memphis, TN, United States

Gianluca Terrin, Maria Di Chiara, Giovanni Boscarino, Paolo Versacci, Violante Di Donato, Antonella Giancotti, Elisabetta Pacelli, Francesca Faccioli, Elisa Onestà, Chiara Corso, Alessandra Ticchiarelli and Mario De Curtis
Department of Maternal and Child Health, University of Rome La Sapienza, Rome, Italy

Tim Hundscheid, Esther J. S. Jansen and Willem P. de Boode
Division of Neonatology, Department of Paediatrics, Radboud Institute for Health Sciences, Amalia Children's Hospital, Radboud University Medical Centre, Nijmegen, Netherlands

Wes Onland
Department of Neonatology, Amsterdam University Medical Centers, VU University Medical Center, Emma Children's Hospital, University of Amsterdam, Amsterdam, Netherlands

Elisabeth M. W. Kooi
Division of Neonatology, University Medical Center Groningen, Beatrix Children's Hospital, University of Groningen, Groningen, Netherlands

Peter Andriessen
Department of Neonatology, Máxima Medical Center Veldhoven, Eindhoven, Netherlands
Department of Applied Physics, School of Medical Physics and Engineering, Eindhoven University of Technology, Eindhoven, Netherlands
Máxima Medical Center, Veldhoven, Netherlands

Alain Fraisse
Pediatric Cardiology Services, Royal Brompton Hospital, London, United Kingdom
Imperial College London, National Heart and Lung Institute, London, United Kingdom

Carles Bautista-Rodriguez and Mary Lane
Pediatric Cardiology Services, Royal Brompton Hospital, London, United Kingdom
National Heart and Lung Institute, Imperial College London, London, United Kingdom

Margarita Burmester
National Heart and Lung Institute, Imperial College London, London, United Kingdom
Pediatric Cardiac Intensive Care Unit, Royal Brompton Hospital, London, United Kingdom

Fahri Ovalı
Division of Neonatology, Department of Pediatrics, Istanbul Medeniyet University, Istanbul, Turkey

Sven C. Weber and Natalie Timme
Department of Pediatric Cardiology, Charité University Medical Center, Berlin, Germany

Hannes Sallmon
Department of Pediatric Cardiology, Charité University Medical Center, Berlin, Germany
Department of Congenital Heart Disease/Pediatric Cardiology, Deutsches Herzzentrum Berlin (DHZB), Berlin, Germany

Georg Hansmann
Department of Pediatric Cardiology and Intensive Care Medicine, Medizinische Hochschule Hannover, Hanover, Germany

Elaine L. Shelton
Department of Pediatrics, Vanderbilt University Medical Center, Nashville, TN, United States
Department of Pharmacology, Vanderbilt University Medical Center, Nashville, TN, United States

Roy M. Nilsen
Department of Health and Functioning, Western Norway University of Applied Sciences, Bergen, Norway

Merete S. Engeseth
Department of Health and Functioning, Western Norway University of Applied Sciences, Bergen, Norway
Department of Clinical Science, University of Bergen, Bergen, Norway

Ola D. Røksund
Department of Health and Functioning, Western Norway University of Applied Sciences, Bergen, Norway
Department of Pediatrics and Adolescent Medicine, Haukeland University Hospital, Bergen, Norway

Mette Engan, Hege Clemm, Maria Vollsæter and Thomas Halvorsen
Department of Clinical Science, University of Bergen, Bergen, Norway
Department of Pediatrics and Adolescent Medicine, Haukeland University Hospital, Bergen, Norway

Trond Markestad
Department of Clinical Science, University of Bergen, Bergen, Norway

Eui Kyung Choi, Kyu Hee Park and Byung Min Choi
Department of Pediatrics, Korea University College of Medicine, Seoul, South Korea

Johan C. A. de Klerk, Floor van Beek, Irwin K. M. Reiss and Sinno H. P. Simons
Division of Neonatology, Department of Pediatrics, Erasmus UMC—Sophia Children's Hospital, Rotterdam, Netherlands

Aline G. J. Engbers
Division of Neonatology, Department of Pediatrics, Erasmus UMC—Sophia Children's Hospital, Rotterdam, Netherlands
Division of Systems Biomedicine and Pharmacology, Leiden Amsterdam Center for Drug Research (LACDR), Leiden University, Leiden, Netherlands

Robert B. Flint
Division of Neonatology, Department of Pediatrics, Erasmus UMC—Sophia Children's Hospital, Rotterdam, Netherlands
Department of Hospital Pharmacy, Erasmus UMC, Rotterdam, Netherlands

Swantje Völler
Division of Systems Biomedicine and Pharmacology, Leiden Amsterdam Center for Drug Research (LACDR), Leiden University, Leiden, Netherlands
Division of BioTherapeutics, Leiden Amsterdam Center for Drug Research (LACDR), Leiden University, Leiden, Netherlands

Index